S0-DVT-193

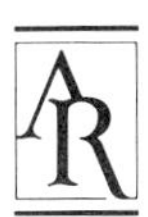

ANNUAL REVIEW OF PUBLIC HEALTH

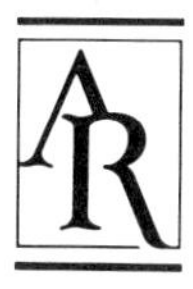

ANNUAL REVIEW OF PUBLIC HEALTH

VOLUME 14, 1993

GILBERT S. OMENN, *Editor*
University of Washington

JONATHAN E. FIELDING, *Associate Editor*
University of California at Los Angeles

LESTER B. LAVE, *Associate Editor*
Carnegie Mellon University

ANNUAL REVIEWS INC. 4139 EL CAMINO WAY P.O. BOX 10139 PALO ALTO, CALIFORNIA 94303-0897

ANNUAL REVIEWS INC.
Palo Alto, California, USA

International Standard Serial Number: 0163–7525
International Standard Book Number: 0–8243–2714-4

♾ The paper used in this publication meets the minimum requirements of American National Standard for Information Sciences—Permanence of Paper for Printed Library Materials, ANSI Z39.48-1984.

Typesetting by Kachina Typesetting Inc., Tempe, Arizona; John Olson, President; Marty Mullins, Typesetting Coordinator; and by the Annual Reviews Inc. Editorial Staff

PRINTED AND BOUND IN THE UNITED STATES OF AMERICA

PREFACE

The year 1993 offers renewed hope for a major advance in health policy in the United States. Those who believe in long-cycle theories of social policy-making may cite the 30-year pattern of Social Security in 1935, Medicare in 1965, and the prospect for action from the 103rd Congress, which most likely takes effect in 1995, for comprehensive health care and public health reform! Any further delay will leave far too many Americans without adequate coverage and will further burden our economy with the continuing upward spiral of health care costs.

From the public health and preventive medicine community, we have an opportunity and an obligation to assure certain elements of the reform package. President Clinton has been steadfast during the campaign and in the early period of his presidency in including "prevention" as one of the primary elements of health policy. We must assure that prevention embraces both clinical preventive services (office-based and community-based) and the population-based public health programs that correspond broadly to the objectives of the Healthy People 1990 and Healthy People 2000 reports. A private/public sector organization, the Partnership for Prevention, the new Advisory Committee to the Director of the Centers for Disease Control, and the academic and practice organizations participating in the Council for Linkages Between Academia and Public Health Practice all endorsed the concept that private and public payers for medical care should also join to support the "traditional" public health services, strengthened and modified to increase their effectiveness. Enactment of comprehensive health reform with universal access, even with adequate appropriations under cost control, will not obviate the need for organized outreach to vulnerable populations. A voucher will not suffice. While the national debate is joined, several individual states have mounted their own programs; in each of these, a similar bridging of medicine and public health is desirable, both for the states' programs and as models for the nation.

For clinical preventive services, we must advocate broad coverage of those services demonstrated to be effective and must target them to groups in the population for whom they are appropriate. A good example of this challenge is the article in this volume by Jacobs about lowering of serum cholesterol. The evidence indicates that regular cholesterol testing and the increasingly common practice of prescribing pharmacologic intervention may be unnecessary or even undesirable for most women and most older people. That article also reflects the commitment of the *Annual Review of Public Health* to bridge the laboratory science underpinning public health and the methods and outcomes of epidemiologic investigations and prevention trials. Two articles from the Centers for Disease Control likewise emphasize the roles of the public health laboratory in public health practice.

Finally, as we debate the multiple reasons for the high cost of medical care, we should not accept the chorus of complaints about the costs of effective medical technologies as any reason to disinvest in research. For too many common diseases our present treatments are palliative; for too many diseases we lack preventive interventions. We should not stop progress in biomedical, behavioral, and health outcomes research. We should, however, redouble our commitment to evaluate the efficacy and the cost-effectiveness of all diagnostic, therapeutic, and preventive services and the corresponding community actions to prevent hazardous exposures to people and the environment.

We note with sadness the passing of Richard Remington during the past year. Dick was our colleague on this Editorial Board and a major contributor to biostatistics and public health policy.

Gilbert S. Omenn, M.D., Ph.D.
Editor

Annual Review of Public Health
Volume 14, 1993

CONTENTS

Behavioral Aspects of Health

Public Health Practice

Indexes

SOME RELATED ARTICLES IN OTHER *ANNUAL REVIEWS*

From the *Annual Review of Genetics*, Volume 26 (1992):

Genetics of Legionella Pneumophila Virulence, A. Marra and H. A. Shuman
Genetic Analysis Using the Polymerase Chain Reaction, H. A. Erlich and N. Arnheim
Mammalian Genes Induced by Radiation: Activation of Genes Associated with Radiation, A. J. Fornace Jr.

From the *Annual Review of Medicine*, Volume 44 (1993):

Atherosclerosis Regression, Plaque Disruption, and Cardiovascular Events: A Rationale for Lipid Lowering in Coronary Artery Disease, B. G. Brown, X.-Q. Zhao, D. E. Sacco, and J. J. Albers
Antioncogenes and Human Cancer, D. P. Carbone and J. D. Minna
Human Herpesvirus-6, M. T. Caserta and C. B. Hall
The Molecular Biology of Cystic Fibrosis, T. J. Sferra and F. S. Collins
Aging—Causes and Defenses, G. R. Martin, D. B. Danner, and N. J. Holbrook
Methods, Successes, and Failures of Smoking Cessation Programs, E. B. Fisher, Jr., E. Lichtenstein, D. Haire-Joshu, G. D. Morgan, and H. R. Rehlberg
Special Aspects of Neuropsychiatric Illness in Women: With a Focus on Depression, J. A. Hamilton and U. Halbreich
Pathogenesis and Pathophysiology of Bacterial Meningitis, A. R. Tunkel and W. M. Scheld

From the *Annual Review of Nutrition*, Volume 13 (1993):

Genetics of Obesity, C. Bouchard and L. Pérusse
Regulation of Plasma LDL-Cholesterol Levels by Dietary Cholesterol and Fatty Acids, D. K. Spady, L. A. Woollett, and J. M. Dietschy
Aluminum Metabolism, J. L. Greger
Nutritional Factors in Osteoporosis, R. P. Heaney
Fungal Toxins in Foods: Recent Concerns, R. T. Riley, W. P. Norred, and C. W. Bacon
Iron Deficiency and Cognitive Function, E. Pollitt

From the *Annual Review of Psychology*, Volume 44 (1993):

Psychoneuroimmunology: Conditioning and Stress, R. Ader and N. Cohen
Child Care Research: Issues, Perspectives, and Results, S. Scarr and M. Eisenberg

Social and Community Interventions, M. Levine, P. A. Toro, and D. V. Perkins
Attitudes and Attitude Change, J. M. Olson and M. P. Zanna
Program Evaluation, L. Sechrest and A. J. Figueredo

From the *Annual Review of Sociology,* Volume 19 (1993):

The Sociology of Work and Occupations, A. Abbott
Perspectives on Organizational Change in the US Medical Care Sector, J. A. Alexander and M. L. Fennell
Social Organization and Risk: Some Current Controversies, L. Clarke and J. F. Short
Comparative Patterns in Retirement, A.-M. Guillemard
Developments in Research on Minority Identity and Self-Esteem, J. R. Porter and K. E. Washington
Sex Segregation in the Workplace, B. F. Reskin

ANNUAL REVIEWS INC. is a nonprofit scientific publisher established to promote the advancement of the sciences. Beginning in 1932 with the *Annual Review of Biochemistry,* the Company has pursued as its principal function the publication of high quality, reasonably priced *Annual Review* volumes. The volumes are organized by Editors and Editorial Committees who invite qualified authors to contribute critical articles reviewing significant developments within each major discipline. The Editor-in-Chief invites those interested in serving as future Editorial Committee members to communicate directly with him. Annual Reviews Inc. is administered by a Board of Directors, whose members serve without compensation.

ANNUAL REVIEWS OF
Anthropology
Astronomy and Astrophysics
Biochemistry
Biophysics and Biomolecular Structure
Cell Biology
Computer Science
Earth and Planetary Sciences
Ecology and Systematics
Energy and the Environment
Entomology
Fluid Mechanics
Genetics
Immunology
Materials Science
Medicine
Microbiology
Neuroscience
Nuclear and Particle Science
Nutrition
Pharmacology and Toxicology
Physical Chemistry
Physiology
Phytopathology
Plant Physiology and Plant Molecular Biology
Psychology
Public Health
Sociology

SPECIAL PUBLICATIONS

Excitement and Fascination of Science, Vols. 1, 2, and 3

Intelligence and Affectivity, by Jean Piaget

For the convenience of readers, a detachable order form/envelope is bound into the back of this volume.

Annu. Rev. Publ. Health 1993. 14:1–17

DIET, HORMONES, AND CANCER

David P. Rose

Division of Nutrition and Endocrinology, American Health Foundation, Valhalla, New York 10595

KEY WORDS: dietary fat, dietary fiber, estrogens, breast cancer, vegetarian diets and cancer risk

---

INTRODUCTION

Despite some continuing controversy, there is mounting evidence that diet can influence the risk of two sex hormone-related cancers, those of breast and endometrium, and that this relationship may also extend to carcinomas of the ovary and prostate. Although the biological mechanisms are under continuing investigation, it is clear that both dietary fat and fiber affect the circulating levels and metabolic fate of the estrogens in women and that similar effects probably apply to the androgenic steroids in men. Moreover, obesity is a risk factor for postmenopausal breast cancer, as well as for carcinoma of the endometrium, and most likely operates through the modification of estrogen synthesis and metabolism.

In this review, we focus on diet-estrogen interactions and breast and endometrial cancer risk. In doing so, however, we should recognize that many constituents of the diet, both macro- and micronutrients, most likely interact in enhancing or suppressing the carcinogenic process.

THE SEX STEROID HORMONES

There are two sources of blood estrogens. Before menopause, these steroids are largely produced and secreted by the ovary. After menopause, however, they are derived almost exclusively from the aromatization of androstenedi- one, a C_{19} steroid that is secreted by both the adrenal glands and the ovaries. This metabolic transformation occurs largely in the stromal cells of adipose tissue and is thus enhanced in obese women, so that there is a consequent elevation in circulating estrogen concentrations (78). Therefore, we might anticipate that

0163-75235/93/0510-0001$02.00

obesity-associated endometrial cancer is accompanied by increased plasma estrogen levels (34) and androstenedione aromatization rates (48).

The immediate estrogenic product of androstenedione aromatization is estrone, but this may be converted to the more biologically potent estradiol. Beranek et al (15) assayed the responsible enzyme, 17-hyroxysteroid dehydrogenase, in breast adipose tissue. The authors observed a positive correlation with body weight and postulated that the increased local production of estradiol provides a stimulus to mammary cell growth and cancer promotion.

Most of the estradiol circulating in the blood is bound to serum proteins, and the relative distribution is believed to govern its biological activity. The proportion that is bound with a high affinity to sex hormone-binding globulin (SHBG), normally 30–50%, is unable to undergo tissue uptake and binding to the cellular estrogen receptors; the albumin-bound fraction is considered to be biologically available, as is the 1–2% of the total blood estradiol that circulates free of any protein binding (54). It follows that changes in plasma SHBG concentration affect estrogen bioactivity. For example, SHBG levels are inversely correlated with body weight (21), which may provide an additional mechanism whereby obesity adversely influences breast and endometrial cancer risks.

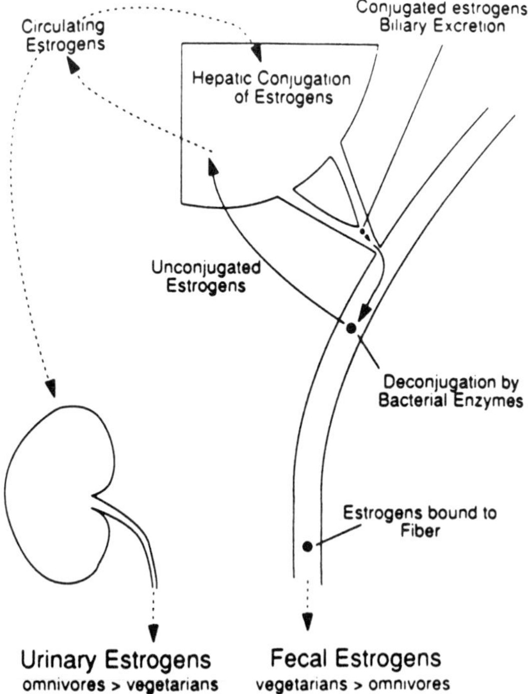

Figure 1 The enterohepatic circulation of estrogens.

Blood estrogens are conjugated in the liver to form glucuronides and sulfoglucuronides, and 20–50% of estrogen metabolites are excreted in the bile as these water soluble, biologically inactive metabolites (10). Within the lumen of the bowel, these conjugates are available for hydrolysis by enzymes of the intestinal microflora, and the resulting deconjugated estrogens are, to some extent, reabsorbed into the circulation and contribute to the total body pool of estrogens that determines the level of both the blood and urinary estrogens (Figure 1). Sterilization of the gut by orally administered ampicillin suppresses this enterohepatic circulation of estrogens with a resulting reduction in their excretion in urine (11). Moreover, as we discuss later, dietary fat and fiber also influence the enzyme deconjugation process, and so affect the process of estrogen excretion.

Estrone also circulates in the blood as the sulfate ester, which is not biologically active but can be converted to the unconjugated steroid by sulfatases present in breast (27, 61) and endometrial (77) tissues. Estrone sulfate is quantitatively the major circulating estrogen in nonpregnant women; after menopause, it is present in the plasma at concentrations that are frequently ten times that of unconjugated estrone (32). The plasma estrone sulfate concentration is increased in obesity, but the elevations that occur in postmenopausal endometrial cancer (32) and breast cancer (61) are independent of body size.

In addition to obesity's effects on estrogen bioavailability and the sulfation

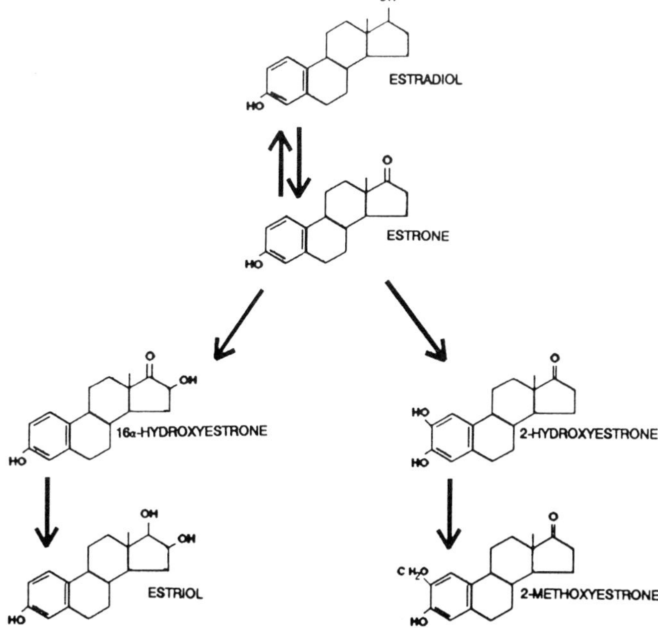

Figure 2 The metabolism of estrogen to catechol and 16α-hydroxy derivatives.

of estrone, it also results in a redistribution of estradiol metabolism into the two competing pathways that involve, respectively, the formation of 16α-hydroxy and catechol derivatives (Figure 2). Obesity is associated with a reduction in 2-hydroxylated metabolite production in the liver, compounds that are rapidly cleared from the circulation and have little estrogenicity. Hydroxylation at the 16α-position, however, remains unchanged in obesity; thus, there is increased availability of the biologically active 16α-metabolite (71). Elevated 16α-hydroxylation of estradiol has been reported in both breast cancer patients (72) and women with a family history of the disease; it has also been proposed as a marker of risk (53).

INTERNATIONAL COMPARISONS OF DIET AND PLASMA HORMONE LEVELS

There are large differences in the breast, endometrial, ovarian, and prostate cancer incidence and mortality rates between different countries of the world. In general, countries with a high incidence of one tumor type have a high incidence for all four, and the rates are highest in northern Europe and North America and lowest in the Asian countries, notably Japan.

Several groups of investigators have noted the positive correlation between estimated per capita fat consumption in different countries and breast (and prostate) cancer incidence and mortality rates (13, 19, 28, 66, 67). Although the validity of these comparisons is sometimes challenged on the basis of the variable quality of the reported cancer registry data and the crude approximation of the estimates of dietary intakes, they have prompted some valuable studies into diet-hormone interrelationships that were located in countries with widely different risks for specific types of cancer.

In contrast to the urban areas, the diet in rural Japan has not become westernized, and fat consumption may still be only 10–20g/day; less than one-fifth the fat content of the typical American diet (84). Shimizu et al (74) determined the serum estrogens in rural-dwelling postmenopausal Japanese women and postmenopausal American white women and found that both the serum estradiol and estrone concentrations were considerably lower in the Japanese women, with a low breast cancer risk, compared with the American women who were at high risk for breast cancer. In Japan as a whole, however, both dietary fat consumption and postmenopausal breast cancer incidence have increased over the past 30–40 years. These changes have occurred in the urbanized centers, and so it is particularly noteworthy that no differences were observed when plasma estrogen concentrations were compared in Japanese women from Tokyo and British women (18).

Key, Wang, and colleagues (38, 79) performed a similar comparison of serum estrogen concentrations in pre- and postmenopausal Chinese and British women. Once again, the Chinese were recruited from rural areas of the country, and a dietary survey had shown that in these locations the mean percentage of energy derived from dietary fat was 15%; in Britain, it is approximately 40%. This was a very large population study involving 3250 Chinese and 300 British women. The final data were stratified on the basis of age, which showed that for the postmenopausal groups, aged 55–64 years, the British women had an average plasma estradiol concentration that was 171% higher than their Chinese counterparts. For perimenopausal women, aged 45–54 years, the corresponding difference was 90%, and for premenopausal women it was 36%. Plasma SHBG levels were also assayed and found to be significantly lower, which implies an elevation in the biologically active estradiol fractions in blood, only in the postmenopausal British compared with the postmenopausal Chinese women. This emphasis on differences in plasma estradiol and SHBG in postmenopausal women is consistent with the belief that diet influences both breast cancer risk (85) and prognosis (69) predominantly in those who are beyond the menopause.

In another international comparison, Moore et al (51) examined the distribution of estradiol in the sera of healthy British and Japanese women and found that the Japanese had significantly more of their bound estradiol associated with SHBG and less with albumin. In this case, the difference was evident regardless of menopausal status.

Goldin et al (26) compared the plasma estradiol and estrone concentrations of white American women resident in Hawaii and recent immigrants from Southeast Asia. The plasma estradiol concentration was 44% less in the premenopausal Asian women; the difference in the plasma estrone levels was less marked. Estimates of dietary intake were also performed in the two groups of premenopausal women, and, although the Asian women were not vegetarians, their diets did contain considerably less fat and more fiber than those of the corresponding American women. When the data from the two groups of women were combined for statistical analysis, a positive correlation was found between dietary fat and plasma estradiol, and an inverse one between dietary fiber and the plasma estradiol concentration. Both the premenopausal and postmenopausal Asian women excreted less estrogens in their urine and more in their feces than their American counterparts, a finding consistent with dietary fat enhancing, and fiber suppressing, the enterohepatic circulation of estrogens (see below).

OMNIVORES AND VEGETARIANS

Phillips (56) originally reported that Seventh-Day Adventist (SDA) women, many of whom conform to their church's doctrine that its members follow a vegetarian dietary regimen, had lower breast and endometrial cancer rates than did other women of similar ethnic and socioeconomic backgrounds. Although subsequent experience has called into question the extent to which a vegetarian diet affects breast cancer risk (22, 57), several investigators have compared the plasma hormone concentrations of vegetarians and omnivores and demonstrated differences that might provide a mechanistic explanation for any observed divergence in cancer risks.

Armstrong et al (12) determined plasma SHBG and urinary estrogen excretions in 50 SDA vegetarian postmenopausal women, aged 50–79 years, and 50 nonvegetarian women of similar age. When alcohol drinkers were excluded from the nonvegetarian group, the vegetarians, none of whom consumed alcoholic drinks, were found to have significantly higher levels of plasma SHBG. This confounding effect of alcohol on the SHBG concentration correlated with the previously described (50) elevating action of alcohol on plasma HDL-cholesterol. The vegetarians also had lower urinary estrogen excretions, which, combined with their higher SHBG estrogen-binding capacity, suggests that they were exposed to less estrogenic activity on target tissues than were the omnivores.

Goldin et al (25) compared the plasma, urinary, and fecal estrogen levels of ten vegetarian and ten omnivorous premenopausal healthy American women. The vegetarian diets contained an estimated average 28g of fiber and 30% of total calories as fat per day, whereas the nonvegetarian diets provided 12g of fiber and 40% of calories as fat. The vegetarians excreted two to three times the amounts of estrogens in their feces as did the omnivores and significantly lower levels in the urine. There was a trend, which did not reach statistical significance, for the vegetarians to have lower plasma estradiol and estrone concentrations, and the plasma estrogen levels were negatively correlated with the fecal excretion of estrogens.

A study of vegetarian and omnivorous premenopausal women, carried out in Helsinki by Adlercreutz et al (2), examined in detail the profile of estrogens excreted in the urine. The authors found that the total dietary fiber intake and the grain fiber intake were negatively associated with the excretion of 10 of the 13 estrogens assayed, but usually only when fiber intake was expressed in terms of body weight. In the context of the location of this study, it is worth noting that breast cancer incidence is increasing in Finland, but at a faster rate in urban Helsinki and in association with a reduction in fiber intake than in the rural parts of the country (3). Moreover, it would be of considerable interest to observe the effect of a dietary intervention aimed at reducing coronary artery disease in Finnish men on the future breast cancer risk of the female family members.

More than one factor may contribute to the differences in estrogen levels observed between vegetarians and omnivores. Fecal β-glucuronidase activity was assayed in the study of premenopausal women performed by Goldin et al (25) and found to be lower in the vegetarians than in the nonvegetarians.

This result is consistent with a suppressive effect of a high-fiber/low-dat diet on fecal bacterial deconjugating enzyme activity, which is at least partly attributable to a dilutional effect resulting from increased fecal bulk and a consequent reduction in the enterohepatic recirculation of estrogens. Direct binding of steroids by fiber within the intestinal lumen may also prevent estrogen reabsorption. Schultz and colleagues (75, 81) showed that unconjugated estrogens bind to various types of fiber and that samples of foods consumed by vegetarians contain more water-insoluble fiber with high estrogen-binding capacity than do typical omnivorous diets. Estrone-3-glucuronide was poorly bound, which implies that binding to fiber within the gut lumen selectively enhances the fecal excretion of estrogens that have been deconjugated by bacterial enzyme activity, so limiting their reabsorption from the bowel.

Studies of the effects of diet on the distribution and bioavailability of estradiol in the plasma have produced conflicting results. Fentiman et al (23) performed a careful investigation of 25 vegetarian and 21 nonvegetarian healthy premenopausal British women from whom serial blood samples were collected every two hours over a 24-hour period. No difference was found in the plasma SHBG or free estradiol fraction between the two groups, but the vegetarians showed a greater proportion of estradiol bound to albumin; consequently, less was bound to SHBG. These results are difficult to reconcile with the hypotheses that elevated levels of bioavailable estrogens are associated with an increased breast cancer risk, but that a vegetarian dietary lifestyle is accompanied by a reduced risk of this disease. A confounder here may be that all forms of dietary fiber do not have the same biological effects and that an important factor influencing the distribution of estradiol in the plasma is the source of dietary fiber. Adlercreutz et al (7, 8) did find a positive correlation between the intake of fibers present in vegetables, fruits, and berries and the serum SHBG level, and a negative association between these same fiber sources and the percentage of unbound estradiol of the plasma. These fiber sources, which are lacking in the diets of British (and American) vegetarians, may provide dietary phytoestrogens necessary for the stimulation of SHBG synthesis in the liver (see below).

Adlercreutz et al (6) have also studied groups of postmenopausal omnivorous and vegetarian healthy women, and postsurgery, disease-free breast cancer patients. The plasma SHBG levels were lower in the breast cancer patients compared with those of the healthy omnivores; nonobese vegetarian women had higher SHBG concentrations than either of the other two groups. Dietary analysis showed that postmenopausal women who consumed a diet rich in fats and proteins, but low in fiber and carbohydrates, had relatively high levels of total and nonprotein bound testosterone and of androstenedione, but low SHBG concentrations, in their plasma. The importance of the elevated levels of C_{19} androgenic steroids to breast cancer risk may lie in the capacity for testosterone to be converted to estradiol, and androstenedione to estrone.

As might be anticipated, the changes in the hormonal status of premenopausal women associated with a vegetarian diet affect the menstrual cycle itself. In one study of premenopausal white American women reported by Pedersen et al (55), menstrual irregularities were noted in 4.9% of 41 nonvegetarians, but 26.5% of 34 vegetarians of similar weight and body mass index. Of particular interest was the finding that the likelihood of having regular cycles was inversely associated with increasing dietary fiber consumption, which is in keeping with the negative relationship between fiber intake and blood estrogen concentrations. In a follow-up study (44), these investigators measured the urinary estradiol excretions of premenopausal omnivorous and vegetarian women and found considerably lower outputs in irregularly menstruating vegetarians compared with normally cycling vegetarians or nonvegetarians.

Whether breast cancer risk is lower in women with irregular, frequently anovulatory menstrual cycles remains uncertain, but, in contrast to the situation in postmenopausal women, obesity has been associated with a reduced risk in premenopausal women (30, 46). This condition may be accompanied by irregular menstrual periods (82) and amenorrhea (62). The low luteal phase plasma progesterone levels that are also present may result in lower proliferative activity in the mammary tissue, thus reducing risk (40). However, by permitting the action of "unopposed" estrogen, this same deficiency in the uterus may increase the risk for endometrial cancer (39).

LOW FAT/HIGH FIBER DIETS

Several studies have been published in which volunteers were transferred from their regular high-fat, low-fiber diet, to one providing a specified intake of fat and/or fiber. Rose et al (65) employed dietary counseling to reduce the fat consumption from an average of 35% to approximately 20% of total calories in 16 American premenopausal women with cystic breast disease. There was no significant change in dietary fiber intake, and the ratio of polyunsaturated to saturated fats (P/S) remained at approximately 0.5. After three months, the estradiol and estrone concentrations were significantly reduced in serum samples obtained at the midluteal stage of the menstrual cycle. Woods et al (83) fed a typical Western ("control") diet, which provided 40% of total calories from fat and 12g of dietary fiber a day, to 17 healthy premenopausal women for four weeks, and then changed them to a low-fat (25% total calories) and high-fiber (40g/day) diet with an accompanying shift in the P/S ratio from 0.5 to 1.0. In this study, the serum samples were collected in the early follicular phase of the menstrual cycle before changing from the control diet, and again after feeding the low-fat/high-fiber diet for eight to ten weeks, at which time the estrone sulfate levels were reduced by an average of 36%. No changes in serum estradiol or estrone were observed in this study; however, in the low-fat intervention experiment performed by Rose et al (65), the levels of these two estrogens were not altered significantly eight weeks into the low-fat experimental period.

The type, as well as the quantity, of dietary fat may be important. Taylor et al (76), in a preliminary report, have described how the follicular phase plasma estradiol concentration in 31 premenopausal women was reduced when they were fed low-fat diets, with P/S ratios of 0.3 or 1.0, for four months. However, during the luteal phase of the menstrual cycle, the plasma estrogen reduction was evident only in those fed the 0.3 P/S low-fat diet.

Dietary modification also alters the serum estrogens in postmenopausal women. Prentice et al (59) obtained a significant reduction in plasma estradiol, averaging 17%, when 73 postmenopausal women, judged on epidemiological or pathological grounds to be at an increased risk for breast cancer, were placed on a low-fat (20% of total calories) diet for 10–22 weeks. In addition to the total plasma estradiol, the albumin-bound fraction was also reduced, but the estrone and estrone sulfate concentrations were unchanged. The lack of an effect of a low-fat diet on the plasma estrone sulfate levels of postmenopausal women reported by Prentice et al (59), and confirmed by Rose in an on-going unpublished study, is puzzling. One possibility is that the critical change with respect to estrone sulfate in the diets of the premenopausal women studied by Woods et al (83) was the doubling of their fiber intake, rather than the reduction in fat consumption.

Rose et al (68) performed an experimental study in which the fiber intake of premenopausal women was increased without any significant change in the level of dietary fat consumption. The women were fed a supplement of either wheat, corn, or oat bran to increase their total dietary fiber consumption to approximately 30g/day. After two months on this regimen, the wheat bran-supplemented group showed significant reductions in serum estrone and estradiol, whereas the women whose diets were supplemented with one of the other two brans showed no change. Feces were also collected for bacterial enzyme assays, and the results showed that wheat bran-supplementation produced a significant reduction in β-glucuronidase activity; oat bran had a lesser effect, and no change was seen in feces from the corn bran-supplemented women. These results showed directly that dietary fiber can alter the blood estrogens. In a study that has been summarized (20), but not yet published in full, Woods and colleagues found independent and reducing effects of a low-fat diet or a high-fiber diet on the plasma estrone sulfate levels of premenopausal women.

Rose (63, 64) has summarized the evidence in support of the hypothesis that dietary fiber has a protective effect against breast cancer. This work includes the observation that the breast cancer incidence in Finland, where the diet is typically high in fat but also high in fiber, is considerably lower than in Western countries where fat consumption is equally high, but the diet contains only approximately half the amount of fiber. Several case-control studies also suggest a specific, protective role for dietary fiber in breast cancer (31, 47), and we have already noted that the diets of women from rural China and Southeast Asia, who have relatively low levels of circulating estrogens, are high in fiber as well as low in fat.

Not only have changes in dietary fat and fiber consumption been associated with reductions in the plasma estrogen concentrations, but a low-fat diet has also been shown to alter estradiol metabolism in a manner that may favorably influence breast cancer risk. Longcope et al (45) examined the metabolism of estradiol to 16α-hydroxylated derivatives and catechol estrogens before and after six healthy premenopausal women were transferred from a typically Western high-fat diet, which provided 40% of the total calories consumed, to one with 25% of the calories as fat; fiber intakes were not reported, but they were not deliberately modified during the two-month experimental period. The low-fat diet resulted in a decreased urinary excretion of 16α-hydroxylated glucuronides and sulfates, but only small, statistically insignificant increases in the other urinary metabolites.

In addition to the level of fat intake, the type of fat consumed may affect breast cancer risk. Both epidemiological (36, 41, 52) and experimental (16, 17, 35, 37) data suggest that the omega-3 fatty acids exert a protective effect. Osborne et al (53) reported a pilot study in which women at high breast cancer risk, because of their family history or the presence of epithelial atypia in benign breast biopsy tissue, were randomized to receive either a fish oil, omega-3 fatty acid-rich dietary supplement or a placebo preparation. Although the controls showed no change in estradiol metabolism, those given the omega-3 fatty acids showed a significant reduction in 16α-hydroxylation.

PHYTOESTROGENS AND LIGNANS

Phytoestrogens are chemical compounds that are generally produced in the intestine by bacterial action from precursors present in a variety of plants and vegetables. One phytoestrogen with a relatively high degree of biological activity is equol, which is formed from the isoflavonic compound formononetin and has been detected in the urine of various animals, including sheep and humans (64). Equol is also present in cow's milk, and so may be consumed as part of the human diet (60). Although such phytoestrogens possess weak estrogenic activity, investigators have suggested that by competing with the more biologically potent estradiol for target cell binding sites, they may actually exert a net suppressive, antiestrogenic effect (24, 49).

Soya is a source of equol precursor, and a diet that contains cooked soy protein usually causes a pronounced increase in urinary equol excretion. Setchell et al (73) observed increases that ranged from 50- to 1000-fold above the basal equol excretion when volunteers were fed textured soya for five days. The authors suggested that, despite the low affinity of equol for estrogen receptors relative to that of estradiol, the high (3.5–7.0 mg/day) concentrations of the phytoestrogen produced when a dietary precursor like soya is eaten may exert a dampening effect on total estrogenic bioactivity at target cell sites, and so have a beneficial effect on hormone-related breast cancer risk.

There is some epidemiological and experimental support for the hypothesis that phytoestrogens derived from constitutents of soy have a protective role in breast cancer. For example, the traditional Japanese diet is not only low in fat, but also includes considerable amounts of soy products, which results in high urinary excretions of phytoestrogens, including equol (9). Furthermore, a case-control study from Singapore indicated that breast cancer risk was inversely related to the consumption of soya-containing foods (43). Baggott et al (14) used a chemically induced, estrogen-dependent rat mammary tumor model to demonstrate inhibitory effects of soybean paste on the carcinogenic process. Although the extent of tumor suppression was of marginal statistical significance, these results do point the way to future studies of this interesting approach to breast cancer chemoprevention.

The lignans form a family of chemical compounds with similar origins and properties to the classical phytoestrogens; they are also formed in the intestine by bacterial action on plant-derived precursors and possess both estrogenic and antiestrogenic biological properties. They are excreted in the urine at concentrations that are directly related to the dietary fiber intake (4, 5). Their chemical structures are similar to that of diethylstilbestrol, the synthetic nonsteroidal estrogen (Figure 3). Enterolactone and enterodiol are the major lignans in human urine, and both bind, although with a relatively low affinity, to estrogen receptors and exert some weak estrogenic bioactivity (3). However, the lignans, like equol, may also compete with estradiol for binding sites and, in so doing, cause antiestrogenic effects (80). Another interesing property of enterolactone is its capacity to inhibit placental aromatase, the enzyme responsible for the conversion of the C_{19} steroid androstenedione to estrone (1). Aromatase inhibitors are finding a place in breast cancer endocrine therapy (70), and so one may speculate as to whether the role of lignans in breast cancer prevention includes attenuation of both estrogen biosynthesis and bioactivity.

Adlercreutz (1) has discussed the typical Finnish and American diets as sources of phytoestrogens and lignans, and postulated that the variation in breast cancer risk in the two countries arises, at least in part, from the much

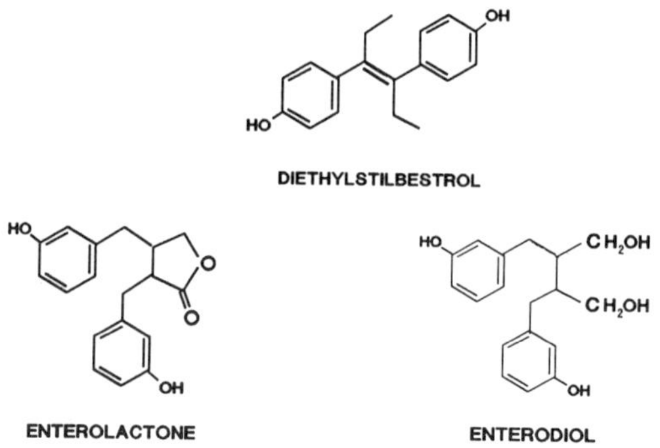

Figure 3 The chemical structure of lignans: similarity to the nonsteroidal estrogen diethylstilbestrol.

higher intake of whole-grain products in Finland. In this context, the intake of wheat bran, which has been reported to reduce the blood estrogens in premenopausal women (68), has no effect on the excretion of lignans in urine. This reduction results only from the consumption of whole grains that have been milled without separating the different components and mixing them again (1).

One study of dietary influences on the lignans was performed in Helsinki and the rural area of North Karelia, Finland, and in Boston (3). Women in Helsinki who consumed a mixed diet had somewhat higher urinary lignan excretions than the American omnivores, whereas the North Karelia omnivores excreted enterolactone at levels that approached those of lactovegetarians in Helsinki. This result is consistent with a shift away from the consumption of whole grains in urban Finland, even in lactovegetarians, and with the observed increase in breast cancer risk noted earlier. In Boston, the omnivores excreted very low levels of urinary enterolactone; lactovegetarians, and particularly a group who followed a "macrobiotic" diet, had much higher levels.

A breast cancer case-control study was also performed in Boston (5). The urinary enterolactone excretion was lower in postmenopausal breast cancer patients compared with normal postmenopausal omnivorous or vegetarian women, but enterodiol excretion was reduced only in comparison to the vegetarian controls.

COMMENTARY AND CONCLUSIONS

There is now convincing evidence that relatively high levels of estrogen bioactivity are associated with increased breast cancer risk. In this chapter, we have seen that elevations in circulating estrogens (61) and altered estrogen metabolism (72) are evident in case-control studies, as are increases in the biologically available estrogen fractions (33, 42). Moreover, similar differences are observed when comprisons are made between women with differing levels of breast cancer risk (18, 38, 51, 72, 74, 79).

It follows logically from these findings that if dietary factors modulate estrogenic stimulation of target tissues, they will, by this mechanism, influence breast cancer risk. As we have discussed and summarized in Table 1, high levels of intake of dietary fat and fiber have opposing effects on circulating estrogens; the former results in higher levels of serum estradiol, estrone, and estrone sulfate; the latter produces reductions in the major blood estrogenic steroids. Moreover, the level of estrogen 16α hydroxylation in women appears to correlate with fat intake (29), and transfer to a low-fat diet results in a shift in estrogen metabolism away from the biosynthesis of 16α hydroxy-derivatives (45), a modification that may also have a favorable effect on breast cancer risk.

These observations, which have been confirmed by several independent groups of investigators, provide biological plausibility for the proposition that a dietary modification, with a reduction in fat intake to 20% of total calories

Table 1 Summary of the interactions between dietary fat and fiber, and circulating estrogen levels in women relative to breast cancer risk

Study design	Dietary factors	Estrogen effects
International comparisons	Postive correlations between estimates of fat consumption and breast cancer risk in different countries: e.g. both are high in US and England and low in Japan.	Lower serum estrogens in women in breast cancer low-risk compared with high-risk locations (rural Japan and China versus US and England).
Special dietary groups	Vegetarians have higher fiber and somewhat lower fat intakes than omnivores.	Higher fecal and lower urinary estrogen excretions in vegetarians, and trend for lower serum levels, compared with omnivores.
		Higher serum SHBG in vegetarians. More frequent menstrual irregularities in vegetarians, and associated with high fiber intakes.
Low fat/high fiber interventions	Low fat (≤20% total calories) or high fiber (wheat bran supplement for total intake of approximately 30g/day) diets.	Reduction in luteal phase serum estradiol and estrone.
	Low fat plus high fiber intervention.	Reduction in follicular phase serum estrone sulphate.
	Low fat diet in postmenopausal women.	Reduction in serum estradiol.

or less and an increase in fiber intake to 25–30g/day, be recommended to reduce the risk of developing breast cancer in the Western countries, where the incidence of this disease is so high. In this context, the endocrine studies reviewed here add support to epidemiological data presented by Prentice & Sheppard (58) that also suggest that a reduction in dietary fat could result in major reductions in breast cancer, and perhaps prostate and ovarian cancer, in the United States and elsewhere.

ACKNOWLEDGMENT

As always, the author is most grateful to Ms. Arlene Banow for her help in preparing the manuscript.

Literature Cited

1. Adlercreutz, H. 1990. Diet, breast cancer and sex hormone metabolism. *Ann. NY Acad. Sci.* 595:281–90
2. Adlercreutz, H., Fotsis, T., Bannwart, C., Hämäläinen, E., Bloigu, S., Ollus, A. 1986. Urinary estrogen profile determination in young Finnish vegetarian and omnivorous women. *J. Steroid Biochem.* 24:289–96
3. Adlercreutz, H., Fotsis, T., Bannwart, C., Wähälä, K., Mäkelä, T., et al. 1986. Determination of urinary lignans and phytoestrogen metabolities, potential antiestrogens and anticarcinogens, in urine of women on various habitual diets. *J. Steroid Biochem.* 25:791–97
4. Adlercreutz, H., Fotsis, T., Heikkinen, R., Dwyer, J. T., Goldin, B. R., et al. 1981. Diet and urinary excretion of lignans in female subjects. *Med. Biol.* 59:259–61
5. Adlercreutz, H., Fotsis, T., Heikkinen, R., Dwyer, J. T., Woods, M., et al. 1982. Excretion of the lignans enterolactone and enterodiol and of equol in omnivorous and vegetarian postmenopausal women and in women with breast cancer. *Lancet* 2:1295–99
6. Adlercreutz, H., Hämäläinen, E., Gorbach, S. L., Goldin, B. R., Woods, M. N., Dwyer, J. T. 1989. Diet and plasma androgens in postmenopausal vegetarian and omnivorous women and postmenopausal women with breast cancer. *Am. J. Clin. Nutr.* 49:433–42
7. Adlercreutz, H., Höckerstedt, K., Bannwart, C., Bloigu, S., Hämäläinen, E., et al. 1987. Effect of dietary components, including lignans and phytoestrogens, on enterohepatic circulation and liver metabolism of estrogens and on sex hormone binding globulin (SHBG). *J. Steroid Biochem.* 27:1135–44
8. Adlercreutz, H., Höckerstedt, K., Bannwart, C., Hämäläinen, E., Fotsis, T., Bloigu, S. 1988. Association between dietary fiber, urinary excretion of lignans and isoflavonic phytoestrogens, and plasma nonprotein bound sex hormones in relation to breast cancer. In *Progress in Cancer Research and Therapy*, ed. F. Bresciani, R. J. B. King, M. E. Lippman, J. P. Raynaud, 35:409–12, New York: Raven
9. Adlercreutz, H., Honjo, H., Higashi, A., Fotsis, T., Hämäläinen, T., et al. 1988. Lignan and phytoestrogen excretion in Japanese consuming traditional diet. *Scand. J. Clin. Lab. Invest.* 48(Suppl.):190 (abstr.)
10. Adlercreutz, H., Martin, F. 1980. Biliary excretion and intestinal metabolism of progesterone and estrogens in man. *J. Steroid Biochem.* 13:231–44
11. Adlercreutz, H., Martin, F., Pulkkinen, M., Dencker, H., Rimér, U., et al. 1976. Intestinal metabolism of estrogens. *J. Clin. Endocrinol. Metab.* 43: 497–505
12. Armstrong, B. K., Brown, J. B., Clarke, H. T., Crooke, D. K., Hähnel, R., et al. 1981. Diet and reproductive hormones: a study of vegetarian and nonvegetarian postmenopausal women. *J. Natl. Cancer Inst.* 67:761–67
13. Armstrong, B. K., Doll, R. 1975. Environmental factors and cancer incidence and mortality in different coun-

tries, with special reference to dietary practices. *Int. J. Cancer* 15:617–31
14. Baggott, J. E., Ha, T., Vaughn, W. H., Juliana, M. M., Hardin, J. M., Grubbs, C. J. 1990. Effect of miso (Japanese soybean paste) and NaCl on DMBA-induced rat mammary tumors. *Nutr. Cancer* 14:103–9
15. Beranek, P. A., Folkerd, E. J., Ghilchik, M. W., James, V. H. T. 1984. 17-Hydroxysteroid dehydrogenase and aromatase activity in breast fat from women with benign and malignant breast tumours. *Clin. Endocrinol.* 20:205–12
16. Borgeson, C. E., Pardini, L., Pardini, R. S., Reitz, R. C. 1989. Effects of dietary fish oil on human mammary carcinoma and on lipid-metabolizing enzymes. *Lipids* 24:290–95
17. Braden L. M., Carroll, K. K. 1985. Dietary polyunsaturated fat in relation to mammary carcinogenesis in rats. *Lipids* 21:285–88
18. Bulbrook, R. D., Swain, M. C., Wang, D. Y., Hayward, J. L., Kumaoka, S., et al. 1976. Breast cancer in Britain and Japan: plasma oestradiol-17, oestrone and progesterone, and their urinary metabolites in normal British and Japanese women. *Eur. J. Cancer* 12:725–35
19. Carroll, K. K. 1975. Experimental evidence of dietary factors and hormone-dependent cancers. *Cancer Res.* 35: 3374–83
20. Crossette, L. B. 1991. Evidence of protective effects of wheat fiber grows. *J. Natl. Cancer Inst.* 83:1614–15
21. DeMoor, P., Joosens, J. V. 1970. An inverse relation between body weight and the activity of the steroid binding globulin in human plasma. *Steroidologia* 1:129–36
22. Dwyer, J. T. 1988. Health aspects of vegetarian diets. *Am. J. Clin. Nutr.* 48:712–38
23. Fentiman, I. S., Caleffi, M., Wang, D. Y., Hampson, S. J., Hoare, S. A., et al. 1988. The binding of blood-borne estrogens in normal vegetarian and omnivorous women and the risk of breast cancer. *Nutr. Cancer* 11:101–6
24. Folman, Y., Pope, G. S. 1969. Effect of norethisterone acetate, dimethylstilboestrol, genistein and coumestrol on uptake of [^{3}H]oestradiol by uterus, vagina, and skeletal muscle of immature mice. *J. Endocrinol.* 44:213–18
25. Goldin, B. R., Adlercreutz, H., Gorbach, S. L., Warram, J. H., Dwyer, J. T., et al. 1982. Estrogen excretion patterns and plasma levels in vegetarian and omnivorous women. *N. Engl. J. Med.* 307:1542–47
26. Goldin, B. R., Adlercreutz, H., Gorbach, S. L., Woods, M. N., Dwyer, J. T., et al. 1986. The relationship between estrogen levels and diets of Caucasian American and Oriental immigrant women. *Am. J. Clin. Nutr.* 44:945–53
27. Hawkins, R. A., Thomson, M. L., Killen, E. 1985. Oestrone sulphate, adipose tissue, and breast cancer. *Breast Cancer Res. Treat.* 6:75–87
28. Hems, G. 1978. The contributions of diet and child-bearing to breast cancer rates. *Br. J. Cancer* 37:974–82
29. Herschcopf, R. J., Fishman, J., Bradlow, H. L., Karmali, R., Michnovicz, J. J., et al. 1988. Extent of estrogen 16-alpha hydroxylation correlates with dietary saturated fat in women. *Proc. Annu. Meet. Endocrine Soc.*, 70th 1332 (Abstr.)
30. Hislop, T. G., Coldman, A. J., Elwood, J. M. 1986. Childhood and recent eating patterns and risk of breast cancer. *Cancer Detect. Prev.* 9:47–58
31. Howe, G. R., Hirohata, T., Hislop, T. G., Iscovich, J. M., Yuan, J.-M., et al. 1990. Dietary factors and risk of breast cancer: combined analysis of 12 case-control studies. *J. Natl. Cancer Inst.* 82:561–69
32. Jasonni, V. M., Bulletti, C., Franceschetti, F., Bonavia, M., Bolelli, G., et al. 1984. Estrone sulfate plasma levels in postmenopausal women with and without endometrial cancer. *Cancer* 53:2698–2700
33. Jones, L. A., Ota, D. M., Jackson, G. A., Jackson, P. M., Kemp, K., et al. 1987. Bioavailability of estradiol as a marker for breast cancer risk assessment. *Cancer Res.* 47:5224–29
34. Judd, H. L., Lucas, W. E., Yen, S. S. C. 1976. Serum 17-estradiol and estrone levels in postmenopausal women with and without endometrial cancer. *J. Clin. Endocrinol. Metab.* 43:272–78
35. Jurkowski, J. J., Cave, W. T. Jr. 1985. Dietary effects of menhaden oil on the growth and membrane lipid composition of rat mammary tumors. *J. Natl. Cancer Inst.* 74:1145–50
36. Kaizer, L., Boyd, N. F., Kriukov, V., Tritchler, D. 1989. Fish consumption and breast cancer risk: an ecological study. *Nutr. Cancer* 12:61–68
37. Karmali, R., Marsh, J., Fuchs, C. 1984. Effect of omega-3 fatty acids on growth of a rat mammary tumor. *J. Natl. Cancer Inst.* 73:457–61

38. Key, T. J. A., Chen, J., Wang, D. Y., Pike, M. C., Boreham, J. 1990. Sex hormones in women in rural China and in Britain. *Br. J. Cancer,* 62:631–36
39. Key, T. J. A., Pike, M. C. 1988. The dose-effect relationship between "unopposed" estrogens and endometrial mitotic rate: its central role in explaining and predicting endometrial cancer risk. *Br. J. Cancer* 57:205–12
40. Key, T. J. A., Pike, M. C. 1988. The role of oestrogens and progestogens in the epidemiology and prevention of breast cancer. *Eur. J. Cancer Clin. Oncol.* 24:29–43
41. Kromann, N., Green, A. 1980. Epidemiological studies in the Upernavik District, Greenland: incidence of some chronic diseases 1950–1974. *Acta Med. Scand.* 208:401–6
42. Langley, M. S., Hammond, G. L., Bardsley, A., Sellwood, R. A., Anderson, D. C. 1985. Serum steroid binding proteins and the bioavailability of estradiol in relation to breast diseases. *J. Natl. Cancer Inst.* 75:823–29
43. Lee, H. P., Gourley, L., Duffy, S. W. Esteve, J., Lee, J., Day, N. E. 1991. Dietary effects on breast cancer risk in Singapore. *Lancet* 337:1197–1200
44. Lloyd, T., Schaeffer, J. M., Walker, M. A., Demers, L. M. 1991. Urinary hormonal concentrations and spinal bone densities of premenopausal vegetarian and nonvegetarian women. *Am. J. Clin. Nutr.* 54:1005–10
45. Longcope, C., Gorbach, S., Goldin, B., Woods, M., Dwyer, J., et al. 1987. The effect of a low fat diet on estrogen metabolism. *J. Clin. Endocrinol. Metab.* 64:1246–50
46. Lubin, F., Ruder, A. M., Wax, Y., Modan, B. 1985. Overweight and changes in weight throughout adult life in breast cancer etiology: a case-control study. *Am. J. Epidemiol.* 122:579–88
47. Lubin, F., Way, Y., Modan, B. 1986. Role of fat, animal protein, and dietary fiber in breast cancer etiology: a case control study. *J. Natl. Cancer Inst.* 77:605–12
48. MacDonald, P. C., Edman, C. D., Hemsell, D. L., Porter, J. C., Siiteri, P. K. 1978. Effect of obesity on conversion of plasma androstendione to estrone in postmenopausal women with and without endometrial cancer. *Am. J. Obstet. Gynecol.* 130:448–55
49. Martin, P. M., Horwitz, K. B., Ryan, D. S., McGuire, W. L. 1987. Phytoestrogen interaction with estrogen receptors in human breast cancer cells. *Endocrinology* 103:1860–67
50. Masarei, J. R., Armstrong, B. K., Skinner, M. W., Ratajczak, T., Hähnel, R., et al. 1980. HDL-Cholesterol and sex hormone status. *Lancet* 1:208
51. Moore, J. W., Clark, G. M. G., Takatani, O., Wakabayashi, Y., Hayward, J. L., Bulbrook, R. D. 1983. Distribution of 17-estradiol in the sera of normal British and Japanese women. *J. Natl. Cancer Inst.* 71:749–54
52. Nielsen, N. H., Hansen, J. P. H. 1980. Breast cancer in Greenland-selected epidemiological, clinical and histological features. *J. Cancer Res. Clin. Oncol.* 98:287–99
53. Osborne, M. P., Karmali, R. A., Hershcopf, J., Bradlow, H. L., Kourides, I. A., et al. 1988. Omega-3 fatty acid: modulation of estrogen metabolism and potential breast cancer prevention. *Cancer Invest.* 6:629–31
54. Pardridge, W. M. 1981. Transport of protein-bound hormones into tissues in vivo. *Endocrinol. Rev.* 2:103–23
55. Pedersen, A. B., Bartholomew, M. J., Dolence, L. A., Aljadir, L. P., Netteburg, K. L., Lloyd, T. 1991. Menstrual differences due to vegetarian and nonvegetarian diets. *Am. J. Clin. Nutr.* 53:879–85
56. Phillips, R. L. 1975. Role of life-style and dietary habits in risk of cancer among Seventh-Day Adventists. *Cancer Res.* 35:3513–22
57. Phillips, R. L., Snowdon, D. A. 1983. Association of meat and coffee use with cancers of the large bowel, breast and prostate among Seventh-Day Adventists: preliminary results. *Cancer Res.* 43(Suppl.):2403s–8s
58. Prentice, R. L., Sheppard, L. 1990. Dietary fat and cancer: consistency of the epidemiologic data, and disease prevention that may follow from a practical reduction in fat consumption. *Cancer Causes Control* 1:81–87
59. Prentice, R. L., Thompson, D., Clifford, C., Gorbach, S., Goldin, B., Byar, D. 1990. Dietary fat reduction and plasma estradiol concentration in healthy postmenopausal women. *J. Natl. Cancer Inst.* 82:129–34
60. Price, K. R., Fenwick, G. R. 1985. Naturally occurring oestrogens in foods—a review. *Food Addit. Contam.* 2:73–106
61. Prost, O., Turrel, M. O., Dahan, N., Craveur, C., Adessi, G. L. 1984. Estrone and dehydroepiandrosterone sulfatase activities and plasma estrone

sulfate levels in human breast carcinoma. *Cancer Res.* 44:661–64

62. Rogers, J., Mitchell, G. W. 1952. The relation of obesity to menstrual disturbances. *N. Engl. J. Med.* 247: 53–55
63. Rose, D. P. 1990. Dietary fiber and breast cancer. *Nutr. Cancer* 13:1–8
64. Rose, D. P. 1992. Dietary fiber, phytoestrogens and breast cancer. *Nutrition* 8:47–51
65. Rose, D. P., Boyar, A. P., Cohen, C., Strong, L. E. 1987. Effect of a low-fat diet on hormone levels in women with cystic breast disease. I. Serum steroids and gonadotropins. *J. Natl. Cancer Inst.* 78:623–26
66. Rose, D. P., Boyar, A. P., Wynder, E. L. 1986. International comparisons of mortality rates for cancer of the breast, ovary, prostate, and colon, and per capita food consumption. *Cancer* 58:2363–71
67. Rose, D. P., Connolly, J. M. 1992. Dietary fat, fatty acids and prostate cancer. *Lipids* 27:798–803
68. Rose, D. P., Goldman, M., Connolly, J. M., Strong, L. E. 1991. High-fiber diet reduces serum estrogen concentrations in premenopausal women. *Am. J. Clin. Nutr.* 54:520–25
69. Sakomoto, G., Sugano, H., Hartman, W. H. 1979. Comparative clinicopathological study of breast cancer among Japanese and American women. *Jpn. J. Cancer Clin.* 25:161–70
70. Santen, R. J. 1987. Current status of aromatase inhibitors for treatment of breast cancer: new perspectives. In *Hormonal Manipulation of Cancer: Peptides, Growth Factors, and New (Anti) Steroidal Agents,* ed. J. G. M. Klijn, R. Paridaens, J. A. Foekens, pp. 71–80. New York: Raven. 535 pp.
71. Schneider, J., Bradlow, H. L., Strain, G., Levin, J., Anderson, K., Fishman, J. 1983. Effect of obesity on estradiol metabolism: decreased formation of nonuterotropic metabolites. *J. Clin. Endocrinol. Metab.* 56:973–78
72. Schneider, J., Kinne, D., Fracchia, A., Pierce, V., Anderson, K. E., et al. 1982. Abnormal oxidative metabolism of estradiol in women with breast cancer. *Proc. Natl. Acad. Sci. USA* 79:3047–51
73. Setchell, K. D., R., Borriello, S. P., Hulme, P., Kirk, D. N., Axelson, M. 1984. Nonsteroidal estrogens of dietary origin: possible roles in hormone-dependent disease. *Am. J. Clin. Nutr.* 40:569–78
74. Shimizu, H., Ross, R. K., Bernstein, L., Pike, M. C., Henderson, B. E. 1990. Serum oestrogen levels in postmenopausal women: comparison of American whites and Japanese in Japan. *Br. J. Cancer* 62:451–53
75. Shultz, T. D., Howie, B. J. 1986. In vitro binding of steroid hormones by natural and purified fibers. *Nutr. Cancer* 8:141–47
76. Taylor, P. R., Judd, J. T., Jones, D. Y., Nair, P. P., Campbell, W. S. 1992. Influence of type and amount of dietary fat on plasma estradiol (E) in premenopausal women. *Am. J. Clin. Nutr.* (Suppl.) Am. Soc. of Clin. Nutr. Annu. Meet. 1992, abstr. 130
77. Tseng, L., Stolee, A., Gurpide, E. 1972. Quantitative studies on the uptake and metabolism of estrogens and progesterone by human endometrium. *Endocrinology* 90:390–404
78. Vermeulen, A., Verdonck, L. 1978. Sex hormone concentrations in postmenopausal women. *Clin. Endocrinol.* 9:59–66
79. Wang, D. Y., Key, T. J. A., Pike, M. C., Boreham, J., Chen, J. 1991. Serum hormone levels in British and rural Chinese females. *Breast Cancer Res. Treat.* 18:S41–S45
80. Waters, A. P., Knowler, J. T. 1982. Effect of a lignan (HPMF) on RNA synthesis in the rat uterus. *Reprod. Fertil.* 66:379–81
81. Whitten, C. G., Shultz, T. D. 1988. Binding of steroid hormones in vitro by water-insoluble dietary fiber. *FASEB J.* 1:A862
82. Willett, W. C., Browne, M. L., Bain, C., Lipnick, R. J., Stampfer, M. J., et al. 1985. Relative weight and risk of breast cancer among premenopausal women. *Am. J. Epidemiol.* 122:731–40
83. Woods, M. N., Gorbach, S. L., Longcope, C., Goldin, B. R., Dwyer, J. T., Morrill-LaBrode, A. 1989. Low-fat, high-fiber diet and serum estrone sulfate in premenopausal women. *Am. J. Clin. Nutr.* 49:1179–83
84. Wynder, E. L., Fujita, Y., Harris, R. E., Hirayama, T., Hiyama, T. 1991. Comparative epidemiology of cancer between the United States and Japan. *Cancer* 67:746–63
85. Wynder, E. L., Rose, D. P., Cohen, L. A. 1986. Diet and breast cancer in causation and therapy. *Cancer* 58: 1804–13

Annu. Rev. Publ. Health 1993. 14:19–42

INFLUENCE OF HIV INFECTION ON MANIFESTATIONS AND NATURAL HISTORY OF OTHER SEXUALLY TRANSMITTED DISEASES

Anna Wald[1,2], *Lawrence Corey*[1,2], *H. Hunter Handsfield*[2], *and King K. Holmes*[2]

Departments of [1]Laboratory Medicine and [2]Medicine, University of Washington, Seattle, Washington 98195

KEY WORDS: genital ulcer disease, herpes simplex, hepatitis, Kaposi's sarcoma

---

INTRODUCTION

Human immunodeficiency virus (HIV) is the most devastating sexually acquired infection. As sexual transmission of HIV continues to occur worldwide, the concomitant presence of other sexually transmitted diseases (STDs) in HIV-infected persons is being seen with increasing frequency. The profound effects on host immunity that HIV exerts appear to influence the clinical course of numerous bacterial, protozoal, and viral pathogens. These problems have recently been explored by Wasserheit (123), who coined the term "epidemiologic synergy" to describe the interrelationships between HIV infection and STDs, including the effects of STDs on HIV transmission and progression, as well as the effects of HIV on progressive STD transmission and in the clinical course of STDs. This paper addresses specifically the influence of HIV on each of the major STDs.

0163-7525/93/0510-0019$02.00

SEXUALLY TRANSMITTED VIRAL INFECTIONS

Genital Herpes

Almost all HIV-infected patients are coinfected with either herpes simplex type-1 (HSV-1) or herpes simplex type-2 (HSV-2), or both. Herpes simplex type-1 infection is universal in the developing world and is found in 80–100% of HIV-infected adults. Herpes simplex type-2 antibodies have been found in 40–100% of HIV-infected adults and are especially frequent among those with sexually acquired HIV. Several cross-sectional studies of both homosexually active men and heterosexually active men and women attending STD clinics have shown that HSV is an independent risk factor for acquisition of HIV (49, 57, 115). For example, among sex workers in Nairobi, 100% have serological evidence of infection with HSV-1; 84% have evidence of infection with HSV-2 (67). Such a high frequency may be a marker for sexual behaviors that are risky for both HIV and HSV infections, such as large numbers of casual sexual partners or anal intercourse among homosexual men.

Alternations in cellular immunity have long been recognized to increase the severity and frequency of HSV recurrences. Nonhealing perianal ulcerative herpes simplex was among the initial opportunistic infections described in homosexual men with acquired immunodeficiency (111). Mucocutaneous herpes that persists for more than one month is sufficient for a diagnosis of AIDS. In persons with low CD4 counts, HSV appears to cause persistent mucocutaneous ulcerative lesions, often in atypical anatomic sites. Among homosexual men, perianal reactivation is particularly common. Chronic herpetic ulcers may persist for months and crust over, which gives an impetigenous quality to the lesions, thus making correct diagnosis difficult, although HSV can be easily isolated from scrapings of the ulcer.

In addition to chronic genital ulcers, facial herpetic infections, extensive herpetic whitlow, esophagitis, transverse myelitis, and meningoencephalitis have been reported (44, 90, 111). Nevertheless, disseminated HSV infection in HIV-infected persons is uncommon.

Although formal studies are not available, a wealth of clinical experience indicates that most mucocutaneous herpetic infections respond well to treatment with oral acyclovir. As in other immunocompromised patients, experts recommend a higher dose than used in normal hosts (31) and prophylactic treatment to decrease the frequency of HSV reactivation.

Several investigators have reported AIDS patients with lesions caused by herpetic isolates resistant to acyclovir (40, 44, 90). Almost all of the patients received previous acyclovir therapy, either intermittently or continuously; for many of these patients, the lesions have healed before the appearance of acyclovir-resistant strain. Most of these mutants appear to be thymidine kinase-deficient and phosphorylate acyclovir poorly. Occasionally, the lesions resolve with intravenous therapy, but in our experience alternative treatment is usually needed. Foscarnet has been used successfully in patients with mucocutaneous acyclovir-resistant herpes virus (26, 106), although resistance to foscarnet has been noted (11). After successful healing with foscarnet, recurrences with both acyclovir-sensitive and acyclovir-resistant herpes strains have been observed (106). Other alternative therapy includes topical trifluorothymidine.

At present, we do not know whether resistance is more likely to occur with intermittent or continuous acyclovir regimens. The probability of spontaneous mutations resulting in acyclovir resistance may be greater with the use of intermittent, as compared with suppressive, therapy (3).

Cytomegalovirus

Cytomegalovirus (CMV) is a ubiquitous infection worldwide, acquired in a variety of ways, including perinatal exposure, breast milk, salivary contact, and sexual transmission. Most persons acquire CMV infection in childhood, but a substantial number become infected in adolescence or adulthood through sexual contact. In women, young age at initiation of sexual activity, number of sexual partners, presence of other STDs, and nonwhite race all correlate with seropositivity of CMV (25, 29). Among homosexual men, the prevalence of CMV infection approaches 95%. In one study, the acquisition of new infection in susceptible gay men over a nine-month period was 71% and correlated closely with receptive anal intercourse (86). Sexual transmission probably results from the persistent shedding of CMV in the semen and endocervical secretions (30, 38). Injection drug users (IDUs) may also be at increased risk for acquiring CMV infection through contaminated needles (15). Thus, CMV spreads by a variety of ways, and serologic surveys show evidence of past infection with CMV in most HIV-infected adults.

Reactivation of CMV in patients with AIDS occurs as the immunosuppression increases; as effective treatment prolongs life in HIV-infected persons, CMV has emerged as one of the major pathogens. A detailed review of clinical syndromes caused by CMV and their treatment is beyond the scope of this paper.

Whereas most other immunocompetent patients experience only intermittent subclinical reactivations of CMV, HIV has profound effects on CMV infection. The most frequently recognized manifestation is a progressive retinitis, which affects about 25% of patients with AIDS and occurs almost exclusively in those with CD4 counts below 50/μL (54). As immunosuppression worsens, the prevalence of CMV viremia increases from 0% of those with normal CD4 count to about 50% of those with CD4 count below 50/μL (45). Asymptomatic viremia often precedes development of symptomatic disease in the retina; gastrointestinal tract, especially colitis and esophagitis;

and central nervous system (CNS), especially encephalitis and radiculopathy (6, 37, 39).

Treatment with ganciclovir is effective in remitting CMV retinitis, but patients require life-long maintenance therapy, and, in most, retinitis eventually recurs (53). Furthermore, the drug is administered intravenously and causes myelosuppression, thus often requiring interruption of antiretroviral therapy with zidovudine. Ganciclovir has not been shown to be as effective for CMV infection of other sites, although treatment is often attempted. A recent comparison of ganciclovir and foscarnet showed a survival advantage in patients with CMV retinitis who received foscarnet, which has a broader antiviral spectrum (114). Because the rate of progression of retinitis was similar in both groups, the prolonged survival may have been mediated by foscarnet's additional activity against HIV.

Hepatitis B

Sexual transmission of hepatitis B virus (HBV) accounts for nearly half of all cases of acute hepatitis B attributable to a recognized risk factor in the United States, with most of the remaining cases attributable to injection drug use. In southern Europe and the newly industrialized countries of Asia and Latin America, perinatal and childhood transmission of hepatitis B is apparently decreasing, such that a growing proportion of the population reaches puberty susceptible to HBV, and sexual transmission may grow in importance in these regions. In parts of Africa, the infection still occurs primarily in the perinatal or childhood periods, and the prevalence of serum HBV markers reaches 50–100% by young adulthood. Serologic markers of past infection with hepatitis B are detectable in approximately 90% of HIV-infected homosexual men; similarly, about 90% of IDUs have been infected, most likely by sharing needles.

Studies suggest that HIV-infected persons 1) have less prominent biochemical and histologic evidence of inflammation; 2) display higher levels of viral markers, such as HBeAg, which suggests increased hepatic production of virus and increased infectivity; 3) progress from acute infection to chronic carriage state more frequently; 4) may reactivate quiescent hepatitis B infection; 5) show an impaired immune response to hepatitis B vaccine; 6) and show little benefit from α-interferon therapy for chronic hepatitis B. These observations are consistent with the hypothesis that intact cellular immunity contributes both to recovery from chronic hepatitis B and to sustained hepatic damage in chronic hepatitis B carriers.

The effect of prior HIV infection on the clinical manifestations of acute hepatitis B is not clear. HIV infection may predispose to more frequent clinical illness during acute hepatitis B infection (51), although patients appear less likely to be icteric (12, 51). Other studies found no difference in the clinical and biochemical profiles during the acute infection (87). Chronic hepatitis B infection tends to be less severe in HIV-seropositive patients with lower transaminase elevations (51, 68); in one group, however, lower serum alanine aminotransferase levels were limited to HBeAg-negative men (13). Histologic grading of liver biopsies also tends to be milder in HIV-infected patients (82). Another study, however, found no difference in serum aspartate aminotransferase between HIV-seropositive patients with various degrees of immune impairment and HIV-seronegative patients (98). Whether the incidence of hepatocellular carcinoma is influenced by concomitant HIV infection has not been addressed.

Studies have found that prior HIV infection increased the hepatitis B carriage rate from 4–7% in HIV-seronegative men to 20–23% in HIV-seropositive men (12, 116). When HIV and HBV are acquired in close temporal sequence, the carrriage rate of HBsAg may approach 40% (12).

Additionally, HIV-infected hepatitis B carriers are more likely to be HBeAg positive (13) and to have lower rates of seroconversion to anti-HBeAg, when compared with HIV-uninfected carriers (68). They tend to have high levels of HBV DNA in serum, large quantities of DNA polymerase on liver biopsy, and increased numbers of hepatocytes staining for HBcAg and HBeAg (68, 82). Severe T-cell depletion associated with HIV may lead to reactivation of "dormant" HBV (71). For example, three patients with AIDS, previously reactive for anti-HBsAg, had clinical and biochemical evidence of acute hepatitis, fatal in one case, with detectable HBsAg and loss of anti-HBsAg (120). Serologic markers for hepatitis D replication also appear to be increased in HIV-infected men with concurrent chronic hepatitis B and D infections (16, 48).

In a therapeutic trial of recombinant $\alpha-$interferon for chronic active hepatitis B infection, one third of HIV-seronegative patients improved, as defined by sustained loss of HBV DNA and HBeAg, compared with none with HIV infection (81).

HIV infection is associated with decreased responsiveness to hepatitis B vaccine (28). HIV-seropositive persons who fail to respond to the vaccine, or who become infected with HBV before completing all doses of the vaccine, appear at greatest risk of becoming chronic carriers, 31% and 55–80%, respectively (51). This surprisingly detrimental effect of partial immunization underscores the importance of safer sex behavior during the immunization schedule.

In the United States, the advent of safer sex practices has been associated with a decrease in hepatitis B infection in homosexual men (2). Unfortunately, this decrease has been offset by a substantial increase in the incidence of hepatitis associated with intravenous drug use and heterosexual activity. As the HIV epidemic shifts to involve those same risk groups, which are not currently targeted in vaccination programs, the prevalence of persons with contagious hepatitis B is likely to be sustained at higher rates (65). Current strategies for routine infant HBV immunization are important, and most practical, to achieve high levels of vaccine usage on a global basis. However, in the United States, this strategy will have almost no impact on hepatitis B morbidity for 20 years. To protect the current generation of children and young adults, a concurrent strategy of immunizing high risk groups and adolescents in high risk settings has been advocated by the World Health Organization (WHO) and the Centers for Disease Control (CDC) (21, 124).

Genital and Anorectal Warts

Human papillomavirus (HPV) infection is one of the most common sexually transmitted infections in the United States. HPV infection has reached critical public health importance, because epidemiologic and laboratory evidence has linked it to cervical cancer, the leading type of cancer in young women in most developing countries (100). Furthermore, HPV is associated with vulvar, vaginal, penile, and anal cancer, each of which is about one-tenth as common as cervical cancer in the United States.

EFFECT OF HIV INFECTION ON GENITAL AND CERVICAL WARTS Because cervical carcinoma arises more frequently in immunosuppressed women, several studies have addressed the influence of HIV infection on the natural history of cervical and anal HPV infection. The prevalence of cervical intraepithelial neoplasia (CIN) in HIV-infected women exceeds community levels tenfold, depending on the techniques used for detection of HPV (77, 107, 110). For example, 23 of 33 women (70%) with symptomatic HIV disease had HPV DNA demonstrated in specimens from the cervix, as compared with 4 of 18 (22%) asymptomatic and 10 of 45 (22%) HIV-seronegative women with similar demographic and behavioral profiles (121). CIN was found in 52% of women with symptomatic HIV infection who had concurrent HPV infection, compared with 18% of women with either virus alone. This effect was especially pronounced in black and Latino women with symptomatic HIV infection. Of women with cytologic evidence of HPV infection, 78% of HIV-positive women had CIN, compared with 57% of HIV-negative IDUs and 33% of outpatients in general (107). CIN was often high grade and involved a greater portion of the cervix, or multiple genital sites, in women with HIV infection (75). The prevalence of dysplasia rose significantly as the lymphocyte count diminished and defects in the lymphoproliferative response developed; four of five invasive cervical carcinomas among HIV-seropositive women were found in women with CD4 lymphocyte count below 50/μl (107).

Therapy of warts appears more difficult in women with HIV infection, as the lesions tend to persist or recur. Resistance to local therapy occurred in 5 of 12 (42%) HIV-seropositive, versus 6 of 50 (12%) HIV-seronegative, women (80). Yearly cytologic examination of the cervix has been recommended for HIV-infected women; semi-annual examination has been recommended for those with CD4 counts below 200/μl (24, 121). However, the usefulness of cytologic smears for detection of abnormal lesions demonstrable by biopsy in HIV-infected women is unclear (76). In one study of 32 HIV-infected women evaluated by both cytology and colposcopy with biopsy, only three had abnormalities detected by cytology, whereas 13 had CIN evident on biopsy.

Because most studies have been cross-sectional, it is difficult to assess whether the higher prevalence of HPV among HIV-seropositive women is caused by more frequent reactivation, or whether the acquisition of both viruses is associated with similar risk behavior. However, the association of dysplasia with immunosuppression among women with HIV infection is compelling.

EFFECT OF HIV INFECTION ON GENITAL AND ANAL WARTS Epidemiologic studies of heterosexual and homosexual men show that homosexual men who practice anal intercourse have a 33-fold increased risk of anal carcinoma (33). The anorectal squamous columnar junction bears embryologic and histologic similarities to the squamo-columnar transitional zone of the cervix, which suggests the possibility of similarities in the pathogenesis of anal and cervical cancer. Tumor registry in San Francisco shows that the incidence of anal cancer has risen sevenfold in the last decade, which coincides with the HIV epidemic and probably follows epidemic spread of anal HPV infection during the 1960s and 1970s. The incidence of anal cancer in homosexual men now approaches the incidence of cervical cancer before routine cytologic screening was implemented (66). As with cervical dysplasia, the prevalence of anal HPV is higher in HIV-seropositive homosexual men than in HIV-seronegative men, even after adjusting for sexual exposure. Among HIV-seropositive men, the prevalence of HPV DNA increases as immunosuppression increases; among homosexual men with demonstrable HPV DNA, the prevalence of anal dysplasia is higher for those with HIV infection, especially for those with immunosuppression (N. B. Kiviat 1992, personal communication).

For example, in an early study involving 61 healthy homosexual men, anal dysplasia was correlated with history of anal warts, frequency of receptive anal intercourse, HIV infection, and decreased CD4/CD8 ratio (42). Subsequently, Palevsky studied 97 HIV-infected homosexual men in San Francisco and demonstrated anal HPV (by relatively insensitive DNA probe methods then available) in 54%; the risk of anal intraepithelial neoplasia (AIN) was fivefold higher in men with HPV than in those without it (93). Recently, using the more sensitive polymerase chain reaction technique, an even higher proportion of HIV-seropositive men was found to have anal HPV infection.

The association between detection of HPV DNA and HIV infection persists after adjustment for demographic and behavioral variables (66) and becomes stronger in men with low CD4 cell counts (20). In a Danish study of 120 homosexual men, detection of anal HPV rose from 7% of subjects with CD4/CD8 ratio above 1 to 35% of those with ratio below 0.4, whereas anal cytologic abnormalities were present in 20% of the subjects (84).

A recent prospective study of 111 homosexual men in Seattle demonstrated HPV DNA in 50% of HIV-infected and 15% of HIV-uninfected men (32). At enrollment, cytologic smears detected abnormalities in 40% and 14%, respectively. Longitudinal follow-up revealed the development of AIN in an additional 39% of HIV-positive and 24% of HIV-negative men who had normal initial findings; the risk was sevenfold higher in men with anal HPV.

A comparative trial of intralesional α-interferon in the treatment of anogenital warts showed that the efficacy of interferon was limited to the HIV-negative group (11/21 versus 0/9) (36). Warts treated with topical agents also appear to require longer courses of therapy in HIV-positive than HIV-negative men (83). Routine anal cytologic screening of homosexual men with HIV infection, with treatment of the lesions detected, is under active consideration.

In summary, in the presence of HIV infection, HPV of the cervix and anus apparently progresses more rapidly or more often than in a normal person to dysplasia. Whether this leads to increased risk of cervical and anal invasive cancer remains to be determined. The time for progression of HPV-related CIN and AIN to invasive cancer is thought to be 10–20 years. Whether this period is substantially shortened in HIV-infected women and men, especially with the advent of antiretroviral therapy, is unknown.

Molluscum Contagiosum

Molluscum contagiosum, a poxvirus, causes a viral eruption that usually has a benign course and resolves spontaneously. Few data are available on the rates of infection in the general population, because the infection is usually asymptomatic and of little consequence in healthy persons. Several case reports have associated widespread, recurrent molluscum contagiosum infection with impaired immunity.

Systematic surveys of cutaneous manifestations of HIV infection have noted a high prevalence of molluscum lesions, especially in persons with clinically overt immunosuppression. Among unselected homosexual patients with AIDS, molluscum contagiosum was noted in 6 of 34 (18%), compared with 0 of 25 asymptomatic seropositive men and 1 of 75 seronegative homosexual men (78); another survey of 117 adult men and women with symptomatic

HIV infection, predominantly IDUs, showed molluscum contagiosum in 10% of patients with AIDS and 7% of those with AIDS-related complex (47). In contrast, a study of 100 consecutive HIV-infected patients found an overall prevalence of molluscum of 8% that did not vary with the clinical stage (27).

Molluscum contagiosum infections in patients with AIDS are usually marked by extensive lesions involving predominantly the face and neck (63, 99). Frequently, the lesions are abundant, recur rapidly in spite of therapy, and represent a substantial cosmetic problem. Umbilicated papules, considered morphologically "typical" for molluscum contagiosum, may be seen with cutaneous cryptococcal infections in AIDS patients (85, 102). The similar appearance has delayed diagnosis and institution of systemic antifungal therapy. Thus, confirmation of molluscum lesions by biopsy and staining for molluscum bodies appears prudent, especially in HIV-infected patients with CD4 counts less than 200/μL.

SEXUALLY TRANSMITTED BACTERIAL INFECTIONS

Syphilis

As with the viral STDs, HIV appears to affect the epidemiology, clinical manifestations, and treatment of many bacterial STDs. The rates of syphilis rose dramatically in the United States in the late 1980s, especially among the inner-city African-American communities, often in connection with crack cocaine use and exchange of sex for drugs. Control has been complicated by the apparent failure of contact tracing and partner notification (4). At the same time, rates of syphilis in homosexually active men declined dramatically, which reflects the adoption of safer sex behavior in response to the HIV epidemic. In parts of Africa and other developing countries, the prevalence of syphilis remains extremely high (14). As with other genital ulcers, *Treponema pallidum* infection appears to be an independent risk factor for HIV infection.

Unusual or severe manifestations of syphilis have been reported increasingly in HIV-infected patients, but the extent to which these case reports represent a true increase in rates of complications in those with HIV infection, or a renewed interest in reporting treponemal infections, is unclear (72). Dermatologic manifestations of syphilis consistent with precocious tertiary syphilis, or gummas, have occurred in persons with recently acquired or previously treated infection (5, 34). Although no population-based studies are available, the number of anecdotally reported patients strongly suggests a true increase in neurosyphilis in the presence of HIV infection. The hypothesis that the natural course of syphilis is adversely affected by HIV infection is indirectly supported by the clinical and pathogenic parallels between syphilis and tuberculosis, for which such interactions are well documented. Both *T. pallidum* and *Mycobacterium tuberculosis* are slow-growing intracellular pathogens, and cell-mediated immunity is important in containment (72). Both syphilis and tuberculosis are characterized by mild or subclinical primary infections accompanied by silent bacteremia with seeding of multiple organs and systems, followed by prolonged subclinical infection and later destructive, granulomatous lesions if cell-mediated immunity wanes. These facts enhance the plausibility of the existing case reports, despite the lack of definitive epidemiologic documentation that neurological complications are more common in the presence of HIV infection.

The clinical aspects of neurosyphilis in HIV-infected patients have recently been reviewed (89). Classic late neurosyphilis (tabes dorsalis, general paresis) appears to be rare; almost all reports have involved meningitis, meningovasculitis, or ocular or otologic infection, with presentations of stroke, cranial nerve dysfunction, syphilitic meningitis, transverse myelitis, polyradiculopathy, asymptomatic neurosyphilis, uveitis, optic neuritis and chorioretinitis, hearing loss, and tinnitis (9, 10, 62, 113). These manifestations are predominantly complications of early syphilis, occurring most commonly in the first year of infection. In many patients, the neurological involvement occurred after prior standard therapy for primary or secondary syphilis (10, 62). The predominant effect of HIV infection appears to be an increased incidence of early neurosyphilis, rather than occurrence of new or previously unrecognized manifestations of neurosyphilis (58).

Invasion of the CNS by *T. pallidum* occurs in most cases of early syphilis, even in persons without HIV infection (73). In most patients with an intact immune system, treatment with benzathine penicillin G seems to be sufficient for cure. Immunodeficiency induced by HIV appears to render the benzathine penicillin G treatment ineffective in a substantial proportion of cases. In the pre-antibiotic era, the incidence of early syphilitic meningitis and ocular infection, but not that of tabes or paresis, was higher in patients who received partial treatment for primary or secondary syphilis than in untreated patients (58, 89). It was believed that this occurred because arsenicals and other drugs failed to eradicate *T. pallidum* from the CNS or the eye, but that killing the organism at other sites resulted in an attenuated immune response that subsequently permitted renewed or accelerated growth in sites where the organism persisted. The same effect may occur when benzathine penicillin, which does not achieve treponemicidal levels in cerebrospinal fluid (CSF), is used to treat syphilis in persons with impaired cellular immunity due to HIV. The effect might also explain the predominance of meningitis, meningovasculitis, and ocular infection.

Data on the effect of HIV infection on the serological diagnosis of syphilis are conflicting. Investigators have hypothesized and occasionally reported that the prevalence and titers of both nontreponemal (cardiolipin) and treponemal antibodies might be reduced, thus increasing the risk of false-negative test results (41, 55). In contrast, others report that HIV-infected patients may manifest unusually high nontreponemal test titers (22, 59). In a study of over 300 patients with secondary syphilis, the geometric mean rapid plasma reagin titer was significantly higher in HIV-seropositive patients than in HIV-seronegative controls (59). Other studies assert that the serological responses to syphilis in HIV-infected patients were the same as in persons without HIV infection (79, 117).

Haas et al (50) reported the loss of *T. pallidum*-specific antibody with increasing frequency as HIV infection progressed in patients previously treated for syphilis. Eight of 21 (38%) patients with advanced HIV disease had negative fluorescent treponemal antibody absorbed (FTA-ABS) or microhemagglutination assays for *T. pallidum* (MHA-TP), compared with 5 of 69 (7%) patients with asymptomatic HIV disease and 0 of 19 without HIV infection. However, despite a common perception that specific antibody tests remain reactive indefinitely following successful treatment of syphilis, a recent study confirmed older data that showed that the MHA-TP and FTA-ABS tests reverted to negative within 36 months in 13% and 24%, respectively, of HIV-uninfected patients following treatment for primary syphilis (103).

The diagnosis of neurosyphilis is especially difficult in HIV-seropositive patients, because both HIV and syphilis can cause a mononuclear pleocytosis and elevated protein in CSF, and the CSF VDRL can be negative in persons with neurosyphilis (41). In the largest series comparing CSF findings in HIV-infected and HIV-negative patients with syphilis, CSF mononuclear pleocytosis, elevated protein, VDRL reactivity, and isolation of *T. pallidum* by rabbit inoculation were not significantly different in about 15 HIV-infected and 25 HIV-uninfected patients with primary or secondary syphilis (73). As most of the patients had early HIV infection, the applicability of these findings to advanced HIV disease and late syphilis is unknown.

Although atypical serological responses to syphilis clearly occur in the presence of HIV infection, the large majority of HIV-infected persons with syphilis mount normal, and perhaps even accelerated, serological responses. Similarly, if seroreversion is more frequent in HIV-infected than in HIV-uninfected patients with past syphilis, the difference probably is quantitatively small.

The more severe manifestations of treponemal infection and the concern about the therapeutic response to benzathine penicillin G have convinced many experts to advocate more intensive therapy for HIV-infected persons with syphilis. Routine examination of CSF is also advocated by some experts for patients with concomitant HIV infection who have any form of syphilis (72, 89). However, these recommendations are controversial because definitive data are lacking and no studies have been done to assess the efficacy of alternative regimens, such as use of daily procaine penicillin plus probenecid, intravenous penicillin G, ceftriaxone, or high-dose oral amoxicillin. All experts agree, however, that close serologic and clinical follow-up of HIV-infected persons with syphilis is clearly indicated, regardless of the therapy provided, with particular attention to neurological symptoms and signs. Clear consensus also exists that all patients with syphilis should be tested for HIV infection to assist in clinical management and that serological tests for syphilis are indicated in all HIV-seropositive patients.

Chancroid and Genital Ulcer Disease

Sexually transmitted genital ulcers are common throughout the world, but are especially frequent in many developing countries. Because of the technical difficulties surrounding laboratory confirmation and precise diagnosis in developing countries, clinicians often apply the term "genital ulcer disease" (GUD) without further specifying microbiologic etiology. In general, genital herpes, syphilis, and chancroid all are common in many areas of the world. Where HIV infection is common, genital herpes appears to be a relatively important cause of GUD, perhaps because of the effects of HIV infection and immunosuppression that cause recurrent genital herpes. Uncommon causes of genital ulcers are donovanosis (granuloma inguinale), which causes a high proportion of GUD in only a few settings, such as the Indian subcontinent, Papua, New Guinea, and South Africa, and lymphogranuloma venereum, which is a rare cause of overt GUD in most settings, even where the causative serovars of *Chlamydia trachomatis* are prevalent. Lack of circumcision has been reported as possibly increasing susceptibility to chancroid and perhaps to syphilis.

Chancroid, caused by *Hemophilus ducreyi,* is among the most common etiologic agents of GUD in many developing countries (14). In the United States, it was relatively infrequent until a dramatic rise in incidence occurred in the mid-1980s, associated with crack cocaine use, prostitution, and migrant workers (109). Chancroid appears to be more closely related to prostitution or substance abuse than even syphilis, perhaps because asymptomatic carriage of *H. ducreyi* is uncommon; an outbreak of chancroid may require a population of infected persons willing, because of economic incentives or addiction, to continue sexual activity in the presence of painful genital ulcers.

Several studies have reported associations between most causes of GUD and acquisition of HIV (19, 49, 96, 115). Most of these reports were based on case-control studies, and definitive control for number of sexual partners and other indices of sexual behavior, which might have independently explained both HIV infection and GUD, was not always possible. More recently, however, prospective cohort studies have shown independent associations between GUD (principally chancroid) and both acquisition and transmission of HIV in men and women (19, 96). Recovery of HIV from genital ulcers in Nairobi sex workers further supports a role for genital ulcers in the sexual transmission of HIV (67). In addition to providing a mechanical portal for shedding and entry of HIV, genital ulcers may biologically enhance transmission. Activated CD4 lymphocytes, monocytes, and macrophages are prevalent in genital ulcers and are susceptible to HIV infection, and activation of CD4 lymphocytes with latent HIV infection results in expression of virus.

Since the advent of HIV infection in Africa, several studies suggest a change in the natural history of chancroid. Among HIV-infected persons, genital ulcers tend to be larger and persist longer (70). A trial of condoms among sex workers in Kenya demonstrated their effectiveness in prevention of GUD, as the acquisition of ulcers fell from 45% of women who did not use condoms to 16% of those who used them consistently (17). Unfortunately, the benefit was negated by a 3.7-fold greater incidence of genital ulcers among HIV-seropositive women than among HIV seronegatives, when controlled for condom use, which suggests that HIV-seropositive women are more susceptible to infections with *H. ducreyi*.

Studies from Nairobi indicate that otherwise effective single-dose therapies have unacceptably high failure rates among HIV-infected men. A single dose of trimethoprim-sulfonamide or of a quinolone failed to cure chancroid in 12 of 39 HIV-seropositive men, compared with 5 of 116 seronegative men [odds ratio (OR) = 10] (18). Similarly, single-dose fleroxacin showed microbiologic failure in 2 of 8 seropositive men and 2 of 37 seronegative men (OR = 6) (74). Other single-dose therapies, such as azithromycin and ceftriaxone, also have been associated with a three- to fourfold higher failure rate in the treatment of chancroid among HIV seropositive when compared with seronegative men (118, 119). Lack of circumcision further increases the failure rate.

In summary, HIV infection appears to result in increased ease of acquisition of chancroid; larger, more persistent ulcers; and increased resistance to single-dose treatment. As a result, the prevalence of chancroid is increased among HIV seropositive patients. Because many persons continue to be sexually active in spite of genital ulcerations, the development of single-dose, cheap, and effective treatments for chancroid in persons with HIV infection is an urgent priority in controlling the spread of both HIV and chancroid.

Gonorrhea, Chlamydia, and Pelvic Inflammatory Disease

Recent investigations suggest that both gonococcal and chlamydial infections also increase the risk of acquisition and transmission of HIV infection, perhaps by causing cervical and vaginal inflammation and microulcerations. A prospective cohort study of HIV seroconversion rates among sex workers from Zaire demonstrated that the OR for HIV seroconversion was 3.5 for women with gonorrhea, 3.2 for women with chlamydial infection, and 2.7 for those with vaginal trichomoniasis (69). The presence of cervical ectopy also appears to be a specific risk factor for HIV acquisition, which perhaps partly explains the enhanced risk associated with these conditions and with oral contraceptive use (88). If the increased risk of HIV acquisition among women who have these infections or who are exposed to men with these infections is confirmed by prospective studies, the population attributable risk may outweigh that of ulcerative STDs.

EFFECT OF HIV INFECTION ON GONORRHEA In a cohort of sex workers from Kenya followed for 18 months, the incidence of gonorrhea and gonococcal salpingitis was significantly greater among HIV-seropositive than seronegative women, with ORs of 2.8 and 7, respectively. In another study of sex workers, the frequency of gonorrhea decreased with the duration of prostitution, which suggests the development of partial immunity (97). HIV-infected women were significantly more likely than controls (OR = 3.8) to acquire new gonococcal infections with a previously experienced strain.

Data on the influence of HIV infection on gonococcal infections are scanty. In a cross-sectional study from Kenya, gonococcal infections in HIV-infected men and women were more likely to be caused by penicillinase-producing *N. gonorrhoeae* than infections in controls (91). However, the standard therapy with ceftriaxone or ciprofloxacin continues to result in high cure rates.

EFFECT OF HIV INFECTION ON PELVIC INFLAMMATORY DISEASE Emerging evidence suggests that HIV infection may alter the frequency and clinical spectrum of pelvic inflammatory disease (PID) among HIV-infected women. In a study in Brooklyn, New York, HIV-seropositive women were more apt to have PID than seronegative women, 14% versus 2%, respectively (56). Significantly fewer HIV-infected women had leucocytosis on admission and tubo-ovarian abscess, and surgical interventions were required more frequently among HIV-seropositive women. The length of hospitalization was similar. An outpatient study of PID in Nairobi suggested that women with concurrent HIV infection were considerably less likely to present with abdominal pain (OR = 0.3), but more likely to have an adnexal mass (OR = 5.7) (C. Okumu 1991, personal communication). The influence of HIV on chlamydial infections has not been assessed. Although the data are sparse, they suggest that HIV infection may aggravate the clinical course of gonococcal infection in women, with increased risk of more severe PID, and may increase the susceptibility to gonococcal infection or reinfection per se.

OTHER SEXUALLY TRANSMITTED INFECTIONS

Vulvovaginal Candidiasis, Trichomonal Vaginitis, and Bacterial Vaginosis

Abnormal vaginal discharge is a frequent complaint in gynecology clinics and STD clinics; most common causes are bacterial vaginosis, vulvovaginal candidiasis, or trichomoniasis.

Two studies have addressed the impact of HIV infection on the course of vaginal candidiasis. Chronic vaginal yeast infection was the presenting complaint in 7 of 29 women with HIV infection (101). None had other predisposing conditions to yeast infections, and all had recurrent episodes that lasted more than one year and required almost continual antifungal therapy. At presentation, all three women also had oral candidiasis of more recent onset than the vaginitis. Half of the women with HIV infection followed at another center noted new onset or increased frequency of vaginal candidiasis before other evidence of immunodeficiency appeared (60). The development of candidal vaginitis predated candidal mucosal infections at other sites and occurred in women whose CD4 lymphocyte counts were lower than those without any candidal infections, with mean values of 506/μL versus 741/μL, respectively. Although vaginal candidiasis obviously affects women with normal immune function, recurrent and severe episodes, especially of new onset, should alert clinicians to the possibility of HIV-related immune impairment. The revised CDC definition of AIDS includes recurrent vaginal candidiasis as a manifestation of AIDS-related illness specific to women (23).

No information is available on the changes induced by HIV in the presentation of bacterial vaginosis or trichomoniasis. The latter has been identified as a possible risk factor for acquisition of HIV, as noted above (69).

Kaposi's Sarcoma

Classic Kaposi's sarcoma (KS) is a rare, indolent tumor of the lower extremities, which affects primarily older men in North America and Europe. A more aggressive, often lymphadenopathic or visceral form, is endemic in equatorial Africa, where it predominates among male youth. In the early 1980s, clusters of disseminated KS, now termed epidemic KS, were noted in young homosexual men in New York and California (43). Recent evidence suggests KS associated with HIV may be a sexually transmitted opportunistic malignancy.

As the HIV epidemic continues, evidence suggests that the epidemiologies of KS and HIV differ. The changes in the epidemiology of AIDS-related KS over the last decade suggest that a cofactor, such as another sexually transmitted agent, may be necessary for the development of KS. In San Francisco, the proportion of patients presenting with KS as the initial AIDS-defining illness declined from 59% in 1981 to 19% in 1987 (104). Similar trends have been noted nationwide: Initially, one third of AIDS cases had been diagnosed with KS; the proportion declined to 8.6% in 1991 (T. A. Green 1992, personal communication). In the United States, the proportion of AIDS cases diagnosed with KS has been higher in the urban centers, where the disease was first noted, than in the rest of the country. Furthermore, KS appears significantly more frequently among homosexual and bisexual men (21%) and heterosexuals born in the Caribbean and Africa (6%) than among persons with other risk factors; the disease is rare among hemophiliacs (1%) (52). Among women who acquired HIV through heterosexual contact, the risk of developing KS was fourfold higher if the male partner were bisexual than if he were an IDU (8). These epidemiologic trends have also been noted in Canada and in Europe (108) and suggest that another agent, which is transmitted more efficiently through sexual activity than parenterally and is promoted, induced, or unmasked by HIV infection, may be implicated in the etiology of KS. This hypothesis, put forth by Beral (8), can explain the decline in KS incidence; the adoption of safer sex practices in the gay community resulted in subsequent decreased acquisition of the causative agent of KS. Reports of KS in sexually active homosexual men without HIV infection and no significant immunologic abnormalities have further supported this hypothesis (1).

Recent investigation of sexual practices of men with AIDS revealed significant association between the development of KS and sexual practices involving oral-anal contact ("rimming") (7). Kaposi's sarcoma developed in 18% of men who never engaged in rimming, as opposed to 75% for those who engaged in it regularly (OR = 13.5), which supports the notion that KS is transmitted by fecal-oral contact.

In spite of advances in understanding the epidemiology of AIDS-related KS, the pathogenesis is unclear. Initial studies implicating CMV and nitrite inhalants as the cause of KS have not been confirmed. In addition, the origin of cells that give rise to KS is controversial, and the reasons for KS's predilection for males—evident both in classic and epidemic form, as well as in the animal model—is unknown (122).

Scabies

Norwegian, or crusted, scabies is an unusual, highly contagious, variant of infestation with the mite *Sarcoptes scabiei,* which produces minimal itching. Initially described in patients with leprosy, subsequent reports identified immunosuppression, institutional settings, and mental retardation as risk factors for development of crusted scabies (92). The combination of diminished immune response and little excoriation results in a very heavy mite burden and a great potential for infectiousness.

Several cases of crusted scabies among patients with HIV infection have been reported. Two presentations of atypical scabetic infestation in HIV-infected individuals have been described: a severe form of common scabies with intensely pruritic maculopapular dermatitis, frequently involving large areas of the body, and a nonpruritic form with widespread hyperkeratotic exfoliative scales. Both manifestations are frequently misdiagnosed initially, and the correct diagnosis is established only after failure to improve with treatment for other dermatitides (61). Microscopic examination of scraped material or skin biopsy confirms the diagnosis. Although patients respond to treatment with lindane, multiple applications may be required, and relapse, at times many months later, occurs (35).

Three reports document the spread of this highly contagious form of scabies to other patients and health-care workers (35, 64, 112). In one hospital, two patients with crusted scabies infected 20 patients, six health providers, and nine relatives in spite of observance of standard precautions. Fortunately, no evidence of HIV transmission by mites has been observed.

The degree of immunosuppression noted in patients with crusted scabies at the time of their dermatologic diagnosis is striking, as most of the patients had a prior AIDS diagnosis or CD4 lymphocyte count under 150 μL (35, 46, 105, 112). The advanced stages of HIV disease described in association with Norwegian scabies suggest that this form of scabies requires profound immunosuppression to develop. Delays in diagnosis increase the chances for complications associated with bacterial superinfection and the potential for nosocomial spread.

CONCLUSION

In summary, HIV infection influences the acquisition rates, severity, transmission, and host response for a variety of STD pathogens. In many situations, rates of acquisition are increased, severity worsened, persistence prolonged, and treatment response impaired in HIV-infected persons. These factors foster the spread of STD agents and result in a higher prevalence of concomitant

STDs in the HIV-infected person and, potentially, increased HIV shedding in the genital tract.

The possible effect of STDs on sexual transmission of HIV has received much attention, but the impact of HIV on other STDs has not. This mutually reinforcing interaction between HIV and STD can profoundly affect the transmission dynamics of HIV (94, 95). Specific research is needed regarding the effects of HIV on *Chlamydia trachomatis,* lymphogranuloma venereum, gonococcal infection, and chancroid, as well as on persistent viral infections. The irony of declining support for STD clinics, or failing to develop STD services where these are entirely lacking, in the face of epidemic sexual transmission of HIV is obvious. A call to action must include research stimulated by National Institutes of Health, CDC, WHO, and other organizations. Greatest support must be given to STD clinics in areas hardest hit by the HIV epidemic, or when worsening of the epidemic is anticipated. The window of opportunity for STD control to prevent HIV transmission is narrow: Once core groups have been saturated with HIV, and those infected become immunosuppressed, it will become much more difficult to deal with chancroid, HSV, hepatitis B, and possibly gonorrhea and chlamydia, with simple and affordable treatment regimens.

ACKNOWLEDGMENT

We thank Ms. Nancy Coomer for expert assistance in the preparation of the manuscript.

Literature Cited

1. Afrasiabi, R., Mitsuyasu, R. T., Nishanian, P., Schwartz, K., Fahey, J. L. 1986. Characterization of a distinct subgroup of high-risk persons with Kaposi's sarcoma and good prognosis who present wih normal T4 cell numbers and Tf:T8 ratio and negative HTLV-III/LAV serologic test results. *Am. J. Med.* 81:969–73
2. Alter, M. J., Hadler, S. C., Marjolis, H. S., Alexander, W. J., Hu, P. Y., et al. 1990. The changing epidemiology of hepatitis B in the United States. *J. Am. Med. Assoc.* 263:1218–22
3. Ambinder, R. F., Burns, W. H., Lietman, P. S., Saral, R. 1984. Prophylaxis: a strategy to minimize antiviral resistance. *Lancet* 1:1154–55
4. Andrus, J. K., Fleming, D. W., Harger, D. R., Chin, M. Y., Bennett, D. V., et al. 1990. Partner notification: can it control epidemic syphilis? *Ann. Int. Med.* 112:539–43
5. Bari, M. M., Shulkin, D. J., Abell, E. 1989. Ulcerative syphilis in acquired immunodeficiency syndrome: a case of precocious tertiary syphilis in a patient infected with human immunodeficiency virus. *J. Am. Acad. Dermatol.* 21: 1310–12
6. Behar, R., Wiley, C., McCutchan A. 1987. Cytomegalovirus polyradiculoneuropathy in acquired immune deficiency syndrome. *Neurology* 37:557–61
7. Beral, V., Bull, D., Darby, S., Weller, I., Carne, C., et al. 1992. Risk of Kaposi's sarcoma and sexual practices associated with fecal contact in homosexual or bisexual men with AIDS. *Lancet* 339:632–35
8. Beral, V., Peterman, T. A., Berkelman, R. L., Jaffe, H. W. 1990. Kaposi's sarcoma among persons with AIDS: a

sexually transmitted infection? *Lancet* 335:123–28

9. Berger, J. R. 1992. Spinal cord syphilis associated with human immunodeficiency virus infection: a treatable myelopathy. *Am. J. Med.* 92:101–3
10. Berry, C. D., Hooton, T. M., Collier, A. C., Lukehart, S. A. 1987. Neurologic relapse after benzathine penicillin therapy for secondary syphilis in a patient with HIV infection. *N. Engl. J. Med.* 316:1587–89
11. Birch, C. J., Tachedjian, G., Doherty, R. R., Hayes, K., Gust, I. D. 1990. Altered sensitivity to antiviral drugs of herpes simplex virus isolates from a patient with the acquired immunodeficiency syndrome. *J. Infect. Dis.* 162: 731–34
12. Bodsworth, N. J., Cooper, D. A., Donovan, B. 1991. The influence of human immunodeficiency virus type 1 on the development of the hepatitis B virus carrier state. *J. Infect. Dis.* 163: 1138–40
13. Bodsworth, N., Donovan, B., Nightingale, B. N. 1989. The effect of concurrent human immunodeficiency virus infection on chronic hepatitis B: a study of 150 homosexual men. *J. Infect. Dis.* 160:577–82
14. Bogaerts, J., Ricart, C. A., Van Dyck, E., Piot, P. 1989. The etiology of genital ulceration in Rwanda. *Sex. Transm. Dis.* 16:123–26
15. Bonetti, A., Weber, R., Vogt, M. W., Wunderli, W., Siegenthaler, W., Luthy, R. 1989. Co-infection with human immunodeficiency virus type 1 (HIV-1) and cytomegalovirus in two intravenous drug users. *Ann. Int. Med.* 111:293–96
16. Buti, M., Esteban, R., Espanol, M. T., Malagelada, A., Jardi, R., et al. 1991. Influence of human immunodeficiency virus infection on cell-mediated immunity in chronic D hepatitis. *J. Infect. Dis.* 163:1351–53
17. Cameron, D. W., Ngugi, E. N., Ronald, A. R., Simonsen, J. N., Braddick, M., et al. 1991. Condom use prevents genital ulcers in women working as prostitutes. *Sex. Transm. Dis.* 18:188–91
18. Cameron, D. W., Plummer, F. A., D'Costa, L. J., Ndinya-Achola, J. O., Ronald, A. R. 1988. *Prediction of HIV by treatment failure for chancRoid, a genital ulcer disease.* 4th Int. AIDS Conf., Stockholm (Abstr. 7637)
19. Cameron, D. W., Simonsen, J. N., D'Costa, L. J., Ndinya-Achola, J. O., Piot, P. 1989. Female to male transmission of HIV in Nairobi. *Lancet* 2:403–408
20. Caussy, D., Goedert, J. J., Palefsky, J., Gonzales, J., Rabkin, C. S., et al. 1990. Interaction of human immunodeficiency and papilloma viruses: association with anal epithelial abnormality in homosexual men. *Int. J. Cancer* 46:214–19
21. Cent. for Dis. Control. 1991. Hepatitis B virus: a comprehensive strategy for eliminating transmission in the United States through universal childhood vaccination. *Morbid. Mortal. Wkly. Rep.* 40:1–25
22. Cent. for Dis. Control. 1988. Recommendations for diagnosing and treating syphilis in HIV-infected patients. *Morbid. Mortal. Wkly. Rep.* 37:600–8
23. Cent. for Dis. Control. 1991. Revised classification system for HIV infection and expanded AIDS surveillance case definition for adolescents and adults. In preparation
24. Cent. for Dis. Control. 1990. Risk for cervical disease in HIV-infected women—New York City. *Morbid. Mortal. Wkly. Rep.* 39:846–49
25. Chandler, S. H., Holmes, K. K., Wentworth, B. B., Gutman, L. T., Wiesner, P. Y., et al. 1985. The epidemiology of cytomegalovirus infection in women attending a sexually transmitted disease clinic. *J. Infect. Dis.* 152:597–605
26. Chatis, P. A., Miller, C. H., Schrager, L. E., Crumpacker, C. S. 1989. Successful treatment with foscarnet of an acyclovir-resistant mucocutaneous infection with herpes simplex virus in a patient with acquired immunodeficiency syndrome. *N. Engl. J. Med.* 320:297–300
27. Coldiron, B. M., Bergstresser, P. R. 1989. Prevalence and clinical spectrum of skin disease in patients infected with human immunodeficiency virus. *Arch. Dermatol.* 125:357–61
28. Collier, A. C., Corey, L., Murphy, V. L., Handsfield, H. H. 1988. Antibody to human immunodeficiency virus (HIV) and suboptimal response to Hepatitis B vaccination. *Ann. Int. Med.* 109:101–5
29. Collier, A. C., Handsfield, H. H., Roberts, P. L., DeRouen, T., Meyers, J. D., et al. 1990. Cytomegalovirus infection in women attending a sexually transmitted disease clinic. *J. Infect. Dis.* 162:46–51
30. Collier, A. C., Meyers, J. D., Corey, L., Murphy, V. L., Roberts, P. L., Handsfield, H. H. 1987. Cytomegalovirus infection in homosexual men.

Relationship to sexual practices, antibody to human immunodeficiency virus, and cell-mediated immunity. *Am. J. Med.* 82:593–600

31. Conant, M. A. 1988. Prophylactic and suppressive treatment with acyclovir and the management of herpes in patients with acquired immunodeficiency syndrome. *J. Am. Acad. Dermatol.* 18:186–88
32. Critchlow, C., Holmes, K. K., Daling, J., Surawicz, C., Sayer, J., et al. 1991. *Development of anal squamous intraepithelial lesions among HIV-seropositive and seronegative homosexual men.* 9th Int. Soc. STD Res., Banff (Abstr. P-17-255)
33. Daling, J. R., Weiss, N. S., Hislop, T. G., Maden, C., Coates, R. J., et al. 1987. Sexual practices, sexually transmitted diseases, and the incidence of anal cancer. *N. Engl. J. Med.* 317:973–77
34. Dawson, S., Evans, B. A., Lawrence, A. G. 1988. Benign tertiary syphilis and HIV infection. *AIDS* 2:315–16
35. Dillon, S. M. 1989. An HIV-infected patient with an extraordinary rash. *Hosp. Pract.* [off]. 24:199–202
36. Douglas, J. M. Jr., Rogers, M., Judson, F. N. 1986. The effect of asymptomatic infection with HTLV-III on the response of anogenital warts to intralesional treatment with recombinant α_2 interferon. *J. Infect. Dis.* 154:331–34
37. Drew, W. L. 1988. Cytomegalovirus infection in patients with AIDS. *J. Infect. Dis.* 158:449–56
38. Drew, W. L., Mintz, L., Miner, R. C., Sands, M., Ketterer, B. 1981. Prevalence of cytomegalovirus infection in homosexual men. *J. Infect. Dis.* 143:188–92
39. Edwards, R. H., Messing, R., McKendall, R. R. 1985. Cytomegalovirus meningoencephalitis in a homosexual man with Kaposi's sarcoma: isolation of CMV from CSF cells. *Neurology* 35:560–62
40. Erlich, K. S., Mills, J., Chatis, P., Mertz, G. J., Busch, D. F., et al. 1989. Acyclovir-resistant herpes simplex virus infections in patients with the acquired immunodeficiency syndrome. *N. Engl. J. Med.* 320:293–96
41. Feraru, E. R., Aronow, H. A., Lipton, R. B. 1990. Neurosyphilis in AIDS patients: initial CSF VDRL may be negative. *Neurology* 40:541–43
42. Frazer, I. H., Medley, G., Crapper, R. M., Brown, T. C., Mackay, I. R. 1986. The association between anorectal dysplasia, human papillomavirus and human immunodeficiency virus infection in homosexual men. *Lancet* 2:657–60
43. Friedman-Kien, A. E., laubenstein, L. J., Rubinstein, P., Buimovici-Klein, E., Marmor, M., et al. 1982. Disseminated Kaposi's sarcoma in homosexual men. *Ann. Int. Med.* 96:693–700
44. Gately, A., Gander, R. M., Johnson, P. C., Kit, S., Otsuka, H., et al. 1990. Herpes simplex virus type 2 meningoencephalitis resistant to acyclovir in a patient with AIDS. *J. Infect. Dis.* 161:711–15
45. Gerna, G., Parea, M., Percivalle, E., Zipeto, D., Silini, E., et al. 1990. Human cytomegalovirus viraemia in HIV-1-seropositive patients at various clinical stages of infection. *AIDS* 4: 1027–31
46. Glover, R., Young, L., Goltz, R. W. 1987. Norwegian scabies in acquired immunodeficiency syndrome: report of a case resulting in death from associated sepsis (letter). *J. Am. Acad. Dermatol.* 16:396–99
47. Goodman, D. S., Teplitz, E. D., Wishner, A., Klein, R. S., Burke, P. G., et al. 1987. Prevalence of cutaneous disease in patients with acquired immunodeficiency syndrome (AIDS) or AIDS-related complex. *J. Am. Acad. Dermatol.* 17:210–20
48. Govindarajan, S., Edwards, V. M., Stuart, M. L., Operskalski, E. A., Mosley, J. W., et al. 1988. Influence of human immunodeficiency virus infection on expression of chronic hepatitis B and D virus infections. In *Viral Hepatitis and Liver Disease,* ed. A. J. Zuckerman, pp. 201–4. New York: Liss
49. Greenblatt, R. M., Lukehart, S. A., Plummer, F. A., Quinn, T. C., Critchlow, C. W., et al. 1988. Genital ulceration as a risk factor for human immunodeficiency virus infection. *AIDS* 2:47–50
50. Haas, J. S., Bolan, G., Larsen, S. A., Clement, M. J., Bacchetti, P., et al. 1990. Sensitivity of treponemal tests for detecting prior treated syphilis during human immunodeficiency virus infection. *J. Infect. Dis.* 162:862–66
51. Hadler, S. C., Judson, F. N., O'Malley, P. M., Altman, N. L., Penley, K., et al. 1991. Outcome of hepatitis B virus infection in homosexual men and its relation to prior human immunodeficiency virus infection. *J. Infect. Dis.* 163:454–59
52. Haverkos, H. W., Drotman, D. P. 1985. Prevalence of Kaposi's sarcoma

among patients with AIDS. *Lancet* 1:1518
53. Henderly, D. E., Freeman, W. R., Causey, D. M., Rao, N. A. 1987. Cytomegalovirus retinitis and response to therapy with ganciclovir. *Ophthalmology* 94:425–34
54. Henderly, D. E., Freeman, W. R., Smith, R. E. 1987. Cytomegalovirus retinitis as the initial manifestation of the acquired immunodeficiency syndrome. *Am. J. Ophthalmol.* 103:316–20
55. Hicks, C. B., Benson, P. M., Lupton, G. P., Tramont, E. C. 1987. Seronegative secondary syphilis in a patient infected with human immunodeficiency virus (HIV) with Kaposi sarcoma. *Ann. Intern. Med.* 107:492–95
56. Hoegsberg, B., Abulafia, O., Sedlis, A., Feldman, J., Des Jarlais, D., et al. 1990. Sexually transmitted diseases and human immunodeficiency virus infection among women with pelvic inflammatory disease. *Am. J. Obstet. Gynecol.* 163:1135–39
57. Hook, E. W., Cannon, R. O., Nahmias, A. J., Lee, F. F., Campbell, C. H., et al. 1992. Herpes simplex virus infection as a risk factor for human immunodeficiency virus infection. *J. Infect. Dis.* 165:251–55
58. Hook, E. W., Marra, C. M. 1992. Acquired syphilis in adults. *N. Engl. J. Med.* 326:1060–69
59. Hutchinson, C. M., Rompalo, A. M., Reichart, C. A., Hook, E. W. 1991. Characteristics of patients with syphilis attending Baltimore STD clinics. *Arch. Intern. Med.* 151:511–16
60. Imam, N., Carpenter, C. C., Mayer, K. H., Fisher, A., Stein, M., et al. 1990. Hierarchical pattern of mucosal candida infections in HIV-seropositive women. *Am. J. Med.* 89:142–46
61. Inserra, D. W., Bickley, L. K. 1990. Crusted scabies in acquired immunodeficiency syndrome. *Int. J. Dermatol.* 29:287–89
62. Johns, D. R., Tierney, M., Felsenstein, D. 1987. Alteration in the natural history of neurosyphilis by concurrent infection with the human immunodeficiency virus. *N. Engl. J. Med.* 316: 1569–72
63. Katzman, M., Carey, J. T., Elmets, C. A., Jacobs, H. H., Lederman, M. M. 1987. Molluscum contagiosum and the acquired immunodeficiency syndrome: clinical and immunological details of two cases: *Br. J. Dermatol.* 116:131–38
64. Kelly, A., Fry, C. 1989. *Outbreak of Norwegian scabies among health-care workers*. 5th Int. AIDS Conf., Montreal (Abstr. M.B.P.308)
65. Kingsley, L. A., Rinaldo, C. R., Lyter, D. W., Valdiserri, R. O., Belle, S. H., et al. 1990. Sexual transmission efficacy of hepatitis B virus and human immunodeficiency virus among homosexual men. *J. Am. Med. Assoc.* 264: 230–34
66. Kiviat, N., Rompalo, A., Bowden, R., Galloway, D., Holmes, K. K., et al. 1990. Anal human papillomavirus infection among human immunodeficiency virus-seropositive and -seronegative men. *J. Infect. Dis.* 162:358–61
67. Kreiss, J. K., Coombs, R., Plummer, F., Holmes, K. K., Nikora, B., et al. 1989. Isolation of human immunodeficiency virus from genital ulcers in Nairobi prostitutes. *J. Infect. Dis.* 160: 380–84
68. Krogsgaard, K., Lindhardt, B. O., Neilsen, J. O., Anderson, P., Kryger, et al. 1987. The influence of HTLV-III infection on the natural history of hepatitis B virus infection in male homosexual HBs Ag carriers. *Hepatology* 7:37–41
69. Laga, M., Nzila, N., Manoka, A. T., Malele, M., Bush, T. J., et al. 1990. *Non-ulcerative sexually transmitted diseases (STD) as risk factors for HIV infection*. 6th Int. AIDS Conf., San Francisco (Abstr. Th.C.97)
70. Latif, A. S. 1989. *Epidemiology and control of chancroid*. 8th Int. Soc. STD Res., Copenhagen (Abstr. 66)
71. Lazizi, Y., Grangeot-Keros, L., Delfraissy, J. F., Boue, F., Dubreuil, P., et al. 1988. Reappearance of hepaiatis B virus in immune patients infected with the human immunodeficiency virus type 1 (letter). *J. Infect. Dis.* 158:666–67
72. Lukehart, S. A. 1990. Syphilis. *Curr. Opin. Infect. Dis.* 3:3–9
73. Lukehart, S. A., Hook, E. W., Baker-Zander, S. A., Collier, A. C., Critchlow, C. W., et al. 1988. Invasion of the central nervous system by *Treponema pallidum:* implications for diagnosis and treatment. *Ann. Intern. Med.* 109:855–62
74. MacDonald, K. S., Cameron, D. W., D'Costa, L. J., Ndinya-Achola, J. O., Plummer, F. A., et al. 1989. Evaluation of fleroxacin (RO 23-6240) as single-oral-dose therapy of culture-proven chancroid in Nairobi, Kenya. *Antimicrob. Agents Chemother.* 33:612–14
75. Maiman, M., Fruchter, R. G., Serur, E., Remy, J. C., Feuer, G., et al. 1990. Human immunodeficiency virus

infection and cervical neoplasia. *Gynecol. Oncol.* 38:377–82
76. Maiman, M., Tarricone, N., Vieira, J., Suarez, J., Serur, E., et al. 1991. Colposcopic evaluation of human immunodeficiency virus-seropositive women. *Obstet. Gynecol.* 78:84–88
77. Marte, C., Cohen, M., Kelly, P., Fruchter, R. 1990. *Pap test and STD findings in HIV positive women at ambulatory care sites*. 6th Int. AIDS Conf., San Francisco (Abstr. T.B.532)
78. Matis, W. L., Triana, A., Shapiro, R., Eldred, L., Polk, B. F., et al. 1987. Dermatologic findings associated with human immunodeficiency virus infection. *J. Am. Acad. Dermatol.* 7: 746–51
79. Matlow, A. G., Rachlis, A. R. 1990. Syphilis serology in human immunodeficiency virus-infected patients with symptomatic neurosyphilis: case report and review. *Rev. Infect. Dis.* 12:703–7
80. Matorras, R., Ariceta, J. M., Rementeria, A., Corral, J., de Teran, G. G., et al. 1991. Human immunodeficiency virus-induced immunosuppression: a risk factor for human papillomavirus infection. *Am. J. Obstet. Gynecol.* 164: 42–44
81. McDonald, J. A., Caruso, L., Karayiannis, P., Scully, L. J., Harris, J. R., et al. 1987. Diminished responsiveness of male homosexual chronic hepatitis B virus carriers with HTLV-III antibodies to recombinant α-interferon. *Hepatology* 7:719–23
82. McDonald, J. A., Harris, S., Waters, J. A., Thomas, H. C. 1987. Effect of human immunodeficiency virus (HIV) infection on chronic hepatitis B hepatic viral antigen display. *J. Hepatol.* 4: 337–42
83. McMillan, A., Bishop, P. E. 1989. Clinical course of anogenital warts in men infected with human immunodeficiency virus. *Genitourin. Med.* 65: 225–28
84. Melbye, M., Palefsky, J., Gonzales, J., Ryder, L. P., Nielsen, H., et al. 1990. Immune status as a determinant of human papillomavirus detection and its association with anal epithelial abnormalities. *Int. J. Cancer* 46:203–6
85. Miller, S. J. 1988. Cutaneous cryptococcus resembling Molluscum contagiosum in a patient with acquired immunodeficiency syndrome. *Cutis* 41: 411–12
86. Mintz, L., Drew, W. L., Miner, R. C., Bratt, E. H. 1983. Cytomegalovirus infections in homosexual men. *Ann. Int. Med.* 99:326–29
87. Monno, L., Angarano, G., Caputo, S. L., Casalino, C., Carbonara, S., et al. 1988. Unfavorable outcome of acute hepatitis B in anti-HIV-positive drug addicts. In *Viral Hepatitis and Liver Disease*, ed. A. J. Zuckerman, pp. 205–6. New York: Liss
88. Moss, G. B., Clemetson, D., D'Costa, L., Plummer, F. A., Ndinya-Achola, J. O., et al. 1991. Association of cervical ectopy with heterosexual transmission of human immunodeficiency virus: results of a study of couples in Nairobi, Kenya. *J. Infect. Dis.* 164: 588–91
89. Musher, D. M., Hamill, R. J., Baughn, R. E. 1990. Effect of human immunodeficiency virus (HIV) infection on the course of syphilis and on the response to treatment. *Ann. Intern. Med.* 113:872–81
90. Norris, S. A., Kessler, H. A., Fife, K. H. 1988. Severe, progressive herpetic whitlow caused by an acyclovir-resistant virus in a patient with AIDS (letter). *J. Infect. Dis.* 157:209–10
91. Ombette, J. J., Ndinya-Achola, J. O., Maitha, G., Emonyi, E., Plourde, P., et al. 1990. *Prevalence of HIV among men and women with* H. ducreyi *and* Neisseria gonorrhoeae *infection in Nairobi, Kenya*. 6th Int. AIDS Conf., San Francisco (Abstr. Th.C.572)
92. Orkin, M., Maibach, H. 1990. Scabies. In *Sexually Transmitted Diseases*, ed. K. K. Holmes, P.-A. Mardh, P. F. Sparling, P. J. Wiesner, W. Cates, et al., 2:473–80. New York: McGraw-Hill
93. Palefsky, J., Gonzales, J., Greenblatt, R. M., Ahn, D. K., Hollander, H. 1990. Anal intraepithelial neoplasia and anal papillomavirus infection among homosexual males with group IV HIV disease. *J. Am. Med. Assoc.* 263:2911–16
94. Pepin, J., Plummer, F. A., Brunham, R. C., Piot, P., Cameron, D. W., et al. 1989. The interaction of HIV infection and other sexually transmitted diseases: an opportunity for intervention. *AIDS* 3:3–9
95. Plummer, F. A. 1991. *Facilitation of HIV transmission by other STD*. 9th Int. Soc. STD Res., Banff (Abstr. PL-02-248)
96. Plummer, F. A., Simonsen, J. N., Cameron, D. W., Ndinya-Achola, O., Kreiss, J. K., et al. 1991. Cofactors in male to female transmission of HIV. *J. Infect. Dis.* 163:233–39
97. Plummer, F. A., Simonsen, J. N.,

Chubb, H., Slaney, L., Kimata, J., et al. 1989. Epidemiologic evidence for the development of serovar-specific immunity after gonococcal infection. *J. Clin. Invest.* 83:1472–76

98. Rector, W. G., Govindarajan, S., Horsburgh, C. R., Penley, K. A., Cohn, D. L., et al. 1988. Hepatic inflammation, hepatitis B replication, and cellular immune function in homosexual males with chronic hepatitis B and antibody to human immunodeficiency virus. *Am. J. Gastroenterol.* 83:262–66
99. Redfield, R. R., James, W. D., Wright, D. C., Brown, C., Salahuddin, S. Z., et al. 1985. Severe Molluscum contagiosum infection in a patient with human T cell lymphtrophic (HTLV-III) disease. *J. Am. Acad. Dermatol.* 13: 821–24
100. Reeves, W. C., Rawles, W. E., Brinton, L. A. 1989. Epidemiology of genital papillomavirus and cervical cancer. *Rev. Infect. Dis.* 11:426–39
101. Rhoads, J. L., Wright, D. C., Redfield, R. R., Burke, D. S. 1987. Chronic vaginal candidiasis in women with human immunodeficiency virus infection. *J. Am. Med. Assoc.* 257:3105–7
102. Rico, M. J., Penneys, N. S. 1985. Cutaneous cryptococcosis resembling Molluscum contagiosum in a patient with AIDS. *Arch. Dermatol.* 121:901–2
103. Romanowski, B., Sutherland, R., Fick, G. H., Mooney, D., Love, E. J. 1991. Serologic response to treatment of infectious syphilis. *Ann. Intern. Med.* 114:1005–9
104. Rutherford, G. W., Schwarcz, S. K., Lemp, G. F., Barnhart, J. L., Rauch, K. J., et al. 1989. The epidemiology of AIDS-related Kaposi's sarcoma in San Francisco. *J. Infect. Dis.* 159:569–71
105. Sadick, N., Kaplan, M. H., Pahwa, S. G., Sarngadharan, M. G. 1986. Unusual features of scabies complicating human T-lymphotropic virus type III infection. *J. Am. Acad. Dermatol.* 15:482–86
106. Safrin, S., Assaykeen, T., Follansbee, S., Mills, J. 1990. Foscarnet therapy for acyclovir-resistant mucocutaneous herpes simplex virus infection in 26 AIDS patients: preliminary data. *J. Infect. Dis.* 161:1078–84
107. Schäfer, A., Friedmann, W., Mielke, M., Schwartländer, B., Koch, M. A. 1991. Increased frequency of cervical dysplasia-neoplasia in women infected with human immunodeficiency virus is related to the degree of immunosuppression. *Am. J. Obstet. Gynecol.* 164:593–99
108. Schecter, M. T., Marion, S. A., Elmslie, K. D., Ricketts, M. N., Nault, P., et al. 1991. Geographic and birth cohort associations of Kaposi's sarcoma among homosexual men in Canada. *Am. J. Epidemiol.* 134:485–88
109. Schmid, G. P., Sanders, L. L., Blount, J. H., Alexander, E. R. 1987. Chancroid in the United States. Reestablishment of an old disease. *J. Am. Med. Assoc.* 258:3265–68
110. Schrager, L. K., Friedland, G. H., Mande, D., Schreiber, K., Adachi, A., et al. 1989. Cervical and vaginal squamous cell abnormalities in women infected with human immunodeficiency virus. *J. Acquired Immuno. Defic. Syndr.* 2:570–75
111. Siegal, F. P., Lopez, C., Hammer, G. S., Brown, A. E., Kornfeld, S. J., et al. 1981. Severe acquired immunodeficiency in male homosexuals, manifested by chronic perianal ulcerative herpes simplex lesions. *N. Engl. J. Med.* 305:1439–44
112. Sirera, G., Rius, F., Romeu, J., Llibre, J., Ribera, M., et al. 1990. Hospital outbreak of scabies stemming from two AIDS patients with Norwegian scabies (letter). *Lancet* 2:1227
113. Smith, M. E., Canalis, R. F. 1989. Otologic manifestations of AIDS: the otosyphilis connection. *Laryngoscope* 99:365–72
114. SOCA. 1992. Mortality in patients with the acquired immunodeficiency syndrome treated with either foscarnet or ganciclovir for cytomegalovirus retinitis. *N. Engl. J. Med.* 326:213–20
115. Stamm, W. E., Handsfield, H. H., Rompalo, A. M., Ashley, R. L., Roberts, P. L., et al. 1988. The association between genital ulcer disease and acquisition of HIV infection in homosexual men. *J. Am. Med. Assoc.* 260: 1429–33
116. Taylor, P. E., Stevens, C. E., de Cordoba, S. R., Pablo Rubinstein. 1988. Hepatitis B virus and human immunodeficiency virus: possible interactions. In *Viral Hepatitis and Liver Disease*, ed. A. J. Zuckerman, pp. 198–200. New York: Liss.
117. Terry, P. M., Page, M. L., Golmeier, D. 1988. Are serological tests of value in diagnosing and monitoring response to treatment of syphilis in patients infected with human immunodeficiency virus? *Genitourin. Med.* 64:219–92
118. Tyndall, M., Agoki, E., Ombetti, J., Ndinya-Achola, J. O., Malisa, M., et

al. 1991. *A randomized, single blinded study of azithromycin versus erythromycin in male patients with culture-proven chancroid*. 9th Int. Soc. STD Res., Banff, (Abstr. A-041)

119. Tyndall, M., Malisa, M., Plummer, F. A., Ombetti, J., Ndinya-Achola, J. O., et al. 1991. *Ceftriaxone in the treatment of chancroid*. 9th Int. Soc. STD Res., Banff, (Abstr. A-042)
120. Vento, S., di Perri, G., Luzzati, R., Cruciani, M., Garofano, T., et al. 1989. Clinical reactivation of hepatitis B in anti-HBs-positive patients with AIDS (lett.). *Lancet* 1:332–33
121. Vermund, S. H., Kelley, K. F., Klein, R. S., Feingold, A. R., Schrieber, K., et al. 1991. High risk of human papillomavirus infection and cervical squamous intraepithelial lesions among women with symptomatic human immunodeficiency virus infection. *Am. J. Obstet. Gynecol.* 165:392–400
122. Vogel, J., Hinrichs, S. H., Reynolds, R. K., Luciw, P. A., Jay, G. 1988. The HIV *tat* gene induces dermal lesions resembling Kaposi's sarcoma in transgenic mice. *Nature* 335:606–11
123. Wasserheit, J. N. 1992. Epidemiological synergy: interrelationships between human immunodeficiency virus infection and other sexually transmitted diseases. *Sex. Transm. Dis.* 19:61–77
124. World Health Org. 1990. *Consultation on Hepatitis B as a Sexually Transmitted Disease*. Geneva: WHO

Annu. Rev. Pub. Health 1993. 14:43–68

REGRESSION ANALYSIS FOR CORRELATED DATA

Kung-Yee Liang and Scott L. Zeger

Department of Biostatistics, Johns Hopkins University, Baltimore, Maryland 21205

KEY WORDS: estimating equations, odds ratio, marginal models, random effects models, transition models

---

INTRODUCTION

Regression analysis is among the most commonly used methods of statistical analysis in public health research. Its objective is to describe the relationship of a response with explanatory variables. One example of a regression problem is to identify factors associated with the racial difference in the risk of low birthweight (29). Regression includes the following as special cases: linear models for measured responses, logistic models for binary responses, and survival analyses for times to events. A basic assumption of regression analysis is that all observations are statistically independent, or at least uncorrelated with each other. In the low birthweight example, this assumption would mean that knowing one child's birthweight status provides no information as to whether another child in the study has a low birthweight. One may argue that the assumption of independence is unlikely to be true if children of the same mother are included in the sample. Due to their common household environment and genes, we would expect a child to have a greater chance of having a low birthweight if his/her sibling had. Data from this hypothetical example can usefully be thought of as being "clustered" into families. Birthweights from different families are likely independent; those from the same cluster are not. This dependence among observations from the same cluster must be accounted for in assessing the relationship between risk factors and health outcomes.

0163-7525/93/0510-0043$02.00

Clustered data are common in public health research. To illustrate the diversity of problems in which clustered data arise, we now briefly summarize seven research problems with dependent responses. The first example also illustrates the statistical methodology appropriate for clustered data.

1. Baltimore eye survey study. More than 5000 persons aged 40 years and older received a visual examination as part of a population-based prevalence study of ocular disorders (31). The objective is to identify demographic variables, such as age, race, education level, and access to medical care, which are associated with vision loss. Data are available on both eyes for all subjects. A single regression model expressing visual impairment in terms of demographic variables addresses the scientific objectives. But, the two eyes from the same person are unlikely to be independent, because many causes of impairment are binocular. This association must be considered.

2. Family study in liver cancer. Information regarding liver cancer on 371 siblings and children of 138 cases of primary hepatic carcinoma in Qi-dong county, Shanghai, was collected as a part of a survey conducted by Dr. F. M. Shen of the Shanghai Medical University (15a). The objective is to determine whether there is a familial aggregation of liver cancer as an important first step for studying the possible genetic explanation of the disease process. To reduce the influence of environmental factors, regression analysis must adjust for household and personal characteristics. The focus, however, is to estimate the degree of association between the liver cancer status for members of the same family.

3. Longitudinal study on numbers of sexual partners. The Multicenter AIDS Cohort Study (12) followed more than 4500 gay/bisexual men in Baltimore, Pittsburgh, Chicago, and Los Angeles since 1984 to study the natural history of AIDS. Investigators are interested in how sexual practice has changed since 1984 and which factors predict continued sexual behaviors that put men at high risk for HIV infection. The primary response variable used in this analysis is the number of sexual partners in the six months before each visit. There are up to 15 visits for each individual.

4. Sister chromatid exchange (SCE) study. A total of 14 hepatocellular carcinoma, 14 nasopharyngeal carcinoma, and 16 cervical cancer patients, and their age-sex-matched controls, were studied to compare the frequency of sister chromatid exchange (SCE) in their peripheral lymphocytes. Sister chromatid changes occur during cell replication when a chromosome duplicates its genetic material, thus forming a pair of chromosomes attached at the centromere (11). Elevated levels of SCEs would indicate that cells have been exposed to a mutagen potentially caused by chemical carcinogens. The hypothesis, which was tested in the study conducted by Dr. C. J. Chen, School of Medicine, National Taiwan University, is that cancer patients may have a higher frequency of SCE in lymphocytes than matched controls. The

outcome variable is the number of SCE per cell where 20 cells from each patient were cultured.

5. Family study on chronic obstructive pulmonary disease (COPD). Literature on obstructive pulmonary disease has suggested that there is a significantly increased risk for this common respiratory disease in relatives of patients with impaired pulmonary function (4, 14). Several studies have also shown that the observed familial aggregation in pulmonary function cannot be explained just by nongenetic risk factors, such as age and smoking (3). As part of a multidisciplinary study of COPD, 613 family members of 158 COPD cases seen at the Johns Hopkins Hospital were examined and given spirometry tests. The objective is to determine the percent of total variance attributable to unobserved genetic factors shared among siblings and their parents.

6. Growth study in Hmong refugee children. More than 1000 Hmong refugee children receiving health care at two Minnesota clinics between 1976 and 1985 were examined for their growth patterns (26). The objective is to study the pattern of growth and its association with the age at entry into the United States. Scientists believe that increases in stature are influenced by both genetic and environmental factors. When the offending environmental factors have been removed, the growth process often progresses at an accelerate rate, known as catch-up growth (36). This study allows investigators to address the questions as to whether there is indeed a period of accelerated growth following remediation, and if so, when this acceleration terminates. To study the growth, repeated observations of heights for each child were collected. The number of visits per child ranged from 1 to 15 and averaged 5. A regression model relating the rate of growth over time to the age at entering the United States will address the main objective. The correlation between repeated observations on height for each child is a nuisance, but cannot be ignored in regression analysis.

7. Indonesian children's health study. Approximately 3000 preschool children in Indonesia were medically examined in early 1980 as part of a survey of children's diseases. An objective of the study was to assess the role of vitamin A deficiency on the risk of respiratory infection and on body mass. A separate regression is needed for each of the two response variables, respiratory infection and weight for height. A secondary question is whether the response variables are correlated with each other, and if so, in what way?

1.1 Characteristics of Examples

Although different in their specific scientific objectives, the above examples have important characteristics in common that allow us to use a unified statistical method, which we present in Sections 3 and 4. Data in each of these examples are organized in clusters. For example, in the longitudinal studies (examples 3 and 6), a cluster comprises the repeated observations for an individual. For family studies (examples 2 and 5), the clusters are formed by families. Table 1 summarizes the clusters for each example.

For a variety of reasons, the responses within a cluster are likely to be dependent, i.e. correlated with one another. In the Hmong study, a child who is smaller than expected at one visit is likely to remain below average at the next visit. This phenomenon is known as "tracking" and is commonly observed in longitudinal studies (5). In the COPD study, the response variable, forced expiratory volume (FEV), is likely to be correlated among siblings because of shared genes and/or shared environments. This notion of familial aggregation has been repeatedly observed in chronic diseases, such as breast cancer (24), and in psychiatric disorders, such as schizophrenia (21).

The second common feature is that the scientific questions for each of the studies above can be formulated as regression analyses. First, one seeks the regression of the mean response on the independent variables. For the eye survey example, we relate the risk of visual impairment to demographic variables, such as age and race; logistic regression is suitable. In the Hmong growth example, we study children's height as a function of age and date of entry to the US by using linear regression. In addition, the regression concept can be applied to the parameters that characterize the within-cluster dependence. For example, researchers in the Baltimore eye survey are interested in knowing whether the degree of correlation of visual impairment between eyes varies by age or race. A more detailed discussion on the choice of measures for within-cluster dependence is given in Section 2.

The studies also differ from another in important ways, such as their type of response variable. We have examples of continuous measurements, such as body weight and FEV, as well as discrete variables that can be either counts, such as number of sexual partners in six months, or dichotomous, such as the presence or the absence of visual impairment for an eye. The studies also

Table 1 Some features of seven examples introduction in Section 1

Example	Cluster	No. of clusters/ cluster size*	Response	Scientific focus Mean	Dependence
Eye survey	individual	5199/2	binary	primary	secondary
Liver cancer	family	138/3*	binary	nuisance	primary
SCE	individual	80/20	count	primary	nuisance
Sexual partners	individual	4500/8*	count	primary	nuisance
COPD	family	158/4*	continuous	nuisance	primary
Hmong growth	individual	1070/5*	continuous	primary	nuisance
Indonesian children	individual	275/2	continuous/ binary	primary	secondary

*Averaged cluster sizes if varied.

differ in the structure of the within-cluster dependence. For example, in the Baltimore eye survey, each cluster (individual) has two responses, visual impairment status for the left and right eyes. If the study included several members of the same family, a more complicated dependence structure would result, because family members would likely have correlated responses. Family studies can present different types of correlation. If first-degree relatives of cases are ascertained, different degrees of correlation would be expected between parents, parents and siblings, or siblings.

Finally, the examples differ from one another with respect to their focus. In some cases, e.g. examples 3 and 6, the regression of the response on explanatory variables is most important, and the within-cluster association is a nuisance. For the family studies (examples 2 and 5), regression for the dependence structure is of primary interest. Even so, regression adjustment for individual and shared household characteristics is crucial in order to separate out the environmental impacts from the genetic ones. Table 1 summarizes both the similarities and the differences among the examples.

1.2 Inadequacy of the Conventional Regression Approach

This section discusses the consequences on regression inferences of totally ignoring the dependence within clusters when it exists. The specific impact of ignoring dependence varies according to the type of response model, the degree of correlation, and other factors. Nevertheless, the patterns are common across a range of problems, which we can illustrate with a simple example.

Let Y_{ij} be the jth observations from the ith cluster, $j = 1, \ldots, n$, $i = 1, \ldots, K$. We assume

$$E(Y_{ij}) = \beta_0 + \beta_1 x_{ij},\ \text{Var}(Y_{ij}) = \sigma^2,$$

$$\text{Cov}(Y_{ij}, Y_{ik}) = \sigma^2\rho,\ j < k = 1, \ldots, n.$$

This model assumes Y is a simple linear function of x and that the correlation between every pair of responses from a cluster is the same value, ρ. Let $\hat{\beta}_1$ be the ordinary least squares estimate of β_1 in which ρ is incorrectly assumed to be zero. Let $\hat{\beta}_1$ be the best possible (weighted least squares) estimate obtained by properly accounting for the correlation. Although $\hat{\beta}_1$ remains unbiased, i.e. $E(\hat{\beta}_1) = \beta_1$, ordinary least squares faces two problems: The estimated variance for $\hat{\beta}_1$ is incorrect, and $\hat{\beta}_1$ may be more variable than $\tilde{\beta}_1$. Each consequence is considered in turn.

1.2.1 VARIANCE ESTIMATE Ignoring the correlation leads to the use of $V_1 = \sigma^2/\Sigma_i\Sigma_j(x_{ij} - \bar{x})^2 = \sigma^2/V_T$ as the variance of $\hat{\beta}_1$. The correct variance, V_2, of $\hat{\beta}_1$ has the form $V_2 = V_1[1 + \rho(n\phi - 1)]$ where

$$\phi = \sum_{i=1}^{K} n(\bar{x}_i - \bar{x})^2/V_T$$

is the fraction of the total variance among the xs that is caused by variation among cluster mean $(\bar{x}_i)$s, rather than variation in xs within clusters. Two important cases of ϕ deserve special attention. When $\phi = 0$, there is no between-cluster variation in x; that is, $\bar{x}_i$ is the same for all clusters. An example would be a longitudinal study in which every person is measured at the same set of times. In this case, β_1 is estimated by using only within-cluster changes in Y. On the other hand, $\phi = 1$ features the between-cluster comparison, because in this case $x_{i1} = \ldots = x_{in}$ for all i. This is typical for cluster-specific covariates, such as the race variable in the Baltimore eye survey example.

Figure 1 shows the plots of

$$f(\rho,n,\phi) = \log(V_1/V_2) = \log[1 + \rho(n\phi - 1)]$$

against ρ for some selected ns and ϕs. The vertical axis is the logarithim of the ratio of incorrect versus correct variance of the ordinary least squares estimate; the horizontal axis is the actual correlation of responses from a cluster. A positive value of f indicates that the naive variance V_1 is too large and, hence, the confidence interval for β_1 based on $\hat{\beta}_1$ and V_1 is too wide. A negative value of f corresponds to confidence intervals for β_1 that are too narrow. The message from the plots is clear. For within cluster-comparisons, i.e. $\phi = 0$, the confidence interval based on V_1 is wider than it should be; the discrepancy between the incorrect and correct variances increases with ρ. On the other hand, the naive confidence interval is too narrow for between-cluster comparisons for which $\phi = 1$. In either case, invalid scientific conclusions may be drawn if V_1 is used as the variance estimate.

1.2.2 EFFICIENCY LOSS The second impact of ignoring the correlation and using $\hat{\beta}_1$ is a loss of efficiency, by which we mean that the uncertainty in $\hat{\beta}_1$ is greater than the uncertainty in the best unbiased estimate, $\tilde{\beta}_1$. The best estimate, $\tilde{\beta}_1$, has variance of the form

$$V_3 = V_1(1 - \rho)[1 + (n - 1)\rho]/[1 - \rho(1 - \phi)].$$

Figure 2 presents plots of

$$g(\rho,n,\phi) = V_3/V_2 = \left\{1 + \frac{n^2\rho^2\phi\,(1 - \phi)}{(1 - \rho)[1 + (n - 1)\rho]}\right\}^{-1}$$

against ρ for selected ns and ϕs. Interestingly, $\hat{\beta}_1$ is fully efficient in this example when either $\phi = 0$ or $\phi = 1$, irrespective of ρ and n. However,

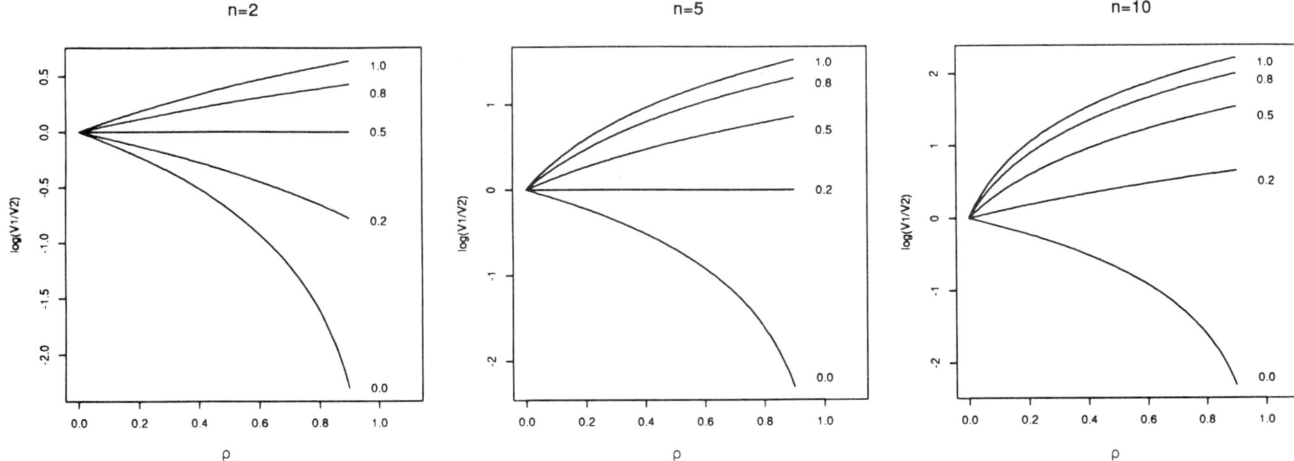

Figure 1 The plot of the logarithm of V_1/V_2 versus ρ for selected cluster sizes $n(2, 5, 10)$ and $\phi(0, 0.2, 0.5, 0.8, 1.0)$. Here, V_1 is the variance of the least squared estimate $\hat{\beta}_1$ when the within-cluster dependence is ignored and V_2 is the correct variance. We have assumed $E(Y_{ij}) = \beta_0 + \beta_1 x_{ij}$ and $\rho = \text{corr}(Y_{ij}, Y_{ik})$, $j < k = 1, \ldots n$; ϕ is the ratio of the between cluster variance to the total variance among the x_{ij}s.

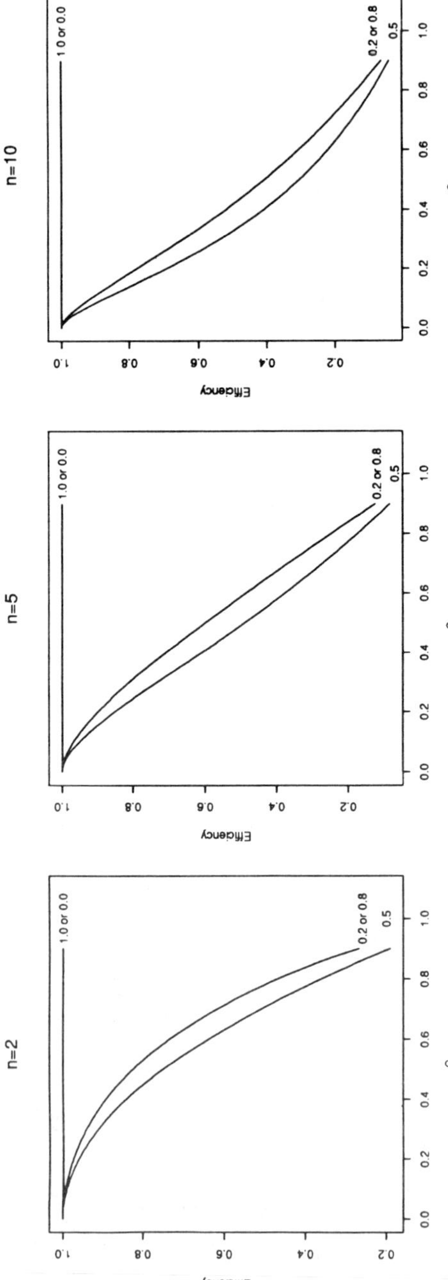

Figure 2 The plot of V_3/V_2 versus ρ for selected n (2, 5, 10) and ϕ (0, 0.2, 0.5, 0.8, 1.0). Here, V_2, ρ, ϕ, and the assumed model are the same as described in Figure 1; V_3 is the variance of the best unbiased estimate of β_1.

efficiency loss is evident when ϕ moves toward 0.5. This phenomenon is more apparent with increased ρ or n. The most important message in Figure 2 is that ignoring correlation can lead to a loss of power when both within-cluster and among-cluster information is being used to estimate β_1.

In Section 2, we provide statistical background for generalized linear models (GLMs) that have unified regression analysis for various types of independent data, and for measures of within-cluster dependence. Section 3 reviews three different approaches to modeling both the regression of Y on x and the within-cluster dependence. Section 4 describes briefly the statistical method called generalized estimating equations (GEE), which was designed to provide valid regression inferences with correlated data. We then illustrate GEE through an analysis of data from the Baltimore eye survey.

2 BACKGROUND

In describing the common features of the examples in Section 1.1, we identified two objectives in the analysis of clustered data: describing the response variable as a function of explanatory variables and measuring within-cluster dependence. In this section, we review briefly how commonly used regression models have been unified under the framework of GLMs when all the data are independent ("univariate case"). We also review two measures of within-cluster dependence: correlation for continuous data and odds ratio (OR) for dichotomous responses.

2.1 Generalized Linear Models

Generalized linear models (20, 22) are a unified class of regression methods for discrete and continuous response variables. Logistic regression for binary responses, linear regression for continuous responses, log-linear models for counts, and some survival analysis methods are special cases. There are two basic parts of a GLM, the systematic component and the random component. For the systematic component, one relates Y to x by assuming the averaged Y among individuals with a common value of x, $\mu = E(Y)$, satisfies

$$g(\mu) = x_1\beta_1 + \ldots + x_p\beta_p,$$

which we write in short-hand notation

$$g(\mu) = x'\beta \qquad 1.$$

where g is a prespecified function known as the "link function." The logistic regression model, frequently used for binary data, is a special case of Equation 1 with

$$\log\left(\frac{E(Y)}{1 - E(Y)}\right) = \log\frac{P(Y = 1)}{P(Y = 0)} = x'\beta.$$

For count data, the familiar log-linear model is a special case that assumes

$$\log E(Y) = x'\beta.$$

Table 2 provides a list of commonly used regression models in public health that are special cases of GLMs.

To account for the variability of the observed responses that is not explained by the systematic component caused by either measurement error or variation between individuals, GLMs assume that Y is generated from a distribution with likelihood function of the form

$$f(y) = \exp\{[y\theta + b(\theta)]/\phi + c(y, \phi)\}, \qquad 2.$$

known as the exponential family. The Poisson distribution is a special case of Equation 2 with

$$\begin{aligned} P(Y = y) &= \mu^y e^{-\mu}/y! \ , y = 0,1,2, \ldots \\ &= \exp\{y \log \mu - \mu - \log y!\}, \end{aligned}$$

so that $\theta = \log \mu$, $b(\theta) = -e^{\theta}$, $c(y) = -\log y!$, and $\phi = 1$. Other commonly used distributions are included in Table 2. The scale parameter ϕ in Equation 2 is called the "overdispersion" parameter. Many biomedical researchers have observed that the variation among count data is beyond that described by the Poisson distribution, which assumes that $\text{Var}(Y) = \mu = E(Y)$. The introduction of ϕ in Equation 2 deals with overdispersion directly by allowing $\text{Var}(Y) = \phi E(Y)$, $\phi > 1$ instead.

When both the systematic component, i.e. the link function, and the random component, i.e. Equation 2, are specified in a GLM, one can estimate the regression coefficients β by solving the estimating equation

$$U(\beta) = \sum_{i=1}^{K} \frac{\partial\mu_i(\beta)'}{\partial\beta} \text{Var}(Y_i)^{-1}[Y_i - \mu_i(\beta)] = 0. \qquad 3.$$

As expected, $U(\beta)$ reduces to $\Sigma_{i=1}^{K} x_i(Y_i - x_i'\beta) = 0$ in the multiple linear regression case, i.e. when $Y_i \sim N(x_i'\beta, \phi^2)$. The form of the estimating equation is intuitively sensible. To estimate β, one equates the observed (Y_i) with the expected (μ_i) for each individual, and these $(O_i - E_i)$s are then combined across individuals with weights that are inversely proportional to the variability of the Y_is. We multiply in front by $\partial\mu_i/\partial\beta$ to change from units of Y to units of x. Because the same equation is solved for the entire class of GLMs, common software, theory, and model checking techniques can be used for logistic, log-linear, linear, and survival models. Finally, we note that the estimating equation above only uses the first two moments of the Ys, i.e. the mean and variance functions (34). This feature of $U(\beta)$ is especially important when one is uncertain about the full distribution for the data.

Table 2 Some commonly used regression models in biomedical applications

Model	Response(Y)	Link function g	Distribution for Y	Scalar parameter (ϕ)	Variance function $\phi V(\mu)$
Linear multiple regression	continuous	Identity	Normal	ϕ	ϕ
		$\mu = x'\beta$	$\frac{1}{\sqrt{2\pi\phi}} e^{-(y-\mu)^2/2\phi}$		
Logistic regression	proportion	logit	Binomial		
	$0, 1/m, 2/m, \ldots, 1$	$\log \frac{\mu}{1-\mu} = x'\beta$	$\binom{m}{my} \mu^{my}(1-\mu)^{m-my}$	$1/m$	$\mu(1-\mu)/m$
Poisson regression (Log-linear)	count	log	Poisson		
	$0, 1, 2, \ldots$	$\log \mu = x'\beta$	$\mu^y e^{-\mu}/y!$	1	μ
Gamma regression	continuous	inverse	Gamma		
	(non-negative)	$\mu^{-1} = x'\beta$	$\frac{1}{\Gamma(1/\phi)(\mu\phi)^{1/\phi}} y^{1/\phi - 1} e^{-y/(\mu\phi)}$	ϕ	$\phi\mu^2$

2.2 Measures of Within-Cluster Dependence

For continuous data, the most commonly used measure of dependence between two responses, Y_1 and Y_2, is the correlation coefficient

$$\rho = \mathrm{Cov}(Y_1,Y_2)/[\mathrm{Var}(Y_1)\mathrm{Var}(Y_2)]^{1/2}$$

where $\mathrm{Cov}(Y_1,Y_2)$ is the covariance. The correlation coefficient is dimensionless, taking values in the range $[-1, 1]$. The correlation ρ is close to 0 when there is little dependence. Strong dependence is indicated when ρ approaches either 1 or -1. A positive correlation indicates that Y_1 tends to be larger than expected if Y_2 is and vice versa. The correlation among observations for the same cluster can take a variety of forms; each can be summarized by the pattern of correlations, as we now illustrate.

In longitudinal studies, each cluster comprises repeated responses over time from an individual. For biological variables, such as blood pressures, cholesterol level, and body weight, the degree of correlation tends to be greater for observations that are closer in time than those that are far apart. One simple assumption is that the correlation between observations at times t_1 and t_2 has the form $\rho^{|t_1-t_2|}$, i.e. decays geometrically with $t_1 - t_2$. An alternate assumption is that correlation is the same for all pairs of observations for the same cluster. In a longitudinal study, this form arises if individuals tend to have their own levels (intercepts) for the response. In family studies, it is important to distinguish within-family correlation that is caused by the shared environment from that caused by shared genes. For families with data from both parents and offspring, one may assume three different correlation coefficients: between parents (ρ_{PP}), between siblings (ρ_{SS}), and between a parent and offspring (ρ_{PS}). Assuming all the relatives share the same environment, a genetic explanation for the trait may be warranted if ρ_{SS} is much greater than ρ_{PP}, as parents do not share genes in common as do siblings. For more details on correlation models, see Laird & Ware (15), Diggle (7), and Diggle et al (8).

For discrete, in particular dichotomous data, the correlation coefficient is a poor measure of association because it is constrained by the mean parameters μ_1, and μ_2. Specifically, for dichotomous variables, Y_1 and Y_2, the correlation is given by

$$\rho = \frac{\Pr(Y_1 = Y_1 = 1) - 2\mu_1\mu_2}{[\mu_1(1 - \mu_1)\mu_2(1 - \mu_2)]^{1/2}}.$$

However, the joint probability, $\Pr(Y_1 = Y_2 = 1)$ is constrained to satisfy

$$\max(0, \mu_1 + \mu_2 - 1) < \Pr(Y_1 = Y_2 = 1) < \min(\mu_1, \mu_2),$$

which narrows considerably the range ρ can take. For this reason, we prefer to use the OR

$$\text{OR}(Y_1, Y_2) = \frac{\Pr(Y_1 = Y_2 = 1)\Pr(Y_1 = Y_2 = 0)}{\Pr(Y_1 = 1, Y_2 = 0)\Pr(Y_1 = 0, Y_2 = 1)},$$

which is not constrained by the means. For the Baltimore eye survey example, Y_1 and Y_2 would represent the visual impairment status for the left and right eyes, respectively, from each individual. An OR of 2 means that the odds of visual impairment for one eye increases twofold if the other eye was impaired.

Different measures of association between discrete variables have been suggested in the literature (9). The OR has been chosen as the primary measure of within-cluster dependence for discrete data, mainly because it is easy to interpret and is familiar to public health researchers.

3. STATISTICAL MODELS FOR CORRELATED DATA

To analyze clustered data, we must model both the regression of Y on x and the within-cluster dependence. If the responses are independent of each other, GLMs, reviewed in Section 2.1, can be used for diverse types of responses. For correlated data, GLMs are not sufficient, as we discussed in Section 1.3, and alternative approaches that address the dependence are needed. We now review three different modeling approaches: marginal, random effects, and observation driven. In marginal models, the regression of Y on x and the within-cluster dependence are modeled separately. The other approaches attempt to address both issues simultaneously through a single model. The public health investigator must select a model based upon one or a combination of these approaches whose parameters most nearly capture the scientific objectives, rather than on the basis of mathematical convenience.

Below, we let $Y_i = (Y_{i1}, \ldots, Y_{ij}, \ldots, Y_{ini})'$ be a $n_i \times 1$ vector of responses from the ith cluster, $i = 1, \ldots, K$. Note that n_i, the cluster size, may vary. In addition to Y_{ij}, one observes a $p \times 1$ vector of explanatory variables, x_{ij}, thought to be related to Y_{ij}. We now consider each modeling approach in turn.

3.1 Marginal Models

In a marginal model, the regression of Y on x and the within-cluster dependence are modeled separately. For the former, we model the marginal expectation $E(Y_{ij})$ as a function of explanatory variables. The marginal expectation is the average response over the population of individuals with a common value of x, just as in the univariate case when $n_i = 1$ for each cluster. Specifically, we assume the following:

1. The marginal expectation or "population-average" of the response, $\mu_{ij} = E(Y_{ij})$ depends on the explanatory variables x_{ij} through $g(\mu_{ij}) = x_{ij}'\beta$,

where g is a known link function, such as the logit for dichotomous responses or log for counts just as in GLMs.
2. The marginal variance depends on the marginal mean by $\text{Var}(Y_{ij}) = V(\mu_{ij})\phi$ where V is a known variance function, such as $V(\mu_{ij}) = \mu_{ij}$ for count data, and ϕ is the overdispersion parameter to be estimated just as in GLMs.
3. The covariance between Y_{ij} and Y_{ik} is a function of the marginal means and perhaps of additional parameters α, i.e. $\text{cov}(Y_{ij}, Y_{ik}) = c(\mu_{ij}, \mu_{ik}; \alpha)$ where c is a known function.

In the Baltimore eye survey study, a marginal model can be used to assess the dependence of visual impairment for either eye on demographic variables, such as sex, age, and race. For simplicity, let x_i indicate the sex (1-male; 0-female) of a subject. A simple marginal model has the form

$$\text{logit}\mu_{ij} = \log[\mu_{ij}/(1 - \mu_{ij})] = \beta_0 + \beta_1 x_i, \; j = 1,2,$$

$$\text{Var}(Y_{ij}) = \mu_{ij}(1 - \mu_{ij}),$$

$$\log \text{OR}\ (Y_{i1}, Y_{i2}) = \alpha_0.$$

The parameter, $\exp(\beta_1)$, is the odds of visual impairment for any eye among males relative to the odds among females. In other words, we have assumed in this model that the difference between men and women in the prevalence of visual impairment is the same for right and left eyes. Note that $\exp(\beta_1)$ is a ratio of population frequencies, so we refer to it as a population-averaged parameter. The degree of correlation between two eyes, measured by the OR, was assumed to be the same for each individual. This simplified assumption may be checked and modified, if necessary, by imposing a regression model on $\text{OR}(Y_{i1}, Y_{i2})$, such as

$$\log \text{OR}(Y_{i1}, Y_{i2}) = \alpha_0 + \alpha_1 x_i.$$

A negative α_1 would suggest that the degree of correlation between two eyes is stronger among females.

Because the marginal model coefficients, β, describe the effects of covariates on the marginal expectation of the response variables, β has the same interpretation regardless of the cluster size, n_i, which may vary among clusters. In particular, the interpretation of β is the same as from a GLM for independent data, which would be appropriate if $n_i = 1$ for all clusters. The interpretation of β is not altered by the magnitude of within-cluster dependence as described by the parameter α.

3.2 Random Effects Models

The essence of the random effects model is the assumption that parameters vary from cluster to cluster, thus reflecting natural heterogeneity caused by unmeasured factors. Suppose Hmong children grow roughly as a linear function of age over the span of our study, so that each child's growth can be summarized by a baseline height (intercept) and growth rate (slope). Children obviously enter the study at different heights and have different growth rates. This heterogeneity in intercepts and slopes is beyond what can be explained by such predictor variables as age and sex. A random effects model is a reasonable description of the data if the collection of intercepts and slopes across children can be thought of as a sample from a distribution. The correlation of repeated observations of heights from the same child arises because of the heterogeneity among children in their true growth curves, which cannot be observed.

To be more specific, suppose a subset of the Hmong data can be described by the following simple model for the height, Y_{ij}, of child i at age j:

1. $Y_{ij} = (\beta_1^* + b_{i1}) + (\beta_2^* \text{age}_{ij} + b_{i2}\text{age}_{ij}) + \beta_3^* \text{sex}_i + \beta_4^*(\text{age}_{ij} \times \text{sex}_i) + \epsilon_{ij}$ where $\text{sex}_i = 1$, if boy and 0 if girl, age_{ij} = the age of the ith child at the jth visit, and $\epsilon_{ij} \sim N(0, \sigma^2)$, $j = 1, \ldots, n_i$.
2. $\epsilon_{i1}, \ldots, \epsilon_{in_i}$ are independent of one another, given $b_i = (b_{i1}, b_{i2})$.
3. b_i follows a bivariate normal distribution with mean = (0,0) and covariance matrix

$$\begin{pmatrix} \delta_{11} & \delta_{12} \\ \delta_{21} & \delta_{22} \end{pmatrix}.$$

In this model, β_1^* and $\beta_1^* + \beta_3^*$ represent the average baseline heights for girls and boys, respectively, whereas β_2^* and $\beta_2^* + \beta_4^*$ describe the average growth rates for girls and boys. A significantly positive β_4^* indicates that, on average, boys grow faster than girls. A negative b_{i2} indicates that the growth rate of the ith child is lower than the average. The random effects variances , δ_{11} and δ_{22}, measure the variability of the initial heights and growth rates among children that cannot be explained by the gender difference. The correlation $\delta_{12}/(\delta_{11}\delta_{22})^{1/2}$ measures the association between the child-specific deviations in initial height and growth rate.

To accommodate the variety of responses seen in public health research, a random effects GLM can be described as follows:

1. Given random effects, b_i, which are specific to the ith cluster, the conditional distribution of Y_{ij} follows a GLM with $g[E(Y_{ij}|b_i)] = x_{ij}^{\prime}\beta^* + z_{ij}^{\prime}b_i$, where z_{ij}, a $q \times 1$ vector of covariates, is a subset of x_{ij}.
2. Given b_i, $Y_{i1}, Y_{i2}, \ldots, Y_{in_i}$ are statistically independent.
3. The b_is are independent observations from a distribution, $F(\cdot;\delta)$, indexed by some possibly unknown parameters, δ. The term "random effects" was coined for b_i, because we treat the b_i as a random sample from F. The key assumption is that a cluster's b_i is not related to the x_{ij}s.

The random effects model is especially useful when the objective is to make inference about individuals, such as the children in the Hmong study, rather than just about the population average, which can be done equally well with the marginal approach. A more detailed discussion on the difference and the connection between β^* in the random effects model and β in the marginal model is given in Zeger et al (41), Neuhaus et al (23), and Zeger & Liang (40).

3.3 Observation-Driven Models

Cox (6) coined the phrase "observation-driven" model for the situation in which the correlation within a cluster arises because one response is explicitly caused by others. An example is infectious disease incidence for children from the same family. If Y_{ij} indicates whether a child j in family i has an incident case, it is likely that Y_{ij} will be directly caused by the responses for the other children, Y_{ik}. $k \neq j$, because infections are often passed among siblings.

Observation-driven models are commonly used in longitudinal and times series studies where they are termed "Markov" or "transition" models (33). Here, the conditional distribution of the response Y_{Ij} at time t_{ij} given the entire past, $Y_{ij-1}, Y_{ij-2}, \ldots, Y_{i1}$, is modeled as a function of the explanatory variables, x_{ij}, and explicitly as a function of the past responses themselves. That is, the past outcomes, or functions thereof, are treated as additional explanatory variables. To simplify the analysis, we commonly assume that only the most recent past observations affect the current response. For example, the probability of respiratory infection for a given child at visit, j, depends only on whether the child had infection at visit, $j - 1$, as well as on explanatory variables, x_{ij}.

The autoregressive model for equally spaced, continuous observations is an example of an observation-driven model. In the simplest first order case, we assume

$$Y_{ij} = x'_{ij}\beta^{**} + \epsilon_{ij}, \qquad 4.$$

where

$$\epsilon_{ij} = \alpha\epsilon_{ij-1} + a_{ij} \qquad 5.$$

and a_{ij} are independent, mean-zero innovations. The residual from the linear regression at time, t_{ij}, depends explicitly on the residual the previous time. Thus, the past directly influences the present. The GLM extension of the transition model is straightforward. We model the conditional distribution of Y_{ij}, given the past as an explicit function of the preceding responses. To illustrate, consider the logistic regression model to study the association between vitamin A deficiency and respiratory infection, using data on children from the Indonesian Children's Health Study. Here, the response is whether a child had infection, and the major explanatory variable is whether the child was vitamin A deficient. But, children infected at one visit are more likely to be infected at the next. An observation-driven model could be written as

$$\text{logit } E(Y_{ij}|y_{ij-1}, y_{ij-2}, \ldots, y_{i1}) = \text{logit } E(Y_{ij}|y_{ij-1}) = x_{ij}'\beta^{**} + \alpha y_{ij-1}. \qquad 6.$$

To specify the general transition model, let $P_{ij} = \{y_{ij-1}, \ldots, y_{i1}\}$ be the past responses at time, t_{ij}, and let $\mu_{ij}^c = E(Y_{ij}|P_{ij})$ and $v_{ij}^c = \text{var}(Y_{ij}|P_{ij})$ be the conditional mean and variance of Y_{ij} given the past responses and the explanatory variables. Analogous to the GLM for independent data, we assume

$$g(\mu_{ij}^c) = x_{ij}'\beta^{**} + \Sigma_{v=1}^{q} f_v(P_{ij}; \alpha)$$

$$v_{ij}^c = V(\mu_{ij}^c).$$

The past outcomes, after transformation by the known functions, f_v, are treated as additional explanatory variables. If the model for the conditional mean is correctly specified, we can treat the repeated transitions for a person as independent events and use standard statistical methods. See Zeger & Qaqish (42), Korn & Whittemore (13), and Ware et al (33) for additional discussion.

When the cluster is formed by a factor, such as family, rather than time, the observations within a cluster do not have a natural, complete ordering. Hence, although it is still possible to specify an observation-driven model in terms of conditional distributions of Y_{ij} given Y_{ik}, $k \neq j$, greater care is required. It is easy to choose apparently sensible conditional models that cannot exist. See Besag (1) for details in the context of spatial data.

With binary responses, Liang & Zeger (17) show that the joint distribution of $Y_{i1}, \ldots, Y_{in_i}$ can be fully specified by n_i logistic models for Y_{ij} given Y_{ik}, $k \neq j$. Rosner (27) has developed beta-binomial models by using this approach. However, it has an inherent limitation. The interpretation for β^{**} is not the same for clusters of different size. For example, in a family study, suppose we regress the response for one member on the responses for others, as well as on explanatory variables. The interpretation of the coefficients for the explanatory variables is different when the number of family members is different. This is a serious problem that limits the use of models that are specified in terms of conditional distributions.

This problem is less acute in longitudinal studies. In the linear regression case, it is possible to specify the model so that the interpretation of the regression coefficients does not change as the number of previous responses used to predict the current value changes. With nonlinear links, such as the log and logit, this is not generally possible. The meaning and values of regression coefficients, β^{**}, change when the model for the dependence on the prior outcomes is changed. This is in contrast to the marginal model, in which the regression of Y on x can be separated from the within-cluster association. In most observation-driven models, the two objectives are intertwined into one modeling equation.

4. STATISTICAL INFERENCE

This section reviews statistical inference for parameters specified by models discussed in Section 3. The focus is centered upon the application of the estimating procedure, GEE (16, 19, 25, 39), to the marginal models for which the GEE method was originated. Extension of the GEE method to the other two models is also briefly reviewed.

4.1 *Marginal Model*

When the regression analysis for the mean is the primary interest, the β coefficients specified in Section 3.1 can be estimated by solving the estimating equation

$$U_1(\beta,\alpha) = \sum_{i=1}^{K} \left(\frac{\partial \mu_i}{\partial \beta}\right)' [\mathrm{Cov}(Y_i;\ \beta,\ \alpha)]^{-1}(Y_i - \mu_i(\beta)] = 0 \qquad 7.$$

where $\mu_i(\beta) = E(Y_i)$, the marginal expectations for Y_i. Note that U_1 in Equation 7 has exactly the same form as $U(\beta)$ in Equation 3, except that Y_i is now a $n_i \times 1$ vector, which comprises the n_i observations from the ith cluster, and the covariance matrix, $\mathrm{cov}(Y_i)$, for Y_i depends not only on β but on α, which characterizes the within-cluster dependence. This additional complication can be alleviated by iterating until convergence between solving $U_1[\beta,\hat{\alpha}(\beta)] = 0$ and updating $\hat{\alpha}(\beta)$, an estimate of α (16). The GEE approach is simply to choose parameter values $\hat{\beta}$ so that the expected $\mu_i(\beta)$ is as close to the observed Y_i as possible, weighting each cluster of data inversely to its variance matrix $\mathrm{var}(Y_i;\ \beta,\ \alpha)$, which is a function of the within-cluster dependence.

Generalized estimating equations have some theoretical and practical advantages. First, no joint distribution assumption for $Y_i = (Y_{i1}, \ldots, Y_{in_i})$ is required to use the method. This is especially important for discrete responses for which there are no simple and sensible classes of joint distributions. Second, $\hat{\beta}$, the solution of $U_1[\beta,\ \hat{\alpha}(\beta)] = 0$, has high efficiency compared with the maximum likelihood estimate of β in many cases studied. Third, White (35), Gourieroux et al (10), and Liang & Zeger (16) proposed use of a a robust variance, $\hat{V_\beta}$, of $\hat{\beta}$, which, in conjunction with $\hat{\beta}$, often provides valid inferences for β, even when the covariance structure $c(\mu_{ij}, \mu_{ik}; \beta, \alpha)$ in Section 3.2 is misspecified. Specifically, suppose the investigators mistakenly assume that the observations from the same cluster are independent of each other. The 95% confidence interval for each regression coefficient β_j, $j = 1, \ldots, p$, based upon

$$\hat{\beta}_j \pm 1.96(V_{\hat{\beta}_j})^{1/2}$$

remains valid. Thus, investigators are protected against misspecification of the within-cluster dependence structure. This is especially appealing when the data set comprises a large number of small clusters, as is the case for nearly all the examples considered in Section 1.

When the within-cluster dependence is the primary interest, as is true for most family studies, this first procedure, which we call "GEE1," has an important limitation (18). In GEE1, we estimate β and α, acting as if they are independent of each other. Consequently, very little information from β is used when estimating α. This can lead to a significant loss of α information. As a remedy, Prentice (25) and Liang et al (18) discuss estimating $\delta = (\beta, \alpha)$ jointly by solving

$$U_2(\beta,\alpha) = \sum_{i=1}^{K} \left(\frac{\partial \mu_i^*}{\partial \delta}\right)' [\mathrm{Cov}(Z_i;\ \delta)]^{-1}(Z_i - \mu_i^*(\delta)] = 0, \qquad 8.$$

where

$$Z_i = (Y_{i1}, \ldots, Y_{in_i}, Y_{i1}^2, \ldots, Y_{in_i}^2, Y_{i1}Y_{i2}, Y_{i1}Y_{i3}, \ldots, Y_{in_i} \ldots, Y_{in_i-1}Y_{in_i})' \qquad 9.$$

and $\mu_i^* = E(Z_i; \delta)$, which is completely specified by the modeling assumptions made in Section 3.1. We call this expanded procedure, which uses both the Y_{ij}s and $Y_{ij}Y_{ik}$s, the "GEE2."

GEE2 appears to have high efficiency for both β and α (18). On the other hand, the robustness property for β of GEE1 is no longer true. Hence, correct inferences about β require correct specification of the within-cluster dependence structure given by $c(\mu_{ij}, \mu_{ik}; \beta, \alpha)$. The same authors suggest using a sensitivity analysis when making inference on β. That is, one may repeat the procedure with different models for the within-cluster dependence structure to examine the sensitivity of $\hat{\beta}$ to choice of dependence structure.

4.2 *Random Effects Models*

The GEE approach can also be used to estimate β^* in some random effects models. For illustration, let us assume that investigators collect count data and use a random intercept model to account for heterogeneity among clusters. That is, they assume the following:

1. Given a scalar random effect b_i, the counts $Y_{i1}, \ldots, Y_{in_i}$ are independent, and each has a Poisson distribution whose mean follows

$$\log E(Y_{ij}|b_i) = x'_{ij}\beta^* + b_i.$$

2. b_i follows a normal distribution with mean zero and variance δ.

To use the GEE method, one needs to compute the marginal expectations of the Z_is given in Equation 9. These computations are tedious yet straightforward. For example,

$$E(Y_{ij}) = E[E(Y_{ij}|b_i)] = E(e^{x'_{ij}\beta^* + b_i}) = e^{\delta/2 + x'_{ij}\beta^*}$$

and for $j \neq k$

$$E(Y_{ij}Y_{ik}) = E[E(Y_{ij}Y_{ik}|b_i)] = E[E(Y_{ij}|b_i)E(Y_{ik}|b_i)]$$
$$= E(e^{x'_{ij}\beta^* + x'_{ik}\beta^* + 2b_i}) = e^{2\delta + x'_{ij}\beta^* + x'_{ik}\beta^*}.$$

Thus, with minor modifications. statistical software that is suitable for fitting marginal models can be used to make inference about the fixed effects, β^*, and the variance of the random effects, δ (41). However, when one is interested in the estimation of the random effects, b_i, a different strategy is needed. Interested readers are referred to Laird & Ware (15), Stiratteli et al (30), Zeger & Karim (38), Breslow & Clayton (2), Schall (28), and Waclawiw & Liang (32).

4.3 *Observation-Driven Models*

As stated above, we treat other responses like explanatory variables in observation-driven models. Hence, we can fit this class using GEE by simply adding the necessary outcomes or functions thereof to the list of predictors for each observation. To illustrate, suppose we assume the logistic model for respiratory infection given in Equation 6. Then, we must add the infection status at the previous visit to vitamin A status in the list of explanatory variables and, in this case, use standard software for fitting a logistic model. If the first order Markov assumption is correct, the inferences will be correct. If the respiratory response at one time, given the entire past, depends on more than the last outcome as assumed, the inferences will be incorrect in much the same way as discussed in Section 1.2.1.

With clusters that are not ordered by time, the same strategy is used, but the repeated conditional events, Y_{ij} given Y_{ik}, $k \neq j$, $j = 1, \ldots, n_i$, will not in general be independent, as was possible for time-ordered data. Hence, the models must be fit by using GEE or some other approach that accounts for the dependence.

5. BALTIMORE EYE SURVEY DATA

As stated earlier, the main objective of the Baltimore eye survey (31) was to identify demographic variables, such as age, race, and education level, that may be associated with the prevalence of visual impairment (VI). Liang et al (18) have provided descriptive statistics on prevalence of VI for both eyes for each race × age combination. In short, the prevalence increases with age and is higher among blacks; the discrepancy between blacks and whites increases with age. In addition, risks of VI were apparently similar between left and right eyes for each race × age combination. Table 3 gives the estimates and the standard errors of regression coefficients when separate logistic regression models have been fit for the right and left eyes. For example, coefficients for the variable "race" reveal that at age 60, the prevalence of VI for left eyes is 43% (= $e^{0.356} - 1$) higher among blacks than whites; similar results held for the right eye: 35% (= $e^{0.314} - 1$) higher among blacks. That the race-associated difference in prevalence is greater for the left eye than for the right appears to have occurred by chance, as the test statistic

$$Z^2 = (0.356 - 0.314)^2/[(0.132)^2 + (0.127)^2 + 0.0056* 2] = 0.039$$

is not significant even at the 0.10 level. Note that the number 0.0056 was produced from the GEE procedure to account for the fact that the data from two correlated eyes for each person were used to compute Z^2. The estimated correlation coefficient 0.334 = 0.0056/(0.132*0.127) between the two estimates of the race effect is indirect evidence of strong within-person dependence between the two eyes.

For the rest of the analyses, we assumed that the logistic regression coefficients for the left and right eyes are the same. We fit a sequence of models that differ only in the manner of modeling the between-eye dependence. In model 1, we incorrectly ignored the dependence to illustrate the consequences. In models 2, 3, and 4, different assumptions about the associa-

Table 3 Regression estimates and standard errors (in parentheses) fitting separate logistic regression models to the right and left eyes from the Baltimore eye survey

	Logistic regression model						
Eye	Intercept	Race	Age-60	(Age-60)^2	Race(Age-60)	Race*(Age-60)^2	Education
Left	−2.870	0.356	0.050	0.0007	−0.003	−0.0009	−0.067
	(0.098)	(0.132)	(0.009)	(0.0004)	(0.011)	(0.0006)	(0.020)
Right	−2.781	0.314	0.048	0.002	0.004	−0.0012	−0.052
	(0.093)	(0.127)	(0.008)	(0.0004)	(0.011)	(0.0006)	(0.020)

tion between eyes were made, as summarized in Table 4. The key features of the results, presented fully in Table 4, can be summarized as follows:

1. Results from model 1, in which the dependence between eyes has been ignored, show the naive variance estimates of $\hat{\beta}$ are, in general, too small. For estimating the race effect, for example, the naive variance estimate is 28% $[= 1 - (0.089/0.105)^2]$ smaller than the correct one. In this example, ignoring dependence does not lead to qualitatively different conclusions. However, ignoring dependence often leads to serious scientific mistakes, as can been seen, for example, in an analysis of a 2 × 2 cross-over trial (40).
2. The frequency of VI increases with age, more rapidly in later life. Blacks have roughly 35% more VI than whites at age 60. Persons with higher education have lower rates of VL.
3. A comparison of the logistic regression coefficients from models 2, 3, and 4 suggests that the regression inferences using GEE are not sensitive to how one models the dependence between eyes. This provides the investigators more confidence in the validity of the results.
4. The last column of Table 4 gives the ratio of the variance estimates from model 2 to the variance estimates where separate regression coefficients were being fitted for each eye. If the data from the two eyes of each person were indeed independent of each other, one would expect the ratio to be close to two because of doubling of the sample size. The ratios presented here (known as the design effect in the context of sample survey) are less than two, which indicates a strong degree of correlation between pairs of eyes.
5. One sees a strong within-person dependence for whites and blacks. For whites, the risk of VI for one eye is inflated by a factor of 9.8 ($e^{2.286}$) should the other eye also be affected. Among blacks, the corresponding OR is estimated as 17.17 ($e^{2.286+0.0557}$). This observation is apparently consistent with the long-standing clinical finding in this country that blacks have higher incidence of glaucoma and of diabetic mellitis, both of which tend to be bilateral diseases.

6. CONCLUDING REMARKS

Clustered data are increasingly common in public health research for many reasons. The search for earlier risk factors, such as biomolecular markers of the disease process, has increased the need for longitudinal studies. The advances in our understanding of the genetic roots of disease have made family studies more attractive. The increased appreciation for the social and behavioral contributions to disease has made multivariate measures neces-

Table 4 Regression estimates and standard errors (in parenthesis) for the visual impairment data for the Baltimore eye survey

Variable	Model 1	Model 2	Model 3	Model 4	Variance ratio†
Intercept	−2.821 (0.076) (0.067)	−2.824 (0.076)	−2.824 (0.076)	−2.824 (0.076)	1.66
Race (1-B;0-W)	0.332 (0.105) (0.089)*	0.334 (0.105)	0.334 (0.015)	0.334 (0.105)	1.58
Age-60	0.049 (0.007) (0.006)*	0.049 (0.007)	0.049 (0.007)	0.049 (0.007)	1.65
$(\text{Age-60})^2$	0.0018 (0.0004) (0.0003)*	0.0018 (0.0003)	0.0018 (0.0003)	0.0018 (0.0003)	1.60
Race*(Age-60)	0.001 (0.0009) (0.0008)*	0.0007 (0.0005)	0.0007 (0.009)	0.0007 (0.009)	1.60
Race*$(\text{Age-60})^2$	−0.001 (0.0005) (0.0004)*	−0.001 (0.0005)	−0.001 (0.0005)	−0.001 (0.0005)	1.43
Education	−0.059 (0.017) (0.013)*	−0.060 (0.017)	−0.060 (0.017)	−0.060 (0.017)	1.39
log-odds ratio					
Intercept	—	2.555 (0.126)	2.286 (0.176)	2.390 (0.205)	
Race	— —	— —	0.557 (0.252)	0.500 (0.256)	
Age	—	—	—	−0.010 (0.011)	

*Naive standard error.
†Ratio of the variance estimates from Table 3 (left eye) to the variance estimates from Model 2.

sary. At the same time, increased computing power has made regression analysis more accessible to public health investigators. Hence, routine analyses attempt to characterize the nature of the dependence of a response on explanatory variables, rather than only asking whether such a relationship exists.

This paper has reviewed approaches to regression analysis of correlated data organized in clusters. We have focused on extensions of GLMs, so that the types of outcomes common in public health—continuous measures, binary indicators of disease counts, or times to events—can be treated in a unified fashion. We believe that marginal, random effects, and observation-driven models, or combinations thereof, provide researchers with many of the tools necessary to infer answers to their scientific questions.

Several issues remain to be addressed. In longitudinal studies, subjects sometimes enter and drop out of cohorts because of factors related to their response variables. Many current methods of analysis give biased inferences in these situations (8, 37). In observation-driven models, the regression inferences depend on the choice of the within-cluster dependence model. Better methods for choosing the best model from a set of candidates are needed. Random effects models are very attractive, but difficult to estimate except in the linear and log-linear case (41). Finally, many of the methods described above have relatively recently been put into practive. We need integrated software that will make it easy for the public health scientist to try different models in an effort to appreciate the sometimes subtle distinctions between them.

ACKNOWLEDGMENTS

This work was partially supported by grants #GM39622 and AI125529 from the National Institutes of Health.

Literature Cited

1. Besag, J. 1974. Spatial interaction and the statistical analyses of lattice systems. *J. R. Stat. Soc. B* 36:192–236
2. Breslow, N. E., Clayton, D. G. 1992. Approximate inference in generalized linear mixed models. *J. Am. Stat. Assoc.* In press
3. Cohen, B. H. 1980. Chronic obstructive pulmonary disease: a challenge in genetic epidemiology. *Am. J. Epidemiol.* 112:274–88
4. Cohen, B. H., Ball, W. C. Jr., Brashears, S., Diamond, E. L., Kreiss, P., et al 1977. Risk factors in chronic obstructive pulmonary disease (COPD). *Am. J. Epidemiol.* 105:223–32
5. Cook, N. R., Ware, J. H. 1983. Design and analysis methods for longitudinal research. *Annu. Rev. Public Health* 4:1–23
6. Cox, D. R. 1981. Statistical analysis of time series, some recent developments. *Scand. J. Stat.* 8:93–115
7. Diggle, P. J. 1988. An approach to the analysis of repeated measurements. *Biometrics* 44:959–72
8. Diggle, P. J., Liang, K.-Y., Zeger, S. L. 1993. *Analysis of Longitudinal Data*. Oxford: Oxford Univ. Press
9. Goodman, L. A., Kruskal, W. H. 1979. *Measures of Association for Cross Classifications*. New York: Springer-Verlag

10. Gourieroux, C., Monfort, A., Trognon, A. 1984. Pseudo maximum likelihood methods: theory. *Econometrica* 52:681–700
11. Hulka, B. S., Wilcosky, T. C., Griffith, J. D. 1990. *Biological Markers in Epidemiology*. New York: Oxford Univ. Press
12. Kaslow, R. A., Ostrow, D. G., Detels, R., Phair, J. P., Polk, F., et al. 1987. The Multicenter Cohort Study: rationale organization and selected characteristics of participants. *Am. J. Epidemiol.* 126: 310–18
13. Korn, E. E., Whittemore, A. S. 1979. Methods for analyzing panel studies of acute health effects of air pollution. *Biometrics* 35:795–802
14. Kueppers, F., Miller, R. D., Gordon, H., Hopper, N. G., Offord, K. 1977. Familial prevalence of chronic obstructive pulmonary disease in a matched prior study. *Am. J. Med.* 63:366–72
15. Laird, N. M., Ware, J. H. 1982. Random effects models for longitudinal studies. *Biometrics* 38:963–74
15a. Liang, K.-Y., Beaty, T. H. 1991. Measuring familial aggregation by using odds-ratio regression models. *Genetic Epidemiol.* 8:361–70
16. Liang, K.-Y., Zeger, S. L. 1986. Longitudinal data analysis using generalized linear models. *Biometrika* 73:13–22
17. Liang, K.-Y., Zeger, S. L. 1989. A class of logistic regression models for multivariate binary time series. *J. Am. Stat. Assoc.* 84:447–51
18. Liang, K.-Y., Zeger, S. L., Qaqish, B. 1991. Multivariate regression analyses for categorical data (with discussion). *J. R. Stat. Soc. B* 54:3–40
19. Lipsitz, S. R. 1989. *Generalized estimating equations for correlated binary data: using the odds ratio as a measure of association,* tech. rep. Boston: Dep. of Biostat. Harvard School of Public Health
20. McCullagh, P., Nelder, J. A. 1989 *Generalized Linear Models*. London: Chapman & Hall. 2nd ed.
21. Murray, R. M., Reveley, A. M., McGuffin, P. 1986. Genetic vulnerability to schizophrenia. *Psychiatr. Clin. North Am.* 9:3–16
22. Nelder, J. A., Wedderburn, R. W. M. 1972. Generalized linear models. *J. R. Stat. Soc. A* 135:370–84
23. Neuhaus, J. M., Kalbfleisch, J. D., Hauck, W. W. 1991. A comparison of cluster-specific and population averaged approaches for analyzing correlated binary data. *Int. Stat. Rev.* 59:25–36
24. Ottman, R., Pike, M. C., King, M. C., Casagrande, J. T., Henderson, B. E. 1986. Familial breast cancer in a population-based series. *Am. J. Epidemiol.* 123:15–21
25. Prentice, R. L. 1988. Correlated binary regression with covariate specific to each binary observation. *Biometrics* 44:1022–48
26. Rorabaugh, M. L. 1990. *Catch-up growth in young Hmong refugee children*. Doctoral thesis. Johns Hopkins School of Hygiene and Public Health, Baltimore
27. Rosner, B. 1984. Multivariate methods in ophthalmology with application to paired data situations. *Biometrics* 40: 961–71
28. Schall, R. 1991. Estimation in generalized linear models with random effects. *Biometrika* 78:719–27
29. Starfield, B., Shapiro, S., Weiss, J., Liang, K.-Y., Ra, K., et al 1991. Race, family income and low birthweight. *Am. J. Epidemiol.* 134:1167–74
30. Stiratteli, R., Laird, N., Ware, J. H. 1984. Random-effects models for serial observations with binary response. *Biometrics* 40:961–71
31. Tielsch, J. M., Sommer, A., Witt, K., Katz, J., Royall, R. M. 1990. Blindness and visual impairment in an American urban population: Baltimore eye survey. *Arch. Ophthalmol.* 108:286–90
32. Waclawiw, M. A., Liang, K.-Y. 1993. Prediction of random effects in the generalized linear model. *J. Am. Statist. Assoc.* In press
33. Ware, J. H., Lipsitz, S., Speizer, F. E. 1988. Issues in the analysis of repeated categorical outcomes. *Stat. Med.* 7:95–107
34. Wedderburn, R. W. M. 1974. Quasi-likelihood function, generalized linear models and the Gaussian method. *Biometrika* 61:439–47
35. White, H. 1982. Maximum likelihood estimation of misspecified models. *Econometrics* 50:1–25
36. Williams, J. P. G. 1981. Catch-up growth. *J. Embryol. Exp. Morphol.* 65: 89–101
37. Wu, M. C., Carroll, R. J. 1988. Estimation and comparison of changes in the presence of informative right censoring by modeling the censoring process. *Biometrics* 44:175–88
38. Zeger, S. L., Karim, M. R. 1991. Generalized linear models with random effects; a Gibbs sampling approach. *J. Am. Stat. Assoc.* 86:79–86
39. Zeger, S. L., Liang, K.-Y. 1986. Longi-

tudinal data analysis for discrete and continuous outcomes. *Biometrics* 42:121–30

40. Zeger, S. L., Liang, K.-Y. 1992. An overview of methods for the analysis of longitudinal data. *Stat. Med.* In press
41. Zeger, S. L., Liang, K.-Y. & Albert, P. 1988. Models for longitudinal data: a generalized estimating equation approach. *Biometrics* 44:1049–60
42. Zeger, S. L., Qaqish, B. 1988. Markov regression models for time series: a quasilikelihood approach. *Biometrics* 44:1019–31

Annu. Rev. Publ. Health 1993. 14:69–93

EXPOSURE MEASUREMENT ERROR: Influence on Exposure-Disease Relationships and Methods of Correction

Duncan Thomas, Daniel Stram, and James Dwyer

Department of Preventive Medicine, University of Southern California, Los Angeles, California 90033-9987

KEY WORDS: exposure measurement, dose-response, biostatistics, diet, radiation

---

INTRODUCTION

Epidemiology, being primarily an observational rather than experimental science, has often encountered problems with measurement of the study variables, which are not under the control of the investigator. Difficulties arise in part because the variables under study are often subjective and often must be ascertained by subjects' self reports or from records of dubious quality, because biological variability and laboratory error can occur, and because studies are often conducted retrospectively, thus requiring information on events that occurred long ago. Epidemiologists have long recognized that measurement errors have been among the major weaknesses of their studies and have gone to great lengths to try to assess the magnitude of such errors and their likely impact on the conclusions. This problem has spurred much methodologic research, initially on understanding the effects of measurement errors on exposure-response relationships and more recently on developing methods to correct for such errors. The results of the former line of research have often been used qualitatively in the interpretation of epidemiologic findings, but the quantitative predictions have seldom been applied. Thus, the latter line of research appears to be particularly promising in terms of practical applications. Because most of this work is relatively

0163-7525/93/0510-0069$2.00

recent, there have been few successful applications to date, but we hope that this review stimulates an interest in the wider application of these methods.

Terminology and Notation

The terms "measurement error," "misclassification," and "errors in variables" refer to any discrepancy between the true value of a variable x and its measured value z, although misclassification is more often used with categorical variables, and measurement error with continuous variables. Most of the epidemiologic literature on this topic has been concerned with a binary disease outcome d or censored survival times (t,d), although many of the same principles apply to continuous outcomes. Except where it is necessary to distinguish a particular type of outcome, we denote the dependent variable as y.

Errors can be "systematic" or "random." Systematic errors are those for which the measured values might not be distributed randomly around the true value; for example, coding a variable so that all exposed persons were classified as unexposed and vice versa, or underestimating everyone's exposure level by a factor of two. The effects of such errors on exposure-response relationships are usually easy to predict. In the former case, the estimated odds ratio (OR) would be the inverse of the true OR; in the latter case, the slope of the exposure-response relationship would be double the true slope. Random errors pose a more difficult problem.

Systematic and random errors can be either "differential" or "nondifferential," depending upon whether the errors in that variable are related to y. If the misclassification of the outcome depends upon exposure status (e.g. because the pathologist confirming the diagnosis of mesothelioma was aware of the subjects' asbestos exposure histories) or the misclassification of the exposure depends upon the disease status (e.g. because of recall bias in a case-control study), then the errors are differential. Such errors can introduce serious and sometimes unpredicatable bias into a study. But, they can often be avoided by good study design, e.g. by blinded assessment of the study variables. However, even nondifferential random errors can bias associations, and this is the primary focus of this paper.

Loosely speaking, exposure errors are nondifferential if their distribution is independent of the outcome, i.e. $\Pr(z-x|y=1) = \Pr(z-x|y=0)$, but this is not a very rigorous definition. If a case and a noncase have the same value of z, the case will generally tend to have had a larger value of x because x, not z, is the true risk factor; thus, $\Pr(x|z,y=1) \neq \Pr(x|z,y=0)$. A more precise definition of nondifferential error is that $\Pr(z|x,y=1) = \Pr(z|x,y=0)$, e.g. no recall bias. This is formally equivalent to requiring that $\Pr(y|x,z) = \Pr(y|x)$, i.e. that the risk of disease depends only on the true exposure x, and given x, the measured exposure does not add any additional information.

In most studies, it is helpful to regard the measurement error problem as consisting of three conceptually distinct modeling tasks (6), which consist of the specification of the disease model—$\Pr(y|x)$; the measurement model—$\Pr(z|x)$; and the distribution of true exposure—$\Pr(x)$. For such probabilities as $\Pr(x)$ to have meaning, we have taken the "structural" view of the measurement error problem, in which the unknown x for each individual is regarded as a random variable having a distribution $\Pr(x)$ among the population of interest. Thus, the characterization of $\Pr(x)$, rather than the direct estimation of each x, is dealt with in the course of analysis. This contrasts with the "functional" approach to measurement errors, in which each subject's value of x is treated as a fixed but unknown parameter to be estimated jointly with the parameters in the disease model. The structural approach is generally more amenable to analysis than the functional, because it yields a large reduction in the number of nuisance parameters to be estimated: Instead of estimating each individual's x, only a few parameters in a prespecified form of $\Pr(x)$ are needed. Of course, uncertainties about the proper form of $\Pr(x)$ are rarely, if ever, fully resolvable.

Overview of the Effects of Measurement Error

In the next sections, we discuss the following effects of measurement error in a variety of settings and describe some currently available methods for correcting for these effects in epidemiological studies:

1. Changes in the observed mean structure, $E(y|z)$ compared with $E(y|x)$. This generally means that there is an attenuation of the observed compared with the true exposure-response relationship.
2. Changes in the observed variance structure, $V(y|z)$ from that of $V(y|x)$. In general, y is more variable ("overdispersed") given z than given x.
3. Distortion of associations and interactions between covariates and outcomes. For example, two outcomes that are independent given x may appear to be associated given z, and the main effect or interaction of a covariate w can be distorted by measurement error in x.

Classical and Berkson Error Models

When $E(y|x)$ is linear in x, a generally applicable approach to providing an unbiased assessment of the regression parameters is to replace the unknown xs in the disease model with their expectations $E(x|z)$. Thus, in many problems, the primary goal of the statistician is to learn enough about the measurement model $\Pr(z|x)$ and the true exposure distribution $\Pr(x)$ that this expectation can be calculated from

$$E(x \mid z) = \frac{\int x \Pr(z \mid x) \Pr(x)\, dx}{\int \Pr(z \mid x) \Pr(x)\, dx}.$$

In fact, the calculation of such expected values of "true given observed" can be said to form the basis of modern approaches to the measurement error problem, beginning with a classic paper by Cochran (7).

Some of the statistical literature distinguishes between measurement models in which $\Pr(z|x)$ can be specified and situations in which it may be more appropriate to specify $\Pr(x|z)$ (1). The classic idealization of the latter situation is in an experiment that uses a machine for delivering doses x, which are randomly distributed around the "dial-setting" z on the machine, the experimenter being free to vary the dial. Such an idealized experiment is often called a "Berkson error" model (3) if the machine has the property that $E(x|z) = z$. Then, if the disease model is also linear in x, no correction for errors in the measured variable is required. In observational epidemiology, exposure measurements sometimes also have this Berkson property, particularly when individuals are classified into groups and all members of group w are assigned a value z that is the mean of x within the group. An example might be an occupational study in which workers with the same job title w are assigned an exposure z based on the mean of area measurements; the true exposures x for individuals with the same job title would differ, but on average would tend to equal the area mean. In this type of study, linear regression of y on z would again lead to an unbiased estimate of the slope parameter if the true dose-response was linear in x.

On the other hand, in the "classical error" model, the observed value z is assumed to be distributed around the true value x with $E(z|x) = x$. As shown below, this model leads to the familiar bias toward the null. In general, the two relations $E(x|z) = z$ and $E(z|x) = x$ cannot both be satisfied except in the trivial situation when there is no measurement error. Although the unbiasedness of the Berkson model is appealing, the model has limited use for several reasons. First, this property applies only in linear disease models. Second, the other features of the measurement error problem—changes in $V(y|z)$, artifactual relationships between multiple outcomes given z, and the residual confounding of covariates given z—all occur for Berkson, as well as classical, measurement error. Finally, in any observational setting, $E(x|z)$ always depends upon the underlying exposure distribution $\Pr(x)$; for example, researchers studying different occupational populations with different distributions of true exposure, but using the same system of job categories, will make different assignments of z to the same job categories, because each will have to average over different underlying distributions of x.

Assessment of Measurement Error Distributions

To put any of these predictions to practical use, an investigator must have an estimate of the distribution of measurement errors. To the extent that subgroups differ in their error distributions, being able to quantify these differences is also helpful. Estimates of error distributions can come from several types of studies, including "validation" and "reproducibility" studies and "pathway uncertainty analysis." Hatch & Thomas (27) provide an extensive discussion of measurement error assessment methods, which we briefly summarize here.

In validation studies, one compares a "gold standard" measurement of x against the flawed measurement z to be used in the main study. This provides a direct estimate of the error distribution, but because the gold standard method is generally prohibitively expensive, it can only be done on a subsample. For example, personal monitors are the gold standard in an occupational study, whereas a room air sampler is the exposure method used. The results of validation studies of categorical exposure variables are easily summarized in terms of the misclassification probabilities $\Pr(z|x)$, which can be used directly in the methods of adjustment described below. For continuous variables, results can be summarized in terms of the variance of the deviations z-x or z/x, depending on the form of the distribution, possibly broken down by important study variables.

If a gold standard is unavailable or infeasible, one can still often obtain indirect information on error distributions by means of a reproducibility study, in which two or more separate assessments of z are performed on the same individuals, e.g. two or more diet assessments at different times. For example, if z_1 and z_2 are independent given x, $z_n \sim N(x,\omega^2)$ and $x \sim N(\mu, \sigma^2)$, then σ^2 can be estimated by $\mathrm{Cov}(z_1,z_2)$ and ω^2 by $V(z) - \hat{\sigma}^2$. For categorical variables, let $\boldsymbol{m}$ be the matrix of misclassification probabilities, $m_{ij} = \Pr(z = j|x = i)$, $\boldsymbol{p}$ be a diagonal matrix of population exposure probabilities [$p_{ii} = \Pr(x = i)$, 0 elsewhere], and $\boldsymbol{Z}$ be the observed matrix of reproducibility data, $Z_{jk} = \Pr(z_1 = j, z_2 = k)$. Again, if z_1 and z_2 are independent given x, then $\boldsymbol{Z} = \boldsymbol{m}^T\boldsymbol{pm}$ and $\boldsymbol{m}$ and $\boldsymbol{p}$ can be estimated as the solution to this matrix equation. Key to both results is the conditional independence assumption. If z_1 and z_2 represent responses to the same question on surveys conducted on consecutive days, then a subject's response on the second day is likely to be influenced by his recollection of the previous day's response, in addition to his true value of x. Because the observed correlation between z_1 and z_2 is thus a combination of the correlation induced by the common $\Pr(z|x)$ and the partial correlation in $\Pr(z_1,z_2|x)$, at most one can say that this provides a means to estimate a lower bound on the misclassification probabilities.

In some studies, exposure estimates are derived by using pathway analysis in which the doses are computed over multiple pathways, each of which may consist of several steps, and each step is subject to various uncertainties. The final dose assignment is then the expectation of this sum over the joint distribution of all the component uncertainties, and a variance of the dose assignment can be similarly computed as the variance over all the component uncertainties. For example, in the studies of cancer in residents downwind of the Nevada Test Site (53), each subject's dose from various radionuclides was computed by summing contributions through external, inhalation, milk, and vegetable pathways from more than 100 detonations. The milk pathway, for example, involved consideration of the yield of each radionuclide from each test, radioactive decay rates, environmental transport and deposition, uptake by vegetation, farming practices, intake by cows and goats, transfer to milk, milk distribution patterns, the family's source of milk (dairy or backyard cow), the subject's (or mother's) consumption, breastfeeding rates and transfer through the mother's breast milk, and finally metabolic processes to the thyroid gland. Each step of this process was characterized by probability distributions, based on available data, expert judgment, the subject's own report, and reliability surveys. Because of the complexity of the dose assignment algorithm, analytic calculation of the expectation and variance of the dose was not feasible, so a Monte Carlo simulation was conducted, which generated 100 dose estimates for each subject by using randomly chosen values of the various parameters and then summarizing the distributions in terms of their means and variances. The unique feature of this approach is that it provides not only a dose estimate for each subject, but also a separate uncertainty estimate for each individual's dose. These individualized uncertainties could then be used to correct dose-response relationships for measurement errors in a way that essentially gives greater weight to the subjects with more precisely estimated doses, as described below.

EFFECTS OF EXPOSURE MEASUREMENT ERRORS

Effects on Mean Structures

CATEGORICAL EXPOSURE VARIABLES The effects of exposure errors are most easily seen for categorical exposure variables, and the early epidemiologic literature was mainly concerned with this situation. The essential points can be made in the case of binary exposure variables $x,z = 0, 1$ with nondifferential misclassification. Hence, following the model specification format outlined above, let

p: $p_i = \Pr(x = \mathrm{i})$, true prevalence of exposure
r: $r_i = \Pr(y = 1|x = i)$, risk of disease in true exposure group i
m: $m_{ij} = \Pr(z = j|x = i)$, misclassification probabilities

where $\Sigma_i p_i = 1$, and $\Sigma_j m_{ij} = 1$. Then the observed disease risks classified by z are

$$\begin{aligned} R_j &= \Pr(y = 1 \mid z = j) \\ &= \sum_i \Pr(y = 1 \mid x = i) \Pr(x = i \mid z = j) \\ &= \sum_i r_i M_{ji} \end{aligned}$$

where $M_{ji} = m_{ij}p_i/P_j$ and $P_j = \Pr(z = j) = \Sigma_i m_{ij} p_i$. Simple algebra shows that any measure of epidemiologic effect (e.g. RR, RD, OR) expressed in terms of the R_js will be biased toward the null compared with the corresponding measure expressed in terms of the r_is (8, 20). Intuitively, this arises because each of the measured exposure groups is contaminated by individuals from the other group. For analogous results in matched studies, see Greenland (22).

However, this argument applies only when individuals are classified in terms of their own exposures, z. In ecologic studies, groups are classified in terms of some other characteristic w, such as place of residence, and the observed disease rates $E(y|w)$ are regressed on the group mean exposures $E(x|w)$. It is easy to see that this regression yields unbiased estimates for linear disease models when exposure is not misclassified. It is also true, but less obvious, that regression on measured group means $E(z|w)$ will yield unbiased estimates under a classical error model. If $E(z|x) = x$ and the measurement error distribution is unaffected by w [i.e. $\Pr(z|x,w) = \Pr(z|x)$], then $E(z|x,w) = E(x|w)$. Consequently, if $E(y|x) = \alpha_0 + \alpha_1 x$, then $E(y|w) = \alpha_0 + \alpha_1 E(x|W) = \alpha_0 + \alpha_1 E(z|w)$. Thus, even though classical error produces a bias toward the null in individual studies, this does not necessarily happen in ecologic studies. In the Berkson error case, a similar argument shows that regression of $E(y|w)$ on $E(z|w)$ is also unbiased, provided one can assume that $E(x|z,w) = z$.

Brenner et al (4) pointed out that if the exposure variable is binary, then neither a classical nor a Berkson error structure can apply, because neither $E(z|x)$ nor $E(x|z)$ can equal 0 or 1, the possible values for individuals. Furthermore, it can be shown that the group means $E(z|w)$ will show less variability than $E(x|w)$. Because the group disease rates are not affected by how the group exposure means are characterized, the resulting slope estimate will be inflated if $E(z|w)$ is used on the x-axis instead of $E(x|w)$.

Returning to analytic studies, the situation is more complex with multilevel categorical exposure variables. Dosemeci et al (11) showed that if three or more groups follow a gradient in disease risk by true exposure, then after nondifferential misclassification, the ORs by measured exposure will not necessarily show a monotonic relationship. This happens because the OR comparing exposure groups 1 and 2, for example, may be corrupted by subjects from group 3; if group 1 is small compared with group 2, the influx of high-risk group 3 subjects will have a proportionally bigger effect on group 1 than on group 2, thus making it appear at higher risk than group 2. The authors further showed that tests of trend can be reversed. In a subsequent paper (55), they showed as a corollary that by collapsing a nondifferentially misclassified $2 \times K$ table, the resulting 2×2 table can show differential misclassification, with ORs biased away from or beyond the null.

CONTINUOUS EXPOSURE VARIABLES If $E(y|x)$ is linear in x, $E(y|x) = \alpha + \beta x$, then the observable exposure-response relationship $E(y|z)$ can be derived by taking expectations over x, so that $E(y|z) = \alpha + \beta E(x|z)$. Consider the special case in which both the population exposure and measurement error models are normal, $x \sim N(\mu, \sigma^2)$ and $z|x \sim N(x, \omega^2)$. Then, the expectation becomes

$$E(x \mid z) = \frac{z/\omega^2 + \mu/\sigma^2}{1/\omega^2 + 1/\sigma^2} = cz + (1 - c)\mu \qquad 1.$$

$$\text{where } c = \sigma^2/(\sigma^2 + \omega^2) < 1 \qquad 1a.$$

so that $E(x|z)$ is a weighted average of the measured exposure and the overall mean. Because this is a linear function of z, the observed exposure-response relationship will still be linear, but its slope will be biased toward the null:

$$E(y|z) = \alpha + \beta(1 - c)\mu + \beta cz = \alpha' + \beta' z \qquad 2.$$

where $\beta' = \beta c$. The intuitive explanation of this effect is that measurement error produces overdispersion of the exposure axis because $V(z) = V(x) + V(z|x)$. By stretching the exposure axis while leaving the disease axis unchanged, the slope of the relationship is reduced. However, this is true only in the special case of an additive model with normal errors, normal x, and a linear relationship for $E(y|x)$. More generally, the shape of the exposure-relationship will also be affected by measurement errors. For example, for linear-quadratic models, $E(y|x) = \alpha + \beta_1 x + \beta_2 x^2$, the mean structure for $y|z$ becomes $E(y|x) = \alpha + \beta_1 E(x|z) + \beta_2 E(x^2|z)$. Thus, the linear-quadratic form of relationship is preserved, but the variables in the regression become the conditional moments $E(x^i|z)$. Berkson error models illustrate the same properties with the slight simplification that $E(x|z) = z$ and $E(x^2|z) = z^2 + V(x|z)$.

Effects on Variance Structures

Consider a response variable y following a statistical model of the form

$$y = \alpha + \beta x + \text{error}. \qquad 3.$$

For a subject with estimated exposure z, Equation 3 can be reexpressed as

$$y = \alpha + \beta E(x|z) + \beta[x - E(x|z)] + \text{error} \qquad \text{3a.}$$
$$= \alpha + \beta E(x|z) + \text{error}^*$$
$$\text{where } V(\text{error}^*) = \beta^2 V(x|z) + V(\text{error}).$$

Thus, for example, if $y|x$ is a Poisson random variable with conditional mean $\mu' = E(y|x) = \alpha + \beta x$, then the conditional variance of $y|z$ is $V(y|z) = \mu' + \beta^2 V(x|z)$. Thus, $y|z$ takes the form of an overdispersed Poisson random variable with variance larger than a true Poisson for which $V(y) = E(y)$. Maximum likelihood techniques consist of iteratively reweighted least squares that use weights $w = 1/V(y|x)$. Thus, efficient estimation of the parameters of the disease model requires us to estimate $V(x|z)$ to compute these weights.

Note that, in the important case of binomial proportions, with mean p and denominator n, Equation 3a needs to be modified so that

$$V(\text{error}^*) = [n/(n-1)]\beta^2 V(x|z) + \text{V (error)}$$

where $\text{V(error)} = p(1-p)/n$. The modification is needed because, in this case, the binomial error in y is not independent of $x - E(x|z)$. The implication is most obvious for binary outcomes (i.e. $n = 1$) where measurement error changes the mean, but does not change the variance structure for y.

For disease models that are not linear in x, the calculation of $E(y|z)$ and $V(y|z)$ becomes more complicated, although it is clear that $y|z$ is generally more variable than $y|x$. In principle, $V(y|x)$ may be calculated from $V(y|z) = V[E(y|x)] + E[V(y|x)]$. For models in which $E(y|x)$ are polynomial functions of x, both the mean and variance of $y|z$ involve linear combinations of $E(x^i|z)$, and it is again computationally feasible to consider the estimation of the parameters in the mean function $E(y|x)$ as an application of iteratively reweighted least squares regression. More complex methods are required for the estimation of nonlinear disease models in the presence of exposure measurement error, as we describe below.

Induced Associations Between Outcomes, Residual Confounding, and Interactions Between Covariates

One topic of interest in the study of the atomic bomb survivors has been whether the presence of early effects of radiation sickness among the survivors, such as loss of hair, bleeding of the mouth and gums, nausea, and vomiting, is predictive of an inherent radiation sensitivity to both early and late effects of radiation exposure. For example, Neriishi et al (38) found that survivors who reported a history of epilation showed a significant twofold higher risk of leukemia than those without epilation at the same estimated dose, which suggests a radiosensitivity shared by early and late effects. If the true doses were observed for each subject, then this would be a simple inference to draw, but because only estimated doses are available, measurement error bias must be considered. Suppose two outcome variables, y_1 and y_2, each have a linear dose-response and are independent given true exposure. Then, the observed covariance between y_1 and y_2 given estimated dose z is $\mathrm{Cov}(y_1,y_2|z) = \beta_1\beta_2 V(x|z)$. The obvious result is that measurement error induces an artifactual association between response variables that would otherwise be seen to be independent if true exposure x was available.

In a similar way, the joint effects of two risk factors x and w can be distorted by measurement errors in either or both of them. Such distortion can arise either because of the association between x and w or because the degree of measurement error in one variable, say x, depends upon the other variable.

In the case of categorical exposures, Greenland (21) showed that misclassification of a confounder can lead to partial loss of control for that variable, e.g. if the crude OR is 4 and the OR adjusted for the true confounder is 2, then the OR adjusted for the measured confounder might be 3. Furthermore, he showed that misclassification of a modifier can mask or introduce spurious effect modification, e.g. if the true OR is 3 in both strata of the modifier, the misclassified data might show ORs of 2 and 4. Such apparent interactions can result from misclassification of either the exposure or the modifying variable. Fung & Howe (19) have examined similar issues in the case where both exposure and confounder were polytomous.

A similar phenomenon was reported for continuous variables by Dwyer et al (13) in a reanalysis of data on coronary heart disease from the Framingham study. By using multivariate adjustment techniques described below, they found that the effect of age (not misclassified) was biased away from the null in the uncorrected analyses as a result of underestimation of the effects of serum cholesterol and blood pressure, which were subject to measurement error. Appropriate adjustment in the multivariate case must allow for the correlation in errors between exposure variables.

Suppose instead that, in the study of the atomic bomb survivors, the precision of the radiation dose estimates depended upon age. Then the slope of the dose-response relationship would appear to be modified by age (spurious interaction), and the magnitude of the age effect might be distorted (residual confounding).

METHODS OF CORRECTING FOR MEASUREMENT ERRORS

In this section, we consider a variety of methods that have been suggested for adjusting exposure-response relationships for measurement error and their relationships. After briefly reviewing methods for categorical exposures, we contrast several basic approaches for the continuous case:

1. Correction of the parameter estimates from the naive regression of y on z for the anticipated degree of bias.
2. A two-stage approach in which $\hat{x}_i = E(x_i|z_i)$ (and similar quantities as needed) are computed first and then used in a simple regression of y on $\hat{x}_i$.
3. Structural equations approaches in which the marginal relationships $y|z$ can be fitted directly in certain restricted situations, such as where all variables are normal and linearly related.
4. Full likelihood treatment, integrating over the unknown xs.
5. Nonparametric specification of $\Pr(x)$ in approaches 2 and 4.
6. Use of additional information w to build a refined model for $\Pr(x|w)$.

Categorical Exposure Variables

Suppose we observe $\boldsymbol{R}$ where $R_{jk} = \Pr(y = k|z = j)$ and also have an independent estimate of the posterior classification probabilities $\boldsymbol{M}$, $M_{ji} = \Pr(x = i|z = j)$ defined earlier, and let $\boldsymbol{r}$ denote the true exposure-response probabilities $r_{ij} = \Pr(y = j|x = i)$. Them, the observed exposure-response relationship can be written in terms of the matrix equation $\boldsymbol{R} = \boldsymbol{Mr}$, and Greenland & Kleinbaum (26) have shown that $\boldsymbol{r}$ can be reconstructed simply as $\boldsymbol{r} = \boldsymbol{M}^{-1}\boldsymbol{R}$. Thus, the basic idea is to replace the counts in the observed tabulation of y by z by the expectations of the counts in the tabulation of y by x, and then compute ORs or other measures of effect on this table of expected counts. This parallels at a grouped level the approach described below for continuous variables, where $E(y|z)$ is computed for each individual in terms of quantities like $E(x|z)$. Greenland (24) further shows how valid interval estimates on effect measures can be derived by incorporating the uncertainties in the estimates of $\boldsymbol{M}$.

Now suppose instead that we have reproducibility data on all subjects, i.e. for each subject we have y, z_1, and z_2. A simple technique proposed by Marshall & Graham (35) is to limit the analysis to the subjects for whom $z_1 = z_2$ and treat that value as x. This only partially eliminates misclassification bias, and there can be a substantial loss of power because of the smaller sample size. Maximum likelihood methods (14, 28) could also be used to fit the observed three-dimensional table to a model involving the OR for the association between x and y, the true exposure prevalence p, and the misclassification probabilities $\boldsymbol{m}$, assuming that z_1 and z_2 are conditionally independent given x and subject to the same misclassification probabilities. A simple way to fit the same model is via the E-M algorithm (9), by using trial estimates of the model parameters to compute the expectations of the numbers of subjects in the four-way table with x as the fourth dimension, conditional on the observed three-way table, and then treating these as known to estimate the model parameters. By using either fitting method, variance estimates are obtained from the Fisher information.

Continuous Exposure Variables

CORRECTION OF ATTENUATED REGRESSION COEFFICIENTS The above discussion of the effects of measurement errors on mean structures suggests a simple method of correction. Suppose $E(y|x)$ is linear in x and both x and $z|x$ are normal. Then Equation 2 shows that $E(y|z)$ is also linear in z with expected slope coefficient given by $\beta' = \beta c$, where the attenuation factor c is given by Equation 1a. Thus, an obvious correction method is simply to estimate β' by regressing y on z and then estimate β as $\hat{\beta}'/c$. By the delta method, the variance of $\hat{\beta}$ is then $V(\hat{\beta}')/c^2 + (\hat{\beta}'/c^2)^2V(c)$.

If both the population exposure variance σ^2 and the measurement error variance ω^2 were known, c could be simply computed from Equation 1a, but in general c must be estimated from validation or reproducibility studies. For validation substudy data, Rosner et al (50) suggest simply regressing x on z, because Equation 1 shows that the coefficient of z in this regression is c. In expectation, this is equivalent to estimating $\hat{\sigma}^2 = V(x)$ and $\hat{\omega}^2 = V(z-x)$ from the substudy data and computing $\hat{c} = \hat{\sigma}^2/(\hat{\sigma}^2 + \hat{\omega}^2)$, although this approach appears to produce somewhat smaller variance in $\hat{\beta}$ than the regression-based approach. Neither approach uses the marginal variance of z in the main study or the relationship between y and z in the estimation of these variances. The structural equations and maximum likelihood approaches described below would therefore be expected to be more efficient. Note also that the delta-method variance estimate given above assumes that the validation study and main studies are independent. If the validation study is a subset of the main study, the variance estimate can be easily corrected to allow for this dependence, but the full structural equations or maximum likelihood treatment described below would make more efficient use of all the data.

The Rosner et al approach is easily generalized to the multivariate case (48). If $\mathbf{x} = (x_1, \ldots, x_p)$ is a vector of true exposures to be related to y and $\mathbf{z}$ is a corresponding vector of measured values, one then regresses $\mathbf{x}$ on $\mathbf{z}$ to obtain a matrix of coefficients $\boldsymbol{C}$ and then estimates $\hat{\beta} = \hat{\beta}'\boldsymbol{C}^{-1}$.

The regression approach depends upon having direct observations of x available on at least a substudy. If instead two independent and replicate measurements z_1 and z_2 were available on all subjects, one would estimate σ^2 from $\mathrm{Cov}(z_1,z_2)$ and ω^2 from $V(z) - \hat{\sigma}^2$, and then proceed as described above.

REPLACEMENT OF Z BY $E(X|Z)$ In linear/normal models, Rosner et al's approach is formally equivalent to regressing y on $\hat{x} = E(x|z) = \hat{c}_o + \hat{c}z$, where $\hat{c}$ is obtained from the regression of x on z in the substudy data. The beauty of this approach is that it is easily generalized to more complex models. For example, for polynomial disease models, one simply replaces x by $E(x|z)$, x^2 by $E(x^2|z)$, etc., where the various expectations can either be computed analytically from knowledge of the underlying distributions of x and $z|x$ or estimated empirically from regressions of x^n on z. In the multivariate case, the corresponding generalization of Equation 1 is

$$\hat{\mathbf{x}} = E(\mathbf{x}|\mathbf{z}) = (\mathbf{z}\Omega^{-1} + \mu\Sigma^{-1})(\Omega^{-1} + \Sigma^{-1})^{-1} \qquad 4.$$

where Ω is the covariance matrix of the measurement errors, and Σ is the covariance matrix of the population distribution of true exposures.

Of course, even for the simplest linear models, efficient estimation requires a weighted regression analysis, so that $V(y|z)$, which involves $E(x^2|z)$ as well as $E(x|z)$, is also needed to provide the regression weights. However, there are several special cases where the calculation of $E(x|z)$ is all that is needed to perform an efficient analysis: the standard additive error model where y, x, and z are jointly multivariate normal; a binary outcome y with a mean that is linear in x; and survival pairs (t,d) where the hazard rate model is linear in x (40, 43). For other types of models, the key step in the correction for measurement error is the calculation of $E(y|z)$ and $V(y|z)$. In general, this is complicated because the functional form of $E(y|z)$ and $V(y|z)$ is inherently nonlinear. For example, in an exponential model, one would need $\hat{e}_n = E[\exp(\beta x_n)|z_n]$, which is a function of the current estimate of β, as well as μ and σ^2.

STRUCTURAL EQUATIONS APPROACHES The approaches described above are somewhat ad hoc in that different pieces of information are used in separate estimations of the different parameters. Structural equations attempt to fit the model in a single stage, by estimating all the parameters simultaneously using all relevant information. The basic idea is to compute the "marginal model" that describes the joint distribution of all the observable variables as a function of the model parameters, after integrating over the unknown xs. This is generally possible only for certain restricted classes of models, the most important of which is where all variables are normally distributed and linearly related to each other.

To illustrate the approach, consider again the situation in which two measurements z_1 and z_2, together with y, are available on all subjects. Suppose the conditional relationships were given by the general set of equations

$$y = \alpha + \beta x + \epsilon \qquad 5.$$

$$z_j = \gamma_j + \lambda_j x + \eta_j \qquad \text{for } j = 1,2. \qquad 6.$$

The classical error model $E(z|x) = x$ discussed above is a special case of this model where $\gamma_j = 0$, $\lambda_j = 1, E(\eta_j) = 0$, $\text{Cov}(x, \eta_j) = 0$, and $\text{Cov}(x, \epsilon) = 0$. Obviously, some constraints would be needed to identify the parameters in the general model 5 and 6 uniquely. One such set of assumptions is that all covariances involving the measurement errors η_j are zero, and that $\lambda_1 = \lambda_2 = 1$. By including y in the model, one can show that the assumption $\lambda_2 = 1$ can be relaxed. Assumptions can be further relaxed in the case where more than two measurements z or more than one x are available, thus allowing estimation of covariances among measurement errors (12).

With these constraints, the corresponding marginal model would then be given by

$$\begin{aligned} V(z_j) &= \lambda_j^2 V(x) + V(\eta) \\ \mathrm{Cov}(z_1,z_2) &= \lambda_1\lambda_2 V(x) \\ V(y) &= \beta^2 V(x) + V(\epsilon) \\ \mathrm{Cov}(y,z_j) &= \beta\lambda_j V(x). \end{aligned}$$

The model is then fitted by finding the values of the parameters for which the predicted covariance matrix Σ of the observed data are closest to their observed values $\boldsymbol{S}$. This is generally done by maximizing the multivariate normal likelihood.

$$L = \ln[\det(\hat{\Sigma})] - \ln[\det(\boldsymbol{S})] + tr(\boldsymbol{S}\hat{\Sigma}^{-1}) - p. \qquad 7.$$

When different subsets of variables are observed in different samples, it is desirable to estimate separately those parameters that are identifiable in each sample. The covariance matrices from each sample can then be pooled in the ML estimation, thus constraining parameters to be equal across the multiple samples. For example, if x and z are measured in a validation sample and y and z in the main sample, all the covariance information from both the validation and main samples can be used for estimation. Fitting these multiple population models can be accomplished with available software in the continuous (31) and categorical (36) cases.

FULL LIKELIHOOD APPROACHES More generally, estimation approaches may be based on maximizing a likelihood obtained by integrating out the unknown xs,

$$L(\beta) = \prod_{n=1}^{N} \int L(y_n|x_n;\ \beta)\ \Pr(z_n|x_n)\ \Pr(x_n)\ dx_n \qquad 8.$$

where $L(y|x)$ is the usual likelihood contribution if the xs were known. This expression is maximized by setting the score statistic, $S_z(\beta) = \partial \ln L/\partial\beta$ to zero and solving for β. The score statistic generally has the form $S_z(\beta) = E_{x|y,z}S_x(\beta)$ where $S_x(\beta)$ is the score statistic for β if x were available. A similar expression for the observed information $I_z(\beta)$ is provided by Louis (34). In principle, the likelihood and score statistic can be extended to include data from validation studies, so that parameters in the measurement error model and the distribution of true exposure can be simultaneously estimated together with β.

SPECIFICATION OF THE DISTRIBUTION OF TRUE EXPOSURE The most difficult part of the specification of a measurement error model is the distribution of true exposures in the population. Because x is not observed, it is difficult to know which form to choose for $\Pr(x)$. A practical approach is to inspect the distribution of z and choose a parametric form that appears appropriate. Once a measurement model $\Pr(z|x)$ is fixed, it is quite possible to consider maximum likelihood estimation of parameters in a model for $\Pr(x)$ on the basis of the z data alone. Alternatively, the estimation of parameters in the distribution of x may be done simultaneously with that of β from the likelihood (8). The calculation of $E(x^n|z)$ can be done by numerical integration once models for both $\Pr(x)$ and $\Pr(z|x)$ are selected.

An alternative to estimating the parameters in a fixed distributional form for $\Pr(x)$ is a nonparametric approach that uses density estimation methods. One assumes that the distribution of x is concentrated at a finite number M of support points with corresponding masses, where $M < N$, the number of subjects. Methods for finding the maximum likelihood value of M and the positions and masses of the support points have been provided (5, 10, 32, 39, 54).

Although the nonparameteric approaches to estimating $\Pr(x)$ are potentially of great interest, it is not known whether they lead to consistent estimates of β, because M generally increases with N, thereby apparently violating the basic asymptotic conditions for the validity of maximum likelihood. The functional approach, where β is estimated by maximizing the likelihood with respect to each x rather than integrating over a prior distribution, gives inconsistent estimates in many measurement error problems (18). The obvious solution is to fix the number of potential support points to be substantially smaller than N. Simulation studies (54) have shown that the bias then declines with increasing N, holding M fixed.

This approach was used in the analysis of dose-response relations in the Utah fallout studies (54). In a case-control study of leukemia, doses were assigned based on residential histories abstracted from Mormon church records, because it was not possible to contact the individuals for more detailed exposure information. The calculated uncertainties on the dose estimates allowed only for variation in deposition rates and incompleteness in some individuals' residence histories. The mean uncertainty was a geometric standard deviation (GSD) of about 1.5 with relatively little variation between individuals. Correction for these errors increased the slope estimate by 12%, but also increased the standard error by 53%, slightly decreasing the significance of the dose-response relation. In the thyroid cohort study, a much more complex dose assignment algorithm was used, and the uncertainty analysis was more comprehensive. The mean uncertainty was a GSD of about 2.7 and varied more between individuals. Correction for these errors increased the slope estimate for thyroid neoplasms about 3-fold and the standard error about 4.6-fold.

MODELING EXPOSURE So far, we have considered the situation in which the information available on x is one or more flawed measurements z. Another important class of information relates to determinants of true exposure, w, which we wish to consider in the exposure model $\Pr(x|\mathrm{w})$. A recent example comes from a study of childhood leukemia and residential electromagnetic fields (EMF) (33). Here, x is some summary of long-term EMF exposure, z is a short-term measurement of EMF, and w represents various characteristics of the electrical wiring in the neighborhood that is the main source of the magnetic fields. A reasonable modeling strategy is to use the marginal model for $z|\mathrm{w}$ to estimate the parameters in $E(x|\mathrm{w})$, and then use these expected values in fitting the disease model. For example, Jiang (30) assumed $x_n \sim N(\mathrm{w}_n^T\gamma,\sigma^2)$ and $z_n \sim N(x_n,\omega_n^2)$ (where x and z are now on a logarithmic scale) and fitted the regression model $z_n \sim N(\mathrm{w}^T\gamma,\sigma^2 + \omega_n^2)$. For exposure-response modeling, the expectation of the true dose is then simply $E(x_n|\mathrm{w}_n) = \mathrm{w}_n^T\hat{\gamma}$. In this approach, the measurements z are used only to develop a prediction model and not to fit the disease model. This is clearly not fully efficient, but one could use $E(x|z,\mathrm{w})$ instead. Thus, in the EMF example,

$$E(x_n \mid \mathrm{w}_n, z_n) = \frac{z_n/\omega_n^2 + \mathrm{w}_u^T\hat{\gamma}/(V_n - \omega_n^2)}{1/\omega_n^2 + 1/(V_n - \omega_n^2)} \qquad 9.$$

where $V_n = V(\mathrm{w}_n^T\hat{\gamma})$, which is the obvious weighted average of the predictions and the measurements.

In Jiang's analysis, a considerably better prediction of z was obtained in the regression on w than for the Wertheimer-Leeper (WL) wiring code that had previously been associated with leukemia risk. However, neither $E(x|\mathrm{w})$ nor $E(x|z,\mathrm{w})$ were associated with leukemia, which suggests that measurement error alone could not explain the lack of association between leukemia and measured EMF. Alternative explanations for the WL-leukemia association, including selection bias or causal effects of some other aspect of EMF than mean intensity, are being explored.

This process is essentially what is done in most occupational mortality studies in which w represents job titles and z area measurements. The means of z by w are computed to develop a "job-exposure matrix," which is then used to compute predicted exposure histories $\hat{x}_n(t)$ for each of the study subjects from their job histories $w_n(t)$. These predicted exposure histories are then treated as the true exposure histories in standard epidemiologic analyses. This process provides an unbiased estimate of the true exposure-response relationship if the assumptions of a linear disease model and a Berkson error structure are true.

In a study of the health effects of air pollution that is currently under way at the University of Southern California (USC) (37), we are using similar approaches to combine area monitoring data on community pollution levels with personal activity data on all subjects and with personal dosimetry and microenvironmental sampling on a subset of subjects. The personal dosimetry, microenvironmental sampling, and activity data are used to develop a model for deviations between the area mean and personal exposures, which can then be applied to all subjects. The analysis of exposure-response relationships involves a combination of individual and ecologic regression analyses, as described below.

Examples

ATOMIC BOMB SURVIVORS An illustration of the techniques under discussion here is provided by recent work on the dosimetry error problem in the cohort study of the Japanese atomic bomb survivors (41). The DS86 dosimetry system (47), which produces dose estimates for approximately 100,000 survivors in Hiroshima and Nagasaki, takes as its input each survivor's location and shielding factors, such as the type of structure they were in and their orientation at the time of the bombing. These input data essentially define a "mathematical box," which contains the survivor, and the distribution of radiation within this box is analyzed on the basis of physical principles. The dose estimates that are assigned are the averages of dose $E(x|\text{input data})$ within each box. Because the primary interest in the analysis of cancer risk is on survival models that are linear or linear-quadratic in x, measurement error correction for these models is based on the calculation of $E(x|z)$ and $E(x^2|z)$ for use in the survival analysis.

To approximate $E(x|z)$ in the cohort, Pierce et al (41) assumed a Weibull distribution of true dose $\Pr(x)$ and a lognormal measurement error model $\Pr(z|x)$ with logarithmic standard deviation σ. They based their choice of true dose distribution principally upon the shape of the distribution of observed dose $\Pr(z)$ for the survivors, which is well described by a Weilbull shape. The two parameters of the Weibull for $\Pr(x)$ were estimated by a simple deconvolution using the z data, based on a specific choice of σ in the measurement error model. The resulting Weibull density for x has a shape that drops off very quickly with increasing dose, which is in conformity both with the geometry of the radiation fields produced by the blasts and with the heavy mortality near the hypocenters. The multiplicative nature of the lognormal error model assumes that errors in doses increase in absolute magnitude with x. Pierce et al investigated the effects of measurement error on estimated cancer risk for a range of values of σ from 0.3 to 0.4, corresponding to a coefficient of variation of $\sqrt{V(z|x)/x}$ of roughly 30–40% of x. In their preferred 35% error model, adjustment for random dosimetry error increased estimates of dose-response slopes for cancer by approximately 7–13%.

Three sources of information underlie this specific choice of measurement error variance. The first is the error analysis provided as a part of the dosimetry system itself, which can be regarded as an estimate of the variance of the dose caused by uncertainties in the physical model; in general, this component of variability is less than the 35% error model specifies. A second component is inaccuracies in the input data, which were only collected by interview five to ten years after the bombing. Estimates of these errors come from analyses of subsets of survivors who were interviewed more than once concerning their location at the time of the bombings (29). The third source of information concerning the variability of estimated dose comes from the analysis of biological outcome data itself. Data on radiation-induced stable chromosome aberrations have been collected on more than 1000 survivors. Typically, 100 cells per survivor are examined, and the fraction of cells showing stable chromosome aberrations is counted. As noted above, the effect of measurement error will be to introduce over-dispersion in such binomial outcomes. The amount of dispersion observed in the chromosome data was used by Sposto et al (52) to provide an estimate of the variance of estimated dose and an analysis of induced association between reports of early effects of radiation, specifically severe epilation, and stable chromosome aberrations. They noted a significant twofold difference in the apparent dose-response for the induction of chromosome aberrations between those survivors who reported severe epilation and those who did not. As noted above, such correlation between multiple endpoints can be produced by dosimetry error alone, even if the actual dose-response for the two groups does not differ. Sposto et al provided a second estimate of the dosimetry measurement error variance, based on the assumption that the observed difference in dose response is caused by measurement error alone. It appeared that at least a 40% lognormal error model would be required to explain both the observed dispersion in the chromosome aberration data and the difference in slope between groups, if there were in fact no heterogeneity in radiosensitivity.

DIET Armstrong et al (2) discussed adjustment for measurement errors in multiple exposure variables by using Equation 4 and illustrated their approach on a study of colon cancer in relation to calories, protein, and fat. Estimates of Ω and Σ came from a multivariate analysis of variance of data from a validation substudy (17). In their analysis, multivariate adjustment for measurement errors had a substantially larger effect on the estimated coefficients than did adjustment for each effect separately in a univariate model. Their analysis also allowed for the possibility that controls might differ by a mean vector δ because of recall bias, which could also be estimated from a validation substudy of cases and controls. In the univariate analyses, adjustment for recall bias reduced the coefficients for all exposure variables; in the multivariate analyses, however, this adjustment increased the coefficient for fat and calories slightly, mainly as a result of the much larger effect on the negative coefficient for protein.

We illustrate the structural equations approach by using data from the Honolulu Heart Program (HHP). An average of seven food records are available for a subsample of 329 men from the larger HHP cohort. A single 24-hour dietary recall is available on all men. The current analysis uses only the data from the 329 men in the validation sample (D. Reed 1992, personal communication). A structural model of the form of Equations 5 and 6 for relating body mass index (BMI) to total caloric intake (Cal) and calories from fat (Fat) can be constructed as follows:

$$\text{BMI} = \alpha + \beta_1 x_1 + \beta_2 x_2 + \epsilon \qquad 10.$$
$$z_1 = \text{Fat}_{24\text{hr}} = \gamma_1 + \lambda_1 x_1 + \eta_1 \qquad 11.$$
$$z_2 = \text{Fat}_{7\text{day}} = \gamma_2 + \lambda_2 x_1 + \eta_2$$
$$z_3 = \text{Cal}_{24\text{hr}} = \gamma_3 + \lambda_3 x_2 + \eta_3$$
$$z_4 = \text{Cal}_{7\text{day}} = \gamma_4 + \lambda_4 x_2 + \eta_4.$$

With $\lambda_j = 1$ for all j and all covariances zero, the fit of the model was poor ($\chi^2 = 303$, $df = 5$), but when the $\text{Cov}(\eta_1, \eta_3)$ and $\text{Cov}(\eta_2, \eta_4)$ were also estimated, the fit was much improved ($\chi^2 = 2.9$, $df = 3$; $p > .05$). The resulting ML estimates were $\hat{\beta}_1 = 0.518$ ($SE = 0.171$) and $\hat{\beta}_2 = .121$ ($SE = 0.036$), where the units of the slopes are kg/1000 kcal. In contrast, regression of BMI on z_1 and z_3 gave $\hat{\beta}_1' = 0.267$ (0.074) and $\hat{\beta}_2' = -.0120$ (0.037), which suggests that a substantial attenuation of slopes occurs when using the 24-hour recall measures. The two-stage estimation procedure gave $\hat{\beta}_1 = 0.889$ and $\hat{\beta}_2 = -0.279$. The ML analysis also gave estimates of $V(x_k)$ and $V(\eta)$ from which the correlations between z and x can be computed. Over 75% of the variance in a single 24-hour recall of fat was estimated to be error, whereas for the average of seven daily records that error was reduced to about 50%.

PRACTICAL IMPLICATIONS

Design Issues

OPTIMAL SAMPLE SIZE ALLOCATION Freedman et al (15) have discussed the impact of measurement error on sample size needs for cohort studies. For example, if the correlation between x and z is 0.65, they found that the sample size would have to be six to eight times larger than if there were no measurement errors.

Traditionally, inference on exposure-response relationships has been based on the naive regression on measured exposures, supplemented with a qualitative discussion of measurement error issues based on separate validation or reproducibility studies. The modern approach advocated here would shift the primary emphasis to error-corrected exposure-response relationships. Because this relies on estimates of measurement error distributions, there is a corresponding shift in emphasis onto validation and reliability studies, even at the expense of resources available for the main study. This naturally raises the problem of optimizing the design of a single study that tries to accomplish both aims within a limited budget. Greenland (23) and Spiegelman & Gray (51) considered the problem of minimizing the variance of an adjusted slope estimate, subject to a constraint on the total cost, the former in the case of a binary exposure variable, the latter for a normally distributed exposure. Both concluded that the optimal design depends in a complex fashion on a number of parameters, but found plausible scenarios under which the most efficient design was a smaller "fully validated" study. Explicit formulae for determining the optimal design can be found in their respective papers. Simulation approaches are being applied in the USC air pollution study to decide upon the most efficient trade-off between area monitoring and personal dosimetry (37).

Rosner & Willett (49) considered the efficient design of studies aimed at estimating correlation coefficients corrected for measurement error estimates derived from reproducibility studies. This involves a similar trade-off between the number of subjects and the number of replicate measurements per subject. They concluded that to minimize the standard error of the corrected correlation, it was generally sufficient to have no more than five replicates per subject, and if the true correlation were large, two replicates would suffice.

ECOLOGIC VERSUS ANALYTIC STUDIES Analytic studies have traditionally been viewed as providing a firmer basis for causal inference than ecologic studies, largely because of concerns about the "ecologic fallacy." Recently, several authors (16, 25, 42, 44) have reexamined this conventional wisdom in the light of measurement error considerations. There are numerous examples in the epidemiologic literature of discrepancies between the inferences based on the two types of designs. In the area of diet and cancer, for example, Prentice & Sheppard (45) have contrasted the strong international correlations between cancer rates and fat consumption rates with the weak relations reported in most case-control and cohort studies. The former is potentially confounded by numerous risk factors that are either unrecognized or not easily measured at the aggregate level, but because a Berkson error structure applies may be less affected by measurement error. The analytic studies are more easily controlled for confounding, but are limited by the restricted range of diets within countries and racial groups and by the difficulties in measuring individual's usual diet. Similar issues have been discussed in the context of air pollution effects (37). Because air pollution levels are geographically determined, it is very difficult to assess exposure-response relations at an individual level, and most studies have relied on between-communities regressions of average health outcomes (e.g. symptom prevalence, mean lung function changes) on average pollution levels.

A multicenter analytic (cohort or case-control) study would appear to incorporate the best features of both designs. By including multiple centers, the problem of restricted variability in exposure can be overcome. By controlling confounders at an individual level, the major concern with the ecologic fallacy can be overcome, at least to the extent that the relevant confounders can be identified and measured. By measuring exposures at an individual level, one can often obtain a better estimate of the relevant population mean exposures for ecologic comparisons than would be possible by using routine data sources. Finally, by analyzing exposure-response relations at the ecologic level, one can overcome the attenuation bias from measurement error, provided a Berkson error structure holds.

To realize all these advantages of the hybrid design, an appropriate analysis must be done to combine the individual and ecologic comparisons. The general approach can be illustrated by using the Harvard Six Cities study of air pollution (56). Letting subscript m denote the centers and n the individuals, we might write the general model as

$$y_{nm} = \alpha + \beta\bar{x}_m + \gamma v_{mn} + \delta_m + \epsilon_{mn}$$

where $\bar{x}_m$ denotes the mean exposure in center m (from area monitoring), v_{mn} denotes the confounding variables assessed at the individual level, and δ_m and ϵ_{mn} are random error terms for unmeasured center and individual effects. To fit the model, a two-stage method was used. In the first stage, an individual-level regression was done, omitting the $\bar{x}_m$ but including a set of indicator variables for center to estimate the δ_m. In the second stage, these estimated center residuals $\hat{\delta}_m$ were then regressed on the $\bar{x}_m$, by using a weighted least-squares analysis that incorporated their estimated variances. This general approach could be extended to incorporate individual-level exposure data with corrections for measurement error. In particular, one might wish to test the hypothesis that the error-corrected regressions on the individual and area exposure data have the same slope. Such approaches are being developed for the USC air pollution study to incorporate the personal dosimetry and microenvironmental sampling data (37) and for the European collaborative study of diet and cancer (42).

Implications for Regulatory Policy

Although epidemiologists have recognized the impact of measurement error on exposure-response relationships, this has not usually carried over into regulatory policy. Government agencies routinely use upper confidence limits on slope coefficients to be health conservative, but the uncorrected slope estimate is always used. This may not, therefore, be conservative. Before concluding that most risk assessments that have ignored measurement errors are inadequate, however, two qualifications must be emphasized. First, many exposure-response relationships are derived from studies in which a Berkson error structure applies (e.g. occupational mortality studies using job-exposure matrices) and thus may not be seriously distorted by measurement error. Second, the attenuation bias applies to the estimation of relations with true exposure, but the agency may not be able to regulate the true exposure. At issue is whether one wishes to predict the change in risk that would result from a change in true exposure or from a change in measured exposure. Because the reliability of measurements change from one setting to another, and because most regulatory policies aim to control average exposure levels rather than individually measured exposures, standards should in most instances be based on error-corrected exposure-response relationships. However, an exception might be when the standard is based on individual exposures that are subject to the same errors as in the epidemiologic data base.

RESEARCH NEEDS

Adjustment for measurement errors has become an active research area only recently. The techniques are still in their infancy and have seldom been applied in routine epidemiologic studies. Nevertheless, the area appears to be very promising, and hopefully the availability of these techniques will encourage epidemiologists to devote greater efforts to quantifying their measurement errors and correcting for them. A high priority for future research is the development of practical procedures and their incorporation into widely available statistical software (46).

On the theoretical level, techniques appear to be much better developed at the individual level than at the ecologic level. Given the considerations discussed above that favor greater use of ecologic studies and exposure models, the development of the approaches for combining individual and aggregate level analyses and incorporating instrumental variables should be a priority. A particularly challenging problem in this context is the case of correlated errors between individuals within the same group.

Finally, only a few papers have addressed the important design issues of optimizing the various trade-offs, such as between validation and main study sample sizes, between numbers of individuals and numbers of replicate measurements in reproducibility studies, and between numbers of individuals and numbers of centers in multicenter studies. Practical methods for sample size and power determination in studies where measurement error correction methods are planned would also be very helpful.

Literature Cited

1. Armstrong, B. G. 1990. The effects of measurement errors on relative risk regressions. *Am. J. Epidemiol.* 132:1176–84
2. Armstrong, D. B., Whittemore, A. S., Howe, G. R. 1989. Analysis of case-control data with covariate measurement error: application to diet and colon cancer. *Stat. Med.* 8:1151–66
3. Berkson, J. 1950. Are there two regressions? *J. Am. Stat. Assoc.* 45:164–180
4. Brenner, H., Savitz, D. A., Jockel, K.-H., Greenland, S. 1992. Effects of nondifferential exposure misclassification in ecologic studies. *Am. J. Epidemiol.* 135:85–95
5. Caroll, R. J., Wand, M. P. 1991. Semiparametric estimation in logistic measurement error models. *J. R. Stat. Soc. Ser. B* 53(3):573–85
6. Clayton, D. G. 1991. Models for the analysis cohort and case-control studies with inaccurately measured exposures. In *Statistical Models for Longitudinal Studies of Health,* ed. J. H. Dwyer, P. Lippert, M. Feinleib, H. Hoffmeister, pp. 301–31. Oxford: Oxford Univ. Press
7. Cochran, W. C. 1968. Errors of measurement in statistics. *Technometrics* 10:637–66
8. Copeland, K. T., Checkoway, H., McMichael, A. J., Holbrook, R. H. 1977. Bias due to misclassification in the estimation of relative risk. *Am. J. Epidemiol.* 105:488–95
9. Dempster, A. P., Laird, N, M., Rubin, D. B. 1977. Maximum likelihood from incomplete data via the EM algorithm. *J. R. Stat. Soc. Ser. B* 39:1–38
10. DerSimonian, R. 1986. Algorithm 221: maximum likelihood estimation of a mixing distribution. *Appl. Stat.* 35:302–9
11. Dosemici, M., Wacholder, S., Lubin, J. H. 1990. Does nondifferential misclassification always bias a true effect toward the mill value. *Am. J. Epidemiol.* 132:746–48
12. Dwyer, J. H. 1983. *Statistical Models.* New York: Oxford Univ. Press
13. Dwyer, J. H., Li, L., Curtin, R., Feinleib, M. 1992. Correction for nonsampling measurement error in risk factors for CHD in women from Framingham. *Circulation* 85:879
14. Elton, R. A., Duffy, S. W. 1983. Correcting for the effect of misclassification bias in a case-control study using data from two different questionnaires. *Biometrics* 39:659–65
15. Freedman, L. S., Schatzkin, A., Wax, Y. 1990. The impact of dietary measurement error on planning sample size required in a cohort study. *Am. J. Epidemiol.* 118:1185–95
16. Freudenheim, J. L., Marshall, J. R. 1988. The problem of profound mismeasurement and the power of epidemiological studies of diet and cancer. *Nutr. Cancer* 11:243–50
17. Friedenreich, C. M., Howe, G. R., Miller, A. B. 1991. An investigation of recall bias in the reporting of past food intake among breast cancer cases and controls. *Ann. Epidemiol.* 1:439–53
18. Fuller, W. A. 1987. *Measurement Error Models.* New York: Wiley
19. Fung, K. Y., Howe, G. R. 1984. Methodological issues in case-control studies III: the effect of joint misclassification of risk factors and confounding factors upon estimation and power. *Int. J. Epidemiol.* 13:366–70
20. Gladen, B., Rogan, W. J. 1979. Misclassification and the design of environmental studies. *Am. J. Epidemiol.* 110:607–16
21. Greenland, S. 1980. The effect of misclassification in the presence of covariates. *Am. J. Epidemiol.* 112:564–69

22. Greenland, S. 1982. The effect of misclassification in matched-pair case-control studies. *Am. J. Epidemiol.* 116: 402–6
23. Greenland, S. 1988. Statistical uncertainly due to misclassification: implications for validation substudies. *J. Clin. Epidemiol.* 41:1167–74
24. Greenland, S. 1988. Variance estimation for epidemiologic effect estimates under misclassification. *Stat. Med.* 7:745–57
25. Greenland, S. 1992. Divergent biases in ecological and individual-level studies. *Stat. Med.* 11:1209–23
26. Greenland, S., Kleinbaum, D. G. 1983. Correcting for misclassification in two-way tables and matched-pair studies. *Int. J. Epidemiol.* 12:93–97
27. Hatch, M., Thomas, D. C. 1992. Measurement of exposure, dose, covariates and outcome in environmental epidemiology. *Environ. Health Perspect.* In press
28. Hui, S. S. L., Walter, S. D. 1980. Estimating the error rates of diagnostic tests. *Biometrics* 36:167–71
29. Jablon, S. 1971. *Atomic Bomb Radiation Dose Estimates at ABCC (TR 23–71).* Hiroshima: At Bomb Casualty Comm.
30. Jiang, F. 1992. *Prediction of Magnetic Fields from Wiring Configurations in a Case-Control Study of Childhood Leukemia.* Los Angeles: USC Dept. of Prev. Med.
31. Joreskog, K. G., Sorbom, D. 1988. *LISREL 7: A Guide to the Program and Applications.* Chicago: SPSS
32. Laird, N. 1978. Nonparametric maximum likelihood estimation of a mixing distribution. *J. Am. Stat. Assoc.* 73:805–11
33. London, S. J., Thomas, D. C., Bowman, J. D., Sobel, E., Cheng, J.-C., Peters, J. M. 1991. Exposure to residential electric and magnetic fields and risk of childhood leukemia. *Am. J. Epidemiol.* 134:923–37
34. Louis, T. A. 1982. Finding the observed information matrix when using the EM algorithm. *J. R. Stat. Soc. Ser. B* 44: 226–33
35. Marshall, J. R., Graham, S. 1984. Use of dual responses to increase validity of case-control studies. *J. Chron. Dis.* 37: 125–36
36. Muthen, B. 1987. *LISCOMP: Analysis of Linear Structural Equations with a Comprehensive Measurement Model.* Mooresville, Ind: Scientific Software
37. Navidi, W. C., Stram, D. O., Thomas, D. C. 1992. *Statistical Methods for Epidemiologic Studies of the Health Effects of Air Pollution (TR 36).* Los Angeles: USC Dep. of Prev. Med.
38. Neriishi, K., Stram, D. O., Vaeth, M., Mizuno, S., Akiba, S. 1991. The observed relationship between the occurrence of acute radiation sickness and subsequent leukemia mortality in the Hiroshima-Nagasaki data. *Radiat. Res.* 125:206–13
39. Pepe, M. S., Fleming, T. 1991. A nonparametric method for dealing with mismeasured covariate data. *J. Am. Stat. Assoc.* 86:108–13
40. Pepe, M. S., Self, S. G., Prentice, R. L. 1989. Further results on covariate measurement errors in cohort studies with time to response data. *Stat. Med.* 8:1167–78
41. Pierce, D. A., Stram, D. O., Vaeth, M. 1990. Allowing for random errors in radiation exposure estimates for the atomic bomb survivor data. *Radiat. Res.* 123:275–84
42. Plummer, M., Clayton, D. 1991. *Assessing measurement errors of dietary survey methods in nutritional epidemiology.* Presented at Stat. and Epidemiol. Aspects of Cancer Res., Nuffeld College, Oxford
43. Prentice, R. L. 1982. Covariate measurement errors and parameter estimation in a failure time regression model. *Biometrika* 69:331–42
44. Prentice, R. L., Sheppard, L. 1990. Dietary fat and cancer: consistency of the epidemiologic data, and disease prevention that may follow from a practical reduction in fat consumption. *Cancer Causes Control* 1:81–97
45. Prentice, R. L., Sheppard, L. 1991. Dietary fat and cancer: rejoinder and discussion of research strategies. *Cancer Causes Control* 2:53–58
46. Prentice, R. L., Thomas, D. C. 1992. Methodologic research needs in environmental epidemiology: data analysis. *Environ. Health Perspect.* In press
47. Roesch, W. C. 1978. *Final Report of US-Japan Joint Reassessment of Radiation Dose Estimates for the Atomic Bomb Survivor Data.* Hiroshima: Radiat. Effects Res. Found.
48. Rosner, B., Spiegelman, D., Willett, W. C. 1990. Correction of logistic regression relative risk estimates and confidence intervals for measurement error: the case of multiple covariates measured with error. *Am. J. Epidemiol.* 132:734–45
49. Rosner, B., Willett, W. C. 1988. Interval estimates for correlation coefficients corrected for within-person variation: implications for study design and hypothesis testing. *Am. J. Epidemiol.* 127:377–86

50. Rosner, B., Willett, W. S., Spiegelman, D. 1989. Correction of logistic regression relative risk estimates and confidence intervals for systematic within-person measurement error. *Stat. Med.* 8:1031–40
51. Spiegelman, D., Gray, R. 1991. Cost efficient study designs for binary response data with Gaussian covariate measurement error. *Biometrics* 47:851–69
52. Sposto, R., Stram, D. O., Awa, A. A. 1991. An estimate of the magnitude of random errors in the DS86 dosimetry from data on chromosome aberrations and severe epilation. *Radiat. Res.* 128: 157–69
53. Stevens, W., Thomas, D. C., Lyon, J. L., et al. 1990. Leukemia in Utah and radioactive fallout from the Nevada Test Site: a case-control study. *N. Engl. J. Med.* 264:585–91
54. Thomas, D. C., Gauderman, J., Kerber, R. 1993. A nonparametric Monte Carlo approach to adjustment for covariate measurement errors in regression. *Biometrics.* In press
55. Wacholder, S., Dosemeci, M., Lubin, J. H. 1991. Blind assignment of exposure does not always prevent differential misclassification. *Am. J. Epidemiol.* 134:433–37
56. Ware, J. H., Ferris, B. G., Dockery, D. W., Spengler, J. D., Strom, D. O., Speizer, F. E. 1986. Effects of ambient sulfur oxides and suspended particles on respiratory health of preadolescent children. *Am. Rev. Respir. Dis.* 133:834–42

Annu. Rev. Publ. Health 1993. 14:95–114

WHY IS LOW BLOOD CHOLESTEROL ASSOCIATED WITH RISK OF NONATHEROSCLEROTIC DISEASE DEATH?

David R. Jacobs, Jr.
Division of Epidemiology, School of Public Health, University of Minnesota, Minneapolis, Minnesota 55454

KEY WORDS: coronary heart disease, cancer

INTRODUCTION

There is strong and congruent evidence that serum cholesterol and its lipoprotein components play a critical role in the development of coronary heart disease (CHD) through a causal role in atherogenesis. Recent evidence shows that reduction of serum total cholesterol (TC), particularly the low-density lipoprotein (LDL) cholesterol fraction, reduces the incidence of CHD (1–14), by arresting or reversing the progression of atherosclerois (15–17). Methodologically and historically, two studies were weighted particularly heavily in development of US TC-lowering policies. The Lipid Research Clinics Coronary Primary Prevention Trial found a 19% reduction in CHD incidence, by reducing TC with a combination of diet plus cholestyramine, compared with TC lowering with diet alone (5). The Helsinki study of TC lowering, which used gemfibrizol compared with placebo, found a 34% reduction in CHD incidence (6). For many years, however, there has been some evidence that total mortality is elevated at low TC levels (18–21) and that all-cause mortality risk may be increased by cholesterol lowering (1–7).

This article reviews evidence concerning these relations and discusses whether the observations can be attributed to confounding or are causal.

0163-7525/93/0510-0095$02.00

Research into low TC level and disease risk should seek to understand the observed relations of low blood cholesterol with a variety of nonatherosclerotic diseases, not just cancers. The epidemiology of blood cholesterol needs to be extended to epidemiologic studies of level and function of cholesterol elsewhere in the body. The connection of laboratory and clinical studies of the cell biology of cholesterol to specific pathogenesis is often weak.

FINDINGS LEADING TO A 1990 CONFERENCE

The National Heart Lung and Blood Institute (NHLBI) sponsored the *Conference on Low Cholesterol: Disease Associations,* held in Bethesda in October 1990 (18). Before this conference, there had been three major examinations of the U-shaped risk curve of TC with total mortality (19–22); the results were synthesized from many cohort studies of TC and cardiovascular disease. Researchers had few biologic hypotheses relating low TC to any disease, as persons with low TC levels appear generally healthy (23) and were known to suffer little from atherosclerotic diseases, a major scourge of affluent society. They reasoned that any biological relations of TC to disease would be as specific as the known relation of TC to atherosclerosis. The most likely set of diseases related to low TC levels was considered to be cancer, a notion bolstered by biologically based ideas concerning colon cancer risk and TC. Cancers are the second leading cause of death in the United States, after CHD. Given that heart disease risk is positively related to TC level, and that total mortality risk is flat or inversely related to TC, it seemed logical that cancer would be inversely related to TC.

A 1981 NHLBI conference on cholesterol and cancer found inconsistent evidence that low TC is associated with increased cancer mortality (19, 20). The report stated: "While there is inconsistent but concerning evidence of a possible increase in cancer risk at very low cholesterol levels (below 180 mg/dl) in men, the magnitude of this risk is generally modest when present. Physicians can feel confident in advising reduction of blood cholesterol levels for all persons with higher than average levels" (19). The conference concluded that the findings represented a scientific, but not a public health, challenge and that the data did not preclude, countermand, or contradict the current public health message for those with elevated TC levels to reduce them through diets lower in saturated fat and cholesterol.

The International Collaborative Group study on TC and cancer (21) pooled cancer mortality data in 61,567 men from ten Western studies and ten years of follow-up, plus a Japanese study with five years of follow-up. Blood TC levels were about 30 mg/dl lower in men dying within one year of baseline of lung, colon, or any other cancers than in survivors. In subsequent follow-up years (except years 6 and 9), blood cholesterol levels were slightly lower in cancer decedents than in survivors. Compared with survivors, a consistently lower TC was seen in lung cancer, but not in colon cancer, decedents in follow-up years 2 through 10. Based on the reduction in mean cholesterol difference between decedents and survivors in years 2 through 10 of follow-up, compared with the first year of follow-up, and the smallness of this difference in years 2–10, the authors concluded that the overall and site-specific findings on cancer death were consistent with the hypothesis that an inverse association between TC and cancer was a reflection of the effect of disease on TC level, and did not substantiate a hypothesis that low TC increases risk of cancer.

Law & Thompson (22) extended the analyses of the International Collaborative Group to a synthesis of cancer case-noncase differences in TC in 22 mortality and 11 incidence studies. They studied cancer at all sites combined, as well as lung, colon, and hematopoietic cancers. Their results closely resembled those of the International Collaborative Group (21): considerably lower TC levels in fatal cases that occurred within five years of blood measurements, or in incident cases within two years of blood measurements, than in survivors. Much smaller, but still statistically significant, differences, on the order of 1–2 mg/dl, were seen in cases occurring later. Law & Thompson interpreted these case-noncase differences for all cancers as corresponding to about a 15% greater incidence in the lowest TC quintile. No evidence of a TC difference was found for late cases of colon cancer, but differences were reported in late cases of lung and hematopoietic cancers. The authors noted that the absolute risk for cancer at low TC, even if causal, is small. They speculated on possible confounding caused by socioeconomic status, smoking, and utilization of cholesterol by growing tumors (22).

The most recent synthesis of cohort studies was motivated by observations in the Multiple Risk Factor Intervention Trial (MRFIT) Screening Follow-up Study concerning epidemiologic correlates of hemorrhagic stroke. The study of hemorrhagic stroke in the MRFIT Screening Follow-up Study was motivated by Japanese epidemiologic (24–30), clinical, laboratory, and pathologic studies (31–34), which suggested that the incidence of intracranial hemorrhage was greater among those who had low levels of TC. The Japanese investigators concluded that low TC level caused arteriolosclerosis and angionecrosis resulting in this type of stroke. Most Western investigators interpreted that the relationship between low TC and hemorrhagic stroke was confounded by some aspect of Japanese life, for instance high salt, low animal protein, or high alcohol intake, coupled with endemic hypertension. If so, an epidemiologic study of Westerners, with lower salt, more animal protein, and lower alcohol intake, coupled with lower blood pressure levels, should find no relationship between low TC and hemorrhagic stroke.

The MRFIT Screening Follow-up Study (not to be confused with the randomized MRFIT study of the effects of multifactor invention on CHD) of fatal stroke was a cohort design in a convenience sample of 361,662 men. The men were initially aged 35–57 years, with TC, blood pressure, smoking, age, history of prior myocardial infarction, and history of diabetes measured or queried at baseline; they were followed for 11–13 years by death certificate linkage (35). Low TC level, defined as <160 mg/dl, was found in about 5% of the population; thus because of the large size of the MRFIT study, the sample included 21,185 men with low TC levels among the 350,977 men with no history of myocardial infarction or diabetes.

In summary, there were 83 hemorrhagic stroke deaths in six years of follow-up, for which hypertension was the predominant risk factor, explaining 32% of the attributable risk. However, 11 of these deaths occurred in men with TC <160 mg/dl, when only three to four were expected, thus constituting a relative risk of 3. Longer follow-up showed a relative risk of 2 (36), with higher mortality rates of hemorrhagic stroke for TC <160 mg/dl, regardless of blood pressure level. The 55 cases of subarachnoid hemorrhage (occurring in larger arteries and at a younger age) showed no relation to TC. The 92 deaths attributed to thromboembolic stroke, or to stroke of uncertain origin, were positively related to TC level.

The 83 deaths attributed to hemorrhagic stroke constituted only a small fraction of the 6902 total deaths in six years of MRFIT follow-up. The finding of elevated risk associated with low TC in this rare condition was considered of little public health importance for the United States. Nevertheless, to put this small excess mortality risk associated with low TC into a public health perspective, the investigators examined the risk of all cause death according to TC level. There was a consistently greater total cardiovascular and coronary heart disease death rate with higher TC levels, except at the very lowest levels of TC. However, the greater risk with greater TC was not the rule in noncardiovascular dieases. In this case, risk was greater at lower levels of TC. Combined cancer and other noncardiovascular diseases comprised more than half of total deaths.

The investigators examined the data by cause of death for total cancer, respiratory disease, trauma, and all other causes combined in unpublished analyses designed to understand these observations better. Mortality due to each of these noncardiovascular causes was greater at low TC levels, even after omission of deaths in the first three years after baseline. The overall result of these opposing epidemiologic findings was a U-shaped curve of TC level with total mortality: higher at the extremes and lower at intermediate values, i.e. 160–219 mg/dl (4.14–5.66 mmol/L).

The MRFIT study on hemorrhagic stroke and low TC (35) concluded that the increased total mortality in the lowest cholesterol-level group of men resulted mainly from an increased risk of death from diseases, particularly cancers, which have the potential to lower serum cholesterol level (37, 38).

However, the need to understand these and other findings led to the NHLBI-sponsored conference in October 1990.

THE OCTOBER 1990 CONFERENCE ON LOW CHOLESTEROL: DISEASE ASSOCIATIONS

A meta-analysis of mortality findings in relation to baseline TC in cohort studies was carried out at the 1990 conference (18). Participants in the meta-analysis were responsible for 19 studies (the MRFIT Screening Follow-up Study and ten others from the United States, one from southern Europe, one from Israel, two from Great Britain, one from Scandinavia, and three from Japan) of 20 invited to participate in the conference. The analyses were done separately for 350,977 men from the MRFIT Screenee Study (21,499 deaths), 172,760 men from other studies (34,026 deaths), and 124,814 women (12,881 deaths in 12 studies), aged 35–69 and free of CHD at baseline. Approximately 45% of deaths were coded to total cardiovascular causes, 33% to total cancer causes, and 22% to noncardiovascular, noncancer causes. The latter category included respiratory, digestive, traumatic, and other causes, comprising 5%, 4%, 6%, and 7% of total mortality, respectively. Length of follow-up ranged from 9 to 30 years. To attempt to account for the potential effects of preexisting illness on the entry TC level and subsequent disease relationships, data on deaths occurring within five years of baseline were excluded. Proportional hazards regressions for mortality on TC level were pooled (39) after adjustment for age, diastolic blood pressure, cigarette smoking, body mass index, and alcohol intake, where available (alcohol intake was available in only 12 studies).

In the meta-analysis (18), risk for 6% of men with TC $<$160 mg/dl or 30% of the men with TC $\geq$240 mg/dl was elevated by about 15% compared with men with TC levels either 160–199 mg/dl or 200–239 mg/dl. For women, the risk curve of all cause mortality was nearly flat across TC levels. There was a graded, increasing risk for CHD death. Relative risks for CHD mortality were 2.2 among MRFIT Screenees, 1.7 among pooled men, and 1.6 among pooled women, comparing those with TC $\geq$240 mg/dl with those with TC in the reference class of 160–199 mg/dl. Intermediate relative risks of 1.5, 1.2, and 1.1, respectively, were reported for those with TC 200–239 mg/dl. In contrast, total cardiovascular disease deaths were higher according to TC in men, but not in women. Relative risks for total cardiovascular disease death in those with TC $\geq$240 mg/dl compared with those in the reference class were 1.9 among MRFIT men, 1.5 among pooled men, but only 1.1 among pooled women. The increased risk for total mortality at lower levels of TC resulted largely from an inverse relation with deaths due to respiratory disease, digestive disease, trauma, and residual deaths in both sexes, and to some cancers in men only (e.g. lung, but not colon). Lesser risk with greater TC was graded for deaths due to lung cancer, respiratory disease, and digestive disease. Greater risk for trauma and residual deaths was seen only for TC <160 mg/dl. Compared with those with TC level 160–199 mg/dl, risk for combined noncardiovascular, noncancer causes of death was 45% higher for men and women whose level was low, <160 mg/dl, and 15% lower in both sexes for those whose level was high, ≥240 mg/dl. Parallel analyses showed that these risk patterns for all-causes, cardiovascular, cancer, and other deaths were similar within smoking and alcohol strata.

Detailed analyses from the MRFIT Screening Followup Study (36) indicated that increased death rates for those men who entered with low TC level occurred especially for hemorrhagic stroke; cancers of the lung, liver, lymphatic system, and hematopoietic systems; chronic obstructive pulmonary disease; cirrhosis of the liver; and suicide. The increased risk at low TC for lung cancer and for chronic obstructive pulmonary disease was far greater in smokers than in nonsmokers, as was also the case in the Whitehall study (40). Other causes of death were less frequent or had less strong associations with low TC levels, for example, stomach and some other digestive and nervous system cancers, other respiratory diseases, and other liver and digestive diseases; alcohol dependence syndrome; and noncancerous diseases of the central nervous system. After all these diseases had been accounted for, all remaining noncardiovascular, noncancer causes of death had excess risk at low levels of TC. Most of these findings held when data on the first five or ten years of deaths after baseline were removed from the analysis. The Honolulu Heart Program (41) was much smaller, and therefore had less power for detailed examination of the data than the MRFIT study. However, the Honolulu Heart Program found excess risk for hemorrhagic stroke (41, 42). Mortality risk at low TC levels persisted for all cancer, chronic obstructive pulmonary disease, benign liver disease, and unknown causes (41), even removing the first ten years of deaths.

RESULTS OF CLINICAL TRIALS

The meta-analysis of clinical trials by Holme (1) considered 19 multi- or single-factor, drug or diet, primary or secondary trials of TC lowering. They showed a clear reduction of CHD occurrence. The greater the net reduction in TC, the greater was the reduction in total mortality. There was, however, greater total mortality with greater reduction of TC in primary prevention trials ($p = 0.05$); there was a similar tendency in single factor studies.

Holme's (1) meta-analysis of secondary prevention trials was in agreement with that of Rossouw et al (43), which, among eight clinical trials of TC lowering, found an odds ratio of 0.78 for treated to control patients for recurrent myocardial infarction ($p < 0.0001$). The odds ratio was 0.88 for cardiovascular deaths ($p = 0.05$), which comprised 82% of all deaths in these studies. Cancer mortality was reduced in the treated groups (odds ratio 0.75, $p = 0.26$). However, no difference was found between treated and control subjects in noncardiovascular, noncancer deaths (44). Not considered was a single secondary prevention trial of TC lowering by partial ileal bypass surgery. This trial found no excess noncardiovascular deaths in the treated group (9).

As Holme (1) noted, three multifactor primary prevention trials found no excess noncardiovascular death among treated subjects (10–13); a recently reported fourth trial showed an excess of cardiac and violent deaths in treated subjects (14). There was extensive use of drugs to lower blood pressure and TC in this latter study.

The meta-analysis by Muldoon et al (3) of six randomized, primary prevention, drug, or diet clinical trials of TC lowering found decreased mortality from CHD in the treated compared with control groups. The meta-analysis showed greater violent and cancer deaths, but not remaining causes of death, in treated versus control groups. They attributed observed increases in cancer deaths to specific effects of clofibrate in the World Health Organization study of this drug (7). Davey Smith & Pekkanen (2) studied primary prevention studies only. They added to Holme's list a nonrandomized diet study, a short follow-up of a trial using lovastatin (45), and extended follow-up from the Helsinki Heart Study (46). They analyzed diet versus drug studies separately. Mortality from CHD was reduced in treated groups in both diet and drug studies. Mortality from cancer, injury, and other noncoronary heart disease causes was greater in treated subjects of drug studies, but differences in rates were small and not statistically significant in diet studies.

Taken as a whole, the evidence for excess noncardiovascular mortality in clinical trials of TC lowering appears in primary prevention studies, in which risk of noncardiovascular disease is relatively greater than in secondary prevention studies. Adverse effects of drugs might also be suspected as a cause of the excess. In principle, interpretation of the noncardiovascular endpoints of randomized clinical trials should use the same rules of inference as interpretation of cardiovascular endpoints; therefore, the greater rates of noncardiovascular death in treated subjects should not be attributable to confounding. The clinical trial evidence should be treated with caution, however, as power is low for study of noncardiovascular disease in these trials; although the evidence is consistent, the level of statistical significance remains marginal in many analyses of studies to date. Only mortality is monitored, and rates are too low for inferences to be made about individual diseases. Several different drugs have been studied; it may be inappropriate to pool drug studies, because different drugs have different actions and side effects. Power is low for combined noncardiovascular causes in diet trials, which comprise many fewer person-years of follow-up than do drug studies.

COULD THERE BE A COMMON BIOLOGICAL BASIS FOR THE OBSERVATIONS IN COHORT STUDIES AND CLINICAL TRIALS?

Low TC measured in cohort studies reflects a history of low TC. This is physiologically different from the relatively brief period of TC lowering in persons with elevated TC in clinical trials. Long-term low TC might have a relatively small effect on each organ system; only after many years, perhaps in conjunction with another disease process, a relative deficiency of cholesterol in cells and tissues may cause a clinical problem. Recently lowered TC in clinical trials might selectively lower cell cholesterol in certain organs, even while TC remains relatively high. Clinical manifestations would depend on which organs were most affected by the particular method of TC lowering.

POTENTIAL SOURCES OF CONFOUNDING AS A BASIS FOR THE OBSERVED RELATIONSHIPS

Although the finding of excess hemorrhagic stroke and excess mortality from noncardiovascular disease in cohort studies is strong and consistent, it may nevertheless be a reflection of epidemiologic confounding. The cohort studies were designed to measure possible confounders for cardiovascular disease, but paid little attention to noncardiovascular diseases and their causes. Several possible confounders have been suggested.

The first confounder is that disease lowers TC levels, so that the excess risk is simply due to a disease that the person already had when TC was measured. Total cholesterol will be lowered by virtually any disease in its final, wasting phases. The first five to ten years of deaths were excluded from analysis in the 1990 NHLBI Conference (18) and related papers (36, 41), in an attempt to eliminate those who might have had unnoticed disease at baseline. This strategy for avoiding confounding appears to be adequate with respect to cancer, which may lower TC four years (47) and possibly as long as ten years, before death (48). However, latent or undetected disease at baseline is a real possibility in these studies; for example, nonlife-threatening liver disease, cholesterol malabsorption, or reduced lung function was not even noted in most cohort studies of the development of CHD. One may survive for many years with a cirrhotic liver, intestinal disease, or reduced lung function. Little is known about when and by how much TC might first be reduced in the course of such diseases.

Any disease risk factor that lowers TC, including cigarette smoking or alcohol intake, can be a confounder. Excessive alcohol intake may lead to malnutrition and/or a compromised liver, either of which might lower TC and cause death by mechanisms independent of TC level. Or, TC may play a role only in certain conditions; for example, low TC may be important in lung disease only among smokers (36, 40). Total cholesterol may affect noncardiovascular disease indirectly, only when a risk factor is present. For example, smoking lowers serum high-density lipoprotein (HDL) cholesterol, which might affect noncardiovascular diseases through its role in steroid hormone production by the ovaries and the adrenal gland (49) and pulmonary surfactant production (50–52).

Dietary factors might lower cholesterol incidentally, while causing disease by mechanisms independent of TC level. For example, vitamin E might influence noncardiovascular disease by affecting cell membrane characteristics. Vitamin E-deficient rat lung microsomes and lipid vesicles (compared with vitamin E sufficient ones) had more cholesterol, more readily oxidized lipids, and decreased fluidity (53). In another example, diets high in vitamin E tend to be high in fruits, vegetables, legumes, and whole grains and are, therefore, likely to result in relatively lower levels of LDL cholesterol. Yet, because LDL lipoprotein is the primary carrier of vitamins E and β-carotene, the resulting low levels of serum LDL cholesterol may carry inadequate amounts of fat soluble antioxidant vitamins E and β-carotene to tissues. Relative antioxidant deficiency may occur when their transport capacity is reduced. That such reduction may have clinical importance is suggested by inhibition of function of fat-soluble drugs, such as cyclosporine, when LDL is low (54).

Low socioeconomic status may be a confounding factor in the low blood cholesterol:disease relationships (22, 40). Many characteristics of poverty, such as infection or violence, predispose to disease. Poverty may also be associated with poor diet quality or alcoholism, both of which may lead to low TC, independent of any effects TC might have on disease risk.

POTENTIAL BIOLOGIC BASES FOR THE OBSERVED RELATIONSHIPS

One may hypothesize that either an excess or a deficiency in functions related to cholesterol metabolism could lead to excess disease risk. There is wide evidence that cholesterol is essential to, and intimately involved with, many aspects of cellular structure and function (55, 56). For example, cholesterol affects the fluidity of cell membranes, membrane permeability, transmembrane exchange, signal transmission, and other cell properties. Cholesterol is a precursor for five major classes of steroid hormones. It affects gluconeogenesis and immune function; its transport forms, the lipoproteins, also serve as vehicles for fat-soluble vitamins, antioxidants, drugs, and toxins. Thus, cholesterol plays general, fundamental, and highly specific roles in the economy of the body.

Cell membrane abnormalities, such as increased or decreased fluidity, are found in many diseases, including atherosclerosis [aortic cell membranes in rabbits (57) and erythrocytes in humans (58)], Type I diabetes [erythrocytes in humans (59)], infection [erythrocytes in sheep (60)], obesity [erythrocytes in children (61)], Crohn's disease [erythrocytes in humans (62)], spinocerebellar degeneration [erythrocytes in humans (63)], chronic liver disease and nephrotic syndrome [erythrocytes in humans (58), and rats (64)], hypothyroidism [erythrocyte and brain subcellular fractions in rats (65)], maternal alcohol use [brain sections in rat pups (66)], and Alzheimer's disease and vascular dementia [white matter in autopsies (67)]. We do not know the causes of these cell membrane abnormalities. Nor do we know whether the abnormalities are in any way related to level of cholesterol in the blood.

Changes in cell membrane cholesterol levels may result in changes in other functional characteristics of the cell membrane. For example, fluidity in porcine pulmonary artery endotheial cells decreased when incubated in cholesterol and transmembrane serotonin transport correspondingly decreased (68). Engelberg (69) speculated that low levels of cerebral serotonin, secondary to low serum cholesterol, may reduce impulse control, thereby increasing likelihood of suicide or aggressive behavior. Some immune functions depend on membrane cholesterol. Roosemond et al (70) studied the effect of altered target cell membrane structure on natural killer (NK) cell-mediated cytotoxicity. Both human and rat NK-resistant cell lines became NK-sensitive (that is, were lysed by NK cells) after fusion with NK-sensitive membrane components. The fusion required the presence of Sendai virus envelope glycoproteins, soybean lecithin, and cholesterol for maximum efficiency. Heiniger et al (71) found that cytolytic function of mice T lymphocytes was strongly suppressed in a medium with an inhibitor of cellular cholesterol synthesis (25-OH-cholesterol). The effect was reversed when cholesterol or mevalonic acid was added to the culture medium. Because similar inhibition of DNA synthesis had no effect on cytolytic activity, the authors concluded that the effect results from inhibition on sterol synthesis, rather than on inhibition of cellular proliferation.

The above authors did not study whether any of these cell membrane abnormalities is related to level or changes in TC. Mistry et al (72) showed that 750 or 1500 mg per day of supplemental dietary cholesterol resulted in higher blood TC and higher levels of cholesterol in leukocytes, but the authors did not specifically study free cholesterol, the form that exists in cell membranes. Shanmugasundaram et al (73) studied 20% [polyunsaturated fatty acid:saturated fatty acid (P:S) ratio 0.6] and 35% fat diets (P:S ratio 0.2) and found that TC was increased on the higher fat diet. The cholesterol was increased in erythrocyte membranes and in whole leucocytes on the higher fat diet; free cholesterol in leucocytes was not studied. Andersen & Dietschy (49) showed that cholesterol in the serum is important in the regulation of cell cholesterol. However, cell cholesterol and cell function may vary at different TC levels, despite the compensatory changes that occur in cell cholesterol synthesis when TC changes. Andersen & Dietschy did not actually show that cell cholesterol level did not change. Phillips et al (74) indicated that the direction of any net transfer of cholesterol between cells and lipoproteins is determined by the molar ratios of free cholesterol/phospholipid of the donor and acceptor particles; cholesterol diffuses down its gradient of chemical potential generally partitioning to the phospholipid-rich particles, independent of any receptor processes. Gotto et al (75) stated that the distribution of LDL to various tissues depends on the rate of transcapillary transport, as well as on the activity of LDL receptors; for example, LDL uptake by the adrenal gland is facilitated by a fenestrated epithelium and cortical cells rich in LDL receptors, whereas adipose tissue and muscle have nonfenestrated capillaries and few LDL receptors and take up LDL slowly. Grundy (76) concluded that one third of cholesterol exchange between cells and serum occurs via nonreceptor mediated pathways; the amount of cholesterol incorporated into the cell via this mechanism may be more susceptible to variation with TC level than the corresponding amount via receptor-mediated pathways.

The level of cholesterol in the cell may be adequate for viability of the cell, yet be inadequate for cell products. Hass & Longmore (50) studied pulmonary surfactant and found that only about 1% of its cholesterol was supplied by synthesis in the Type II pneumocytes that produce lung surfactant. The rest of the cholesterol was supplied by the plasma; receptors for both LDL and HDL cholesterol were found (51). A recent experiment found that both HDL and LDL stimulate pulmonary surfactant secretion (52). Thus, if serum cholesterol were low, surfactant function could possibly be impaired; however, this has not been studied. Longmore and coworkers have found that surfactant chemical composition is altered in acute respiratory distress syndrome (77) and that replacement of surfactant corrects abnormalities caused in rats by experimentally injuring lungs (78). Possible alterations in the biochemical composition of pulmonary surfactant might have relevance to the consistent finding of a graded negative relationship between TC and either lung cancer or chronic obstructive pulmonary disease mortality.

Genetic errors result in low TC. In the classic, extreme example of a low TC:disease association found in the exceedingly rare individuals having homozygous abeta-lipoproteinemia, there are low circulating levels of TC (less than 50 mg/dl) and low-to-absent circulating LDL or apoprotein-B (79). Homozygotes suffer numerous defects, including intestinal malabsorption of fat, progressive degeneration of the central nervous system, retinal pigmentary degeneration, abnormal red blood cells, and cardiomyopathy (79). The underlying biochemical defect probably involves an abnormality in the synthesis or secretion of apoprotein B-containing lipoproteins and results in a functional disturbance of delivery of cholesterol to peripheral tissues (79). Affected persons experience serious disease consequences involving multiple organ systems; however, these consequences are partly correctable by administration of large doses of vitamin E and water-soluble vitamin A and vitamin K (79). These clinical manifestations are most likely due to deficiencies in fat soluble vitamins and/or other lipid soluble factors in the blood, not just to the low LDL level. Granot & Deckelbaum (80) reported that heterozygotes who also have low TC levels, sometimes well below 100 mg/dl, nevertheless appear healthy and may be long-lived. However, Andersen et al (81) found mild impairment of function of long motor and sensory tracks in heterozygotes, which might, with long exposure, predispose to accident.

Another genetic error of metabolism related to cholesterol synthesis in the cell is mevalonic aciduria secondary to mevalonate kinase deficiency. This condition has been identified in ten children (82, 83). The defect is partially countered by increased activities of HMG CoA reductase and of the LDL receptor pathway. Total cholesterol is normal or slightly reduced. There are severe consequences: psychomotor retardation (10/10), hypotonia/myopathy (9/9), ataxia (5/9), failure to thrive (9/10), recurrent crises with fever/diarrhea (8/9), anemia (7/9), hepatosplenomegaly (5/10), cerebellar atrophy (5/7), dysmorphic features (5/10), cataracts (3/10), elevated serum creatine kinase (6/9), decreased tissue and plasma ubiquinone 10 (4/6), and death (4/10). Low doses of lovastatin in two patients worsened their conditions; plasma creatine kinase and ubiquinone worsened. These conditions are similar to those seen in dogs treated with high doses of lovastatin (84–86). Lovastatin in doses used clinically reduces mevalonic acid excretion by the kidney only by one-third (87). Because two patients treated with high doses of vitamin E, vitamin C, and ubiquinone 10 showed some improvement, Hoffmann (83) suggests that the severe multisystem pathology in mevalonic aciduria might be attributed to free radical pathology. However, the extent to which cholesterol in cell membranes or in other functions is involved in either short- or long-term prognosis of these patients is unknown.

Considerable work has been done on the biologic role of low TC in hemorrhagic stroke patients. The inverse relationship between TC level and the risk of hemorrhagic stroke suggests that hypertensive, hypocholesterolemic individuals are more liable to develop this complication than those with either hypertension or low TC level alone (35, 36, 42). Cerebral hemorrhage occurs mostly from penetrating vessels in the basal ganglia of the brain, the intraparenchymal small arterioles of 100–300 microns in diameter. Angionecrosis, the basic pathologic finding, is not a proliferative disorder of the intima like atherosclerosis, but rather involves the disappearance of medial smooth muscle cells. Because these cells are an important component of vascular structure, their loss is thought to lead to vessel wall fragility, hypothesized to be caused by increased permeability of endothelial membranes. Vessel wall fragility, in turn, leads to the formation of microaneurysms. When microaneurysms burst, bleeding occurs. When thrombi are formed and organize in microaneurysms, lacunar infarction occurs. The presence or absence of dietary factors that exert deleterious or protective effects on endothelial and medial elements of the vessels is seen as important. Although it has not been demonstrated whether cholesterol content of endothelial cell membranes is low in humans having a low TC level, men with a history of intracerebral hemorrhage have lower cholesterol content in both serum and erythrocytes than men with no history of stroke (31). Dietary changes have been shown to relate to cell cholesterol content (72, 73). Low TC also may lead to decreased numbers of medial smooth muscle cells, a process accelerated by high blood pressure. Experimental increase of TC level in hypertensive rats from a very low level (mean 114 mg/dl) to a moderately high level (mean 242 mg/dl) was associated with attenuation of the loss of medial smooth muscle cells (32) and risk of development of stroke (33). Some other researchers have shown relationships of low TC to cell membrane function (34, 88, 89) but others have not (90). Brown et al (91) and Goldstein & Brown (92) have emphasized the powerful homeostatic mechanisms controlling cellular content of free cholesterol.

The manifold functions of cholesterol present a fundamental problem in understanding any biologic role of low TC in nonatherosclerotic disease: There are so many places to look for abnormality, yet all critical body functions of cholesterol are homeostatically well controlled. Is homeostasis adequate in all tissues in all people at all ages, even when compromised over many years by the physiologically "degrading" effects that might result from exposure to smoking, infectious agents, alcohol-induced damage, or a variety of drugs? There is a lack of fundamental information about how cholesterol in the plasma effects each of these functions, such as the role of TC level in regulation of cell membrane cholesterol, in transport of antioxidants, or in maintenance of lung surfactant. Each of these roles may be complex and may express problems in an interacting variety of ways, not only by the most obvious routes of reduced cholesterol in the membrane at low serum cholesterol levels, or modified fluidity at low TC levels.

The basis for observed relationships of low TC, or TC lowering, and disease does not appear to be readily at hand. The excess noncardiovascular mortality in TC lowering trials, particularly those using drugs, may be related to blood and cell cholesterol in complex ways. Similarly complex may be the explanation of the excess noncardiovascular mortality at low TC levels in cohort studies. There may, in fact, be no biological connection of these diseases to TC. Confounding may be subtle. The salient epidemiologic needs for understanding this issue are to study TC in relation to morbidity, including the time course of TC change before, during, and after disease onset. The development of epidemiologic information about the relation to disease of cell and tissue cholesterol and its function should be a priority. At the same time, there is enough tantalizing biologic information available to justify vigorous study of the influence of TC on cell and tissue cholesterol and on cholesterol related function.

IMPLICATIONS FOR PUBLIC HEALTH POLICY

Several authors have recently suggested caution in the pursuit of low TC. Frank et al (41) recommended against TC lowering in persons with TC ≤225 mg/dl, based on models that imply that the 60% of persons in the Honolulu Heart Program with this level of TC might be harmed by TC lowering. Hulley et al (93), commenting on the 1990 Bethesda conference (18), suggested limiting TC screening and intervention to the minority for which benefits clearly predominate over harms, that is, those with coronary disease or other reasons for being at a comparable very high risk of CHD death. This recommendation was based on an association between low TC and noncardiovascular disease death rates in men and women, the absence of association between high TC and cardiovascular disease death rates in women, and the absence of change in total mortality in primary prevention trials. Kronmal et al (94) recommended caution in initiating any TC lowering treatment in men and women above 65–70 years of age, based on inverse relationships of TC to all-cause and CHD mortality in Framingham data and the absence of clinical trials of TC lowering in the elderly. Hazzard (95) felt that it is an open question whether to treat high TC in the elderly, based on several factors, including the absence of demonstrated efficacy of TC lowering in increasing longevity. Davey Smith & Pekkanen (2) suggested a moratorium on general use of medications to lower TC in primary prevention, pending the results of ongoing trials. This conclusion was based on a meta-analysis of past trials in which drug trials had adverse effects.

The absence of a clear demonstration of efficacy of TC lowering drugs in increasing longevity makes me uncomfortable with heavy reliance on medications as a public health strategy for TC lowering (96), particularly in inadequately studied groups, such as women and the elderly. What, then, of population-wide efforts to lower TC by dietary change? Total cholesterol changes in whole populations tend to be greater at high than at low TC levels (25, 96). Less TC lowering at low TC levels would dampen any adverse effects that might result from TC lowering (96). Although many biologic possibilities are outlined in this review, there is no definite evidence of biologically based adverse consequences, and it appears unlikely that 100% of the observed associations between low TC and nonatherosclerotic disease death is causally mediated by TC. In contrast, a causal relationship of TC level with atherosclerosis and CHD is established. Models for mortality, which consider these points, suggested net benefit from a 20 mg/dl average reduction of population TC by diet (96). These models pertained specifically to men aged 35–57 when TC was measured, starting at a mean TC of 215 mg/dl. The models suggested that the lower the starting average TC level the less the benefit. There is less information on mortality risk in women and the elderly. The Bethesda conference finding (18) of no association between TC and total cardiovascular disease death in women is provocative; in addition, premenopausal women have lower average TC than men.

Nevertheless, I consider current public health recommendations concerning eating patterns sound. Irrespective of effects on TC itself, there are many positive aspects for both men and women in the widely recommended healthy eating patterns for individuals, families, and whole populations. Prevention of CHD in high TC cultures remains a pressing need, and TC lowering has been shown to contribute to prevention. Furthermore, population-wide efforts (i.e. food industry changes, government policy, medical practice) to reduce saturated fat and cholesterol intake are important to any effective program of TC lowering; they also tend to agree with other dietary policies aimed at increasing fruit, vegetable, legume, whole grain, and fish intake (97, 98). Although current population-wide efforts to lower TC by diet should continue, there is minimal absolute benefit for CHD prevention in adults with low TC, e.g. TC <180 mg/dl, who are free of heart disease, and there is potential risk for adults with low TC. A low-risk strategy, in which population-wide policy initiatives continue, is therefore suggested, but those individuals identified with low TC and who are free of heart disease are not advised to take personal steps toward TC lowering. Almost half of the total population of the United States, namely adults with higher TC (perhaps ≥ 200 mg/dl) and those who have heart disease, would continue to be advised to pursue personal TC lowering strategies.

ACKNOWLEDGMENT

This work was done with the support and assistance of two individuals. The author thanks Henry Blackburn for leadership, friendship, and scientific acumen. John Belcher has been generous with his time and knowledge of biochemistry. The syntheses and conclusions of this review are the author's, however.

Literature Cited

1. Holme, I. 1990. An analysis of randomized trials evaluating the effect of cholesterol reduction on total mortality and coronary heart disease incidence. *Circulation* 82:1916–24
2. Davey Smith, G., Pekkanen, J. 1992. Should there be a moratorium on the use of cholesterol-lowering drugs? *Br. Med. J.* 304:431–34
3. Muldoon, M. F., Manuck, S. B., Matthews, K. A. 1990. Lowering cholesterol concentrations and mortality: a review of primary prevention trials. *Br. Med. J.* 301:309–14
4. Yusuf, S., Wittes, J., Friedman, L. 1988. Overview of results of randomized clinical trials in heart disease: II. Unstable angina, heart failure, primary prevention with aspirin, and risk factor modification. *J. Am. Med. Assoc.* 260: 2259–63
5. Lipid Res. Clin. Program. 1984. The Lipid Research Clinics coronary primary prevention trial results: I. Reduction in incidence of coronary heart disease. *J. Am. Med. Assoc.* 251:351–64
6. Frick, M. H., Elo, M. O., Haapa, K., Heinonen, O. P., Heinsalmi, P., et al. 1987. Helsinki Heart Study. Primary prevention trial with gemfibrozil in middle aged men with dyslipidemia; safety of treatment, changes in risk factors, and incidence of coronary heart disease. *N. Engl. J. Med.* 317:1237–45
7. Comm. of Princ. Invest. 1984. WHO co-operative trial on primary prevention of ischaemic heart disease with clofibrate to lower serum cholesterol: final mortality followup. *Lancet* 2: 600–4
8. Dayton, S., Pearce, M. L., Goldman, H., Hamish, A., Plotkin, D., et al. 1969. A controlled trial of a diet high in unsaturated fat. *Circulation* 40:(Suppl. 2) 1–62
9. Buchwald, H., Varco, R. L., Matts, J. P., Long, J. M., Fitch, L. L., et al. 1990. Effect of partial ileal bypass surgery on mortality and morbidity from coronary heart disease in patients with hypercholesterolemia. Report of the Program on the Surgical Control of the Hyperlipidemias (POSCH). *N. Engl. J. Med.* 323:946–55
10. Hjermann, I., Velve Byre, K., Holme, I., Leren, P. 1981. Effect of diet and smoking intervention on the incidence of coronary heart disease. Report from the Oslo Study Group of a randomized trial in healthy men. *Lancet* 2:1303–10
11. Multiple Risk Factor Interv. Trial Res. Group. 1986. Coronary heart disease death, non-fatal acute myocardial infarction and other clinical outcomes in the Multiple Risk Factor Intervention Trial. *Am. J. Cardiol.* 58:1–13
12. Multiple Risk Factor Interv. Trial Res. Group. 1990. Mortality rates after 10.5 years for participants in the Multiple Risk Factor Intervention Trial. Findings related to a prior hypothesis of the trial. *J. Am. Med. Assoc.* 263:1795–1801
13. World Health Org. Eur. Collab. Group. 1986. European collaborative trial of multifactorial prevention of coronary heart disease: final report on the 6-year results. *Lancet* 1:869–72
14. Strandberg, T. E., Salomaa, V. V., Naukkarinen, V. A., Vanhanen, H. T., Sarna, S. J., Miettinen, T. A. 1991. Long-term mortality after 5-year multifactorial primary prevention of cardiovascular diseases in middle-aged men. *J. Am. Med. Assoc.* 266:1225–29
15. Blankenhorn, D. H., Nessim, S. A., Johnson, R. L., Sanmarco, M. E., Azen, S. P., Cashin-Hemphill, L. 1987. Beneficial effects of combined colestipol-niacin therapy on coronary atherosclerosis and coronary venous bypass grafts. *J. Am. Med. Assoc.* 257:3233–40
16. Ornish, D., Brown, S. E., Scherwitz, L. W., Billings, J. H., Armstrong, W. T., et al. 1990. Can lifestyle changes reverse coronary heart disease? The Lifestyle Heart Trial. *Lancet* 336: 129–33
17. Brown, G., Albers, J. J., Fisher, L. D., Schaefer, S. M., Lin, J.-T., et al. 1990. Regression of coronary artery disease as a result of intensive lipid-lowering therapy in men with high levels of Apolipoprotein B. *N. Engl. J. Med.* 323:1289–98
18. Jacobs, D., Blackburn, H., Higgins, M., Reed, D., Iso, H., et al. 1992. Report of the conference on low blood cholesterol: mortality associations, October 9–10, 1990. *Circulation* 86:1046–60
19. Feinleib, M. 1982. Summary of a workshop on cholesterol and noncardiovascular disease mortality. *Prev. Med.* 1:360–67
20. Feinleib, M. 1981. On a possible inverse relationship between serum cho-

lesterol and cancer mortality. *Am. J. Epidemiol.* 114:5–10

21. Int. Collab. Group. 1982. Circulating cholesterol level and risk of death from cancer in men aged 40 to 69 years. *J. Am. Med. Assoc.* 248:2853–59
22. Law, M. R., Thompson, S. G. 1991. Serum cholesterol and cancer: conclusions from an analysis of data from all the prospective studies. *Cancer Causes Control* 2:253–61
23. Glueck, C. J., Gartside, P., Fallat, R. W., Sielski, J., Steiner, P. M. 1976. Longevity syndromes: familial hypobeta and familial hyperalpha lipoproteinemia. *J. Lab. Clin. Med.* 88:941–57
24. Komachi, Y., Iida, M., Shimamoto, T., Chikayama, Y., Takahashi, H., et al. 1971. Geographic and occupational comparisons of risk factors in cardiovascular diseases in Japan. *Jpn. Circ. J.* 35:189–207
25. Shimamoto, T., Komachi, Y., Inada, H. 1989. Trends for coronary heart disease and stroke risk factors in Japan. *Circulation* 79:503–15
26. Blackburn, H., Jacobs, D. R. 1898. The ongoing natural experiment of cardiovascular diseases in Japan. *Circulation* 79:718–20
27. Komachi, Y., Iida, M., Ozawa, H., Shimamoto, T., Ueshima, et al. 1977. Risk factors of stroke (in Japanese). *Saishin Igaku* 32:2264–69
28. Ueshima, H., Iida, M., Shimamoto, T., Konishi, M., Tsujioka, K., et al. 1980. Multivariate analysis of risk factors for stroke: eight-year followup study of farming villages in Akita, Japan. *Prev. Med.* 9:722–40
29. Tanaka, H., Ueda, Y., Hayashi, M., Date, C., Baba, T., et al. 1982. Risk factors for cerebral hemorrhage and cerebral infarction in a Japanese rural community. *Stroke* 13:62–73
30. Konishi, M., Komachi, Y., Iso, H., Iida, M., Naito, Y., et al. 1990. Secular trends in atherosclerosis of the coronary arteries and basal cerebral arteries in Japan: The Akita Pathology Study. *Arteriosclerosis* 10:535–40
31. Konishi, M., Terao, A., Doi, M., Iida, M. 1982. Osmotic resistance and cholesterol content of the erythrocyte membrane in cerebral hemorrhage. (In Japanese) *Igaku no Ayumi* 120:30–32
32. Yamori, Y., Horie, R., Ohtaka, M., Nara, Y., Fukase, M. 1976. Effect of hypercholesterolaemic diet on the incidence of cerebrovascular and myocardial lesions on spontaneously hypertensive rats (SHR). *Clin. Exp. Pharmacol. Physiol.* (Suppl. 3) 205–8
33. Ooneda, G., Yoshida, Y., Suzuki, K., Shinkai, H., Hori, S., et al. 1978. Smooth muscle cells in the development of plasmatic arterionecrosis, arteriosclerosis, and arterial contraction. *Blood Vessels* 15:148–56
34. Yamori, Y., Nara, Y., Horie, R., Ooshima, A. 1980. Abnormal membrane characteristics of erythrocytes in rat models and men with predisposition to stroke. Clin. Exp. Hyperten. 2:1009–21
35. Iso, H., Jacobs, D. R., Wentworth, D., Neaton, J. D., Cohen, J. 1989. Serum cholesterol levels and six-year mortality from stroke in 350,977 men screened for the Multiple Risk Factor Intervention Trial. *N. Eng. J. Med.* 320:904–10
36. Neaton, J. D., Blackburn, H., Jacobs, D., Kuller, L., Lee, D. J., et al. 1992. Serum cholesterol level and mortality. Findings for men screened in the Multiple Risk Factor Intervention Trial. *Arch. Int. Med.* 152:1490–1500
37. Martin, M. J., Hulley, S. B., Browner, W. S., Kuller, L. H., Wentworth, D. 1986. Serum cholesterol, blood pressure, and mortality: implications from a cohort of 361, 662 men. *Lancet* 2:933–36
38. Sherwin, R. W., Wentworth, D. N., Cutler, J. A., Hulley, S. B., Kuller, L. H., Stamler, J. 1987. Serum cholesterol levels and cancer mortality in 361, 662 men screened for the Multiple Risk Factor Intervention Trial. *J. Am. Med. Assoc.* 257:943–48
39. DerSimonian, R., Laird, N. 1986. Meta-analysis in clinical trials. *Controlled Clin. Trials* 7:177–88
40. Smith, G. D., Shipley, M. J., Marmot, M. G., Rose, G. 1992. Plasma cholesterol concentration and mortality. The Whitehall Study. *J. Am. Med. Assoc.* 267:70–76
41. Frank, J. W., Reed, D. M., Grobe, J. F., Benfante, R. 1992. Will lowering population levels of serum cholesterol affect total mortality? Expectations from the Honolulu Heart Program. *J. Clin. Epidemiol.* 45:333–46
42. Yano, K., Reed, D. M., Maclean, C. J. 1989. Serum cholesterol and hemorrhagic stroke in the Honolulu Heart Program. *Stroke* 20:1460–65
43. Rossouw, J. E., Lewis, B., Rifkind, B. M. 1990. The value of lowering cholesterol after myocardial infarction. *N. Engl. J. Med.* 323:1112–19
44. Rossouw, J. E., Lewis, B., Rifkind, B. M. 1992. Deaths from injury, vi-

olence and suicide in secondary prevention trials of cholesterol lowering. *N. Engl. J. Med.* 325:1813

45. Bradford, R. H., Shear, S. L., Chremos, A. N., Dujovne, C., Downtown, M., et al. 1991. Expanded clinical evaluation of lovastatin (EXCEL) study results: 1. Efficacy in modifying plasma lipoproteins and adverse event profile in 8245 patients with moderate hypercholesterolemia. *Arch. Intern. Med.* 151:43–49
46. Warner-Lambert Co. 1991. *Key Answers to Vital Questions: Lipid.* Morris Plains, NJ: Warner-Lambert Co.
47. Kritchevsky, S. B., Wilcosky, T. C., Morris, D. L. Truong, K. N., Tyroler, H. A. 1991. Changes in lipid and lipoprotein cholesterol and weight prior to the diagnosis of cancer. *Cancer Res.* 51:3198–3202
48. Winawer, S. J., Flehinger, B. J., Buchalter, J., Herbert, E., Shike, M. 1990. Declining serum cholesterol levels prior to diagnosis of colon cancer. *J. Am. Med. Assoc.* 263:2083–85
49. Andersen, J. M., Dietschy, J. M. 1977. Regulation of sterol synthesis in 15 tissues of rat. II. Role of rat and human high and low density lipoproteins and of rat chylomicron remnants. *J. Biol. Chem.* 252:3652–59
50. Hass, M. A., Longmore, W. J. 1979. Surfactant cholesterol metabolism of the isolated perfused rat lung. *Biochim. Biophys. Acta* 573:166–74
51. Hass, M. A., Longmore, W. J. 1980. Regulation of lung surfactant cholesterol metabolism by serum lipoproteins. *Lipids* 15:401–6
52. Voyno-Yasenetskaya, T. A., Dobbs, L. G., Erickson, S. K., Hamilton, R. L. 1992. LDL- and HDL-mediated signal transduction and exocytosis in alveolar type II cells. *Mol. Biol. Cell* (Suppl. 3) 354 (abstr.)
53. Patel, J. M., Edwards, D. A. 1988. Vitamin E, membrane order, and antioxidant behavior in lung microsomes and reconstituted lipid vesicles. *Toxicol. Appl. Pharmacol.* 96:101–14
54. de Groen, P. C. 1988. Cyclosporine, low density lipoprotein and cholesterol. *Mayo Clin. Proc.* 63:1012–21
55. Sabine, J. 1977. *Cholesterol.* New York: Marcel Dekker
56. Fielding, C. J., Fielding, P. E. 1982. Cholesterol transport between cells and body fluids. *Med. Clin. North Am.* 66:363–73
57. Gillies, P., Robinson, C. 1988. Decreased plasma membrane fluidity in the development of atherosclerosis in cholesterol-fed rabbits. *Atherosclerosis* 70:161–64
58. Cheng, S., Chen, Y. L. 1988. Study on erythrocyte membrane fluidity by laser Raman spectroscopy. *Cell. Biol. Int. Rep.* 12:205–11
59. Watala, C., Kordacka, M., Loba, A., Jozwiak, Z., Nowak, S. 1987. Analysis of membrane fluidity alterations and lipid disorders in Type I diabetic children and adolescents. *Acta Diabetol. Lat.* 24:141–48
60. Bhat, T. K., Sharma, R. L. 1989. Osmotic fragility of sheep erythrocytes and alterations in their membrane constituents in *Dictyocaulus filaria* infection. *Int. J. Parasitol.* 19:953–55
61. Ferretti, G., Dotti, M., Bartolotta, E., Giorgi, P. L., Curatola, G., Bertoli, E. 1988. Changes of erythrocyte membrane fluidity associated with childhood obesity: a molecular study using fluorescence spectroscopy. *Biochem. Med. Metab. Biol.* 40:101–8
62. Aozaki, S. 1989. Decreased membrane fluidity in erythrocytes from patients with Crohn's disease. *Gastroenterol. Jpn.* 24:246–54
63. Yasuda, Y., Uyesaka, N., Shio, H., Akiguchi, I., Kameyama, M. 1989. Electron spin resonance studies of erythrocyte membrane in spinocerebellar degeneration. *J. Neurol. Sci.* 90:281–90
64. Kawata, S., Chitranukroh, A, Owen, J., S., McIntrye, N. 1987. Membrane lipid changes in erythrocytes, liver and kidney in acute and chronic experimental liver disease in rats. *Biochim. Biophys. Acta* 896:26–34
65. Tacconi, M. T., Cizza, G., Fumagalli, G., Sarzi Sartori, P., Salmona, M. 1991. Effect of hypothyroidism induced in adult rats on brain membrane fluidity and lipid content and composition. *Res. Commun. Chem. Pathol. Pharmacol.* 71:85–103
66. Lalitha, T., Ramakrishnan, C. V., Telang, S. D. 1989. Lipid composition of brain regions during chronic maternal alcohol treatment and withdrawal in the rat. *Indian J. Biochem. Biophys.* 26:259–61
67. Wallin, A., Gottfries, C. G., Karlsson, I., Svennerholm, L. 1989. Decreased myelin lipids in Alzheimer's disease and vascular dementia. *Acta Neurol. Scand.* 80:319–23
68. Block, E. R., Edwards, D. 1987. Effect of plasma membrane fluidity on serotonin transport by endothelial cells. *Am. J. Physiol.* 253:C672–78
69. Engelberg, H. 1992. Low serum cholesterol and suicide. *Lancet* 339:727–29

70. Roozemond, R. C., van der Geer, P., Bonavida, B. 1986. Effect of altered membrane structure on NK cell-mediated cytotoxicity. II. Conversion of NK-resistant tumor cells into NK-sensitive targets upon fusion with liposomes containig NK-sensitive membranes. *J. Immunol.* 136:3921–29
71. Heiniger, H.-J., Brunner, K. T., Cerottini, J. C. 1978. Cholesterol is a critical cellular component for T-lymphocyte cytotoxicity. *Proc. Natl. Acad. Sci. USA* 75:5683–87
72. Mistry, P., Miller, N. E., Laker, M., Hazzard, W. R., Lewis, B. 1981. Individual variation in the effects of dietary cholesterol on plasma lipoproteins and cellular cholesterol homeostasis in man. *J. Clin. Invest.* 67: 493–502
73. Shanmugasundaram, K. R., Visvanathan, A., Dhandapani, K., Srinivasan, N., Rasappan, P., et al. 1986. Effect of high-fat diet on cholesterol distribution in plasma lipoproteins, cholesterol esterifying activity in leucocytes, and erythrocyte membrane components studied: importance of body weight. *Am. J. Clin. Nutr.* 44: 805–15
74. Phillips, M. C., Johnson, W. J., Rothblat, G. H. 1987. Mechanisms and consequences of cellular cholesterol exchange and transfer. *Biochim. Biophys. Acta* 906:223–76
75. Gotto, A. M., Pownall, H. J., Havel, R. J. 1986. Introduction to the lipoproteins, In *Methods in Enzymology: Plasma Lipoproteins Part A: Preparation, Structure and Molecular Biology*, ed. J. P. Segrest, J. J. Albers, 128:3–41. New York: Academic
76. Grundy, S. M. 1978. Cholesterol metabolism in man (medical progress). *West. J. Med.* 128:13–25
77. Gregory, T. J., Longmore, W. J., Moxley, M. A., Whitsett, J. A., Reed, C. R., et al. 1991. Surfactant chemical composition and biophysical activity in acute respiratory distress syndrome. *J. Clin. Invest.* 88:1976–81
78. Harris, J. D., Jackson, F. Jr., Moxley, M. A., Longmore, W. J. 1989. Effect of exogenous surfactant instillation on experimental acute lung injury. *J. Appl. Physiol.* 66:1846–51
79. Molloy, M. J., Kane, J. P. 1982. Hypolipidemia. *Med. Clin. North Am.* 66:469–84
80. Granot, E., Deckelbaum, R. J. 1989. Hypocholesterolemia in childhood. *J. Pediat.* 115:171–85
81. Andersen, G. E., Trojaberg, W., Lou, H. C. 1979. A clinical and neurophysiological investigation of a Danish kindred with heterozygous familial hypobetalipoproteinemia. *Acta Paediatr. Scand.* 68:155–59
82. Hoffmann, G., Gibson, K., Brandt, I. K., Bader, P. I., Wappner, R. S., Sweetman, L. 1986. Mevalonic aciduria—an inborn error of cholesterol and nonsterol isoprene biosynthesis. *N. Engl. J. Med.* 314:1610–14
83. Hoffmann, G., Charpentier, C., Gibson, K., Hübner, C. 1992. Mevalonic aciduria: impaired ubiquinon biosynthesis and model for side effects of HMG-CoA reductase inhibitors. *Pediatr. Res.* (abstr.) In press
84. Hoffmann, G. F., Gibson, K. M. 1990. Regulatory adapatation of cholesterol biosynthesis and the LDL-pathway in mevalonic aciduria. *Pediatr. Res.* (abstr.) 28:282
85. Mann, F. D. 1990. The dynamics of free cholesterol exchange may be critical for endothelial cell membranes in the brain. *Persp. Biol. Med.* 33:531–34
86. Berry, P. H., MacDonald, J. S., Alberts, A. W., Molon-Noblot S., Chen J. S., et al. 1988. Brain and optic system pathology in hypocholesterolemic dogs treated with a competitive inhibitor of 3-hydroxy-3-methyglutaryl coenzyme A reductase. *Am. J. Pathol.* 132:427–43
87. Beil, F. U., Schrameyer-Wernecke, A., Beisiegel, U., Greten, H., Karkas, J. D., et al. 1990. Lovastatin versus bezafibrate: efficacy, tolerability, and effect on urinary mevalonate. *Cardiology* 77(Suppl. 4): 22–32
88. Bruckdorfer, K. R., Demel, R. A., De Gier. J., can Deenen, L. L. 1969. The effect of partial replacements of membrane cholesterol by other steroids on the osmotic fragility and glycerol permeability of erythrocytes. *Biochim. Biophys. Acta* 183:334–45
89. Kroes, J., Ostwald, R. 1971. Erythrocyte membranes—effect of increased cholesterol content on permeability. *Biochim. Biophys. Acta* 249:647–50
90. Marenah, C. B., Lewis, B., Hassall, D., La Ville, A., Cortese, C., et al. 1983. Hypocholesterolemia and noncardiovascular disease: metabolic studies on subjects with low plasma cholesterol concentrations. *Br. Med. J.* 286:1603–6
91. Brown, M. S., Faust, J. R., Goldstein, J. L. 1975. Role of the low density lipoprotein receptor in regulating the content of free and esterified cholesterol in human fibroblasts. *J. Clin. Invest.* 55:783–93

92. Goldstein, J. L., Brown, M. S. 1977. The low density lipoprotein pathway and its relation to atherosclerosis. *Annu. Rev. Biochem.* 46:897–930
93. Hulley, S. B., Walsh, J., Newman, T. B. 1992. Health policy on blood cholesterol. Time to change directions. *Circulation* 86:1046–60
94. Kronmal, R. A., Cain, K. C., Ye, Z., Omenn, G. S. 1993. Total serum cholesterol levels and mortality risk as a function of age: a report based on the Framingham data. *Arch. Int. Med.* In press
95. Hazzard, W. R. 1992. Dyslipoproteinemia in the elderly. Should it be treated? In *Health Promotion in Older Adults,* ed. G. S. Omenn, I, Abrass, E. B. Larson, E. Wagner, 8:89–102. *Clin. Geriatr. Med.* Philadelphia: Saunders
96. Jacobs, D. R., Blackburn, H. 1993. Models of effects of low blood cholesterol on the public health: implications for practice and policy. *Circulation.* In press
97. Nat. Res. Counc. 1989. *Diet and Health: Implications for Reducing Chronic Disease Risk.* Rep. of Comm. on Diet and Health; Food and Nutr. Board. Washington, DC: Nat. Acad. Press
98. *The Surgeon General's Report on Nutrition and Health.* 1988. DHHS (PHS) Publ. No. 88-50210. Public Health Serv., US Dep. of Health and Hum. Serv. Washington, DC: GPO. 712 pp.

Annu. Rev. Publ. Health 1993. 14:115–36

GLOBAL CHANGE: Ozone Depletion, Greenhouse Warming, and Public Health

John M. Last
Department of Epidemiology and Community Medicine, University of Ottawa, Ottawa, Canada K1H 8M5

KEY WORDS: global warming, environmental ethics, population dynamics

INTRODUCTION

Mass media (1–3), the Worldwatch Institute (4), technical reports (5, 6), international expert groups (7, 8), the World Health Organization (9, 10), international conferences (11, 12), and science journals (13, 14) have all depicted damage to the biosphere caused by human activity. The topic has also received some attention in the medical press (15–21). This paper is partly speculative, but it is based on the observations and judgment of scientists, in many fields, who agree that the global environment is changing in ways that could have serious consequences for human health. Public health workers face new challenges and responsibilities in coming decades.

COMPONENTS OF GLOBAL CHANGE

Global change is a complex process; many interconnected factors can be regarded as either causes or consequences. There is controversy about several aspects, particularly those that have economic and political implications. Since the late 1970s, attention has been focused on stratospheric ozone depletion, which is leading to increased ultraviolet (UV) radiation of the biosphere (22), and on accumulation of atmospheric greenhouse gases, which many authorities believe to be inducing global warming (23–25).

Ozone depletion and global warming and their health effects are discussed in some detail in this paper. Related features of global change include environmental contamination with pesticides (26) and toxic chemicals (27)

0163-7525/93/0510-0115$02.00

and damage to aquatic ecosystems, agriculture, certain kinds of vegetation, and building materials due to acidic deposition (28). Like ozone depletion and global warming, these features are associated with industrial development and energy use, especially fossil fuel combustion and dispersal into the air, water and soil of industrial products, and toxic wastes. Other features of global change are depleted supplies of arable land, fresh water, and renewable and nonrenewable resources (29), and species extinction that reduces biodiversity (30, 31). Underlying all of these phenomena are rising population pressure and increased migration, which lie at the root of many armed conflicts (32) (Table 1).

Table 1 Components of global change

Phenomenon	Cause	Consequences
Ozone depletion	Anthropogenic	UV Radiation-related biological effects
	CFCs	
	Other halons	
	NO_x	
Greenhouse warming	Atmospheric gases	Climate change
	CO_2	Sea-level rise
	CH_4	Threats to food security
		Other health effects (see Table 4)
	N_2O	
	H_2O	
Acid deposition	Anthropogenic	Ecosystem damage
	SO_2	Respiratory system damage
	NO_x	Perhaps other health effects
Environmental pollution	Anthropogenic	Ecosystem damage
	Many chemicals	Various adverse health effects
	Pesticides	
	Radioactive waste and leaks	
Resource depletion	Population pressure	Shortages
Agricultural land	Mismanagement	Conflict
Fresh water		War
Nonrenewable resources		
Petroleum		
Coal		
Natural gas		
Minerals		
Population growth	Inadequate family planning	Migration
		Periurban slum development
		Conflict
		War
Climate, ecosystem, and other variation	Natural	Variable

STRATOSPHERIC OZONE DEPLETION

Ionizing and UV radiation act on oxygen to produce ozone. In the troposphere, ozone is a toxic constituent of photochemical smog, created by interaction of UV radiation with automobile and other exhaust fumes; ozone also occurs in some industrial emissions. In the stratosphere, ozone shields the biosphere from what otherwise would be lethal amounts of UV radiation. The stratospheric ozone layer is situated at an altitude of 12–45 km; the ozone moiety would be only a few millimeters thick at surface pressure and temperature, but of course expands greatly at high altitudes.

Ultraviolet radiation comprises UV-A, with a wavelength of 320–400 nm; UV-B, which is 290–320 nm; and UV-C, which is 200–290 nm. The most dangerous, UV–C, is prevented from reaching the earth's surface by stratospheric ozone. The least harmful UV-A passes through the stratosphere; it contributes to tanning of fair-skinned persons. Biologically harmful UV-B reaches the earth's surface in amounts inversely proportional to the concentration of atmospheric ozone. UV-B is impeded by urban air pollution, suspended particulates, aerosols, and ozone in the troposphere, as well as by stratospheric ozone.

The stratospheric ozone layer is a fragile shield. Among the chemicals that destroy ozone are chlorine monoxide, which began to accumulate in the atmosphere following the development and widespread use of refrigerants, and volatile solvents containing chlorofluorocarbons (CFCs). Chlorofluorocarbons are stable, lighter-than-air chemicals, but break down to release chlorine monoxide when exposed to UV radiation. In 1979, an expert panel of the National Academy of Sciences concluded that CFCs would damage the ozone layer, with serious consequences for human health and other adverse biological effects (33). The panel recommended restricting the use of CFCs.

The ozone layer has been under observation from satellites, high-altitude balloons, and surface stations for many years. Some thinning was observed in the 1970s (34). In 1985, observations in Antarctica showed severe attenuation, often described as a "hole" (35, 36); since then, seasonal fluctuations have been observed, with maximum attenuation in the Antarctic spring. These fluctuations have become more pronounced and widespread each year; in 1990 and 1991, they extended into southern regions of Chile, Argentina, New Zealand, and Australia (37). In the northern hemisphere, ozone depletion was first observed more recently (38); there was significant seasonal thinning over parts of Asiatic Russia in 1990–1991 and the northeastern region of North America in 1992. In early 1992, NASA air quality monitoring revealed high concentrations of CFCs and chlorine monoxide in the atmosphere above New England and eastern Canada (39). These high concentrations are expected to persist for decades and cause further deterioration of the ozone layer. The upper limit of the ozone layer, at an altitude of 45 km, declined by about 7% in 1980–1989, which suggests that chlorine monoxide or other ozone-destroying chemicals have already diffused to very high altitudes (40).

Quality and Coherence of Evidence

Measurements include atmospheric concentrations of CFCs and chlorine monoxide; stratospheric ozone density; UV radiation flux; quantitative and qualitative changes in small organisms, such as phytoplankton; and data from epidemiological and other studies of adverse human health effects that may be attributable to UV radiation. Atmospheric physics and chemistry are arcane sciences: Only miniscule proportions of the huge atmospheric volume can be examined. Instruments to measure UV radiation (expensive UV spectrophotometers and relatively cheap Robertson-Berger meters) are sparsely distributed; only 25 US recording stations existed in 1990 (41). The readings have uncertain validity in relation to human exposure. No increase in surface-level UV-B was observed in the US during 1974–1985 (42), but the measuring stations are in urban areas where air pollution confounds the readings. Some increase has been observed at a high-altitude measuring station in Switzerland (43) and Antarctica (44). Use of personal dose-meters would resolve uncertainty about human exposure in urban areas.

The 1991 Update of the United Nations Environment Programme (UNEP) Report on the Environmental Effects of Ozone Depletion (44) summarized the situation. Seasonal fluctuations continue, but there is a long-term trend toward further attenuation of stratospheric ozone; regions that will be vulnerable as attenuation progresses include populated parts of the northern hemisphere in the mid-latitudes. A reduction in total ozone of about 3% has occurred over the last ten years (45), associated at least in some places in the southern hemisphere with increased UV-B radiation readings at ground level (44). Anthropogenic tropospheric ozone and aerosols have masked the effect of ozone depletion on UV-B radiation readings in urban areas, but little or no such compensation occurs in places that are remote from industrial emissions.

Biological Effects of UV Radiation

UV-B has harmful effects on a wide range of biological systems (44, 46, 47). It causes DNA damage proportional to the intensity and duration of exposure; small, delicate organisms suffer more damage than large robust species, such as humans. UV-B impairs the growth and photosynthesis of certain plants, e.g. seedlings of maize, rye, and sunflowers. UV-B impairs the motility and reproductive capacity of phytoplankton. Change is evident in the composition of phytoplankton in aquatic ecosystems; these ecosystems are already under UV-B stress, and further increases in UV radiation are expected to cause detrimental effects, including disruption of some food chains. Moreover, marine phytoplankton metabolize a great deal of atmospheric CO_2 (48); reduction of phytoplankton would decrease the uptake of CO_2 and thus aggravate the greenhouse effect, as I discuss later. In short, the ecological effects of increased surface level UV-B radiation, although not fully predictable, are likely to be widespread and harmful. We need more studies of the effects of UV-B radiation on forestry, marine and fresh-water ecosystems, and food production.

Effects of UV Radiation on Human Health

The effects of UV radiation on human health are summarized in Table 2.

IMMUNOSUPPRESSION Induction of immunosuppression by UV radiation has been demonstrated in animals and humans (49–51). This is independent of skin pigmentation, so all people everywhere are at risk from potential adverse effects on the immune system, including increased incidence and severity of infectious disease and enhanced risk of malignant changes.

Table 2 Biological effects of ozone depletion/ultraviolet irradiation

Ecologically important	
DNA damage	Maximum effect on small and single-cell organisms
Impaired growth and photosynthesis	Poor crop yields
Phytoplankton: impaired motility	Reduced uptake of CO_2
impaired reproductive capacity	
Nitrogen-fixing soil bacteria	Reduced, damaged
Human health effects	
Immunosuppression	Enhanced susceptibility to infection
	Cancer proneness
Dermatological	Sunburn
	Loss of skin elasticity
	("Premature aging")
	Photosensitivity
Neoplasia	Melanocytic (malignant melanoma)
	Squamous cell skin cancer
	Basal cell skin cancer
	? Cancer of lip
	? Salivary gland cancer
Ocular	Cataract
	Pterygium

DERMATOLOGICAL EFFECTS Acute exposure to UV-B causes sunburn; chronic exposure leads to loss of elasticity and accelerated aging of the skin (52). Some fair-complexioned persons experience photo-allergy, which can be severe.

CANCER The most serious effect of UV-B is the enhanced risk of malignant melanoma and nonmelanoma skin cancer (53). Increased risk of other malignancies, e.g. cancer of the lip and salivary glands and intra-ocular melanoma, is uncertain. The relationship of UV radiation to cancer is discussed in detail in a current International Agency for Research on Cancer monograph (54), which concludes that there is convincing evidence for a causal relationship of malignant melanoma and nonmelanoma skin cancer to UV radiation. Case-control studies (55–57) suggest a higher risk of malignant melanoma related to a few episodes of acute sunburn, especially in childhood, than to prolonged low-level exposure with tanning. Cancer registry statistics demonstrate that the incidence rates of malignant melanoma have been rising and the age at onset has been declining for some years. Many, if not all, of these trends are almost certainly attributable to the popularity of sunbathing, rather than to exposure to rising concentrations of UV radiation; incidence rates can be expected to rise even more, perhaps rapidly, under the influence of higher concentrations of UV radiation. Mortality rates, however, have remained unchanged or have declined (58, 59); this probably reflects early detection and efficacious treatment.

OCULAR DAMAGE Ultraviolet radiation increases the risk of postcapsular and nuclear cataract and probably macular degeneration (60–62). Pterygium also occurs more frequently. Whether these effects are directly caused by UV radiation or by the combined effects of sunlight, heat, and dust is uncertain. Many other factors contribute to the risk of cataract formation; the role of UV radiation requires more careful risk assessment.

A sustained 10% decrease in atmospheric ozone has been estimated to increase the risk of cataract by 5% per annum (1.6–1.75 million additional cases worldwide). The risk of malignant melanoma has increased by 10%, and the risk of nonmelanoma skin cancer by 26% (44).

The Response to Ozone Depletion

Several kinds of response to the situation are warranted.

TREND ASSESSMENT Measurements of stratospheric ozone and surface-level UV radiation flux are needed, in relation to incidence rates of skin cancer and cataract; this should be feasible in selected sentinel communities.

Observations of UV radiation flux would be improved by installing measuring stations both in and close to urban areas and in ecologically sensitive regions remote from population centers.

RESEARCH NEEDS More research is needed on the biological effects and on the effects on human health of exposure to UV radiation. Research is needed on attitudes toward sunbathing and use of protective measures. Protective measures, such as sunscreen ointments and creams, require rigorous evaluation. There are published reports of the protective effect of sunscreen against sunburn (63, 64), but their efficacy in preventing skin cancer and malignant melanoma remains unclear. Randomized controlled trials could, over many years, answer this question, but ethical objections will arise if sunscreens are widely believed to be efficacious.

EPIDEMIOLOGICAL STUDIES Both descriptive and analytic studies are needed and should include surveillance of incidence and mortality rates from malignant melanoma and nonmelanoma skin cancer. Cohort analyses (58) are especially useful, because they reveal incidence and mortality trends in relation to generation of birth; rising incidence rates in recently born generations would suggest increased exposure to risk. Randomized controlled trials of population screening for malignant melanoma have been proposed (54), but there are ethical concerns, comparable to ethical objections to randomized controlled trials of cervical cytology for cancer of the cervix. Because UV radiation also contributes to cataract formation, we need more information on, for example, age-specific incidence rates of cataract, particularly varieties strongly associated with UV radiation, such as postcapsular cataract. Large case-control studies and serial incidence studies in sentinel communities, where data on UV flux are also available, would help to assess the risk of cataract specifically associated with UV exposure. We should maintain rigorous surveillance of infectious diseases because of the role of UV radiation in immunosuppression.

We also need surveillance of UV-related damage to other vulnerable species, e.g. phytoplankton and mammals that live at high latitudes, such as sheep in Patagonia and Iceland. There have been press reports of eye disease among sheep in Patagonia, but such information has not appeared in scientific journals. Veterinary epidemiologists could conduct studies of animal herds and wildlife populations as sentinels of human health outcomes. Skin cancer has been reported among sheep in Australia (65), which suggests that sheep might be a useful sentinel population (65).

PUBLIC HEALTH ACTION Strategic and tactical public health responses are required (66, 67). Weather advisory messages warning about safe exposure levels have been routinely used on Australian radio and television for some years, and started in Canada in early 1992; such advisories are not part of routine weather reports in the US. Advisories should include messages about avoiding severe sunburn, especially for children, and recommendations about clothing, sun glasses, and sunscreen ointments and creams that may protect against excessive exposure to UV radiation. Suncreams and lotions are assessed for toxicity and potential carcinogenicity by government agencies, such as the Bureau of Chemical Hazards in Canada. There are no Occupational Safety and Health Act standards for protection against UV radiation, and permissable exposure limits only for short-term, high-intensity exposure. Health education might help to change attitudes back to those that prevailed in western societies from late Victorian times through the end of World War I, when a pale complexion, rather than a "healthy tan," was considered attractive. Should we try to convert persons with fair skins to this view and away from the notion that suntan is desirable? If so, research is needed to identify and evaluate ways to do this. An Institute of Medicine workshop in 1990 offered some ideas (68).

PUBLIC POLICY The goal is to reduce, as rapidly as possible, the contamination of the atmosphere by ozone-destroying chemicals, notably CFCs. This requires political action. Most of the industrial nations in which CFCs are produced and used have signed the Montreal protocol (69), thus agreeing to eliminate the production and use of CFCs as soon as possible. In early 1992, the Bush administration undertook to phase out CFCs by 1995; however, even if production and use of CFCs ceases worldwide, they will continue to accumulate in the atmosphere for up to 100 years (70). Many developing nations have just begun to use CFCs; their economies will suffer more than those of industrial countries if eliminating CFCs leaves them with no alternative to these useful solvents and refrigerants (71). Moreover, CFC substitutes (hydrochlorofluorocarbons) may have deleterious effects on the ozone layer that are almost as bad as CFCs (72).

CONCLUSION There is convincing evidence that the stratospheric ozone layer has been damaged by human action, that the damage is progressive, and that this poses serious threats to biological systems and human health. Action to limit the damage has begun and must continue. In addition, public health action to mitigate risks to human health is needed.

GREENHOUSE GASES, AMBIENT TEMPERATURE, CLIMATE, AND WEATHER

In 1896, Svante Arrhenius pointed out that atmospheric CO_2 permits the passage of short wavelength radiant heat to the earth's surface and traps reflected longer wavelength radiant heat (73). In 1937, Trewartha (74) used the term "greenhouse effect" to describe how atmospheric gases stabilize the earth's temperature by allowing the passage of visible and UV radiation from the sun, which warms the earth's surface, but block the escape to space of reflected infrared radiation. Thus, the biosphere preserves a temperature range that sustains life. Without the greenhouse effect, most of the radiant heat from the sun would be reflected back into space, and the surface temperature in the shade would fall to many degrees below freezing. The surface temperature does fall if solar radiation is blocked by dust or gases, e.g. SO_2, in the stratosphere (76). Volcanic eruptions, such as those of Mount Pinatubo in the Philippines in 1991, can thus have a moderating effect on average global temperature; this appears to have happened in 1992.

Greenhouse Gases and Temperature Trends

The principal greenhouse gases are CO_2, water vapor, oxides of nitrogen, methane (CH_4), CFCs, ozone (not to be confused with stratospheric ozone), and miscellaneous others. The greenhouse gases are mainly caused by human activity, especially exhaust emissions from internal combustion engines, coal-burning electric power generators, and innumerable other industrial processes (77). There are some puzzling features of the CO_2 cycle: It remains unclear where all the CO_2 comes from and where it goes. CH_4 also comes from boreal peatlands, rice cultivation, and the flatus of cattle (78).

Since accurate recording began, the concentration of these gases in the atmosphere has risen because of the greatly increased scale of fossil fuel combustion (Table 3). Average global temperatures rose by an estimated 0.3–0.6C from 1880 to 1990, more rapidly in the last ten years than in earlier periods. However, the increase has been erratic rather than smooth, in contrast to the increase in atmospheric concentration of greenhouse gases, and it is not possible to determine whether this is part of a natural fluctuation associated with solar activity, such ocean currents as el Niño, or a consequence of the greenhouse effect.

Atmospheric scientists are concerned about the rising concentrations of greenhouse gases, and many believe that the temperature of the biosphere will rise (7, 8, 11, 23–25). There are a few dissenting views (78, 79), but the model proposed by one of these (79) was soon refuted by empirical observations (80). A temperature rise in the range of 1–5C in the next 50–100 years has been predicted; at the upper end of the range, this is greater and faster than at any time in the last 140,000 years. It could overwhelm the capacity of many species to adapt. Recent predictions (25) are for a smaller increase of 0.5–1C by 2050, but this is a global "average" that predicts a greater temperature rise, perhaps 4–5C, in mid-latitudes and a smaller increase at the equator and poles.

Table 3 Historical trends of anthropogenic greenhouse gases

	CO_2	CH_4	CFC-11	CFC-12	N_2O
Preindustrial atmospheric concentration	280 ppmv	0.8 ppmv	0	0	288 ppbv
1990 concentration	353 ppmv	1.72 ppmv	280 pptv	484 pptv	310 ppbv
Current rate of atmospheric accumulation	1.8 ppmv (0.5%)	0.015 ppmv (0.9%)	9.5 pptv (4%)	17 pptv (4%)	0.8 ppbv (0.25%)
Atmospheric lifetime (years)	50–200	10	65	130	150

ppmv = parts per million by volume.
ppbv = parts per billion by volume.
pptv = parts per trillion by volume.
Source: World Meteorological Association 1990, as quoted by National Academy of Sciences (54).

A Global Warming Scenario

In this section, I offer some speculation and opinions based on several recent accounts (3, 15–21, 81–84). A temperature rise of 5C would affect local, regional, and global ecosystems; sea levels and ocean currents; prevailing winds; fresh water supplies; agriculture; forests; fisheries; industry; transport; urban planning; demographics; and human health. Some effects are mutually reinforcing, so a small increment in an existing trend could induce massive change, in accordance with the mathematics of catastrophe theory. Such a sequence would have economic and political consequences, security implications, and direct and indirect effects on human health (15–21, 81–85). The smaller temperature rise of 0.5–1C, which is more likely, will have milder but perceptible effects.

Some of these changes may already be in progress. Six of the ten hottest summers since record-keeping began occurred in the 1980s. The summer of 1988 was not only unusually hot, grain crops everywhere suffered, which led to a reduction in world grain reserves from about 100 to 55 days (86).

WEATHER Apart from temperature rise, global warming is expected to change the configuration of jet streams and ocean currents. This will alter the distribution of rainfall, thus making some regions wetter, others drier. Weather disturbances, such as hurricanes, might become more violent.

VEGETATION AND FOOD SUPPLIES Global warming will change the distribution of vegetation. The capability of grain crops and trees to "migrate" from hot to cooler zones is uncertain (87). Some productive agricultural regions, the American midwest for instance, are more likely to get drier than wetter, which would reduce grain production, perhaps drastically. As grasslands and prairies get hotter, they dry out and become even hotter; the self-correcting effect of vegetation on microclimates is lost. This is one of several feedback loops that accentuate climate change. Temperate zone warming leads to a decline in soil moisture that impairs grain production. Ultimately these areas could become desertified, the topsoil lost in dust storms. The distribution of grasses, weeds, and allergens will also shift, as will the distribution of the myriad species of insects whose habitats are related to specific vegetation.

Food crops can be damaged in other ways. Warm climates provide a favorable habitat for insects, fungus, and microorganisms that cause diseases of grain, fruits, and vegetables.

Forests are disappearing now because of human depredation. Tropical rain forests are being cleared for agriculture or cut for commercially useful hardwood. In temperate zones, such as the high-rainfall areas of the Pacific slopes of North America, forests have been subjected to clear-cut logging. Slash-burning of tropical rain forests contributes to the atmospheric burden of CO_2 and leads to the loss of many species of plants and animals, thus reducing biodiversity as well as the amount of vegetation available to metabolize CO_2. In high latitudes, the warming could thaw permafrost, thus releasing frozen rotting vegetation in arctic bogs and ponds. This would lead to emission of large amounts of CH_4 and add to the burden of greenhouse gases.

SEA LEVEL RISE Another consequence of global warming is sea level rise, caused by melting of ice-caps and thermal expansion of the seawater mass. The extent of polar and alpine ice-melt is difficult to predict. Alpine ice-melt has been going on for many years, as shown in photographs of glaciers at intervals since the 1890s (88). In a worst-case scenario, the Antarctic ice-shelf would melt, thus causing a sea level rise of 5–7 meters. This scenario is unlikely: Recent estimates (25) predict a rise of 0.5 meters or less in the next 50 years, which would be enough to submerge many coastal wetlands and disrupt their ecosystems. This process is aggravated by other factors. For example, the annual monsoon in Bangladesh is made worse by Himalayan deforestation, which leads to torrential floods, in contrast to more gentle run-off when vegetation impedes the flow.

Many of the world's important fishing grounds are dependent on ecosystems involving coastal wetlands, so coastal flooding contributes to depletion of fish stocks. In some areas, e.g. the Humboldt current off Chile and the Newfoundland Grand Banks, fish stocks have already fallen sharply because of over-fishing in past years, perhaps aggravated by marine ecosystem changes. Ecological disasters, such as massive oil spills, are another danger to fishing grounds.

FOOD SECURITY All the above phenomena threaten food security. Severe food shortages, perhaps famines, could occur early in the twenty-first century. On the other hand, a warmer agricultural region with higher atmospheric CO_2 could become more productive (89).

COASTAL FLOODING A sea level rise of 0.5 meters would flood many coastal communities, especially in the poorest developing countries, such as Bangladesh. Sea level rise, therefore, would increase the number of environmental refugees.

DRINKING WATER Fresh water supplies are threatened by salination of coastal estuaries. Potable fresh water supplies are further reduced when seawater infiltrates subterranean water tables, as in parts of Florida. Moreover, water supplies are often polluted by toxic wastes, domestic refuse, human excreta, or all of these.

VECTOR-BORNE DISEASES Insect vectors of disease become more abundant as ambient temperatures rise. Most vector-borne pathogenic organisms flourish in warm climate zones; both the pathogens and their vectors survive better in warm climates than in cool ones; as the climate warms, temperate zones become more hospitable to ticks and hematophagous insects, such as anophelene and culicine mosquitoes. The range of bats that carry rabies also extends more widely as the climate gets warmer (90, 91). With warmer ambient temperatures, such pathogens as viruses and plasmodia remain viable for longer periods, and both they and their vectors breed more vigorously. Consequently, vector-borne diseases extend over a wider range. If enhanced UV radiation impairs immune responses, humans will be more susceptible to infection, thus further increasing the probability of epidemics.

DIRECT EFFECTS OF HEAT Over the next 50 years, the average annual number of very hot days could double in the temperate zone cities of the world. The "heat island" phenomenon, which makes cities warmer than surrounding rural areas, will lead to longer and more severe heat waves than now. In temperate zones, a sustained hot-spell increases the incidence of heat-related illness: heat stroke and heat exhaustion, which affect especially the very young, the old, and those already weakened by chronic cardiovascular or respiratory disease (92, 93).

Cities are getting larger, and many have extensive periurban slums (94).

Acts of domestic violence and civil disturbances, such as riots, occur more often in hot than cold weather. Heat waves strain utilities and essential services, such as fire departments. Heat waves increase the demand for air conditioning, but unless solar energy is used, the extra fuel consumption contributes to the burden of greenhouse gases. Climatic emergencies can be a stressor, even to stable political systems, and often contribute to a breakdown of law and order. Public health services are difficult to maintain in such situations. Other indirect effects include breakdown of sanitary services, if sewage treatment plants are inactivated by floods.

MIGRATION Depletion of resources in regions of climatic extremes, poor agricultural resources, and high birth rates have led to regional food scarcity and much population movement since the end of World War II (95). The migrants are sometimes described as environmental or ecological refugees; their predicament is often complicated by regional conflicts attributed to political, religious, or ethnic strife, but really caused by competition for living space (32). Some indirect health effects of global change are related to migration: Migrants carry the diseases of their place of origin to their destinations and, once there, they may be susceptible to diseases that they had not previously experienced. Often they live outside the established social system and may not have access to adequate health-care services.

OTHER HEALTH EFFECTS The combination of allergenic vegetation, dust, polluted water, and reduced resistance to infection (due to chronic undernutrition or UV radiation induced immune disorders) increases the risk of epidemic respiratory and gastrointestinal infections. Some commentators (16, 17, 20, 84) regard epidemics as the most serious risk associated with global change.

Overall Impact of Global Warming on Human Health

The above account conveys a sense of urgency or unreality depending upon one's point of view. The main health implications are the threat to food security, i.e. food shortages, perhaps famines, and epidemic disease. An alternative view is that warming will enhance the productivity and duration of the growing season in subarctic regions where food now grows poorly (89, 96). This sounds attractive, but assumes the presence of suitable soil, soil bacteria, and sunlight to foster more productive growing seasons. An increase in ambient temperature of permafrost to levels around 0C would not enhance plant growth. These effects of global warming are summarized in Table 4.

CONCLUSION The evidence on global warming due to greenhouse gases is confusing and equivocal. Much of it relies on models with little or no empirical demonstration that the models are valid. Uncertainty about CO_2 circulation

Table 4 Health effects of global warming

Related to temperature rise	
Heat stress illnesses	Urban areas Vulnerable groups: very young, very old, hypertensives, cardiovascular, respiratory disease
Violent behavior (?)	Domestic violence Riots, civil disturbances
Related to ecosystem changes	
Grasses, pollens	Respiratory disease Allergic conditions
Insect vectors	Vector-borne diseases
Related to weather emergencies	Natural disasters Floods, hurricanes, etc.
Related to altered precipitation	
Water-borne diseases	Diarrhea, dysentery
Related to food shortages	
Undernutrition, perhaps famine	
Increased migration	Diseases of migrants

complicates interpretation of the models. However, articles in such journals as *Nature* and *Science* that present arguments and evidence to support the global warming hypothesis have greatly outnumbered those refuting the case; empirical evidence is accumulating in support of the global warming scenario. Moreover, global warming is just part, albeit a prominent part, of a wider complex of global change. I believe the situation is serious and that public health specialists would be justified in preparing to deal with the predictable health consequences.

RESPONSE TO GLOBAL CHANGE

International Responses

Concern about the deteriorating global environment has evoked responses from several international agencies. The World Meteorological Organization (WMO) and the International Council of Scientific Unions (ICSU) have focused on climate change (97). UNEP has coordinated studies of atmospheric change (11, 44) and, with WMO and many national agencies, supports the Global Climate Observing System (98), an international collaborative endeavor coordinated by the UK Meteorological Office. UNEP was a prime mover in the United Nations Conference on Environment and Development (UNCED) in Rio de Janeiro in July 1992. Although political pressure from several directions influenced the agenda and resolutions, and although

President Bush refused to sign the Biodiversity Treaty, UNCED was not a fiasco. All nations represented at UNCED signed the protocol on greenhouse emissions. Canada and the European community are committed to lowering emissions to 1990 levels by the year 2000. Japan will hold CO_2 emissions at year 2000 levels. The US is committed to an unspecified reduction without target dates. Some statesmen, e.g. Albert Gore of the US (99), and concerned groups in many nations have proposed a more drastic reduction in carbon emissions. The arguments in favor of this are cogent; US emissions could be reduced by 10–40% at relatively low cost, perhaps even with net savings (76, 100).

National Programs

Some nations have set up multidisciplinary scientific programs to monitor the effects of global change and to plan strategic and tactical responses. These include the Canadian Global Change Program (101) and similar programs in the Netherlands (102) and Australia (103). The Canadian Global Change Program is coordinated by a working group of scientists from many disciplines and sectors. Its areas of attention include the Arctic, critical zones, climate, oceans and hydrology, culture and values, data and information systems, energy, human health, ecosystem research and monitoring, past environments, renewable resources, and security. Each of these areas has a research committee that is responsible for defining research questions, setting priorities, and encouraging research programs.

THE PUBLIC HEALTH RESPONSE

Some actions, summarized in Table 5, are appropriate despite the equivocal evidence and uncertainty about scenarios.

Surveillance

Assuming global warming scenarios are valid (or even if they are not), it would be useful to monitor the distribution and abundance of insect vectors, such as anophelene and culicine mosquitoes, ticks, and sandflies, and of the pathogens that they carry. Surveillance would work best in combination with comprehensive reporting of diseases caused by these pathogens. Monitoring of food supplies is also required, in combination with development of national food policies similar to those of Britain during World War II. Surveillance of heat-related illness, using a method similar to that used by the Centers for Disease Control for surveillance of influenza, could reveal outbreaks of heat-related illnesses and deaths.

Table 5 Public health response to ozone depletion and global warming

Action	Target
Surveillance	Water quality
	Vectors
	Pathogens
	Infectious diseases
	Fecal-oral
	Respiratory
	Vector-borne
	Cancer
	Melanoma
	Nonmelanoma skin cancer
	Other cancer
	Cataract
	Skin lesions, sunburn
Monitoring	Food production, supplies
Surveys	Behavior, attitudes towards sun exposure
	Heat-related illness
Epidemiological studies	Case-control and cohort studies (to measure risks of UV-related disease)
Evaluative studies	Sunscreen ointments, creams
	UV-filtering sunglasses
Public health action	Advisory messages about sun exposure
	Standard-setting and advice on protective clothing, etc.
	Health education directed at behavior change
	Health care of migrant populations
	Disaster preparedness
Public health policy	Development of national food and nutrition policies

Health Protection of Migrants

Whether because of changing global climate or other factors, considerable international migration is occurring. This has predictable health implications, and public health authorities in all nations affected by migration should be preparing to cope with the increasing impact of these migrations.

Disaster Preparedness

Weather disturbances could become more violent, e.g. severe floods could occur if stable weather systems are disrupted, as predicted in global warming scenarios. The mass movement of environmental refugees is a human disaster, and the scale of this movement will increase if more habitats, especially in developing countries, become unable to sustain their populations. The public health response to such emergencies is better worked out ahead of time than during a disaster.

Education, Awareness, and Advocacy

Scientists (104) and health workers (105) in many countries have discussed the implications of global change. Some have advised their national leaders to take action to limit the burden of greenhouse gases. So far, however, action has been limited and localized.

POPULATION GROWTH

The worrisome aspects of global change result from human activity. The world's population is increasing now at a rate of more than 90 million a year and is expected to pass 6 billion before the year 2000. This proliferation has been likened to a cancer of the planet: Aerial photographs and maps of urban areas at intervals resemble the appearance of neoplastic growths (106). The rate of global change is enhanced by population growth, which cannot continue indefinitely in a closed, finite system, the biosphere. Like bacterial colonies, flour beetles, field mice, shoals of fish, and roving herds of caribou, humanity must strike a balance between reproductive rates and available supplies of nutriment and other essential resources. The exponential population growth of the past eight to ten generations must be followed eventually by one of only two outcomes: leveling off or crashing into reverse. A population crash is more likely if we take no action now.

Aspirations to have children are encouraged by favorable economic conditions, by deeply held beliefs that are integral parts of the world's religions, by almost universally held moral and social values, and in some nations by pronatalist policies. There are troubling ethical dilemmas. Endeavors by health workers from industrial nations to establish family planning programs in some of the world's poorest and most crowded nations may be perceived locally as genocidal (71). But the hopes of people in nations that are emerging into industrialization to achieve the level of affluence enjoyed by Western Europeans and North Americans, with automobiles and other heavy users of fossil fuels for every family, threaten further detrimental global change.

HUMAN VALUES AND GLOBAL CHANGE

Anxiety and concern are expressed in many mass media discussions of global change. Scientific journals are more restrained: the evidence does not warrant the conclusion that the effects of global change will be calamitous. The caution of scientists in the absence of certainty has encouraged governments and many influential commercial interest groups to take minimal action aimed at reducing harmful emissions, despite campaigns by environmental interest groups. Governments in the industrial nations have mostly resisted pressure from these quarters, with backing from the energy industry. I believe there is an element of denial in this, akin to a person's reluctance to accept a diagnosis of incurable cancer or an adolescent's faith in immunity from the consequences of risky behavior.

It is helpful to recall the evolution of attitudes toward the public health that have shaped public health practice and law in the past 100 years (107). The sequence is penetration of scientific knowledge about the nature and cause of a health problem through mass media to the general public, followed by a change in values, thus leading to political pressure for legislation aimed at control of the underlying cause of the health problem. Examples of the sequence include the nineteenth century sanitary revolution and changes in social values that led to increasingly stringent regulation of tobacco use in many countries in the second half of the twentieth century.

This sequence may be beginning with growing public concern about the implications of global change for humanity. There have been proposals for a code of environmental conduct (108, 109) and for laws dealing with crimes against the environment (110). Public health organizations are mobilizing for advocacy (111), which may encourage a shift in values and might lead to the evolution and adoption of an environmental ethic that recognizes the need for sustainable development (112, 113).

If population pressure is the ultimate cause of all the other problems, we have to limit population growth. The ethical and moral conflicts involved are very difficult to resolve. After the development of the atom bomb, Albert Einstein remarked that everything had changed and that humanity required an entirely new way of thinking. The same can be said about the problems of population and the environment, the most challenging problems we face in the future. Public health workers, along with all other thoughtful members of the human race, must wrestle with these difficult issues.

Literature Cited

1. Sancton, T. A., Linden, E., Lemonick, M. D., et al. 1989. Earth, planet of the year. *Time* Jan. 2: 2–65
2. Stevens, W. K. 1989. Governments start preparing for global warming disasters. *NY Times* Nov. 14: C1, C13
3. *It's a Matter of Survival.* Canadian Broadcasting Corp., five-part radio document.; publ. as Gordon, A., Suzuki, D. 1990. *It's a Matter of Survival.* Toronto: Stoddart
4. Brown, L. R. and others. 1984 et seq. *State of the World.* Worldwatch Inst. Annu. Rep. New York: Norton
5. *Preparing for Climate Change.* 1987. Proc. of the 1st North Am. Conf. on Preparing for Climate Change, the Climate Inst. Washington DC: Gov. Inst. Inc.
6. Russell-Jones, R., Wigley, T., eds. 1989. *Ozone Depletion; Health and Environmental Consequences.* Chichester: Wiley
7. Intergov. Panel on Climate Change.

1990. *Scientific Assessment of Climate Change*. Rep. to IPCC from Working Group No. 1. Geneva: WMO/UNEP
8. Intergov. Panel on Climate Change. 1990. *Impact Assessment*, Rep. to IPCC from Working Group No. 2. Canberra: Aust. Gov. Print. Off.
9. World Health Org. 1990. *Potential Health Effects of Climatic Change*. Geneva: WHO/PEP/90.10
10. World Health Org. 1992. *Rep. of the WHO Comm. on Health and the Environ*. Geneva: WHO/EHE/92.1
11. *Rep. of the Int. Conf. on the Assess. of the Role of Carbon Dioxide and other Greenhouse Gases in Climatic Variations and Assoc. Impacts*. 1985. Villach, Austria, UNEP/WMO/ICSU Villach Conf. Statement. Geneva: World Meteorol. Assoc. WMO/NO661
12. World Meteorol. Org. 1988. *Proc. of the Changing Atmosphere Conf.* Toronto; Geneva: WMO 1989 conf. statement.
13. *Science*. 1989. Issues in atmospheric science. 243:709–81
14. *Sci Am*. 1989. Issue on Managing Planet Earth. 261:3
15. Editorial. 1989. Health in the greenhouse. *Lancet* 1:819–20
16. Leaf, A. 1989. Potential health effects of global climatic and environmental changes. *N. Engl. J. Med.* 321:1577–83
17. McCally, M., Cassel, C. K. 1990. Medical responsibility and global environmental change. *Ann. Int. Med.* 113:467–73
18. Last, J. M., Guidotti, T. L. 1990. Implications for human health of global ecological changes. *Public Health Rev.* 18:49–67
19. Haines, A., Fuchs, C. 1991. Potential impacts on health of atmospheric change. *J. Public Health Med.* 13:69–80
20. Ewan, C., Bryant, E. A., Calvert, G. D., Marthick, J., Condon-Paoloni, D. 1991. Potential health effects of greenhouse effect and ozone layer depletion in Australia. *Med. J. Aust.* 154:554–59
21. Hayes, R. L., Husain, S. T., Socci, A. D. 1992. Human health in a warmer world. *World Resourc. Rev.* 4: In press
22. NASA. 1987. *Rep. of the Ozone Trends Panel*. Washington DC
23. Schneider, S. H. 1989. The greenhouse effect; science and policy. *Science* 243: 771–81
24. Rind, D., Rosenzweig, C., Goldberg, R. 1992. Modelling the hydrological cycle in assessments of climate change. *Nature* 358:119–22
25. Wigley, T. M. L., Raper, S. C. B. 1992. Implications for climate and sea level of revised IPCC emissions scenarios. *Nature* 357:293–300
26. Carson, R. 1962. *Silent Spring*. Boston: Houghton Mifflin
27. Commoner, B. 1971. *The Closing Circle*. New York: Knopf
28. Natl. Acid Precip. Assess. Project. 1990. *Final Report*. Washington, DC
29. World Bank. 1992. World Development Reports, 1985–1992, *Development and the Environment*. New York: Oxford Univ. Press
30. Wilson, E. O. 1989. Threats to biodiversity. *Sci. Am.* 261(3):108–16
31. Wilson, E. O., Myers, N., Ehrenfeld, D. 1991. Species diversity and extinction. In *Ecology, Economics, Ethics*, ed. F. H. Bormann, S. R. Kellert, pp. 3–39. New Haven:Yale Univ. Press
32. Homer-Dixon, T. F. 1991. Environmental changes as causes of acute conflict. *Int. Secur.* 16(2):76–116
33. Panel on Stratos. Chem. and Transp., Comm. on Impacts of Stratos. Change, Natl. Acad. of Sci. 1979. *Stratospheric Ozone Depletion by Halocarbons: Chemistry and Transport*. Washington DC: Natl. Acad. Sci.
34. McElroy, M. B., Salawitch, R. J. 1989. Changing composition of the global stratosphere. *Science* 243:763–70
35. Farman, J. C., Gardiner, B. G., Shanklin, J. D. 1985. Large losses of total ozone in Antarctica reveal seasonal ClO_x/NO_x interaction. *Nature* 315:207–10
36. Watson, R. T. 1989. Stratospheric ozone depletion; Antarctic processes, in Ozone Depletion, Greenhouse Gases and Climate Change. Proc. of Joint Symp. by Board on Atmos. Sci. and Climate and Comm. on Global Change, pp. 19–32. Washington, DC: Natl. Acad. Sci.
37. Solomon, S. 1990. Towards a quantitative understanding of Antarctic ozone depletion. *Nature* 347:347–54
38. Kerr, R. A. 1992. New assaults seen on ozone shield. *Science* 255:747–48
39. Kerr, R. A. 1992. Ozone hole not over the Arctic—for now. *Science* 256:734
40. Hilsenrath, E., Cebula, R. P., Jackman, C. H. 1992. Ozone depletion in the upper stratosphere estimated from satellite and Space Shuttle data. *Nature* 358:131–33
41. Cotton, G. F. 1990. Robertson-Berger UV meter. In Summ. Rep., 1989, *Climate Monitoring and Diagnostics Laboratory*, Rep. No. 18. Boulder, Colo: Natl. Oceanic and Atmos. Adm.

42. Scotto, G., Cotton, G., Urbach, F., Berger, D., Fears, T. 1988. Biologically effective UV radiation; surface measurements in the US, 1974–1985. *Science* 239:762–64
43. Blumthaler, M., Ambach, W. 1990. Indications of increasing solar ultraviolet-B radiation flux in Alpine regions. *Science* 248:206–8
44. United Nations Environ. Programme. 1991. *Environmental Effects of Ozone Depletion,* 1991 update. Nairobi: UNEP
45. Stolarski, R. S., Bloomfield, P., McPeters, R. D., Herman, J. R. 1991. Total ozone trends deduced from Nimbus 7 TOMS data. *Geophys. Res. Lett.* 18:1015–18
46. Frank, A. L., Slesin, L. 1991. Ultraviolet radiation. In *Maxcy-Rosenau-Last Public Health and Preventive Medicine,* ed. J. M. Last, R. B. Wallace, pp. 513–15. Norwalk, Conn: Appleton & Lance. 13th ed.
47. Health and Welf. Canada, Environ. Health Dir. Health Prot. Branch. 1992. *Global Climate Change—Health Issues and Priorities*. Ottawa: Health & Welf. Canada
48. Smith, R. C., Prezelin, B. B., Baker, K. S., et al. 1992. Ozone depletion, ultraviolet radiation and phytoplankton biology in Antarctic waters. *Science* 255:952–58
49. Morison, W. L. 1989. Effects of ultraviolet radiation on the immune system in humans. *Photochem. Photobiol.* 50:4:515–24
50. Roberts, L. K., Smith, D. R., Seilstad, K. H., Jun, J.-D. 1988. Photoimmunology; the mechanisms involved in immune modulation by UV radiation. *J. Photochem. Photobiol.* 21(8):149–77
51. Kripke, M. L. 1990. Photoimmunology. *Photochem. Photobiol.* 52(4): 919–24
52. Young, A. R. 1990. Cumulative effects of ultraviolet radiation on the skin; cancer and photoageing. *Semin. Dermatol.* 9:25–31
53. Elwood, J. M., Whitehead, S. M., Gallagher, R. P. 1989. Epidemiology of human malignant skin tumours with special reference to natural and artificial ultraviolet radiation exposures. *Carcinog. Compr. Surv.* 11:55–84
54. Int. Agency for Res. on Cancer. 1992. *IARC Monographs on the Evaluation of Carcinogenic Risks to Humans: Ultraviolet Radiation*. IARC Monogr. No. 55. Lyon: IARC
55. English, D. R., Armstrong, B. K. 1988. Identifying people at high risk of cutaneous malignant melanoma: results from a case-control study in Western Australia. *Br. Med. J.* 91:114–16
56. Evans, R. D., Kopf, A. W., Lew, R. A., et al. 1988. Risk factors for the development of malignant melanoma: a review of case-control studies. *J. Dermatol. Surg. Oncol.* 14:393–408
57. Elwood, J. M., Whitehead, S. M., Davison, J., Stewart, M., Galt, M. 1990. Malignant melanoma in England: risks associated with naevi, freckles, social class, hair colour and sunburn. *Int. J. Epidemiol.* 19:801–10
58. Scotto, J., Pilcher, H., Lee, J. A. H. 1991. Indications of future decreasing trends in skin melanoma mortality among whites in the United States. *Int. J. Cancer* 49:490–97
59. Rousch, G. C., McKay, L. Holford, T. R. 1992. A reversal of the long-term increase in deaths attributable to malignant melanoma. *Cancer* 69:1714–20
60. Taylor, H. R., West, S. K., Rosenthal, F. S., et al. 1988. Effect of ultraviolet radiation on cataract formation. *N. Engl. J. Med.* 319:1429–33
61. Dolezal, J. M., Perkins, E. S., Wallace, R. B. 1989. Sunlight, skin sensitivity and senile cataract. *Am. J. Epidemiol.* 129:559–68
62. Bochow, T. W., West, S. K., Azar, A., Munoz, B., Sommer, A., Taylor, H. R. 1989. Ultraviolet light exposure and risk of posterior subcapsular cataracts. *Arch. Ophthalmol.* 107:369–72
63. Diffey, B. L., Farr, P. M. 1991. Sunscreen protection against UVB, UVA and blue light: an in vivo and in vitro comparison. *Br. J. Dermatol.* 124:258–63
64. Gilmore, G. D. 1989. Sunscreens: a review of the skin cancer protection value and educational opportunities. *J. School Health* 59:210–13
65. Ladds, P. W., Entwhistle, K. W. 1977. Observations on squamous cell carcinomas of sheep in Queensland, Australia. *Br. J. Cancer* 35:110–14
66. Am. Med. Assoc. Counc. on Sci. Aff: 1989. Harmful effects of ultraviolet radiation. *J. Am. Med. Assoc.* 262:380–84
67. Lab. Cent. for Dis. Control, Health and Welf. Canada. 1992. Rep. of symp. on ultraviolet radiat. and health, Ottawa, Mar. 1992. *Chron. Dis. Canada.* 13 (Suppl.):5
68. *Translating Knowledge into Behavioral Change: Lessons To Be Learned from Skin Cancer*. Rep. of Inst. of Med. workshop. Apr. 1990
69. United Nations Environ. Programme. 1989. *Action on Ozone*. Nairobi: UNEP

70. Environ. Prot. Agency. 1987. *Assessing the Risks of Trace Gases that Can Modify the Stratosphere,* EPA 400/1-87/001A-H. Washington DC: GPO
71. *For Earth's Sake: A Report from the Commission on Developing Countries and Global Change.* 1992. Ottawa: IDRC
72. Solomon, S., Albritton, D. L. 1992. Time-dependent ozone depletion potentials for short- and long-term forecasts. *Nature* 357:33–37
73. Arrhenius, S. 1896. On the influence of carbonic acid in the air upon the temperature on the ground. *Philos. Mag.* 41:237–76
74. Trewartha, G. T. 1937. *An Introduction to Weather and Climate,* p. 25,.London: Macmillan
75. Hansen, J. E., Lacis, A. A. 1990. Sun and dust versus greenhouse gases: an assessment of their relative roles in global climate change. *Nature* 346:713–19
76. Natl. Acad. of Sci. 1991. *Policy Implications of Greenhouse Warming.* Washington, DC: Natl. Acad. Press
77. Harriss, R. C. 1989. Historical trends in atmospheric methane concentration and the temperature sensitivity of methane outgassing from Boreal and polar regions. In *Ozone Depletion, Greenhouse Gases and Climate Change,* pp. 79–84. Washington, DC: Natl. Acad. Press
78. Lindzen, R. S. 1990. Some remarks on global warming. *Environ. Sci. Technol.* 24:424–26
79. Ramanathan, V., Collins, W. 1991. Thermodynamic regulation of ocean warming by cirrus clouds deduced from observations of the 1987 El Niño. *Nature* 351:27–32
80. Fu, R., DelGenio, A. D., Rossow, W. B., Liu, W. T. 1992. Cirrus cloud thermostat for tropical sea surface temperatures tested using satellite data. *Nature* 358:394–97
81. Abrahamson, D. E., ed. 1989. *The Challenge of Global Warming.* Washington, DC: Island Press
82. Last, J. M. 1991. Homo sapiens—a suicidal species? *World Health Forum* 12:121–39
83. Ewan, C., Bryant, E., Calvert, D. 1991. *Health Implications of Long-Term Climatic Change.* Canberra: Natl. Health and Med. Res. Counc.
84. McMichael, A. J. 1991. Global warming, ecological disruption and human health. *Med. J. Aust.* 154: 499–501
85. Brown, L. R., Durning, A., Flavin, C., et al. 1991. *State of the World 1991.* New York: Norton
86. Brown, L. R. 1989. Feeding six billion. *Worldwatch* 2:5:32–40
87. Roberts, L. 1989. How fast can trees migrate? *Science* 243:735–37
88. Houghton, R. A., Woodwell, G. M. 1989. Global climatic change. *Sci. Am.* 260(4):36–44
89. Simon, J. L., Kahn, H. 1984. *The Resourceful Earth: A Response to Global 2000.* Oxford: Blackwell
90. Dobson, A. P., Carper, E. R. 1989. Global warming and potential changes in host-parasite and disease-vector relationships. In *Consequences of Global Warming for Biodiversity,* ed. R. Peters. New Haven: Yale Univ. Press
91. Shope, R. 1990. Global warming and the public health. *Health Environ. Digest* 4:9:1–3
92. Kalkstein, L. S., Davis, R. E. 1989. Weather and human mortality: an evaluation of demographic and interregional response in the United States. *Ann. Assoc. Am. Geogr.* 79:44–64
93. Kilbourne, E. M., et al. 1982. Risk factors for heat stroke: a case control study. *J. Am. Med. Assoc.* 247:3332–36
94. World Bank. 1986. *World Development Report, 1986.* New York: Oxford Univ. Press
95. World Health Org. 1986. *Migration and health; towards an understanding of the health care needs of ethnic minorities.* Proc. of consult. group on ethnic minorities. Geneva: WHO
96. Brookes, W. T. 1989. The global warming panic. *Forbes,* 144(14):96–102
97. World Meteorol. Assoc. and Int. Counc. of Sci. Unions. 1990. *Global Climate Change.* Geneva: WMO/ICSU
98. *The Global Climate Observing System. 1991. Winchester, UK: The Meteorol. Off.*
99. Gore, A. 1992. *Earth in the Balance.* Boston: Houghton Mifflin
100. Rubin, E. S., Cooper, R. N., Frosch, R. A., et al. 1992. Realistic mitigation options of global warming. *Science* 257:148–49, 261–66
101. Canadian Global Change Program. R. Soc. of Canada (P.O. Box 9734, Ottawa, Canada K1G 5J4)
102. *Global Change.* 1991. Dutch Natl. Res. Programme on Global Air Pollut. and Climate Change. Rep. No. 00-02. (In English)
103. Natl. Health and Med. Res. Counc. 1991. *Ecologically Sustainable Development—The Health Perspective.* Canberra: GPO

104. United Nations Educ. Sci. and Cultural Org. 1990. *Final Report of the UNESCO Symposium on Science and Culture for the 21st Century: Agenda for Survival* (The Vancouver Declaration). Canadian Commission for UNESCO
105. Health workers unite for global security. 1992. *Br. Med. J.* 304:798
106. Hern, W. M. 1990. Why are there so many of us? Description and diagnosis of a planetary ecopathological process. *Popul. Environ.* 12(1):9–37
107. Last, J. M. 1993. Epidemiology, society and ethics. In *Principles of Health Care Ethics,* ed. R. Gillon, Chap. 80. Chichester: Wiley
108. Shrader-Frechette, K. 1991. Ethics and the environment. *World Health Forum* 12(3):311–21
109. *Environment and Health: The European Charter and Commentary*. 1990. Copenhagen: WHO Region. Off. for Europe
110. Law Reform Commission of Canada, Working Paper No. 44. 1985. *Crimes Against the Environment*. 1985. Ottawa: Supply and Serv. Canada
111. Canadian Public Health Assoc. 1991. *Human and Ecosystem Health; Canadian Perspectives, Canadian Action*. Ottawa: CPHA
112. UN World Commission on Environ. and Dev. 1987. *Our Common Future (the Brundtland Report)*. Oxford/New York: Oxford Univ. Press
113. World Conserv. Union, United Nations Environ. Programme and World Wildlife Fund. 1991. *Caring for the Earth. A Strategy for Sustainable Living*. Gland, Switzerland

Annu. Rev. Publ. Health 1993. 14:137–57

PUBLIC POLICY TOWARD MUNICIPAL SOLID WASTE

James V. DeLong
Olsson, Frank & Weeda, Washington, DC 20036

KEY WORDS: trash, landfills, recycling, disposal, garbage

INTRODUCTION

This paper covers three topics. The first part reviews the history and evolution of public policy toward municipal solid waste (MSW). The second sets forth the basic facts about MSW in the US—its amount and composition and the special characteristics of its discrete components. The third section analyzes the options for dealing with MSW and critiques current policy trends.

THE EVOLUTION OF POLICY ON MUNICIPAL SOLID WASTE[1]

The history of MSW goes back to about 10,000 BC, when formerly nomadic hunter-gatherers, abandoning a life-style in which people simply left their wastes, adopted sedentary habits. As cities grew, MSW, combined with the even more serious problem of sewage disposal, became a problem.

Some cities made progress. Trash bins and rubbish chutes were used in the Indus Valley as early as 2500 BC. Athens had the first municipal dumps in about 500 BC. Both China and the cities of Islam developed sanitation systems. Ancient Rome had extensive, but only partially successful, regulations that created both public and private responsibilities for cleanup efforts.

On the whole, however, these efforts were exceptions. In ancient times, in the medieval city, and on into the nineteenth century, trash and garbage were usually thrown out of windows onto the city streets, where they mixed with the tons of horse excrement (about 20 pounds of manure and several gallons

[1]The facts in this section are, unless otherwise noted, from the work of Martin V. Melosi, who manages to be erudite, enlightening, and entertaining, all at once (7).

0163-7525/93/0510-0137$02.00

of urine per horse) deposited each day. The offal was collected by scavengers, eaten by the dogs, pigs, and swans that ran loose, or allowed to pile up, sometimes to the point at which the level of the streets had to be raised.

A modern sensibility wonders why people did not care more about MSW before the nineteenth century. One obvious answer is that our ancestors' system was not as bad as it seems in hindsight. Those staples of modern life and modern waste, the daily newspaper and the suburban lawn, had not yet been invented, and containers were almost entirely made of reusable pottery or wood, rather than metal, glass, or plastic. Most waste was from food, and animals were an efficient solution.

Furthermore, until the twentieth century the average annual amount of trash and garbage in a city was probably 100 or 200 pounds per capita, at most. For a city of 20,000, which was the size of medieval Rome or colonial Philadelphia, this would amount to 2000–4000 tons per year, or 5.5 to 11 tons per day. As a problem, this amount of waste would have been totally submerged (so to speak) by the far more important problems presented by accumulation of human and animal wastes. In terms of volume, the major MSW problem must have been the disposal of 1000–1500 pounds of ashes per year generated by an urban household that burned coal and wood, a now extinct category of waste. When one considers that ashes and cinders would actually improve a muddy street surface, the practice of throwing trash out the window becomes more understandable.

Between 1840 and 1920, the total US urban population grew from 1.8 million (10% of the population) to 54 million (51%), and the number of urban areas grew from 131 to 2722. This increase in both the size and concentration of population, combined with the pollutive by-products of the industrial revolution and the steady growth of the horse problem (by 1900, New York dealt with the wastes of 120,000 horses, and scavengers removed 15,000 carcasses per year) required the radical transformation of the infrastructure of the city during the nineteenth century. Municipal solid waste was perceived as a problem, but it was down the priority list, behind organizing police and fire departments, tapping sources of pure water, and constructing sewage lines. By the 1870s, when these higher priority tasks were completed or under way, municipal reformers turned their attention to solid waste, and a nationwide movement began to establish municipal waste collection services.

From the outset, three intertwined issues have dominated decisions about MSW policy. The first is source separation—the feasibility of separating wastes according to their potential for reuse or their optimum means of disposal. Treating "solid waste" as a single, undifferentiated category conceals significant distinctions. With reference to the waste stream of the late nineteenth century, for example, cinders could be used instead of gravel on paths and roads, or could be disposed of almost anywhere without posing a threat to the public health. Garbage would breed flies and vermin if dumped haphazardly, but would ultimately biodegrade, again with little threat to public health. Tin or steel—and, eventually, aluminum—cans had valuable reuses. Rags were needed to make paper. Wood and paper could be burned as fuel, or simply for disposition. The questions, then and now, are whether source separation is valuable enough to justify its costs, and how to get it done.

The next issue is collection. Urban Americans, so accustomed to curbside pickup, forget that this is not an inalienable right. Two basic arguments favor it, though. First, pickup encourages citizens to get waste out of the home quickly, which reduces opportunities for vermin. Second, the more effort citizens must make to dispose of waste, the more likely they are to dispose of it improperly. By 1915, 89% of cities had collection service; in the late 1930s, all cities of more than 100,000 offered it.

Collection was the most expensive part of the operation, costing, circa 1910, two to eight times as much as disposal. In fact, the cost of collection was probably a principal reason for the abandonment of efforts to encourage source separation. It is far easier, and cheaper, to collect MSW if it can all be tossed into one truck than if the collectors have to keep different types of waste pure.

The third issue is the method of disposal. Separation affects the volume of trash to be disposed of by pulling out reusable materials and allows a city to use a variety of options, such as incineration and dumping, as opposed to dumping alone. However, the basic problem of what to do with tons of waste remains.

An obvious possibility, quickly adopted by municipalities in the nineteenth century, was to dump the trash in the nearest body of water and watch it sink or float away. This practice caused objections when the water was a river and there were downstream communities to consider, or when the waste washed back up onto a lakeshore. Ocean dumping was used on a massive scale by several cities, including New York. The practice continued in some places until outlawed by the Ocean Dumping Act of 1972. New York was not forced to cease the practice until 1934 (2, 7).

Another possibility was incineration, which boomed around the turn of the century, with about 30% of MSW burned in 1902. Some cities even had mobile incinerators that burned trash in the street at the point of generation. The movement toward combustion was aborted by a proliferation of technical difficulties, and by the problems of air pollution and disposition of the residues. Of the 180 incinerators built between 1880 and 1908, 102 had been abandoned by 1909. In 1913, only 7% of MSW was incinerated.

Other methods involved making garbage productive—finding "gold in garbage" was the phrase used. A process called "reduction" compressed garbage to extract oils and other valuable by-products. "Waste-to-energy" plants were constructed to utilize waste as fuel, and pig farming was voguish during and after World War I. Waste was used as landfill for construction, or to fill in swamps. Costs, noxiousness, disease, or technical problems undid all these efforts, as each went through a similar cycle of enthusiasm, precipitous implementation, reevaluation, and abandonment; over time, the dominant solution became simply to dump the waste somewhere. By 1970, the US contained 15,000 authorized, and an estimated 150,000 unauthorized, land-disposal sites.

The median age of the US population is now 33, so the majority of Americans have probably never seen that hallowed national institution, the city dump. For a big city, the disposal site was indeed a scene out of Hieronymus Bosch. A stream of public and private trucks tipped strange-looking and often odorous loads. Scanvengers pawed through the heaps looking for salable items. The smoke from the inefficient fires set to burn off anything flammable permeated everything and everyone. Bulldozers crushed down piles of ashes and refuse. Wildlife, such as cats, dogs, and mosquitos, teemed, and boys hunted rats with .22 rifles.

Not surprisingly, people came to object to the noxious odors, the vermin, and the whole gestalt. Engineers promoted the idea of the sanitary landfill, in which each day's accumulation of trash was covered with a layer of dirt to suppress smells and vermin, and practices improved slowly over the years. As environmental consciousness increased in the 1960s and 1970s, concern also arose about the effect of the open dump on air pollution and, especially, on both surface and groundwater. Municipal waste is not formally classified as "hazardous waste" under federal law, but it certainly contains many hazardous substances, ranging from used oil to old paint thinner to the toxic metals in printing inks. Many municipal waste dumps were also indiscriminate about the sources of their trash, and substantial quantities of industrial waste, sometimes including hazardous chemicals, were put into dumps over the years. All of these sources can combine to produce an obnoxious leachate. In 1986, 184 of the 850 sites proposed for inclusion on the Superfund National Priorities List were municipal landfills (11).

Location was also a problem. City dumps were put on land that was convenient for dumping but worthless for development, such as swamps or marshes. The characteristics of this property facilitated the development of leachate and the escape of contaminants. Further, attitudes changed, and formerly worthless "swamps" are now regarded as precious "wetlands."

This rise in environmental concern resulted in a series of improvements in waste sites and restrictions on methods of disposal. Numerous state restrictions were imposed over the years, and federal requirements intensified in the 1970s and 1980s. Ocean dumping was proscribed, disposal in rivers eliminated, open burning prohibited, and open dumps banned. In the 1980s, the federal government focused on eliminating air pollution and protecting groundwater. Environmental Protection Agency (EPA) rules governing MSW disposal sites, effective in 1992, establish criteria for site selection and require liners, leachate collection systems, environmental monitoring, and control of air emissions in all new landfills and extensions of old ones. These rules have caused the usual teeth-gnashing in the regulated community, but in fact the impact should not be undue. The EPA estimates that the rules will raise the average cost of disposing of MSW from $46 per ton to $48 and will cost an average of $4 per household annually (9).

The EPA has not stopped with imposing tighter control on land disposal, though. In the late 1980s, both the Agency and its state and local satellites began to regard the generation of waste, not simply its improper disposal, as the evil to be fought. They have also fostered a crusade against land disposal, arguing that if waste is generated at all it should be burned. These positions are embodied in a structure called "the Waste Hierarchy," which is a set of options for dealing with waste arrayed in descending order of desirability:

1. Source reduction. Waste can be reduced by using bulk items instead of packaged, which would mean eliminating excess packaging, avoiding certain products, or using products made of recycled or recyclable materials. Consumers can also choose reusable products over throwaway items, such as cloth diapers instead of paper/plastic or European-style durable shopping bags.
2. Recycling. Such items as glass bottles, aluminum cans, newspapers, and the many other materials that can be recycled do not take up space in landfills. Recycling has the additional advantage of conserving raw materials necessary for production from virgin sources. The EPA has initiated a major campaign to encourage recycling and to develop new techniques and markets for recycling such materials as paper, plastics, and metals. At present, about 10% of MSW is recycled.
3. Composting. This process converts organic waste into soil-enriching humus, and the EPA classifies it as a subcategory of recycling. Active management is necessary to ensure proper temperature, oxygen levels, and other favorable conditions.
4. Burning for energy. Some types of waste, particularly paper and plastic, have energy value that can be recaptured through combustion.
5. Thermal destruction. This process is appropriate when a waste, albeit flammable, does not itself generate recoverable energy and requires additional fuel, or when high temperatures are needed to destroy toxic components.

6. Landfilling. Even in a properly situated, constructed, and maintained disposal site, landfilling is at the bottom of the Waste Hierarchy.

Ocean dumping and uncontrolled land disposal are regarded as so far beyond the bounds of acceptable behavior that they are not included in the hierarchy at all. The official position is that all of the included elements are necessary for a satisfactory integrated waste management system, but that each option is to be favored over all options listed beneath it. Guided by the Waste Hierarchy, various levels of government are considering a long list of further control measures. At the federal level, proposed amendments to the laws governing wastes would put numerous recycling requirements on MSW. The figure "25%" has assumed shibboleth status as the percentage of MSW that should be recycled, but its rational justification (if any) is unclear. States have enacted laws to forbid the disposition within their borders of solid waste from other states. Although the Supreme Court recently held that such provisions violate the Commerce Clause of the US Constitution (5), there is a movement in Congress to legalize them. States are active in other areas, as well. Plastic packaging is regarded as particularly nefarious, and many localities have imposed or are considering restrictions on it. Local requirements for source separation and recycling have become common, and arbitrary recycling percentage requirements are promoted for newspapers, plastics, glass, and metal. Compulsory composting of yard wastes is also a popular regulatory proposal. Some states are proposing special taxes designed to force the incorporation of the cost of a product's ultimate disposition into its initial price. Other proposals target more directly components of the waste stream thought to present particular hazards. Efforts to collect and recycle used oil and other hazardous consumer products are under way, as are efforts to find nontoxic substitutes for materials that may produce toxic leachate.

THE WASTE PROBLEM

The Waste Stream and Its Components

As of 1988, the nation's 250 million people generated about 180 million tons of MSW, an average of about 1440 pounds per person per year, or about 3.9 pounds per person per day.[2] This figure includes residential and commercial waste (i.e. from stores, hotels, and so on), but not the waste generated by industry, agriculture, or mining. Nor does it include the special waste stream of junked automobiles, which is handled by a system of collection and disposal

[2]All discussions of MSW, including this one, rely on the numerical estimates of waste quantities contained in a report prepared for the EPA by Franklin Associates (6).

separate from the normal MSW process. Of this 180 million tons, (MT), 23.5 MT (13%) are recycled and 25.5 MT (14%) are incinerated. The rest go into landfills.

The amount of MSW generated in the US has increased steadily in recent years, from 88 MT in 1960, to 122 MT 1970, to 150 MT in 1980, to the 180 MT of 1988. Official extrapolations are for 216 MT in 2000 and 251 MT in 2010. (6). Table 1 presents the estimated composition of 1988's 180 MT of MSW, categorized by type of material and by weight.

A more detailed breakdown, shown in Table 2, classifies the waste stream by product, as well as by substance, to the extent possible. Subtotals for types of waste (i.e. paper, plastics, etc.) are not given in Table 2. These subtotals would not equal the totals for those categories in Table 1, because of the existence of mixed wastes. Disposable diapers, for example, are about two-thirds paper and one-third plastic. Furniture is wood, plastic, and textiles in uncertain percentages.

Weight is not the only important characteristics of MSW. Volume also has important effects on costs of transportation and, most crucially, determines the rate at which the capacity of a landfill will be exhausted. There is little data on waste volume, largely because it is difficult to define and measure and it varies with the degree of compression to which the trash is subjected. For example, how do we measure the volume of a milk carton—the carton in its original shape, after complete crushing, or after the partial crushing that might occur in a truck or a disposal site? Or, how about a glass bottle, which might break in a landfill, as about half do and half do not?

The only comprehensive analysis of this issue was performed for the EPA

Table 1 Weight of municipal solid waste generated, 1988, by type of material[1]

	Amount (millions of tons)	Percentage
Paper and paperboard	71.8	40
Yard waste	31.6	18
Metals	15.3	9
Plastics	14.4	8
Food waste	13.2	7
Glass	12.5	7
Wood	6.5	4
Rubber and leather	4.6	3
Textiles	3.9	2
Other	5.8	3
Total	179.6	100

[1] From Ref. 6.

Table 2 Weight of municipal solid waste generated, 1988, by type of product[1]

	Amount (millions of tons)	Percentage
Paper and paperboard		
Corrugated boxes	23.1	12.9
Newspaper	13.3	7.4
Office paper	7.3	4.1
Books and magazines	5.3	3.0
Paper toys and games	5.2	2.9
Folding cartons	4.4	2.4
Junk mail	4.1	2.3
Paper tissue and towels	3.0	1.7
Paper bags	2.9	1.6
Paper plates and cups	0.7	0.4
Paper milk cartons	0.5	0.3
Yard waste	31.6	17.6
Metals		
Large appliances	3.0	1.7
Steel food cans	2.5	1.4
Aluminum beer and soft drink cans	1.4	0.8
Plastics		
Misc. plastic products	1.7	0.9
Plastic wraps	1.1	0.6
Plastic bags	0.8	0.4
Plastic soft drink bottles	0.4	0.2
Plastic milk bottles	0.4	0.2
Food waste	13.2	7.3
Glass		
Glass beer and soft drink bottles	5.4	3.0
Glass jars	3.9	2.2
Glass wine and liquor bottles	2.0	1.1
Wood		
Wood crates and pallets	2.1	1.2
Rubber and leather		
Rubber tires	2.2	1.2
Rocks and dirt	2.7	1.5
Mixed wastes		
Consumer electronics	10.6	5.9
Furniture	7.5	4.2
Clothing and shoes	4.0	2.2
Disposable diapers	2.7	1.5
Lead-acid batteries	1.6	0.9
Other	9.0	5.0
Total	179.6	100.0

[1] From Ref. 6.

Table 3 Weight and volume of MSW actually discarded in landfills, 1988, by type of material[1]

Type of waste	Weight (1988)		Volume (1988)	
	Million Tons	% Total	Million Cubic Yards	% Total
Paper	53.4	34.2	136.2	34.1
Plastics	14.3	9.2	79.7	19.9
Yard waste	31.0	19.9	41.3	10.4
Ferrous metals	10.9	7.0	39.0	9.8
Rubber/leather	4.4	2.9	25.7	6.4
Textiles	3.8	2.5	21.1	5.3
Wood	6.5	4.2	16.3	4.1
Food wastes	13.2	8.5	13.2	3.3
Other	5.6	3.6	10.0	2.5
Aluminum	1.7	1.1	9.3	2.3
Glass	11.0	7.1	7.9	2.0
	156	100	400	100

[1] From Ref. 6.

by Prof. William L. Rathje and his University of Arizona Garbage Project.[3] His estimates of the volume of different kinds of wastes actually placed in landfills as of 1988, after removals for recycling and burning, are presented in Table 3. The researchers note that measurement problems may skew these volume estimates up somewhat; earlier unpublished data developed by the Garbage Project found that plastics and metals accounted for 12% and 3%, respectively, of the volume of materials found (11).

Characteristics of the Components of the Waste Stream

Different components of the waste stream vary widely in importance, risks presented, amenability to recycling, and methods of disposal.

PAPER AND PAPERBOARD Various types of paper and paperboard make up the largest single segment of the waste stream. In 1988, 71.8 MT of waste paper were generated, divided roughly into the categories shown in Table 2.

Most kinds of paper lend themselves to recycling (the 2 MT of paper in disposable diapers are an exception), but it is difficult to generalize. The technical and economic feasibility of using waste paper differs for the production of newsprint, tissue, printing and writing paper, corrugated paper, construction paper, and the several different kinds of paperboard (11).

[3]Prof. Rathje's project has involved a series of archaeological-style digs into landfills and has produced important information on the composition of MSW, its rate of degradation (which is almost zero), and other questions. Everyone interested in the field is greatly indebted to Rathje and his team. He also writes with humor, wit, and perspective (10).

In general, recycling technology, and thus the quality of recycled paper, is improving, but there are some inherent limitations on the reuse of paper. Wet paper, paper/food residue mixtures, disposable diapers, and multi-material products are not easily separated out from recyclable streams. De-inking, often absolutely necessary, is not cheap. The recycling process shortens paper fibers, which decreases strength and makes consumers avoid recycled paper for uses where strength is important.

Because of the importance of newspapers in the waste stream, many communities are making special efforts to collect old newspapers (ONP, in the trade jargon). The US now uses about 14.7 MT of newsprint annually, of which 1.4 MT is made from ONP. Major barriers to expansion of recycling are contamination, the expense of de-inking, and the limitations imposed by competition from low-cost virgin pulp in a highly competitive industry. Recycling capacity, also expensive to build, is currently limited (about 1.5 MT per year as of 1987). Municipal collection efforts may have outstripped capacity; the price paid for ONP went from \$6/ton in early 1990 to zero a few months later; as of mid-1991, the price was about \$4/ton (9).

Newspaper is highly combustible, with a BTU value of about 7500 per pound (8). Other papers are similar. If incineration is the treatment of choice for nonrecycled MSW, then removing the paper for recycling complicates this process by removing the bulk of the most combustible waste. In fact, if all paper were removed, additional coal, oil, or gas would have to be added to compensate.

Paper, like other organic material, may decompose in a landfill, thus producing organic acids and other chemicals and either carbon dioxide or methane, depending on whether the decomposition is aerobic or anaerobic. It is considered undesirable to allow these products to pass into groundwater, so some form of leachate collection system is required. This, in turn, necessitates a liner to catch and channel the leachate. Even if the products from decomposing paper itself were not harmful, inks contain metals and other hazardous substances.

The significance of biodegradability is actually small. It used to be thought that most waste placed in a landfill would degrade. In particular, it was assumed that yard waste, paper, food, and other organic substances would return to nature. The work of the Arizona Garbage Project has thrown doubt on this, because most landfilled garbage mummifies rather than decomposes, and 20-year-old newspapers can be perfectly readable. As a practical proposition, land disposal is usually long-term waste storage.

Efforts at source reduction for paper focus on excess packaging of consumer goods. Packages for compact disks, for example, are twice as big as they need to be, and many other forms of packaging are directed at sales rather than product protection. However, packaging of this sort is such a small part of the waste stream that even heroic efforts to eliminate the excess would produce only minuscule gains in saved landfill space.

YARDWASTE Yard waste is the second largest category of MSW, comprising about 18% by weight. It is biodegradable, and the products of decomposition are not usually considered harmful to groundwater. Yard waste is burnable, but the heat value is low—about 2000–3000 BTU per pound—so it cannot serve as fuel for waste-to-energy facilities. Fuel must be added to make it burn.

Yard waste is called recyclable, because it can be used for compost, which can be used by municipal facilities or sold to gardeners and landscapers. Interest in composting has increased greatly in recent years, and an estimated 1000 composting projects are operating in 31 states. Thirteen states have banned yard waste from their landfills (9).

Source reduction is not very seriouly suggested for yard waste, although it is sometimes proposed that grass clippings could be left to rot rather than raked.

METALS The EPA numbers show this category as the third largest, at 15.5 MT, but identifiable product categories (large appliances, steel food cans, aluminum cans, and lead-acid batteries) add up to only 8.5 MT. (The breakdown is large appliances, 3.0 MT; steel food cans, 2.5 MT; aluminum cans, 1.4 MT; lead-acid batteries, 1.6 MT.) The balance comes from the large, amorphous, product categories of consumer electronics (10.6 MT), furniture (7.5 MT), and other (9.0 MT).

Metals are recyclable. Aluminum cans are the major example of recycling success—about 44 billion (64% of the total used each year) are recycled—because the economics are favorable. Refining bauxite into aluminum takes many times the energy needed to melt down used cans.

Lead from lead-acid batteries is also recovered at a rate of about 90%, partly because of its value and partly because old batteries tend to come into the hands of the automotive service industry, which can handle them more efficiently than householders can. Other metals, primarily steel, are recyclable from a technical point of view, but, unlike aluminum, do not have economic advantages over virgin product.

PLASTICS The EPA lists plastics as composing 14.4 MT of waste annually (4). The specific product categories listed in Table 2 add up to only 5.3 MT, with the remaining plastic in the catch-all categories of consumer electronics (10.6 MT), furniture (7.5 MT), and other (9.0 MT).

Plastics have become a particular target of the environmental movement, primarily because their use has been growing and they are a convenient target.

The difficulty is that the issues presented by plastics are complicated and conflicting, and complaints are not necessarily consistent. The first complaint is that some plastics are not degradable and thus become a permanent part of the landscape when disposed of improperly on land or in water. Nondegradable plastics can also be harmful in more serious ways; plastic six-pack rings can strangle wildlife, for example. Nondegradable plastics used to be criticized for failure to decompose when placed in a landfill; this argument is heard less often since the Arizona Garbage Project found that nothing else degrades either.

The second problem is that some plastics are degradable. This raises a fear that decomposing plastic will release toxic substances into groundwater. The third problem is that plastic products tend to be bulky, thus occupying disproportionate space in a landfill unless they are compressed. If one assumes that the nation is running out of land in which to dispose of trash, bulk is a problem.

At present, there is enthusiasm for recycling plastic, and rates are rising steadily. In 1990, about 0.26 MT of plastics packaging were recycled, out of a total of 13.35 MT of plastic products produced, including about 9.4% of all plastic bottles. Recycling is not simple, though, because the broad category "plastics" encompasses numerous resins that cannot be mixed together for recycling. No single resin constitutes more than about one quarter of the 14.4 MT of plastics in the MSW stream, and 15 different major resins account for 92% of the waste, with the remaining 8% divided among numerous other types (4).

Plastics are highly combustible, with a BTU per pound of 15,000–20,000. As with paper, removing them from the waste stream for recycling has a deleterious effect on efforts to promote combustion.

FOOD WASTES Food wastes, which comprise 9% of MSW, are similar to yard wastes. They are biodegradable and burnable, with heat value comparable to yard waste. Theoretically, food waste could be composted, but this is not the usual practice.

MIXED AND MISCELLANEOUS WASTES Most other components of the waste stream present no novel issues. For the most part, such materials as consumer electronics, furniture, clothing and shoes, and disposable diapers are composed of combinations of paper, plastics, and metals, or of textiles, and exhibit the characteristics of those substances. The 234 million rubber tires discarded each year are a special problem, because they resist compression, provide homes for vermin, and, if collected in one spot, can provide fuel for stubborn and noxious fires. As of 1990, 31 states had addressed tires, and most required shredding or chipping before disposal.

HOUSEHOLD HAZARDOUS WASTE (HHW) The MSW stream also contains numerous chemical substances regarded as hazardous (11). Common household products include more than 100 substances that would be formally classified as "hazardous waste" if generated by industry, including pesticides, used motor oil, household cleaners, fingernail polish remover, batteries, paint, and similar substances. In relative terms, the amount is not overwhelming, as it constitutes less than 1% of all MSW, but these substances present the greatest danger to human health and the environment if they end up in the leachate from a landfill and the leachate escapes. In addition, business generators of small quantities of hazardous waste, who are exempt from rules governing large-scale generators, create an estimated 197,000 tons per year. An unknown fraction of this becomes municipal waste.

Although some segregation of HHW from the waste stream is feasible, complete separation is difficult. In some cases, a hazardous substance is an integral part of the basic product. In others, a hazardous substance is a small residual in an almost empty container, or, like a flashlight battery, is not considered hazardous by a consumer.

PUBLIC POLICY RECONSIDERED

Starting from this review of the composition of the waste stream and the characteristics of its specific components, the Waste Hierarchy and the policies on which it is based can be reexamined.

Disposal on Land or Water Under Minimal Restrictions

As noted earlier, disposing of waste in unlined, unmonitored landfills or dumping it into the ocean are not even on the list of options encompassed by the Waste Hierarchy. Such a total taboo seems more a product of ideology than of serious analysis, because it is far from clear that no forms of MSW can be safely dumped into the ocean. Yard waste and possibly newspapers (depending on the effects of the inks) are good examples. Other kinds of papers, metals, heavy plastics, construction debris, and glass would also be candidates. Wise policy might dictate that the dumping occur much further out than had previously been allowed, which could make the practice uneconomical. However, deciding that ocean dumping cannot be done economically is far different from outlawing it completely.

Similarly, the case against the classic big-city dump is solid, on public health, economic, and aesthetic grounds. Our medieval ancestors may have been willing to share their living space with vermin and foul odors, but modern

Americans are more squeamish. They also object to the depressing effects dumps have on property values.

The case that MSW poses a serious threat to ground or surface water is far less certain, and is usually asserted rather than demonstrated. The oft-cited statistic that municipal waste sites constitute 22% of the sites of the Superfund National Priorities List means little. Much industrial waste, including substantial quantities of hazardous waste, was placed in municipal dumps over the years. If one examines the components of the waste stream, the possible sources of serious groundwater contamination are surprisingly nebulous, except for the impact of hazardous chemicals discarded by consumers or small quantity generators. For example

1. Plastic resins do not seem to foul groundwater, and the situation vis-a-vis additives in plastics is unsettled. There is no strong evidence that they create problems, but the possibility cannot be ruled out.
2. Yard and food wastes are sometimes referenced as a source of water contamination. This might be correct, but millions of tons of organic matter decay every year in forests, fields, lakes, and streams. It is not clear why yard or food wastes would be more harmful than these natural organic substances.
3. Glass does not degrade. Nor, so far as present information indicates, do tires.
4. Paper is the largest category of waste. Some authorities think that anaerobic processes convert some components of paper into hazardous substances, but there is no consensus on the matter. There is also a question about the impact of printing inks, but, again, no consensus.
5. Incinerator ashes may present the most acute concern, because they tend to contain heavy metals.

In the light of these characteristics of the most important relevant waste streams, it may well be that threats to ground and surface water from MSW would be rendered small indeed if hazardous chemicals were extracted from the waste stream. The question is not settled, certainly, but current policy rests on dubious assumptions.

This issue may appear academic. The EPA only recently issued regulations requiring landfills to have liners and leachate collection systems when there is any possibility of a threat to groundwater, and the probability that this requirement will change in the foreseeable future is zero. Public policy will continue to be based on the assumption that disposal in unlined landfills presents unacceptable risks. However, the issue is important to the next step in the Waste Hierarchy, which is disposal in protected landfills, because it is relevant to the consequences of any failure in the system of protection. The risk from a liner failure cannot be considered apart from the risks presented by the contents of the landfill.

Landfilling

Land disposal, even if carried out with the full protection of liners, leachate collection, covers, methane gas control, and competent management, is at the bottom of the Waste Hierarchy. The EPA concedes that landfills must be used for noncombustibles, some nonrecyclables, and ash residues from incineration, but it regards this as the last resort, behind combustion (for waste that is unavoidable), recycling, and source reduction.

This conclusion rests on two major arguments, neither of which is persuasive. The first argument is that the US is running out of land space and must conserve this valuable resource by minimizing the amount of disposed waste. This argument is spurious. At the current level of compaction, which is about 30 pounds per cubic foot, the 180 MT of MSW generated in the US in 1988 could be accommodated in a pile two square miles in area and 215 feet high. Such a mound would be an impressive pile of trash, but in a country more than 3 million square miles in area, not counting Alaska, it would be no more than a minor irritant, and certainly not a national crisis. If the rate of disposal remained at 180 MT per year, it could be accommodated for the next century by finding a patch of barren waste 10 miles on a side (100 square miles) and piling compacted trash on it to a depth of 430 feet. This would be a truly awesome heap of trash, and perhaps a major tourist attraction, but it would hardly be a national crisis. If the nation did this for several millennia, it might become noticeable, but panic about a minor land use problem that might arise in a thousand years or so is a ludicrous distortion of national priorities. In any event, landfills whose capacity is exhausted can be covered over and used as parks, as is happening in—wouldn't you know it?—Japan (11).

Furthermore, even the above assessment is too gloomy. It assumes trash compaction at the pressures currently prevalent in landfills, which is about eight or nine pounds per square inch (6). Home trash compactors produce pressures of double this and can compact 60–80 gallons of household trash (8–10 cubic feet, before any compression) into about 1.3 cubic feet. Some new models produce 5000 pounds of pressure over a surface area of 136 square inches, which is 37 pounds per square inch. (Personal communications between author and applicance manufacturer.) Compacting trash before discard might well reduce the size of the National Trash Mountain considerably. The exact amount is not a calculation that can be found in any of the government publications, however.

The "running out of land" argument has a political basis. Given the NIMBY (Not-In-My-Backyard) syndrome, municipal officials have difficulty finding acceptable locations for landfills anywhere near population centers. Also, EPA rules are making landfills more expensive and are increasing the size that a landfill must reach if it is to attain reasonable economies of scale (3). Large dumps are even harder to site than small ones.

These factors create strong incentives for municipal officials to try to reduce the amount of MSW that must be put into existing facilities, thus postponing the politically risky decisions about siting new facilities. Waste reduction, by prolonging the operating lives of existing landfills, will prolong the political lives of the municipal officials.

In the longer run, the landfill problem is a transportation problem, not a shortage-of-land problem. The challenge is the efficient removal of MSW to the ample supply of existing land suitable for waste disposal. This problem could be well on the way to solution through the combination of compression, which increases transportation efficiency; containerization, which prevents the escape of wastes and odors; and railroad or truck transportation to landfill sites well away from urban areas. Massive sites exist in the Western US, and the more crowded East has ample room if the free movement of trash is allowed.

The second comprehensive argument against land disposal is that any landfill, no matter how carefully constructed, is certain to develop leaks, given enough time. Consequently, a groundwater contamination problem could develop.

From a theoretical perspective, this argument has some basis. Given enough time, some sharp object in a landfill will puncture a plastic liner and create a path for the escape of leachate, or leachate will permeate a clay liner. It may take aeons, of course. In addition, the fact of a release does not mean that the release will be harmful or irremediable, that it will actually reach groundwater, that any groundwater it reaches will be a drinking water source, that the contamination cannot be remediated, or that human ingestion cannot be avoided if the contamination is irremediable. Many steps lie between the casual assumption that "all landfills leak" and the conclusion that protection of human health requires that landfills be eliminated.

In any event, careful site-selection combined with transportation is also a response to the "all landfills leak" contention. Landfills can be located on sites where the groundwater is well-protected and the weather conditions are such that leachate formation is minimized.

On balance, the fundamental concept underlying the approach embodied in the Waste Hierarchy, which assumes that land disposal must be minimized, does not withstand analysis. It certainly cannot be justified as a matter of public health.

COMBUSTION The next step up the Waste Hierarchy is combustion, which can involve either pure destruction or waste-to-energy facilities. The pros and cons of this method of disposal are quickly stated.

On the plus side, burning trash reduces the need for land disposal. It also reduces the costs of transporting wastes. If waste-to-energy is involved, then the heat value of such wastes as paper and plastic is captured rather than lost, a benefit that had considerably more weight when oil prices seemed headed for $80 per barrel than it has today. The basic economics of combustion are not analyzed in the government documents, but, based on the some of the numbers available, they appear mediocre.

The EPA, perhaps made myopic by its own assumption that land is scarce, has promoted waste-to-energy enthusiastically, usually in conjunction with municipal governments and marauding bands of engineering consultants. As of 1989, 155 municipal waste combustors were in operation, with a capacity of 78,700 tons per day, which is enough to burn about 16% of the municipal waste stream.

This policy has brought the Agency into conflict with the environmentalist community, which is concerned about air pollution, ash disposal (ashes constitute 10–25% of the weight of the original trash and contain high concentrations of hazardous substances), and the loss of recyclable paper and plastic. The merits of these concerns are debatable. On balance, the pollution problems are apparently controllable, and the risks to human health from incineration minimal. These outcomes are heavily dependent on continuing investment in equipment and on a high quality of operations and management, however, and the populace is skeptical that municipal governments will provide these.

RECYCLING Recycling is next step up the EPA's Waste Hierarchy. Yard waste can be composted, paper can be recycled into more paper, all kinds of metal from cans and other sources, and even plastics, can be reused. Special wastes, such as used oil, tires, and batteries, can be reclaimed or converted into fuel.

Recyling involves three major steps. The first is collecting the waste and separating it into its components, the second is transferring the waste to a recycler, and the third is the actual recycling.

The biggest hurdle is source separation, which is a labor-intensive activity. This was true in the nineteenth century, and it remains so. Machines can be used to a limited degree—magnets can extract steel, for example—but there is no substitute for human sorting. Furthermore, the sorting must be done well because recycling processes are sensitive: Small amounts of the wrong color glass can ruin a batch of glass. Plastic recycling is sensitive to the presence of mixed resins. Food-contaminated or wet newspapers are useless.

Throughout history, the principal method of source separation has been to have a class of people poor enough to be willing to undertake the dirty and low-value-added work of garbage picking. Medieval scavengers were in this category, and nineteenth-century New York relied on external or internal migrants or destitute children. To the extent that the growth of the "MSW problem" is caused by the absence of this class of people, it is a measure of social progress. As Prof. Rathje has said, "[E]fficient disposal is not always compatible with . . . human dignity and economic modernization" (10).

If human scavengers are lacking, then the most obvious (and cheapest) approach is to force or induce generators of trash to separate it. This was tried repeatedly in the US in the late nineteenth and early twentieth centuries, but the effort was always abandoned, partly because of the sloppy habits of the public and partly because of the availability of cheap alternatives. The problem, then and now, is that a comprehensive system requires the generator to sort the waste into myriad categories. Newspapers, other papers of different grades, bottles of disparate colors, containers made of assorted metals, plastics made of different resins, yard waste, various special wastes (e.g. batteries, tires), and household chemicals must all be segregated. Such a system is unworkable. People will not keep 30 separate receptacles in a kitchen, even if they could be trained to identify all the different plastic resins. Such a system also significantly increases the costs of municipal collection, which is already the highest cost part of the system.

Realistically, a community might compel separation of one or two items. This means, though, that its recycling programs will either be limited to these few items or that it must incur the expense of source separation anyway, which would largely obviate the point of requiring it of householders in the first place. If household separation is not feasible, then the only alternative is for the municipality to take on the chore and make the pay and working conditions good enough to compete for workers. This is technically straightforward, but building and operating the facilities is expensive.

Once the MSW is sorted, it must still be transported to a recycling center and transformed into useful products. The industrial process required varies with the substance involved, but one important generalization can be made: It is rarely certain that recycling makes either economic or environmental sense. The bottom line is a complex result of the nature of the feedstocks involved; the amount of energy needed to transform virgin material into product, as compared with the energy required by recycling; the waste products generated by the alternative processes and the costs of their disposal, capital, and operating costs; and substitution effects among products.

For some products, such as aluminum cans, some scrap paper, and lead from automobile batteries, recycling is clearly beneficial. For most others, the benefits are equivocal or nonexistent. Technological progress might alter the balance, but at present the imposition of arbitrary recycling requirements on the MSW stream is clearly destructive from an economic point of view, and probably in terms of environmental values as well.

With respect to the protection of human health and the environment, the emphasis on recycling clearly distracts attention from the most important area—the control of hazardous household products. From a health policy standpoint, one would like to persuade households to segregate the discards containing hazardous substances from everything else. These items could then be picked up and handled separately. The current emphasis on segregating selected wastes for symbolic recycling crowds out this more desirable option.

SOURCE REDUCTION The acme of the Waste Hierarchy is source reduction. In the abstract, the concept is unexceptionable, but perusing Table 2 shows how difficult it is to achieve significant change. The US discards many corrugated boxes; on the other hand, it is nice to have products arrive unbroken. Some rail against disposable diapers, but these may be people who do not have to deal with the problem. Also, the environmentally correct position on the diaper issue is not straightforward. Collecting and processing reusable diapers uses energy, which generates pollution of its own, and the zinc oxide put on babies' bottoms rubs off on cloth diapers and creates problems for local water-treatment facilities.

Table 2 clearly shows that the current faddish targeting of particular products, such as compact disk boxes and hamburger containers, is a ludicrous kind of symbolism, intended to make people feel active and engaged while systematically doing nothing about any real problem. Source reduction, like so many other social issues, is not susceptible to a magic bullet solution, or to Canute-like decrees. It must be fostered through millions of individual decisions at the micro level.

In the barrens that constitute the public debate on source reduction, one valid point is made. Municipalities have, for the most part, made disposal of MSW free for the public. Payment does not increase with the amount of MSW generated, so no household has an incentive to reduce this amount. Following this logic, the best way to reduce the amount of waste is not through some arbitrary Gosplan, but through incentives for source reduction.

These incentives can be of two types. One, which operates on product sellers, imposes a special Advance Disposal Fee (ADF) that reflects the ultimate costs of disposing of a product and its packaging. As of 1991, 28 state bills that embodied some kind of ADF approach were under considertation, although some of these were no more than reflagged deposit measures (1). If established honestly, ADFs force producers and consumers to factor disposal costs into their decisions about the utility of product and packaging features.

The ADF concept is theoretically elegant and practically nightmarish. Its application requires the collection of fees measured in fractions of one cent from multitudinous products and requires an incredible administrative and accounting mechanism. Often, honest economics would run afoul of political realities—for example, for many products a premium should be charged if they are recycled rather than disposed of. If ADFs are imposed at a state or local level, it is impossible to match fee collection with the actual incidence of disposal costs; a package may be bought one place, discarded in another, and reach a final disposal site in yet another. Which jurisdiction gets what part of a fee that may be less than one cent anyway, and how is it all accounted for? The probabilities that ADFs will be anything other than disguised sales taxes and/or slush funds to support politically correct approaches are small.

The second incentive approach, user fees on households or businesses that vary with their MSW weight and/or volume, is much more promising. These fees would be related directly to the actual burden on the disposal system imposed by a household. Furthermore, because the municipality pays for both collection and ultimate disposition, it can factor the total costs into the amount of the fees. Householder fees also allow the use of the carrot rather than the stick to encourage source separation; a generator may pay if newspapers are tossed into the general trash, for example, but not if they are bundled separately. Finally, household fees provide a mechanism for encouraging the segregation of hazardous household subtances. Many of these are fairly heavy, such as used oil, paint, insecticides, batteries, and tires, and forgiveness of disposal fees in exchange for waste segregation could be effective.

CONCLUSION

The conclusion that grows out of this analysis is that the MSW problem is mundane and solvable, a nuisance and not a crisis. The exact shape of the best long-term resolution is not clear, because it depends on the development of markets and technology in several areas, but the general outlines are obvious. If the healthy processes of society are allowed to work, some materials will be recycled, some incineration will occur once the bugs are worked out, and landfills will remain of major importance. Future landfills will be large, remote, and properly managed. Zoning requirements will keep landfill owners from shifting costs onto their neighbors, and some regulation of transportation will be necessary. Government will also set collection fees that provide incentives for appropriate waste reduction. The heavy machinery of government regulation will be reserved for efforts to pull toxic substances out of the waste stream for more careful disposal.

It is far from clear that the healthy processes of society will be allowed to work, because powerful economic and social forces keep pushing the nation toward a crisis mentality. A crisis does exist, but it is almost totally iatrogenic, and every nostrum prescribed will make things worse. The most aggravating aspect of this crisis is not its economic irrationality, but its moral perversity.

To watch US cities, New York in particular, putting large resources into symbolic action while they squeeze the budgets needed to help desperate people is offensive.

The MSW issue is itself an apt symbol for many of the nation's current problems, which are caused by ourselves and our institutions rather than by our stars, because the dysfunctional character of policymaking is particularly obvious in this area, once we look at the numbers. If we cannot even address the MSW nuisance in an intelligent way, how can we hope to cope with real issues? Let Prof. Rathje have the last word: "Perhaps more than anything else, then, what we need as we confront the garbage problems that do exist in America is a sense of perspective" (10).

Literature Cited

1. A. D. Little, Inc. 1991. *A Report on Advance Disposal Fees*. Washington, DC: Environ. Educ. Assoc. Inc.
2. Blumberg, L., Gottlieb, R. 1989. *War on Waste: Can American Win Its Battle With Garbage?* Washington, DC/Covelo, Calif: Island Press. 301 pp.
3. Environ. Prot. Agency. Oct. 9, 1991. *Final Rule on Solid Waste Disposal Facility Criteria*. 56 Fed. Reg. 50977, 50986–87
4. Environ. Prot. Agency. Feb. 1990. *Methods To Manage and Control Plastic Wastes: Report to Congress*. Washington, DC: EPA/530-SW-89-051. 375 pp.
5. *Fort Gratiot Sanitary Landfill, Inc. v. Michigan Dept. of Natural Resources*, 112 S. Ct. 2019 (1992)
6. Franklin Assoc. June 1990. *Characterization of Municipal Solid Waste in the United States, 1960 to 2000 (1990 Update)*. Washington, DC: US Environ. Prot. Agency (EPA/530-SW-90-042). 109 pp.
7. Melosi, M. V. 1981. *Garbage in the Cities: Refuse, Reform and the Environment, 1880–1980*. Chicago: Dorsey Press. 268 pp.
8. Miller, C. 1992. Newspapers. *Waste Age* June, p. 97
9. Natl. Solid Waste Manage. Assoc. 1992. *Recycling Solid Waste*. 4 pp.
10. Rathje, W., Murphy, C. 1992. *Rubbish: The Archaeology of Garbage*. New York: HarperCollins. 250 pp.
11. US Congress, Off. of Technol. Assess. Oct. 1989. *Facing America's Trash: What's Next for Municipal Solid Waste*, OTA-O-424, p. 284. Washington, DC: GPO. 377 pp.

Annu. Rev. Publ. Health 1993. 14:159–81

MALE-MEDIATED DEVELOPMENTAL TOXICITY

Andrew F. Olshan
Department of Epidemiology, University of North Carolina, Chapel Hill, North Carolina 27599

Elaine M. Faustman[1]
Department of Environmental Health, University of Washington; Child Development and Mental Retardation Center, Seattle, Washington 98195

KEY WORDS: animal, human, abnormalities, germ cells, occupations

---

INTRODUCTION

The etiology of many of the adverse reproductive outcomes among humans is not well understood. Most epidemiologic and laboratory research focuses on maternal factors. Studies of such adverse developmental outcomes as spontaneous abortion, low birthweight, and birth defects have assessed maternal drug, smoking, alcohol, infectious, and occupational exposures. The potential role of paternal exposures has not been extensively investigated, partly because of the prevailing view that male-mediated developmental effects are unlikely (7). Thus, the acquisition of epidemiologic data and the development of a definitive mechanism for male-mediated effects have been hindered. However, recent laboratory and epidemiologic investigations have reinforced earlier animal data, which suggested that paternal exposures may be important.

This review describes potential mechanisms, highlights new data from both laboratory and epidemiologic studies, and points out limitations of previous studies and gaps in knowledge. We review studies that use a variety of developmental endpoints, including gene mutation, chromosomal abnormalities, spontaneous abortion, congenital abnormalities, and cancer. The as yet unclear relationship of these endpoints to effects on sperm production and

[1]For reprints, please contact Dr. Faustman.

0163-7525/93/0510-0159$02.00

sperm abnormalities is not discussed here (see Refs. 49, 89). Finally, we place the findings within a multidisciplinary public health context.

EXPERIMENTAL ANIMAL DATA

Experimental evidence for direct genetic effects on male germ cells has long been recognized (63). However, only recently have sufficient data been obtained from a variety of chemicals to begin to discern patterns. The number is still insignificant when compared with the hundreds of agents examined using short-term tests for mutagenicity. The more commonly utilized mammalian tests and the patterns that have emerged from these findings are presented in the next section.

Mammalian tests can be divided into two general types: those in which the heritable genetic lesions are primarily intragenic mutations or chromosomal aberrations, such as the specific locus test, and those in which the specific nature of the lesion is uncertain, but the developmental outcome is of direct relevance to humans, such as growth retardation, congenital abnormalities, tumors, and neurobehavioral effects. This section provides an overview of each test with a summary of findings.

Specific Locus Test

The specific locus test with visible markers is one of the most widely used test systems (62). A treated test-stock male mouse heterozygous for seven marked recessive loci that result in visible phenotypes is crossed with an untreated homozygous female mouse. If a germ-cell mutation at one of these loci occurs in the treated male, the offspring will express the visible mutant phenotype. The visible loci include changes in coat color, eye color, pigment, and external ear morphology. A variant of the specific locus test uses electrophoretic markers to detect protein variants at 32 loci (31).

The test detects intragenic lesions, deletions of the marked locus, and deletions involving other loci, and researchers can easily score the offspring in a large sample. The test is also highly sensitive because of the substantial historical control sample (801,406 animals) available. The test is most useful for comparative studies of radiation and chemicals and the effects of dose, dose fractionation, and cell-stage sensitivities. Additional studies can provide information on the nature of the mutation itself. Although the specific locus test does not provide an endpoint directly related to human health, it does give a general indication of the mutational damage of the male germ cell caused by different exposures.

Ionizing radiation and several chemicals have yielded positive results in the specific locus test. Recent evaluations of the effects of chemicals in the specific locus test have produced some interesting patterns (60, 61). For example, most chemicals known to induce mutations in mouse germ cells do so after meiosis (61). However, several chemicals have been identified as causing mutations with both pre- and postmeiotic cells (60). Also, there is little overlap of chemicals capable of inducing mutations in differentiating cells that also induce mutations in stem cells. If we add the dramatic differences seen among species to these complex patterns of specific mutagen sensitivity, we can easily understand why prediction of human risk from studies of heritable effects has not been more successful. Thus, studies of atomic bomb survivors and childhood cancer patients that failed to detect induced germinal mutations following stem-cell exposures do not constitute proof of the lack of mutations in differentiating germ cells.

New consideration of the mechanistic implications of mutagenic risk for exposure in the postmeiotic stages is necessary. Recent analysis of the type of mutation produced in the specific locus test has shown that small lesions are produced in the premeiotic stages, whereas large lesions are found in postmeiotic stages (60). The implications of these findings with respect to DNA structure, repair, and phenotypic effects need to be explored.

Dominant Lethal and Heritable Translocation Tests

One of the most commonly used tests involving chromosomal effects, the dominant lethal, is defined as a genetic defect occurring in the germ cell that allows fertilization, but results in embryonic death (62). The genetic basis of these deaths is believed to be structural and/or numerical chromosome abnormalities in the germ cell of the treated male animal. The death occurs either before or after implantation. The test is relatively quick and has been useful for determining the pattern of stage-specific effects. Limitations include reduced sensitivity caused by the high baseline levels of early embryonic loss and the effect of the female genotype.

Green et al (19) recommended that the assay be used to confirm positive results from other chromosomal assays. A positive effect confirms that the agent penetrated gonadal tissue and produced damage. This test is of potential importance to public health evaluation, because it not only detects chromosomal effects, but also early embryonic loss, which is an endpoint not easily measured in humans. The test reveals fetal loss caused by chromosomal abnormalities, a cause of about 40% of human spontaneous abortions (35). Radiation and several chemicals have produced positive results in this assay (6).

The heritable translocation test measures inherited chromosomal rearrangements in viable male F_1 offspring (62). Exposed males are mated to untreated females, and male offspring are evaluated for translocations by using either a fertility or cytologic test. The test is directly relevant to human health, because it specifically measures inherited chromosomal defects in mammals.

Many of the agents positive in the dominant lethal test have also been positive in the heritable translocation tests (6).

A comparative summary of test results for the specific locus, heritable translocation, and dominant lethal tests is provided in Table 1. Table 1 shows a summary of the Environmental Protection Agency-International Agency for Research on Cancer (EPA-IARC) Genetic Activity Computer Program data base, with supplementary data from the EPA Gene-Tox Program. Table 1 lists both positive and negative results from the germ-cell tests. A positive result in any of these gold standard assays is evidence of mammalian germ-cell mutagenicity (86). Most mammalian male germ-cell mutagenicity has been assessed in the mouse. These authors were careful to highlight potential weakness in these reported results. Some results were obtained using inadequate protocols, some have not been replicated, and some need to be evaluated for known test artifacts. Selby (70) highlighted potential pitfalls of many studies of dominant mutations in mammals, by citing the importance of randomizing parents between experimental and control groups, identifying preexisting mutations, doing coded assessments, and acknowledging limitations of small numbers. The accumulated data are strongly biased toward a collection of compounds known to be carcinogenic or mutagenic or structurally related to such compounds.

Of the 69 agents listed in Table 1, 13 were positive in at least one specific locus test, 18 positive in the heritable translocation test, and 48 positive in the dominant lethal tests. Five listed agents have been tested in only two germ-cell tests and have been positive in both. Twelve listed agents report mixed results from two or more tests. Three chemicals have tested positive in three germ-cell tests, and seven have tested positive in four or more individual tests.

Dominant Skeletal and Cataract Tests; Other Congenital Anomalies and Tumors

Several animal tests have been developed that may be especially relevant for risk characterization because of their phenotypic resemblance to human disorders (13, 69). The dominant skeletal test evaluates mutant phenotypes by examination of the prepared skeleton of F_1 offspring of treated males; defects may be caused by gene mutations, small deletions, or translocations. The related dominant cataract tests involves slit-lamp examination of offspring eyes. Heritability of the skeletal and cataract traits has been demonstrated in breeding studies. The inheritance pattern is irregular with incomplete expression in each generation, similar to some genetic disorders in humans. Several mutagens, including radiation and ethylnitrosourea (ENU), have induced these specific defects after paternal exposures (13, 69).

By using a general exam of uterine implants and live and dead fetuses, investigators have studied other congenital anomalies and tumors in offspring of treated males (34, 50, 81, 83).

An excess of skeletal, central nervous system (CNS), and oral cleft malformations has been detected in F_1 offspring after paternal treatment with x-rays, cyclophosphamide, ENU, and other compounds (29, 46, 47, 50, 84). Interestingly, chronic low exposure to cyclophosphamide produced an excess of congenital anomalies without affecting fertility (84). Cyclophosphamide can also produce congenital anomalies in the F_2 progeny of treated males (20). Paternal treatments with radiation, ENU, and urethane have produced tumors in the F_1 and later generations (50, 81, 83). Additional, carefully designed studies are needed to replicate and expand these findings.

Chromosomal Aberrations

The cytogenetic assessment of male germ cells is a useful method of detecting germ-cell mutagens (88). In these experiments, males are exposed to the test agent, and spermatogonia (B-type), stem cell spermatogonia, or preleptotene spermatocytes are collected and assessed cytogenetically at 1–24 hours, 50–100 days, or 12–14 days posttreatment, respectively. In addition, either postmeiotic spermatogenic cells or oocytes can be assessed in the first embryonic mitotic metaphase. Table 1 shows the results for chromosomal aberration assays for the series of chemicals that were reviewed by Waters et al (86) and Shelby et al (73).

Other Endpoints

Although it is often not the major endpoint of interest and not always reported, growth retardation in the F_1 offspring, an easily measured outcome, is important for comparison with human studies. Because growth retardation is probably due to multiple loci, it may occur at higher frequency than other endpoints. Stunted growth ($\pm$ 2 standard deviations below mean of control group) has been reported for the offspring of males exposed to radiation or ENU (71).

The value of studying behavioral endpoints to evaluate male-mediated effects has not been fully appreciated. These behavioral disturbances can provide evidence of morphological or biochemical changes, sometimes subtle, in the CNS. Behavioral effects can be seen without detectable physical anomalies (8), but the potential subjectivity in the tests may be a concern. These behavioral abnormalities can occur at doses lower than those required for other standard germ-cell mutagenicity tests (1). The specific genetic mechanism involved in the transmission of the behavioral defects is unclear, although transmission to the F_2 generation has been shown (15). Five

Table 1 Mammalian germ cell assay results[a]

Chemical	CAS number	Specific locus test[b]	Heritable translocation test[c]	Dominant lethal test[d,e]	Chromosomal aberrations assay[f]
Acetaldehyde	75-07-0				COE
Acrylamide	79-06-1	SLP, (SLO), SLT	MHT	DLM	CGC, CGG
Adriamycin	23214-92-8			(DLM)	CGC
Aflatoxin B_1	1162-65-8			DLM	(CGC)
Azathioprine	446-86-6			DLM	
BCNU	154-93-8				CCC, (CGG), ?CGC
Benzo(a)pyrene	50-32-8	(SLO)		DLM	
Bleomycin	5034-77-5		MHT	(DLM)	CGC
N-Butyl glycidyl ether	142-96-1			DLM	
Captan	133-06-2		(MHT)	DLT	
CCNU	13010-47-4			DLR	
Chlorambucil	305-03-3	SLP, (SLO)	MHT	DLM	
Chloramphenicol	56-75-7			(DLM)	CCC, CGG
Chloromethane	74-87-3			DLR	
Chloroprene	126-99-8			DLM, DLR	
Cisplatin	15663-27-1	(SLP), (SLO)		(DLM)	CCC, CGC
Corn oil	8001-30-7			(DLM)	
Cyclophosphamide	50-18-0		MHT	DLM, DLR	CCC, CGC, CGG, COE
DDT	50-29-3			DLR, (DLM)	CGC
Diazepam	439-14-5			DLM	
Dibromochloropropane	96-12-8	(SLP), (SLO)		DLR, (DLM)	

Diethyl sulphate	64-67-5			DLM	COE
Dimethyl sulphate	77-78-1			(DLM)	
Divinyl sulphone	77-77-0			(DLM)	
Ergotamino tartrate	639-81-6			DLT	
Ethanol	64-17-5			DLR, DLM	COE, (CGG)
Ethyl methanesulphonate	62-50-0	SLT	MHT	DLT	
Ethyl nitrosourea	759-73-9	SLT, SLO	MHT	DLM	
Ethyl nitrosourethane	614-95-9	SLT			
Ethylene bisacrylamide	2956-58-3		MHT	DLM	
Ethylene dibromide	106-93-4	(SLO)		(DLM)	
Ethylene oxide	75-21-8	SLP, (SLO)	MHT	DLM, DLR	CCC
Fotrin	37132-72-2			DLT	
Furosemide	54-31-9				CCC
Hexamethyl phosphoramide	680-31-9	(SLO)		(DLM), DLT	
Hycanthone	3105-97-3			(DLM)	
Hycanthone methanesulphonate	23255-93-8	(SLT)		DLT	
2-Hydroxyethylnitrosourea	13743-07-2	SLT			
Isopropyl methanesulphonate	67-63-0		MHT	DLT	COE
Mephalan	148-82-3	SLP, SLO	MHT	DLM	
6-Mercaptopurine	50-44-2	(SLP), (SLO)	(MHT)	DLM, ?DLR	
Mercuric chloride	7487-94-7			DLR	(CGG), (COE)
Metepa	57-39-6			DLT	
Methyl methanesulphonate	66-27-3	SLT	MHT	DLT	CCC, COE
Methylnitrosourea	70-25-7	SLT, SLO	MHT	(DLT), DLM	

Table 1 (*Continued*)

Chemical	CAS number	Specific locus test[b]	Heritable translocation test[c]	Dominant lethal test[d,e]	Chromosomal aberrations assay[f]
Methyl vinyl sulfone	3680-02-2			(DLM)	
Methylene bisacrylamide	110-26-9		MHT	DLM	
Methotrexate	59-05-2				COE
Mitomycin C	50-07-7	SLT	MHT	DLT	CCC, COE
Myleran	55-98-1	(SLO)		DLM, DLR	(CGC)
Nitrogen mustard	51-75-2			DLM	
Nitrogen mustard, N-oxide	302-70-5			DLT	
Norethisterone acetate	51-98-9			DLM	
Octyl adipate	103-23-1			DLT	
Phenol	108-95-2			(DLM)	
Potassium dichromate	7778-50-9			DLM	
Procarbazine HCl	671-16-9	SLP, SLO	(MHT)	?DLM	
Saccharin, sodium	128-44-9			DLM	(CGG)
Streptonigrin	3930-19-6				COE
Tetrahydrocannabinol	1972-08-3		(MHT)	(DLM)	
Thiotepa	52-24-4		MHT	DLM	CCC, CGG, COE
Triaziquone	68-76-8		MHT	DLM	COE
Triethylenemelamine	51-18-3	SLT	MHT	DLT	CCC, COE
Triethylenephosphoramide	52-24-4		MHT	DLT	
Triflupromazine	2622-37-9			DLT	

Trimethyl phosphate	512-56-1			DLT
Trimustine	817-09-4			DLM
Tris (2-chloroethyl) phosphate	73972-80-2			DLR
Urethane	51-79-6	(SLP), (SLO)		(DLM)

[a] Positive or (negative) results are listed. Conflicting reports are listed as ?; positive or (negative) only listed once, even if multiple reports exist. Summary data table compiled from Ref. 86, based on EPA-IARC Genetic Activity Profile Computer Program and Gene-Tox Program; Ref. 73; Ref. 74; RTECS online. We have not rechecked all original literature sources, but list results as reported in these sources.

[b] SLP = mouse specific locus test, post-spermatogonial; SLO = mouse specific locus test, other stages; SLT = mouse specific locus test (Gene-Tox).

[c] MHT = mouse heritable translocation test.

[d] DLM = dominant lethal test, mice; DLR = dominant lethal test, rats; DLT = dominant lethal test (Gene-Tox).

[e] Some compounds have also been tested in a dominant lethal test in female germ cells. Adriamycin, benzo(a)pyrene, bleomycin, cisplatin, ethylene oxide, ethyl nitrosourea, hexamethyl phosphoramide, hycanthone, and triethylenemelamine gave positive results. 2-Acetyl and 4-acetylaminofluorene, corn oil, dibromochloropropane, diethyl sulfate, dimethyl sulphate, methylmethane sulphonate, nocodozole, and pyrene gave negative results (see Ref. 73).

[f] CCC = chromosomal aberrations, spermatocytes treated in vivo, spermatocytes observed; CGC = chromosomal aberrations, spermatogonia treated in vivo, spermatocytes observed; CGG = chromosomal aberrations, spermatogonia treated in vivo, spermatogonia observed; COE = chromosomal aberrations, oocytes, or embryos treated in vivo.

preweaning and two postweaning tests that evaluate motor and cognitive behaviors in the offspring of exposed rodent males are examined in typical behavioral-testing protocols. These behaviors include surface righting, cliff avoidance, swimming, and avoidance. Behavioral effects have been reported in the offspring of males exposed to morphine, cyclophosphamide, nitrous oxide, triethylenemelamine, ethylene oxide, ethylene dibromide, lead, and ionizing radiation (41).

EPIDEMIOLOGIC FINDINGS

Epidemiologic findings reported to date have primarily involved two categories of exposure: lifestyle factors, such as smoking and alcohol use, and paternal occupational and environmental exposures. Table 2 summarizes the associations reported in one or more published epidemiologic studies that examined paternal exposures and selected developmental endpoints.

Fetal Loss

The first indications that paternal occupational exposures may be linked with an increase in spontaneous abortions were derived from studies of paternal exposure to vinyl chloride, anesthetic gases, and dibromochloropropane (10, 28, 33). Additional studies have suggested that other paternal occupational exposures are associated with the risk of spontaneous abortions (Savitz et al, submitted). We highlight some of the positive associations reported, recognizing that the research to confirm or refute potential causal associations largely remains to be done.

Several studies have examined paternal occupational exposure to metals, with exposure either directly measured or inferred from job title and industry. Positive associations have been reported for smelter workers and plate and steel industry workers, as well as workers exposed to mercury, lead, zinc, or copper. Although some studies (a minority) did not report an association with paternal exposure to these metals, recent studies that actually measured metal exposure reported positive findings for some metals, most consistently for mercury (2, 11, 39).

Community-based and industry-specific studies have found an excess of spontaneous abortions among wives of fathers with occupational exposure to rubber, plastics, and solvents (23, 38, 80). Implicated agents include vinyl chloride, toluene, xylene, gasoline and benzene in petroleum refineries, trichloroethane and methylene chloride in rubber manufacturing, and general trichloroethane exposure.

The relationship between paternal exposure to anesthetic gases and occurrence of spontaneous abortion has also been examined (10). Several studies showed a positive effect, including associations with operating room techni-

Table 2 Summary of epidemiologic associations

Occupation/Industry/Exposure	Developmental endpoint
Rubber workers	SA
Petroleum and refinery workers	SA
Textile workers	SB, PM, SGA
Forestry and logging workers	CNS, CHD, OC, GU
Painters	CNS, CHD, OC, LK, CBT, WT
Welders	CNS, OC, WT
Auto mechanics	CNS, OC, LK, WT
Firemen	CHD
Motor vehicle drivers	CNS, CHD, OC, LK, CBT
Sawmill workers	CHD, GU, MS
Machinists	LK, WT
Aircraft industry	CBT
Electronics industry/occupations	CBT, NBL, WT
Toluene	SA
Xylene	SA
Benzene	SA, SB, SGA
Trichloroethane	SA
Anesthetic gases	SA
Vinyl chloride	SA
Lead	SA
Mercury	SA
Rubber, plastics, and synthetics	PM
Paints	LK, CBT, WT
Solvents	LK, CBT, WT
Metals	LK, CBT, WT, HB
Dyes	LK, CBT
Hydrocarbons	LK, CBT, WT
Pesticides	LK
Cigarette smoking	OC, CNS, CHD, GU, LK, CBT
Alcohol	LBW, CHD

SA = Spontaneous abortion
SB = Stillbirth
SGA = Small for gestational age
PM = Premature
LBW = Low birthweight
CNS = Central nervous system anomalies
CHD = Congenital heart defects
OC = Oral clefts
GU = Genitourinary defects
MS = Musculoskeletal defects
LK = Childhood leukemia
CBT = Childhood brain tumors
WT = Wilms' tumor
NBL = Neuroblastoma
HB = Hepatoblastoma

cians, dentists with anesthesia exposure greater than three hours a week, and anesthesiologists. Negative findings have been reported for physicians, who usually have less exposure than the occupations mentioned above (58).

Exposures that have received much attention are pesticides and herbicides. Fourteen studies have evaluated pesticide exposure via employment in chemical manufacturing and agriculture (Savitz et al, submitted). Herbicide exposure during military service in Vietnam has also been studied. The results of studies of 2,4-D, 2,4,5-T, dioxin, and Agent Orange have been mixed (3, 9, 78).

Although not usually the primary focus of the occupational studies, paternal use of tobacco and alcohol have been examined (mostly for their role as confounders) as risk factors for spontaneous abortion. Tobacco has been evaluated in six studies, with mostly negative results; the largest relative risk was reported as 1.5 (Savitz et al, submitted). Alcohol has been assessed in three studies and has produced no association with elevated risk. However, because smoking and alcohol were not the primary factors of interest in these studies, important data on timing and dose were not collected.

Few studies on paternal exposures and stillbirth have been carried out. One study found an increased risk for smelter workers (4). Another indicated an almost twofold elevated relative risk for paternal employment in the textile industry (67).

Prematurity and Low Birthweight

Two relatively large studies of prematurity and low birthweight have been reported. An analysis of 9941 births from the National Natality Survey, a 1980 probability sample of US live births, found associations with preterm delivery (< 37 weeks) and paternal employment in the glass/clay and stone, textile, mining, and rubber/plastics/synthetics industries (67). When small-for-gestational-age births (lowest tenth percentile) were considered, fathers' employment in construction and textile industries showed elevated relative risk estimates (67).

The other study (64, 87) utilized prenatal care visit and birth discharge records for Scotland (1981–1984). Their analysis of 252,147 births did not reveal strong associations with paternal occupation for either preterm birth (<36 weeks) or low birthweight (<2500 g). Slightly elevated risk ratios were reported for preterm birth and occupations involving ceramics and textiles. Slightly increased risk ratios were noted for low birthweight among children of men employed in textile, leather, and rubber occupations.

An interesting report by Little & Sing (40) indicated that fathers' use of alcohol in the month before conception was related to a reduction in birthweight of the offspring. Based upon the study of 377 infants, fathers' use of two or more drinks daily, or at least five drinks on one occasion, was related to an average decrease of 181 g in birthweight. This association remained after adjustment for maternal drinking, parental smoking and drug use, and a variety of other potential confounding factors.

Birth Defects

Paternal occupation and birth defects in the offspring has been examined in several smaller epidemiologic studies, mostly focused on neural tube defects. Only recently has a wider variety of birth defects been explored in larger studies (45, 54). The published studies provide suggestive positive associations with several birth defects [see Table 2 for occupation-defect group results and Olshan et al (54) for comparison of published findings]. In general, occupations reported to be associated with birth defect include forestry and logging workers, painters, motor vehicle operators, welders, printers, farmers, auto mechanics, firemen, janitors, metal workers, plywood mill workers, sawmill workers, and carpenters and wood workers. Janitors, mechanics, farm workers, and metal workers reportedly have an excess of children with Down syndrome (53). Olshan et al (54) found suggestive relationships with solvents, wood and wood products, metals, and pesticides.

Only a few studies have examined the relationship between a father's smoking and use of alcohol and birth defects in his offspring. An analysis of data from the Child Health and Development Study of 14,685 births during 1959–1966 to members from the Kaiser Foundation Health Plan in San Francisco showed that father's cigarette smoking was associated with cleft lip and cleft palate, hydrocephalus, ventricular septal defect, and urethral stenosis (66). Alcohol use was related to increased risk of ventricular septal defects. An analysis of 1012 cases of birth defects from Shanghai, China, detected elevated risks for paternal smoking and anencephalus and spina bifida (93).

Childhood Cancer

More than 30 published studies have examined the relationship between paternal occupation and childhood cancer in the offspring (see Refs. 52, 65). Some earlier, relatively small studies relied on birth certificate or other vital records data to obtain information of father's occupation. Recently, larger case-control interview studies of specific childhood cancer types with collection of detailed information on occupational exposures and potential confounding factors have shown some patterns of association with certain occupations, industries, and related exposures.

Childhood leukemia and brain tumors have been investigated in most of the studies. Associations with childhood leukemia have been reported for painters, mechanics, machinists, and motor vehicle drivers. Exposures of interest include hydrocarbons (broadly defined), paints, solvents, petroleum products, pesticides, metals, and dyes. Similarly, childhood brain tumors have been associated with painters, motor vehicle-related occupations, metal processing, aircraft industry, ionizing radiation-related industries, and electrical assembling, installing, and repairing occupations. Related exposures include hydrocarbons, solvents, paints, metals, and dyes. Wilms' tumor has been examined in several studies, with associations reported for auto mechanics, machinists, welders, auto body repairmen, and painters, and related exposure to hydrocarbons, metals, paints, and solvents. Paternal employment in the electronics industry has been associated with an increased risk of neuroblastoma.

Paternal lifestyle factors in relation to childhood cancer have been examined, although it is difficult to assess the results of many published studies in which these factors are not the main focus and detailed results are not presented. An excess risk due to paternal cigarette smoking has been reported for childhood brain cancer, rhabdomyosarcoma, acute lymphocytic leukemia, and lymphoma, but not all studies have replicated these associations (30).

Recent media and scientific attention has been drawn to a report of paternal exposure to ionizing radiation and leukemia in offspring near the Sellafield nuclear plant in England (16). Gardner et al conducted a case-control study, including all cases of leukemia and lymphoma diagnosed in persons under 25 years of age in the West Cumbria Health Authority (the area containing Sellafield) between 1950 and 1985 (16). Although based upon small numbers, the authors reported a strong association between childhood leukemia and paternal employment at Sellafield (based upon a review of work records). For example, among fathers with more than 10 mSv cumulative radiation exposure in the six months before conception, the relative risk of leukemia among offspring was 8.2 (95% CI = 1.6–41.7), based on 4 (3 born in Seascale) of 46 cases and 3 of 276 controls.

Gardner et al's study has provoked much discussion and critical review (5, 14, 42, 48, 57, 82). The concerns raised generally involve inconsistency with other epidemiologic studies, alternative mechanisms, inconsistency with animal evidence, and mutation theory. The finding of paternal radiation exposure and increased risk of childhood cancer is supported by some (17, 75), but not all (26), epidemiologic studies. Studies of childhood cancer occurrence around nuclear facilities in other countries have not provided strong evidence of an increased risk (42). Other explanations include biased definition of study areas and selection of cluster boundaries, exposure to other agents at work, accumulation of radionuclides in reproductive organs, contaminated clothes brought home, and such exposures as infectious agents (42, 57). Direct evidence for paternal germ-cell effects due to ionizing radiation and leukemia in offspring is lacking (although see Ref. 51). In addition, compared with results from animal studies, the minimum dose of radiation needed to double the rate of a variety of genetic defects in the mouse is about 150–300 mSv, which is 15–30 times greater than the dose received by Sellafield workers in the six months before conception (14). Although the Gardner et al study has been criticized on epidemiologic and genetic grounds, it has provoked new interest in paternal exposures and disease in offspring.

Atomic Bomb Survivors

Two unique cohorts with relatively large and well-documented exposures are the survivors of the atomic bombs in Japan and survivors of childhood cancer. These are certainly groups with high-dose exposures in which one would expect to see an effect, if it exists. No association with an increased risk of leukemia, birth defects, or other adverse pregnancy outcomes among the offspring of Japanese men who survived the bomb have been found (55, 85, 91, 92). Among the 7387 men exposed (mean radiation dose of 492 mSv), 5 cases of leukemia among offspring were found compared with 5.2 expected. An important consideration is that the number of conceptions just after the bomb was limited and Gardner et al's study found the highest risk for the period of exposure in the six months before conception. As noted above, the most important exposure period may involve the postmeiotic germ-cell stages. The nature of the radiation exposure, i.e. the high-dose, acute exposure of the bomb and a chronic, lower-dose occupational exposure, may be related to some of the differences in results (51, 82).

Childhood Cancer Survivors

Another group of uniquely exposed individuals is childhood cancer survivors. Studies have generally found no association with reproductive endpoints, such as fetal death, low birth weight, neonatal death, congenital anomalies, and childhood cancer, among offspring of male survivors (24, 37). These studies all had limited power to detect an association with developmental endpoints, such as congenital anomalies and childhood cancer among offspring. A recent single hospital study had only 38 children of male childhood cancer survivors who received chemotherapy (18). The detailed, multi-institutional study of Wilms' tumor survivors (37) ascertained only 34 pregnancies of wives of male survivors. A large British study, based on 1078 male survivors, had only 300 reported offspring, and only 48 of those were considered to have been exposed to either radiotherapy or chemotherapy (24, 25). Thus, although the published studies may have ruled out extremely large relative risks, until larger, multi-institutional studies with an adequate number of survivors are conducted, the potential association with adverse reproductive outcomes remains an open question.

Methodologic Issues

The epidemiologic findings summarized above, for the most part, have been published only recently, since 1980. They provide valuable clues that can serve as a basis for further evaluation. One of the most important sources of potential bias is the misclassification of exposure. This is especially problematic for the majority of studies of paternal exposures, because most have examined paternal occupational exposures. A potential source of misclassification involves the use of birth certificates as the primary means to ascertain parental job title and industry at the time of birth (72). This type of error is nondifferential with respect to case or control status.

Uncontrolled confounding due to factors associated with outcome and the risk factor may also bias the results. Studies using the birth certificate have only limited information on potentially confounding factors. Because at present there are very few definitive risk factors for most adverse developmental outcomes, the role of confounding cannot be fully evaluated.

Given the rarity of these outcomes, epidemiologic studies are often hindered by limited sample sizes. This limitation has often led to the use of very broad groupings of outcome, occupation, and other exposures, thus providing an additional source of misclassification. Additionally, small samples have, for the most part, precluded the analysis of subgroups, such as the pathogenetic subgroups of spontaneous abortions, birth defects, and childhood cancer.

In sum, the epidemiologic studies of paternal exposures and developmental endpoints are limited by the usual imperfections of epidemiologic research. It is probably true that many of the published studies suffer to some degree from misclassification of paternal occupational exposures. This would result in a bias of the relative risk estimates toward the null, that is, these studies may have yielded underestimates of the actual relative risk (59). Nonetheless, other potential biases are probably at play to a varying degree and with unpredictable effects.

POTENTIAL MECHANISMS

The mechanisms proposed for male-mediated effects on offspring are of two general types: direct germ-cell effects by either genetic or epigenetic mechanisms and indirect effects by transmission of agents to the mother via the seminal fluid and maternal exposure to toxicants brought home by the father.

Seminal fluid transfer of chemicals has been known for many years and has been implicated in male-mediated developmental effects for methadone, trimethaprin, phenytoin, cyclophosphamide, sulfamethodoxozole, and valproic acid (44, 77). In fact, some agents, such as thalidomide, tetracycline, and cocaine, bind directly to sperm (90). Information on concentrations of the agent in the semen, solubility, and half-life are central in determining the contribution of these exposure pathways to adverse developmental outcome. Hales and coworkers (21, 56) reported a twofold increase in preimplantation loss, presumably through seminal fluid transfer of cyclophosphamide. Replication of these suggestive findings is warranted.

Another possible route of maternal exposure in humans is by household contamination with substances brought home by the father. Examples include lead, beryllium, tetrachlorodibenzodioxin, and polychlorinated biphenyls (36). The role of household contamination in adverse pregnancy outcome is uncertain at present.

Direct germ-cell effects by genetic mechanisms are the basis for the heritable mutation assays described earlier. Thus, this mechanism of paternally mediated effects has already been shown to result in a myriad of manifestations that encompass all endpoints of developmental toxicity, including growth retardation, specific malformations, behavioral and functional abnormalities, and carcinogenesis.

The recent research literature has provided intriguing clues on unconventional mechanisms that might explain paternal influences on development. Recent investigations demonstrating a key role for parent-of-origin differences in phenotype have supported the view that genomic imprinting may be an important biologic process (22). Initial clues have been provided by early developmental work with pronuclear transplantation and parthenogenetic experiments (76). These studies showed differing patterns of embryonic and placental growth dependent upon the parent of origin. Varying the contribution of maternally and paternally derived chromosomal material can produce a variety of adverse developmental outcomes, including early miscarriage, intrauterine growth retardation, and placental overgrowth (79). Chemicals administered to the male before fertilization can mimic the effects observed with paternally derived zygotes. A recent study demonstrated that cyclophosphamide treatment of male rats before mating can cause a selective loss of inner cell mass-derived cells in postimplantation sites without apparent effects on trophoblast development (32).

Studies of human deletion syndromes and embryonal tumors have provided additional data on paternally mediated effects. The phenotype of the Prader-Willi syndrome, in which the paternally derived chromosome 15 has deletions, is markedly different from the Angelman Syndrome cases, in which the deletions are in the maternally derived chromosome 15 (43). Several childhood tumors, such as Wilms' tumor and retinoblastoma, have shown parent-of-origin differences (12, 68). For many cases, the maternally derived chromosome is apparently lost during tumorigenesis, which implies that the maternal chromosome harbors tumor suppressor gene(s). In most cases of retinoblastoma, the new mutations are of paternal origin (94). Other lines of evidence for phenotypic differences due to genomic imprinting include uniparental disomy and disorders with a modified inheritance pattern (22).

These clues from the animal and human literature point to epigenetic mechanisms, that is, changes in gene activity during development (for example, methylation or addition or removal of proteins that control imprinting), as being the basis for differential gene-activity patterns (27). Epigenetic imprinting-like differences could occur through paternally mediated developmental toxicity. The chemical 5-azacytidine is not mutagenic, but has been shown to modify the methylation pattern of genes and thus alter gene activity pattern by an epigenetic mechanism. This chemical is incorporated into DNA and inhibits normal methylase activity. Such an exposure in vitro has caused 10–30% of previously inactive genes to become reactivated. This effect represents about a 1 millionfold increase over spontaneous reversion rates (27).

It is not difficult to imagine that agents that cause paternally mediated effects could potentially function via these epigenetic pathways to cause adverse paternally mediated developmental outcomes. Obviously, much more work is needed to define the role that changes in methylation patterns and imprinting may play in defining developmental outcome after chemical exposure of the male.

CONCLUSIONS: A MULTIDISCIPLINARY PERSPECTIVE

This review has presented information from both the animal and human literatures of chemical and radiation-induced, male-mediated developmental toxicity. Unfortunately, both literatures are plagued with incomplete reports characterized by either biases, incomplete exposure assessments, or small numbers of experimental units to evaluate. Nevertheless, enough scientific information exists to suggest potential associations and mechanisms for both genetic and epigenetic mechanisms of action. Several chemicals and other agents can induce mutations in the male germ cell and produce such outcomes as pregnancy loss, growth retardation, congenital anomalies, tumors, and neurobehavioral effects. As data continue to accumulate, investigators will be able to examine the patterns relating to concordance among test system results, the relationship between chemical structure and test results, germ-cell stage specificity, and the specific nature of the genetic damage induced.

Initial epidemiologic studies have identified certain paternal environmental, occupational, and lifestyle exposures that may increase the risk of pregnancy loss, preterm delivery, intrauterine growth retardation, birth defects, and childhood cancer. At present, many of these findings await confirmation. More work is needed to evaluate and attempt to synthesize these findings, describe limitations, and propose potentially fruitful areas of further investigation. In addition, evaluation of epidemiologic studies should incorporate consideration of laboratory results and biologic models. Direct comparison with results of laboratory studies is difficult at present, because the epidemiologic findings mostly involve association with a broad array of occupations and industries. This makes it difficult to compare directly specific agents listed in Table 1 with exposures listed in Table 2.

The public health relevance of male-mediated developmental toxicity currently cannot be fully evaluated. More basic experimental animal and human data, as well as elaboration of possible mechanisms, are needed. At a fundamental level, the available data do indicate that paternal exposures can produce adverse developmental outcomes. The developmental endpoints discussed here are of public health importance; given that most do not have a known etiology, male-mediated pathways should not be ignored. Hopefully, this review will stimulate the combined community of toxicologists, epidemiologists, and geneticists to evaluate further this pathway of toxicity.

ACKNOWLEDGMENTS

This work was supported by National Institute of Environmental Health Sciences Grant 01357 and a grant from the Charles A. Dana Foundation. We thank Drs. David Savitz and Michael Shelby for their helpful review and comments, as well as Zamyat Kirby for editorial assistance and Lynn Welson and Anne Crumpler for secretarial support. We also thank Drs. Michael Waters, Bryn Bridges, and Michael Shelby for providing copies of their unpublished manuscripts.

Literature Cited

1. Adams, P. M., Shabrawy, O., Legator, M. S. 1984. Male-transmitted developmental and neurobehavioral deficits. *Teratog. Carcinog. Mutagen* 4:149–69
2. Alcser, K. H., Brix, K. A., Fine, L. J., Kallenbach, L. R., Wolfe, R. A. 1989. Occupational mercury exposure and male reproductive health. *Am. J. Ind. Med.* 15:517–29
3. Aschengrau, A., Monson, R. R. 1989. Paternal military service in Vietnam and risk of spontaneous abortion. *J. Occup. Med.* 31:619–23
4. Beckman, L., Nordstrom, S. 1982. Occupational and environmental risks in and around a smelter in northern Sweden. IX. Fetal mortality among wives of smelter workers. *Hereditas* 97:1–7
5. Beral, V. Leukaemia and nuclear installations. 1990. *Br. Med. J.* 300:411–12
6. Bishop, J. B., Shelby, M. D. 1990. Mammalian heritable effects research in the National Toxicology Program. In *Biology of Mammalian Germ Cell Mutagenesis*, ed. J. W. Allen, B. A. Bridges, M. F. Lyon, M. J. Moses, L. B. Russell, 34:425–35. Cold Spring Harbor, New York: Cold Spring Harbor Lab. Press. 461 pp.
7. Brown, N. A. 1985. Are offspring at risk from their father's exposure to toxins? *Nature* 316:110
8. Butcher, R. E. 1976. Behavioral testing as a method for assessing risk. *Environ. Health Perspect.* 18:75–78
9. Cent. for Dis. Control Vietnam Exp. Study. 1988. Health status of Vietnam Veterans, III. Reproductive outcomes and child health. *J. Am. Med. Assoc.* 259:2715–19
10. Cohen, E. N., Brown, B. W., Wu, M. L., Whitcher, C. E., Brodsky, J.

B., et al. 1980. Occupational disease in dentistry and chronic exposure to trace anesthetic gases. *J. Am. Dent. Assoc.* 101:21–31
11. Cordier, S., Deplan, F., Mandereau, L., Hemon, D. 1991. Paternal exposure to mercury and spontaneous abortions. *Br. J. Indust. Med.* 48:375–81
12. Dryja, T. P., Mukai, S., Peterson, R., Rapaport, J. M., Walton, D., Yandell, D. W. 1989. Parental origin of mutations of the retinoblastoma gene. *Nature* 339:556–58
13. Ehling, U. H. 1985. Induction and manifestations of hereditary cataracts. In *Assessment of Risk from Low-Level Exposure to Radiation and Chemicals,* ed. A. Woodhead, C. Shellaburger, V., Pavel, A. Hallaender, pp. 345–61. New York: Plenum
14. Evans, H. J. 1990. Ionising radiations from nuclear establishments and childhood leukaemias—an enigma. *BioEssays* 12:541–49
15. Friedler, G. 1985. Effects of limited paternal exposure to xenobiotic agents on the development of progeny. *Neurobehav. Toxicol. Teratol.* 7:739–43
16. Gardner, M. J., Snee, M. P., Hall, A. J., Powell, C. A., Downes, S., Terrell, J. D. 1990. Results of case-control study of leukemia and lymphoma among young people near Sellafield nuclear plant in West Cumbria. *Br. Med. J.* 300:423–29
17. Graham, S., Levin, M. L., Lilienfeld, A. M., Schuman, L. M., Gibson, R., et al. 1966. Preconception, intrauterine and postnatal irradiation as related to leukemia. *Natl. Cancer Inst. Monogr.* 19:347–71
18. Green, D. M., Zevon, M. A., Lowrie, G., Seigelstein, N., Hall, B. 1991. Congenital anomalies in children of patients who received chemotherapy for cancer in childhood and adolescence. *N. Eng. J. Med.* 325:141–46.
19. Green, S., Auletta, A., Fabricant, J., Kapp, R., Manandhar, M., et al. 1985. Current status of bioassays in genetic toxicology—the dominant lethal assay: a report of the US Environmental Protection Agency Gene-Tox Program. *Mutat. Res.* 154:49–67
20. Hales, B. F., Crosman, K., Robaire, B. 1992. Increased postimplantation loss and malformations among the F_2 progeny of male rats chronically treated with cyclophosphamide. *Teratology* 45: 671–78
21. Hales, B. F., Smith, S., Robaire, B. 1986. Cyclophosphamide in the seminal fluid of treated males: transmission to the female during mating and effect on pregnancy outcome. *Toxicol. Appl. Pharmacol.* 84:423–38
22. Hall, J. G. 1990. Genomic imprinting: review and relevance to human diseases. *Am. J. Hum. Genet.* 46:857–73
23. Hamill, P. V. V., Steinberger, E., Levine, R. J., Rodriguez-Rigau, L. J., Lemeshow, S., Avrunin, J. S. 1992. The epidemiologic assessment of male reproductive hazard from occupational exposure to TDA and DNT. *J. Occup. Med.* 24:985–94
24. Hawkins, M. M. 1991. Is there evidence of a therapy-related increase in germ cell mutation among childhood cancer survivors? *J. Natl. Cancer Inst.* 83:1643–50
25. Hawkins, M. M., Smith, R. A., Curtice, L. J. 1988. Childhood cancer survivors and their offspring studied through a postal survey of general practitioners: preliminary results. *J. R. Coll. Gen. Pract.* 38:102–5
26. Hicks, N., Zack, M., Caldwell, G. G., Fernbach, D. J., Falletta, J. M. 1984. Childhood cancer and occupational radiation exposure in parents. *Cancer* 53:1637–43
27. Holliday, R. 1987. The inheritance of epigenetic defects. *Science* 238:163–70
28. Infante, P. F., Wagoner, J. K., McMichael, A. J., Waxweiler, R. J., Falk, H. 1976. Genetic risks of vinyl chloride. *Lancet* 1:734
29. Jenkinson, P. C., Anderson, D., Gangolli, S. D. 1987. Increased incidence of abnormal fetuses in the offspring of cyclophosphamide-treated male mice. *Mutat. Res.* 188:57–62
30. John, E. M., Savitz, D. A., Sandler, D. P. 1991. Prenatal exposure to parents' smoking and childhood cancer. *Am. J. Epidemiol.* 133:123–32
31. Johnson, F. M., Lewis, S. E. 1981. Electrophoretically detected germinal mutations induced in the mouse by ethylnitrosourea. *Proc. Natl. Acad. Sci. USA* 78:3138–41
32. Kelly, S. M., Robaire, B., Hales, B. F. 1992. Paternal cyclophosphamide treatment causes postimplantation loss via inner cell mass-specific cell death. *Teratology* 45:313–18
33. Kharrazi, M., Potashnik, G., Goldsmith, J. R. 1980. Reproductive effects of dibromochloropropane. *Isr. J. Med. Sci.* 16:403–6
34. Kirk, K. M., Lyon, M. F. 1984. Induction of congenital malformations in the offspring of male mice treated with x-rays at pre-meiotic and post-meiotic stages. *Mutat. Res.* 125:75–85

35. Kline, J., Stein, Z., Susser, M. 1989. *Conception to Birth. Epidemiology of Prenatal Development,* pp. 83. New York: Oxford Univ. Press. 433 pp.
36. Knishkowy, B., Baker, E. L. 1986. Transmission of occupational disease to family contacts. *Am. J. Ind. Med.* 9:543–50
37. Li, F. P., Gimbrere, K., Gelber, R. D., Sallan, S. E., Flamant, F., et al. 1987. Outcome of pregnancy in survivors of Wilms' tumor. *J. Am. Med. Assoc.* 257:216–19
38. Lindbohm, M.-L., Hemminki, K., Bonhomme, M. G., Anttila, A., Rantala, K., et al. 1991. Effects of paternal occupational exposure on spontaneous abortions. *Am. J. Pub. Health* 81:1029–33
39. Lindbohm, M.-L., Sallmen, M., Anttila, A., Taskinen, H., Hemminki, K. 1991. Paternal occupational lead exposure and spontaneous abortion. *Scand. J. Work Environ. Health* 17: 95–103
40. Little, R. E., Sing, C. F. 1987. Father's drinking and infant birth weight: report of an association. *Teratology* 36:59–65
41. Lowery, M. C., Au, W. W., Adams, P. M., Whorton, E. B. Jr., Legator, M. S. 1990. Male-mediated behavioral abnormalities. *Mutat. Res.* 229:213–29
42. MacMahon, B. 1992. Leukemia clusters around nuclear facilities in Britain. *Cancer Causes Control* 3:283–88
43. Magenis, R. E., Toth-Fejel, S., Allen, L. J., Black, M., Brown, M., et al. 1990. Comparison of the 15q deletion in Prader-Willi and Angelman Syndromes: specific regions extent of deletions, parental origin and clinical consequences. *Am. J. Med. Genet.* 35:333–49
44. Mann, T., Lutwak-Mann, C. 1982. Passage of chemicals into human and animal semen: mechanisms and significance. *CRC Crit. Rev. Toxicol.* 11:1–14
45. McDowall, M. E. 1985. *Occupational Reproductive Epidemiology,* Ser. SMPS 50. London: Her Majesty's Stationery Off.
46. Nagao, T. 1988. Congenital defects in the offspring of male mice treated with ethylnitrosourea. *Mutat. Res.* 101:25–33
47. Nagao, T., Fujikawa K. 1990. Genotoxic potential in mouse spermatogonial stem cells of triethylenemelamine, mitomycin C, ethylnitrosourea, procarbazine, and propyl methanesultonate as measured by F_1 congenital defects. *Mutat. Res.* 229:123–28
48. Narod, S. A. 1990. Radiation, genetics and childhood leukemia. *Eur. J. Cancer* 26:661–64
49. Natl. Res. Counc. 1989. *Biologic Markers in Reproductive Toxicology.* Washington, DC: Natl. Acad. Press. 395 pp.
50. Nomura, T. 1982. Parental exposure to x-rays and chemicals induces heritable tumours and anomalies in mice. *Nature* 296:575–77
51. Nomura, T. 1990. Of mice and men? *Nature* 345:671
52. O'Leary, L. M., Hicks, A. M., Peters, J. M., London, S. 1991. Paternal occupational exposures and risk of childhood cancer: a review. *Am. J. Ind. Med.* 20:17–35
53. Olshan, A. F., Baird, P. A., Teschke, K. 1989. Paternal occupational exposures and the risk of Down Syndrome. *Am. J. Hum. Genet.* 44:646–51
54. Olshan, A. F., Teschke, K., Baird, P. A. 1991. Paternal occupation and congenital anomalies in offspring. *Am. J. Ind. Med.* 20:447–75
55. Otake, M., Schull, W. J., Neel, J. V. 1990. Congenital; malformations, stillbirths, and early mortality among the children of atomic bomb survivors: a reanalysis. *Radiat. Res.* 122:1–11
56. Qiu, J., Hales, B. F., Robaire, B. 1992. Adverse effects of cyclophosphamide on progeny outcome can be mediated through post-testicular mechanisms in the rat. *Biol. Reprod.* 46:926–31
57. Roman, E., Beral, V. 1991. Possible aetiological factors in childhood leukaemia. *Arch. Dis. Child.* 66:179–80
58. Rosenberg, P. H., VanHinen, H. 1978. Occupational hazards to reproduction and health in anaesthetists and paediatricians. *Acta Anaesth. Scand.* 22:202–7
59. Rothman, K. J. 1986. *Modern Epidemiology.* Boston: Little Brown. 358 pp.
60. Russell, L. B. 1990. Patterns of mutational sensitivity to chemicals in poststem-cell stages of mouse spermatogenesis. In *Mutation and the Environment. Part C: Somatic and Heritable Mutations, Adduction, and Epidemiology,* ed. M. L. Mendelsohn, R. J. Albertini, pp. 101–13. New York: Wiley-Liss.
61. Russell, L. B., Russell, W. L., Rinchik, E. M., Hunsicker, P. R. 1990. Factors affecting the nature of induced mutations. In *Biology of Mammalian Germ Cell Mutagenesis,* ed. J. W. Allen, B. A. Bridges, M. F. Lyon,

M. J. Moses, L. B. Russell, 34:271–85. Cold Spring Harbor, New York: Cold Spring Harbor Lab. Press. 461 pp.

62. Russell, L. B., Shelby, M. D. 1985. Tests for heritable genetic damage and for evidence of gonadal exposure in mammals. *Mutat. Res.* 154:69–84

63. Russell, W. L. 1951. X-ray-induced mutations in mice. *Cold Spring Harbor Symp. Quant. Biol.* 16:327–36

64. Sanjose, S., Roman, E., Beral, V. 1991. Low birthweight and preterm delivery, Scotland, 1981–84: effect of parents' occupation. *Lancet* 338:428–31

65. Savitz, D. A., Chen, J. 1990. Parental occupation and childhood cancer: review of epidemiologic studies. *Environ. Health Perspect.* 88:325–37

66. Savitz, D. A., Schwingle, P. J., Keels, M. A. 1991. Influence of paternal age, smoking, and alcohol consumption on congenital anomalies. *Teratology* 44: 429–40

67. Savitz, D. A., Whelan, E. A., Kleckner, R. C. 1989. Effect of parents' occupational exposures on risk of stillbirth, preterm delivery, and small-for-gestational-age infants. *Am. J. Epidemiol.* 129:1201–18

68. Schroeder, W. T., Chao, L. Y., Dao, D. D., Strong, L. C., Pathak, S., et al. 1987. Non-random loss of maternal chromosome 11 alleles in Wilms' tumour. *Am. J. Hum. Genet.* 40:413–20

69. Selby, P. B. 1982. Dominant skeletal mutations: applications in mutagenicity testing and risk estimation. In *Mutagenicity: New Horizons in Genetic Toxicology*, ed. J. A. Heddle, pp. 385–406. New York: Academic

70. Selby, P. B. 1990. Experimental induction of dominant mutations in mammals by ionizing radiations and chemicals *Issues Rev. Teratol.* 5:181–253

71. Selby, P. B., Raymer, G. D., Hunsicker, P. R. 1988. High frequency of dominant mutations causing stunted growth is induced in spermatogonial stem cells by ENU. *Environ. Mol. Mutagen.* 11(Suppl. 11):93

72. Shaw, G. M., Malcoe, L. H., Croen, L. A., Smith, D. F. 1990. An assessment of error in parental occupation from the birth certificate. *Am. J. Epidemiol.* 131:1072–79

73. Shelby, M. D., Bishop, J. B., Mason, J. M., Tindall, K. R. 1993. Fertility, reproduction and genetic disease: Studies on the mutagenic effects of environmental agents on mammalian germ cells. *Environ. Health Perspect.* In press

74. Shepard, T. H. 1992. *Catalog of Teratogenic Agents*. Baltimore: Johns Hopkins Univ. Press. 534 pp. 7th ed.

75. Shu, X. O., Gao, Y. T., Brinton, L. A., Linet, M. S., Tu, J. T., et al. 1988. A population based case-control study of childhood leukemia in Shanghai. *Cancer* 62:635–44

76. Solter, D. 1988. Differential imprinting and expression of maternal and paternal genomes. *Annu. Rev. Genet.* 22:127–46

77. Soyka, L. F., Joffe, J. M. 1980. Male mediated drug effects on offspring. *Prog. Clin. Biol. Res.* 36:49–66

78. Stellman, S. D., Stellman, J. M., Sommer, J. F. 1988. Health and reproductive outcomes among American Legionnaires in relation to combat and herbicide exposure in Vietnam. *Environ. Res.* 47:150–74

79. Surani, M. A., Kothary, R., Allen, N. D., Singh, P. B., Fundele, R., et al. 1990. Genome imprinting and development in the mouse. *Development* Suppl. 89–98

80. Taskinen, H., Anttila, A., Lindbohm, M-L., Sallmen, M., Hemminki, K. 1989. Spontaneous abortions and congenital malformations among the wives of men occupationally exposed to organic solvents. *Scand. J. Work Environ. Health* 15:345–52

81. Tomatis, L., Cabral, J. R. P., Likhackev, A. J., Ponomarkov, V. 1981. Increased cancer incidence in the progeny of male rats exposed to ethylnitrosourea before mating. *Int. J. Cancer* 28:475–78

82. Tomatis, L., Narod, S., Yamasaki, H. 1992. Transgeneration transmission of carcinogenic risk. *Carcinogenesis* 13: 145–51

83. Tomatis, L., Turusov, V. S., Cardis, E., Cabral, J. P. R. 1990. Tumour incidence in the progeny of male rats exposed to ethylnitrosourea before mating. *Mutat. Res.* 229:231–37

84. Trasler, J. M., Hales, B. F., Robaire, B. 1985. Paternal cyclophosphamide treatment of rats causes fetal loss and malformations without affecting male fertility. *Nature* 316:144–46

85. Upton, A. C., Shore, R. E., Harley, N. H. 1992. The health effects of low-level ionizing radiation. *Annu. Rev. Publ. Health* 13:127–50

86. Waters, M. D., Stack, H. F., Jackson, M. A., Bridges, B. A. 1993. Hazard identification—efficiency of short-term

tests in identifying germ cell mutagens and putative nongenotoxic carcinogens. *Environ. Health Perspect.* In press

87. Whelan, E. A., Savitz, D. A. 1991. Parental occupation and risk of prematurity. *Lancet* 338:1082

88. Working, P. K. 1989. Germ cell genotoxicity: methods for assessment of DNA damage and mutagenesis. In *Toxicology of the Male and Female Reproductive Systems,* ed. P. K. Working. pp. 231–55. New York: Hemisphere

89. Wyrobek, A. J., Gordon, L. A., Burkhart J. G., Francis, M. W., Kapp, R. W. Jr., et al. 1983. An evaluation of human sperm as indicators of chemically induced alterations of spermatogenic function. A report of the US Environmental Protection Agency Gene-Tox Program. *Mutat. Res.* 115: 73–148.

90. Yazigi, R. A., Odem, R. R., Polakoski, K. L. 1991. Demonstration of specific binding of cocaine to human spermatozoa. *J. Am. Med. Assoc.* 266:1956–59

91. Yoshimoto, Y. 1990. Cancer risk among children of atomic bomb survivors. A review of RERF epidemiologic studies. *J. Am. Med. Assoc.* 264:596–600

92. Yoshimoto, Y., Neel, J. V., Schull, W. J., Kato, H., Soda, M., et al. 1990. Malignant tumors during the first two decades of life in the offspring of atomic bomb survivors. *Am. J. Hum. Genet.* 46:1041–52

93. Zhang J., Savitz, D. A., Schwingl, P. J., Cai, W.-W. 1992. A case-control study of paternal smoking and birth defects. *Int. J. Epidemiol.* 21: 273–78

94. Zhu, X., Dunn, J. M., Phillips, R. A., Goodard, A. D., Paton, K. E., et al. 1989. Preferential germline maturation of the paternal allele in retinoblastoma. *Nature* 340: 312–13

Annu. Rev. Publ. Health 1993. 14:183–203

RISK PERCEPTION AND COMMUNICATION

Baruch Fischhoff
Department of Engineering and Public Policy, Department of Social and Decision Sciences, Carnegie Mellon University, Pittsburgh, Pennsylvania 15213

Ann Bostrom
School of Public Policy, Georgia Institute of Technology, Atlanta, Georgia 30332-0345

Marilyn Jacobs Quadrel[1]
Carnegie Mellon University, Pittsburgh, Pennsylvania 15213

KEY WORDS: health behavior, judgment, decision making

INTRODUCTION

Role of Risk Perceptions in Public Health

Many health risks are the result of deliberate decisions by individuals consciously trying to get the best deal possible for themselves and for those important to them. Some of these choices are private ones, such as whether to wear bicycle helmets and seatbelts, whether to read and follow safety warnings, whether to buy and use condoms, and how to select and cook food. Other choices involve societal issues, such as whether to protest the siting of hazardous waste incinerators and half-way houses, whether to vote for fluoridation and "green" candidates, and whether to support sex education in the schools.

In some cases, single choices can have a large effect on health risks (e.g. buying a car with airbags, taking a dangerous job, getting pregnant). In other

[1]Dr. Quadrel's current address is Decision Analysis Group, Battelle Pacific Northwest Laboratories, Richland, Washington 99352.

0163-7525/93/0510-0183$02.00

cases, the effects of individual choices are small, but can accumulate over multiple decisions (e.g. repeatedly ordering broccoli, wearing a seatbelt, using the escort service in parking garages). In still other cases, choices intended to affect health risks do nothing at all or the opposite of what is expected (e.g. responses to baseless cancer scares, adoption of quack treatments).

To make such decisions wisely, individuals need to understand the risks and the benefits associated with alternative courses of action. They also need to understand the limits to their own knowledge and the limits to the advice proffered by various experts. In this chapter, we review the research base for systematically describing a person's degree of understanding about health risk issues. We also consider some fundamental topics in designing and evaluating messages that are intended to improve that understanding. Following convention, we call these pursuits risk perception and risk communication research, respectively. In practice, the beliefs and messages being studied might deal with the benefits accompanying a risk, with the individuals and institutions who manage it, or with the broader issues that it raises (e.g. who gets to decide, how equitably risks and benefits are distributed).

The Role of Perceptions about Risk Perceptions in Public Health

The fundamental assumption of this chapter is that statements about other people's understanding must be disciplined by systematic data. People can be hurt by inaccuracies in their risk perceptions. They can also be hurt by inaccuracies in what various risk managers believe about those perceptions. Those managers might include physicians, nurses, public health officials, legislators, regulators, and engineers—all of whom have some say in what risks are created, what is communicated about them, and what role laypeople have in determining their fate.

If their understanding is overestimated, then people may be thrust into situations that they are ill-prepared to handle. If their understanding is underestimated, then people may be disenfranchised from decisions that they could and should make. The price of such misperceptions of risk perceptions may be exacted over the long run, as well as in individual decisions. The outcomes of health risk decisions partly determine people's physical and financial resources. The processes of health risk decisions partly determine people's degree of autonomy in managing their own affairs and in shaping their society.

In addition to citing relevant research results, the chapter emphasizes research methods. One conventional reason for doing so is improving access to material that is scattered over specialist literatures or part of the implicit knowledge conveyed in professional training. A second conventional reason is to help readers evaluate the substantive results reported here, by giving a feeling for how they were produced.

A less conventional reason is to make the point that method matters. We are routinely struck by the strong statements made about other people's competence to manage risks, solely on the basis of anecdotal observation. These statements appear directly in pronouncements about, say, why people mistrust various technologies or fail to "eat right." Such claims appear more subtly in the myriad of health advisories, advertisements, and warnings directed at the public without any systematic evaluation. These practices assume that the communicator knows what people currently know, what they need to learn, what they want to hear, and how they will interpret a message.

Even the casual testing of a focus group shows a willingness to have those (smug) assumptions challenged.[1] The research methods presented here show the details needing attention and, conversely, the pitfalls to casual observation. The presentation also shows the limits to such research, in terms of how far current methods can go and how quickly they can get there. In our experience, once the case has been made for conducting behavioral research, it is expected to produce results immediately. That is, of course, a prescription for failure, and for undermining the perceived value of future behavioral research.

Overview

ORGANIZATION The following section, Quantitative Assessment, treats the most obvious question about laypeople's risk perceptions: Do they understand how big risks are? It begins with representative results regarding the quality of these judgments, along with some psychological theory regarding reasons for error. It continues with issues in survey design, which focus on how design choices can affect respondents' apparent competence. Some of these methodological issues reveal substantive aspects of lay risk perceptions.

The next section, Qualitative Assessment, shifts the focus from summary judgments to qualitative features of the events to which they are attached. It begins with the barriers to communication created when experts and laypeople unwittingly use terms differently. For example, when experts tell (or ask) people about the risks of drinking and driving, what do people think is meant regarding the kinds and amounts of "drinking" and of "driving"? The section continues by asking how people believe that risks "work," on the basis of which they might generate or evaluate control options.

The next section provides a general process for developing communications

[1]Focus groups are a popular technique in market research. In them, survey questions, commercial messages, or consumer products are discussed by groups of laypeople. Although they can generate unanticipated alternative interpretations, focus groups create a very different situation than that faced by an individual trying to make sense out of a question, message, or product (44).

about health risks. That process begins with identifying the information to be communicated, based on the descriptive study of what recipients know already and the formal analysis of what they need to know to make informed decisions. The process continues by selecting an appropriate format for presenting that information. It concludes with explicit evaluation of the resulting communication (followed by iteration if the results are wanting). The process is illustrated with examples taken from several case studies, looking at such diverse health risks as those posed by radon, Lyme disease, electromagnetic fields, carotid endarterechtomy, and nuclear energy sources in space.

EXCLUSIONS We do not address several issues that belong in a full account of their own, including the roles of emotion, individual differences (personality), culture, and social processes in decisions about risk. This set of restrictions suits the chapter's focus on how individuals think about risks. It may also suit a public health perspective, where it is often necessary to "treat" populations (with information) in fairly uniform ways. Access to these missing topics might begin with Refs. 27, 32, 36, 49, 66, 68, 71, 72.

QUANTITATIVE ASSESSMENT

Estimating the Size of Risks

A common presenting symptom in experts' complaints about lay decision making is that "laypeople simply do not realize how small (or large) the risk is." If that were the case, then the mission of risk communication would be conceptually simple (if technically challenging): Transmit credible estimates of how large the risks are (32, 49, 60, 68). Research suggests that lay estimates of risk are, indeed, subject to biases. Rather less evidence clearly implicates these biases in inappropriate risk decisions, or substantiates the idealized notion of people waiting for crisp risk estimates so that they can run well-articulated decision-making models. Such estimates are necessary, but not sufficient, for effective decisions.

In one early attempt to evaluate lay estimates of the size of risks, Lichtenstein et al (40) asked people to estimate the number of deaths in the US from 30 causes (e.g. botulism, tornados, motor vehicle accidents).[2] They

[2]The "people" in this study were members of the League of Women Voters and their spouses. Generally speaking, the people in the studies described here have been students paid for participation (hence, typically older than the proverbial college sophomores of some psychological research) or convenience samples of adults recruited through diverse civic groups (e.g. garden clubs, PTAs, bowling leagues). These groups have been found to differ more in what they think than in how they think. That is, their respective experiences have created larger differences in specific beliefs than in thought processes. Fuller treatment of sampling issues must await another opportunity.

used two different response modes, thus allowing them to check for the consistency of responses. One task presented pairs of causes; subjects chose the more frequent and then estimated the ratio of frequencies. The second task asked subjects to estimate the number of deaths in an average year; subjects were told the answer for one cause, in order to give an order-of-magnitude feeling (for those without a good idea for how many people live or die in the US in an average year). The study reached several conclusions that have been borne out by subsequent studies:

INTERNAL CONSISTENCY Estimates of relative frequency were quite consistent across response mode. Thus, people seemed to have a moderately well-articulated internal risk scale, which they could express even in unfamiliar response modes.

ANCHORING BIAS Direct estimates were influenced by the anchor given. Subjects told that 50,000 people die from auto accidents produced estimates two to five times higher than those produced by subjects told that 1000 die from electrocution. Thus, people seem to have less of a feel for absolute frequency, rendering them sensitive to the implicit cues in how questions are asked (51).

COMPRESSION Subjects' estimates showed less dispersion than did the statistical estimates. In this case, the result was an overestimation of small frequencies and an underestimation of large ones. However, the anchoring bias suggests that this pattern might have changed with different procedures, which would make the compression of estimates the more fundamental result.

AVAILABILITY BIAS At any level of statistical frequency, some causes of death consistently received higher estimates than others. These proved to be causes that are disproportionately visible (e.g. as reported in the news media, as experienced in subjects' lives). This bias seemed to reflect a general tendency to estimate the frequency of events by the ease with which they are remembered or imagined—while failing to realize what a fallible index such availability is (32, 65).

MISCALIBRATION OF CONFIDENCE JUDGMENTS In a subsequent study (21), subjects were asked how confident they were in their ability to choose the more frequent of the paired causes of death. They tended to be overconfident. For example, they had chosen correctly only 75% of the time when they were 90% confident of having done so. This result is a special case of a general tendency to be inadequately sensitive to the extent of one's knowledge (38, 72).

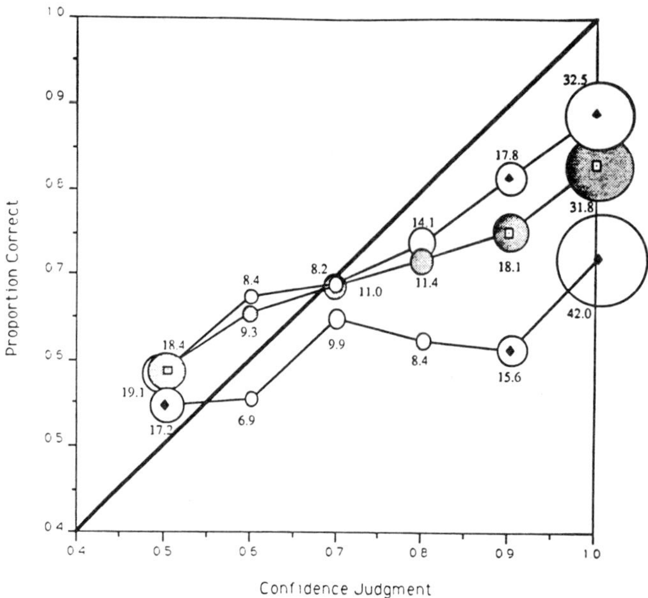

Figure 1 Calibration curves for adults (top, white: $N = 45$), not-at-risk teens (middle, dark: $N = 43$), and at-risk teens (bottom, white: $N = 45$). Each point indicates the proportion of correct answers among those in which subjects expressed a particular confidence level; the size of each circle indicates the percentage of answers held with that degree of confidence. (From Ref. 52.)

Figure 1 shows typical results from such a calibration test. In this case, subjects expressed their confidence in having chosen the correct answer to two-alternative questions regarding health behaviors [e.g. alcohol is (a) a depressant; (b) a stimulant]. The two curves reflect a group of middle-class adults and some of their adolescent children, recruited through school organizations.[3]

Response Mode Problems

One recurrent obstacle to assessing or improving laypeople's estimates of risk is reliance on verbal quantifiers. It is hard for them to know what experts

[3]In other studies comparing individuals drawn from these groups (53), we have also observed little difference in their respective response patterns. These studies suggest that any differences in their risk behaviors cannot be attributed to differences in the sorts of judgments considered in this chapter. If that is the case, and if such adults and teens do differ in their risk behaviors, then it may reflect differences in the benefits that they get from the behaviors (or in the risks and benefits of alternative behaviors).

mean when a risk is described as "very likely" or "rare"—or for experts to evaluate lay perceptions expressed in those terms. Such terms mean different things to different people, and even to the same person in different contexts (e.g. likely to be fatal versus likely to rain, rare disease versus rare Cubs pennant), sometimes even within communities of experts (3, 39, 67).

The Lichtenstein et al study (40) could observe the patterns reported above because it used an absolute response scale. As noted, it provided anchors to give subjects a feeling for how to answer. Doing so improved performance by drawing responses to the correct range, within which subjects were drawn to higher or lower values depending on the size of the anchor. Although most conclusions were relatively insensitive to these effects, they left no clear answer to the critical question of whether people overestimate or underestimate the risks that they face.

PERCEIVED LETHALITY A study by Fischhoff & MacGregor (19) provides another example of the dangers of relying on a single response mode to describe behavior. They used four different response modes to ask about the chances of dying, given that one was afflicted with each of various maladies (e.g. how many people die out of each 100,000 who get influenza; how many people died out of the 80 million who caught influenza last year). Again, there was strong internal consistency across response modes, whereas absolute estimates varied over as much as two orders of magnitude. A follow-up study reduced this range by providing an independent basis for eliminating the response mode that produced the most discrepant results (e.g. subjects were least able to remember statistics reported in that format—estimating the number of survivors for each person who succumbed to a problem).

PERCEIVED INVULNERABILITY Estimating the accuracy of risk estimates requires not only an appropriate response mode, but also credible statistical estimates against which responses can be compared. The studies just described asked about population risks in situations where credible statistical estimates were available. Performance might be different (poorer?) for risks whose magnitude is less readily calculated. Furthermore, people may not see these population risks as personally relevant.

As a partial way to avoid these problems, some investigators have asked subjects to judge whether they are more or less at risk than others in more or less similar circumstances (63, 69). They find that most people in most situations see themselves as facing less risk than average others (which could, of course, be true for only half a population). A variety of processes could account for such a bias, including both cognitive ones (e.g. the greater availability of the precautions that one takes) and motivational ones (e.g. wishful thinking). To the extent that this bias exists in the world outside the experiment and interview, such a bias could prompt unwanted risk taking (e.g. because warnings seem more applicable to other people).[4]

Defining Risk

These studies attempt to measure risk perceptions under the assumption that people define "risk" as the probability of death. Anecdotal observation of scientific practice shows that "risk" means different things in different contexts (8, 23). For some analysts, risk is expected loss of life of expectancy; for others, it is expected probability of premature fatality (with the former definition placing a premium on deaths among the young). Some of the apparent disagreement between experts and laypeople regarding the magnitude of risks in society may be due to differing definitions of risk (20, 62).

CATASTROPHIC POTENTIAL One early study asked experts and laypeople to estimate the "risk of death" faced by society as a whole from 30 activities and technology (62). The experts' judgments could be predicted well from statistical estimates of average-year fatalities—as could the estimates of laypeople given that specific definition. Lay estimates of "risk" were more poorly correlated with average-year fatalities. However, much of the residual variance could be predicted by their estimates of catastrophic potential, the ability to cause large numbers of death in a nonaverage year. Thus, casual observation had obscured the extent to which experts and laypeople agreed about routine death tolls (for which scientific estimates are relatively uncontroversial) and disagreed about the possibility of anomalies (for which the science is typically weaker).

Sensing that there was something special about catastrophic potential, some risk experts have suggested that social policy give extra weight to hazards carrying that kind of threat. One experimental study has, however, found that people may not care more for many lives lost in a single accident than for the same number of lives lost in separate incidents (61).[5] The critical factor in catastrophic potential is not how the deaths are grouped, but the possibility of discovering that a technology is out of control. Such "surprise potential"

[4]In a recent study (53), we derived judgments of relative risk from judgments of the absolute degree of risk that people assigned to themselves and to target others (a close friend, an acquaintance, a parent, a child). On a response scale that facilitated expressing very low probabilities, subjects assigned a probability of less than 1 in 10 million about 10% of the time and a probability of less than 1 in 10,000 about one third of the time. The events involved "a death or injury requiring hospitalization over the next five years" from sources like auto accidents, drug addiction, and explosions. Here, too, middle-class adults and adolescents responded similarly, despite the common belief that teens take risks, in part, because of a unique perception of invulnerability (11).

[5]When accidents involving large numbers of fatalities are easy to imagine, catastrophic potential can be rated high because of availability, even when estimates of average-year fatalities are relatively low, as was the case for nuclear power in this study.

is strongly correlated with catastrophic potential in people's judgments (and, presumably, in scientific estimates). However, the two features represent rather different ethical bases for distinguishing among risks.

DIMENSIONS OF RISK Recognizing that correlated features can confuse the interpretation of risk behaviors, investigators have looked extensively at the patterns of correlations among features (1, 22, 60). Overall, they have found a remarkably robust picture, typically revealing two or three dimensions of risk, which capture much of the variation in judgments of up to 20 aspects of risk. The general structure of this "risk space" is relatively similar across elicitation method, subject population (e.g. experts versus laypeople), and risk domain. Core concepts in these dimensions include how well a risk is understood and how much of a feeling of dread it evokes. The placement of individual hazards in the space does vary with individual and with group, in ways that can predict judgments of risk management policies (e.g. how tightly a technology should be regulated). Relatively little is known about the role of these dimensions in individual risk decisions.

RISK COMPARISONS The multidimensional character of risk means that hazards that are similar in many ways may still evoke quite different responses. This fact is neglected in appeals to accept one risk, because one has accepted another that is similar to it in some ways (8, 18). The most ambitious of these appeals present elaborate lists of hazards, the exposure to which is adjusted so that they pose equivalent risks (e.g. both one tablespoon of peanut butter and 50 years of living at the boundary of a nuclear power plant create a one-in-a-million risk of premature death). Recognizing that such comparisons are often perceived as self-serving, the Chemical Manufacturers Association (6) commissioned a guide to risk comparisons, which presents such lists, but with the attached caution, WARNING! USE OF DATA IN THIS TABLE FOR RISK COMPARISON PURPOSES CAN DAMAGE YOUR CREDIBILITY.[6]

QUALITATIVE ASSESSMENT

Event Definitions

Scientific estimates of risk require detailed specification of the conditions under which it is to be observed. For example, a fertility counselor estimating a woman's risk of an unplanned pregnancy would consider the amount of

[6]The guide also offers advice on how to make risk comparisons, if one feels the compulsion, along with examples of more and less acceptable comparisons. Although the advice is logically derived from risk perception research, it was not tested empirically. In such a test, we found little correlation between the predicted degree of acceptability and the acceptability judgments of several diverse groups of subjects (56).

intercourse, the kinds of contraceptive used (and the diligence with which they are applied), her physiological condition (and that of her partner), and so on. If laypeople are to make accurate assessments, then they require the same level of detail. That is true whether they are estimating risks for their own sake or for the benefit of an investigator studying risk perceptions.

When such investigators omit needed details, they create adverse conditions for subjects. To respond correctly, subjects must first guess the question and then know the answer to it. Consider, for example, the question, "What is the probability of pregnancy with unprotected sex?" A well-informed subject who understood this to mean a single exposure would be seen as underestimating the risk by an investigator who intended the question to mean multiple exposures.

Such ambiguous events are common in surveys designed to study public perceptions of risk. For example, a National Center for Health Statistics survey (70) question asked, "How likely do you think it is that a person will get the AIDS virus from sharing plates, forks, or glasses with someone who had AIDS?" Even if the survey had not used an ambiguous response mode (very likely, unlikely, etc.), it would reveal relatively little about subjects' understanding of disease risks. For their responses to be meaningful, subjects must spontaneously assign the same value to each missing detail, while investigators guess what subjects decided.

We asked a relatively homogeneous group of subjects what they thought was meant regarding the amount and kind of sharing implied by this question (after they had answered it) (16). These subjects generally agreed about the kind of sharing (82% interpreted it as sharing during a meal), but not about the amount (a single occasion, 39%; several occasions 20%; routinely, 28%; uncertain, 12%). A survey question about the risks of sexual transmission evoked similar disagreement. We did not study what readers of the survey's results believed about subjects' interpretations.

Supplying Details

Aside from their methodological importance, the details that subjects infer can be substantively interesting. People's intuitive theories of risk are revealed in the variables that they note and the values that they supply. In a systematic evaluation of these theories, Quadrel (52) asked adolescents to think aloud as they estimated the probability of several deliberately ambiguous events (e.g. getting in an accident after drinking and driving, getting AIDS through sex).

These subjects typically wondered (or made assumptions) about numerous features. In this sense, subjects arguably showed more sophistication than the investigators who created the surveys from which these questions were taken or adapted. Generally speaking, these subjects wre interested in variables that could figure in scientific risk analyses (although scientists might not yet know what role each variable plays). There were, however, some interesting exceptions. Although subjects wanted to know the "dose" involved with most risks, they seldom asked about the amount of sex in one question about the risks of pregnancy and in another question about the risks of HIV transmission. They seemed to believe that an individual either is or is not sensitive to the risk, regardless of the amount of the exposure. In other cases, subjects asked about variables without a clear connection to risk level (e.g. how well members of the couple knew one another).

In a follow-up study, Quadrel (52) presented richly specified event descriptions to teens drawn from the same populations (school organizations and substance abuse treatment homes). Subjects initially estimated the probability of a risky outcome on the basis of some 20 details. Then, they were asked how knowing each of three additional details would change their estimates. One of those details had been provided by subjects in the preceding study; two had not. Subjects in this study responded to the relevant detail much more than to the irrelevant ones. Thus, at least in these studies, teens did not balk at making judgments regarding complex stimuli and revealed consistent intuitive theories in rather different tasks.

Cumulative Risk—A Case in Point

As knowledge accumulates about people's intuitive theories of risk, it will become easier to predict which details subjects know and ignore, as well as which omissions they will notice and rectify. In time, it might become possible to infer the answers to questions that are not asked from answers to ones that are—as well as the inferences that people make from risks that are described explicitly to risks that are not. The invulnerability results reported above show the need to discipline such extrapolations with empirical research. Asking people about the risks to others like themselves is not the same as asking about their personal risk. Nor need reports about others' risk levels be taken personally.

One common, and seemingly natural, extrapolation is between varying numbers of independent exposures to a risk. Telling people the risk from a single exposure should allow them to infer the risk from whatever multiple they face; asking subjects what risk they expect from one amount should allow one to infer what they expect from other amounts. Unfortunately, for both research and communication, teens' insensitivity to the amount of intercourse (in determining the risks of pregnancy or HIV transmission) proves to be a special case of a general problem. Several reviews (9, 48) have concluded that between one third and one half of sexually active adolescents explain not using contraceptives with variants of, "I thought I (or my partner) couldn't get pregnant." Another study (59) found that adults greatly underestimated the rate at which the risk of contraceptive failure accumulates through repeated exposure, even after eliminating (from the data analysis) the 40% or so of subjects who saw no relationship between risk and exposure. One corollary of this bias is not realizing the extent to which seemingly small differences in annual failure rates (what is typically reported) can lead to large differences in the cumulative risk associated with continued use.

After providing practice with a response mode designed to facilitate the expression of small probabilities, Linville et al (41) asked college students to estimate the risks of HIV transmission from a man to a woman as the result of 1, 10, or 100 cases of protected sex. For one contact, the median estimate was .10, a remarkably high value according to public health estimates (14, 33). For 100 contacts, however, the median estimate was .25, a more reasonable value. Very different pictures of people's risk perceptions would emerge from studies that asked just one of these questions or the other. Risk communicators could achieve quite different effects if they chose to describe the risk of one exposure and not the other. They might create confusion if they chose to communicate both risks, thus leaving recipients to reconcile the seeming inconsistency.

Mental Models of Risk Processes

THE ROLE OF MENTAL MODELS These intuitive theories of how risks accumulate were a byproduct of research intended to improve the elicitation and communication of quantitative probabilities. Such research can serve the interests of individuals who face well-formulated decisions in which estimates of health risks (or benefits) play clearly defined roles. For example, a homeowner poised to decide whether to test for radon needs estimates of the cost and accuracy of tests, the health risks of different radon levels, the cost and efficacy of ways to mitigate radon problems, and so on (64).

Often, however, people are not poised to decide anything. Rather, they just want to know what the risk is and how it works. Such substantive knowledge is essential for following an issue in the news media, for participating in public discussions, for feeling competent to make decisions, and for generating options among which to decide. In these situations, people's objective is to have intuitive therories that correspond to the main elements of the reigning scientific theories (emphasizing those features relevant to control strategies).

The term mental model is often applied to intuitive theories that are elaborated well enough to generate predictions in diverse circumstances (24). Mental models have a long history in psychology (7, 50). For example, they have been used to examine how people understand physical processes (26), international tensions (43), complex equipment (57), energy conservation (34), and the effects of drugs (31).

If these mental models contain critical bugs, they can lead to erroneous conclusions, even among otherwise well-informed people. For example, not knowing that repeated sex increases the associated risks could undermine much other knowledge. Bostrom et al (5) found that many people know that radon is a colorless, odorless, radioactive gas. Unfortunately, some also associate radioactivity with permanent contamination. However, this widely publicized property of high-level waste is not shared by radon. Not realizing that the relevant radon byproducts have short half-lives, homeowners might not even bother to test (believing that there was nothing that they could do, should a problem be detected).

ELICITING MENTAL MODELS In principle, the best way to detect such misconceptions would be to capture people's entire mental model on a topic. Doing so would also identify those correct conceptions upon which communications could build (and which should be reinforced). The critical threat to capturing mental models is reactivity, i.e. changing respondents as a result of the elicitation procedure. One wants neither to induce nor to dispell misconceptions, either through leading questions or subtle hints. The interview should neither preclude the expression of unanticipated beliefs nor inadvertently steer subjects around topics (13, 24, 28).

Bostrom et al (5) offer one possible compromise strategy, which has been used for a variety of risks (2, 42, 47). Their interview protocol begins with very open-ended questions: They ask subjects what they know about a topic, then prompt them to consider exposure, effects, and mitigation issues. Subjects are asked to elaborate on every topic mentioned. Once these minimally structured tasks are exhausted, subjects sort a large stack of diverse photographs, according to whether each seems related to the topic, and explain their reasoning as they go.

Once transcribed, the interviews are coded into an expert model of the risk. This is a directed network, or influence diagram (29), which shows the different factors affecting the magnitude of the risk. The expert model is created by iteratively pooling the knowledge of a diverse group of experts. It might be thought of as an expert's mental model, although it would be impressive for any single expert to produce it all in a single session following the open-ended interview protocol. Figure 2 shows the results of coding one subject's interview into the expert model for radon. The subject's concepts were characterized as correct, incorrect, peripheral (technically correct, but only distantly related to the topic), background (referring to general principles of science), evaluative, and nonspecific (or vague).

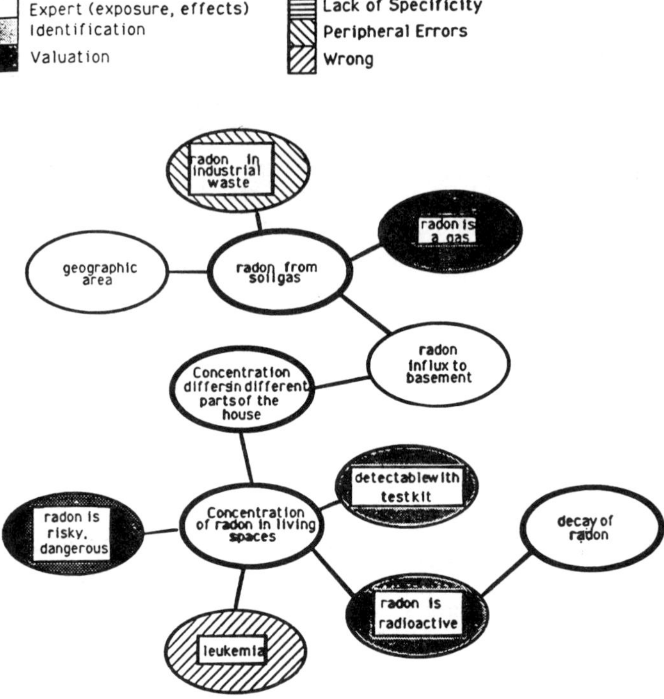

Figure 2 One subject's model of processes affecting radon risk, elicited with an open-ended interview protocol. (From Ref. 5.)

CREATING COMMUNICATIONS

Selecting Information

The first step in designing communications is to select the information that they should contain. In many existing communications, this choice seems arbitrary, reflecting some expert or communicator's notion of "what people ought to know." Poorly chosen information can have several negative consequences, including both wasting recipients' time and being seen to waste it (thereby reflecting insensitivity to their situation). In addition, recipients will be judged unduly harshly if they are uninterested in information that, to them, seems irrelevant. The Institute of Medicine's fine and important report, *Confronting AIDS* (30), despaired after a survey showed that only 41% of the public knew that AIDS was caused by a virus. Yet, one might ask what role that information could play in any practical decision (as well as what those subjects who answered correctly meant by "a virus").

The information in a communication should reflect a systematic theoretical perspective, capable of being applied objectively. Here are three candidates for such a perspective, suggested by the research cited above:

MENTAL MODEL ANALYSIS Communications could attempt to convey a comprehensive picture of the processes creating (and controlling) a risk. Bridging the gap between lay mental models and expert models would require adding missing concepts, correcting mistakes, strengthening correct beliefs, and deemphasizing peripheral ones.

CALIBRATION ANALYSIS Communications could attempt to correct the critical "bugs" in recipients' beliefs. These are defined as cases where people confidently hold incorrect beliefs that could lead to inappropriate actions (or lack enough confidence in correct beliefs to act on them).

VALUE-OF-INFORMATION ANALYSIS Communications could attempt to provide the pieces of information that have the largest possible impact on pending decisions. Value-of-information analysis is the general term for techniques that determine the sensitivity of decisions to different information (46).

The choice among these approaches would depend on, among other things, how much time is available for communication, how well the decisions are formulated, and what scientific risk information exists. For example, calibration analysis might be particularly useful for identifying the focal facts for public service announcements. Such facts might both grab recipients' attention and change their behavior. A mental model analysis might be more suited for the preparation of explanatory brochures or curricula.

Merz (45) applied value-of-information analysis to a well-specified medical decision, whether to undergo carotid endarterectomy. Both this procedure, which involves scraping out an artery that leads to the head, and its alternatives have a variety of possible positive and negative effects. These effects have been the topic of extensive research, which has provided quantitative risk estimates of varying precision. Merz created a simulated population of patients, who varied in their physical condition and relative preferences for different health states. He found that knowing about a few, but only a few, of the possible side effects would change the preferred decision for a significant portion of patients. He argued that communications focused on these few side effects would make better use of patients' attention than laundry lists of undifferentiated possibilities. He also argued that his procedure could provide an objective criterion for identifying the information that must be transmitted to insure medical informed consent.

Formatting Information

Once information has been selected, it must be presented in a comprehensible way. That means taking into account the terms that recipients use for understanding individual concepts and the mental models they use for integrating those concepts. It also means respecting the results of research into text comprehension. That research shows, for example, that comprehension improves when text has a clear structure and, especially, when that structure conforms to recipients' intuitive representation of a topic; that critical information is more likely to be remembered when it appears at the highest level of a clear hierarchy; and that readers benefit from "adjunct aids," such as highlighting, advanced organizers (showing what to expect), and summaries. Such aids might even be better than full text for understanding, retaining, and being able to look up information. Fuller treatment than is possible here can be found in Refs. 12, 25, 35, 54, 58.

There may be several different formats that meet these general constraints. Recently, we created two brochures that presented clear but different structures to explain the risks of radon (4). One was organized around a decision tree, which showed the options facing home owners, the probabilities of possible consequences, and the associated costs and benefits. The second was organized around a directed network, in effect, the expert model of the mental model studies. Both were compared with the Environmental Protection Agency's (EPA) widely distributed (and, to EPA's great credit, heavily evaluated) *Citizen's Guide to Radon* (65a), which uses primarily a question-and-answer format, with little attempt to summarize or impose a general structure. All three brochures substantially increased readers' understanding of the material presented in them. However, the structured brochures did better (and similar) jobs of enabling readers to make inferences about issues not mentioned explicitly and to give explicit advice to others.

Evaluating Communications

Effective risk communications can help people to reduce their health risks, or to get greater benefits in return for those risks that they take. Ineffective communications not only fail to do so, but also incur opportunity costs, in the sense of occupying the place (in recipients' lives and society's functions) that could be taken up by more effective communications. Even worse, misdirected communications can prompt wrong decisions by omitting key information or failing to contradict misconceptions, create confusion by prompting inappropriate assumptions or by emphasizing irrelevant information, and provoke conflict by eroding recipients' faith in the communicator. By causing undue alarm or complacency, poor communications can have greater public health impact than the risks that they attempt to describe. It may be no more acceptable to release an untested communication than an untested drug. Because communicators' intuitions about recipients' risk perceptions cannot be trusted, there is no substitute for empirical validation (17, 20, 49, 55, 60).

The most ambitious evaluations ask whether recipients follow the recommendations given in the communication (37, 68). However, that standard requires recipients not only to understand the message, but also to accept it as relevant to their personal circumstances. For example, home owners without the resources to address radon problems might both understand and ignore a communication about testing; women might hear quite clearly what an "expert" is recommending about how to reduce their risk of sexual assault, yet reject the political agenda underlying that advice (15). Judging the effectiveness of a program by behavioral effects requires great confidence that one knows what is right for others.

A more modest, but ethically simpler, evaluation criterion is ensuring that recipients have understood what a message was trying to say. That necessary condition might prove sufficient, too, if the recommended action is, indeed, obviously appropriate, once the facts are known. Formal evaluations of this type seem to be remarkably rare, among the myriad of warning labels, health claims and advisories, public service announcements, and operating instructions that one encounters in everyday life and work.

Evaluating what people take away from communications faces the same methodological challenges as measuring ambient risk perceptions. To elaborate slightly on a previous section, the evaluator wants to avoid reactivity, changing people's beliefs through the cues offered by how questions and answers are posed; illusory expertise, restricting the expression of inexpert beliefs; and illusory discrimination, suppressing the expression of inconsistent beliefs.

For example, as part of an ambitious program to evaluate its communications regarding the risks of radon, the EPA (10) posed the following question: "What kinds of problems are high levels of radon exposure likely to cause? a. minor skin problems; b. eye irritations; c. lung cancer." This question seems to risk inflating subjects' apparent level of understanding in several ways. Subjects who know only that radon causes cancer might deduce that it causes lung cancer. The words "minor" and "irritation" might imply that these are not the effects of "high levels" (of anything). There is no way to express other misconceptions, such as that radon causes breast cancer and other lung problems, which emerged with some frequency in our open-ended interviews (5).

In principle, open-ended interviews provide the best way to reduce such threats. However, they are very labor intensive. The stakes riding on many risk communications might justify that investment. Realistically speaking, the needed time and financial resources are not always available. As a result, open-ended, one-on-one interviews are better seen as necessary stepping stones to structured questionnaires, suitable for mass administration. Those questionnaires should cover the critical topics in the expert model, express questions in terms familiar to subjects, and test for the prevalence of misconceptions. Worked examples can be found in Ref. 4.

CONCLUSION

Risk perception and risk communication research are complicated businesses, perhaps as complicated as assessing the magnitude of the risks that they consider. A chapter of this length can, at best, indicate the dimensions of complexity and the directions of plausible solutions. In this treatment, we have emphasized methodological issues because we believe that these topics often seem deceptively simple to those not trained in them. Because we all talk and ask questions in everyday life, it seems straightforward to do so regarding health risks. Unfortunately, there are many pitfalls to such amateurism, hints to which can be found in those occasions in life where we have misunderstood or been misunderstood, particularly when dealing with strangers on unfamiliar topics.

Research in this area is fortunate in being able to draw on well-developed literatures in such areas as cognitive, health, and social psychology; survey research; psycholinguistics; psychophysics; and behavioral decision theory. It is unfortunate in having to face the particularly rigorous demands of assessing and improving beliefs about health risks. These often involve complex and unfamiliar topics, surrounded by unusual kinds of uncertainty, for which individuals and groups lack stable vocabularies. Health risk decisions also raise difficult and potentially threatening tradeoffs. Even the most carefully prepared and evaluated communications may not be able to eliminate the anxiety and frustration that such decisions create. However, systematic preparation can keep communications from adding to the problem. At some point in complex decisions, we "throw up our hands" and go with what seems right. Good risk communications can help people get further into the problem before that happens.

Health risk decisions are not just about cognitive processes and cooly weighed information. Emotions play a role, as do social processes. Nonetheless, it is important to get the cognitive part right, lest people's ability to think their way to decisions be underestimated and underserved.

Literature Cited

1. Arabie, P., Maschmeyer, C. 1988. Some current models for the perception and judgment of risk. *Org. Behav. Hum. Decis. Proc.* 41:300–29
2. Atman, C. 1990. *Network structures as a foundation for risk communication.* Doctoral diss. Carnegie Mellon Univ.
3. Beyth-Marom, R. 1982. How probable is probable? Numerical translation of verbal probability expressions. *J. Forecasting* 1:257–69
4. Bostrom, A., Atman, C., Fischhoff, B., Morgan, M. B. 1993. Evaluating risk communications: completing and correcting mental models of hazardous processes. Submitted.
5. Bostrom, A., Fischhoff, B., Morgan, M. G. Eliciting mental models of hazardous processes: a methodology and an application to radon. *J. Soc. Issues.* In press
6. Covello, V. T., Sandman, P. M., Slovic, P. 1988. *Risk Communication, Risk Statistics, and Risk Comparisons: A Manual for Plant Managers.* Washington, DC: Chem. Manuf. Assoc.
7. Craik, K. 1943. *The Nature of Explanation.* Cambridge: Cambridge Univ. Press
8. Crouch, E. A. C., Wilson, R. 1982. *Risk/Benefit Analysis.* Cambridge, Mass: Ballinger
9. Cvetkovich, G., Grote, B., Bjorseth, A., Sarkissian, J. 1975. On the psychology of adolescents' use of contraceptives. *J. Sex Res.* 11:256–70
10. Desvousges, W. H., Smith, V. K., Rink, H. H. III. 1989. *Communicating Radon Risk Effectively: Radon Testing in Maryland.* EPA 230-03-89-408. Washington, DC: US Environ. Prot. Agency, Off. Policy, Plan. Eval.
11. Elkind, D. 1967. Egocentrism in adolescence. *Child Dev.* 38:1025–34
12. Ericsson, K. A. 1988. Concurrent verbal reports on text comprehension: a review. *Text* 8:295–325
13. Ericsson, K. A., Simon, H. A. 1980. Verbal reports as data. *Psychol. Rev.* 87:215–51
14. Fineberg, H. V. 1988. Education to prevent AIDS. *Science* 239:592–96
15. Fischhoff, B. 1992. Giving advice: decision theory perspectives on sexual assault. *Am. Psychol.* 47:577–88
16. Fischhoff, B. 1989. Making decisions about AIDS. In *Primary Prevention of AIDS,* ed. V. Mays, G. Albee, S. Schneider, pp. 168–205. Newbury Park, Calif: Sage
17. Fischhoff, B. 1987. Treating the public with risk communications: a public health perspective. *Sci. Technol. Hum. Values* 12:13–19
18. Fishhoff, B., Lichtenstein, S., Slovic, P., Derby, S. L., Keeney, R.L. 1981. *Acceptable Risk.* New York: Cambridge Univ. Press
19. Fischhoff, B., MacGregor, D. 1983. Judged lethality: how much people seem to know depends upon how they are asked. *Risk Anal.* 3:229–36
20. Fischhoff, B., Slovic, P., Lichtenstein, S., 1983. The "public" vs. the "experts": perceived vs. actual disagreement about the risks of nuclear power. In *Analysis of Actual vs. Perceived Risks,* ed. V. Covello, G. Flamm, J. Rodericks, R. Tardiff, pp. 235–49. New York: Plenum
21. Fischhoff, B., Slovic, P., Lichtenstein, S., 1977. Knowing with certainty: the appropriateness of extreme confidence. *J. Exp. Psychol. Hum. Percept. Perform.* 3:552–64
22. Fischhoff, B., Slovic, P., Lichtenstein, S., Read, S., Combs, B. 1978. How safe is safe enough? A psychometric study of attitudes towards technological risks and benefits. *Policy Sci.* 8:127–52
23. Fischhoff, B., Watson, S., Hope, C. 1984. Defining risk. *Policy Sci.* 17: 123–39
24. Galotti, K. M. 1989. Approaches to studying formal and everyday reasoning. *Psychol. Bull.* 105:331–51
25. Garnham, A. 1987. *Mental Models as Representations of Discourse and Text.* New York: Halsted
26. Gentner, D., Stevens, A. L., eds. 1983. *Mental Models.* Hillsdale, NJ: Erlbaum
27. Heimer, C. A. 1988. Social structure psychology, and the estimation of risk. *Annu. Rev. Soc.* 14:491–519
28. Hendrickx, L. C. W. P. 1991. *How versus how often: the role of scenario information and frequency information in risk judgment and risky decision making.* Doctoral Diss., Rijksuniversiteit Groningen
29. Howard, R. A. 1989. Knowledge maps. *Manage. Sci.* 35:903–22
30. Inst. of Med. 1986. *Confronting AIDS.* Washington, DC: Natl. Acad. Press
31. Jungermann, H., Shutz, H., Thuring, M. 1988. Mental models in risk assessment: informing people about drugs. *Risk Anal.* 8:147–55

32. Kahneman, D., Slovic, P., Tversky, A., eds. 1982. *Judgment Under Uncertainty: Heuristics and Biases*. New York: Cambridge Univ. Press
33. Kaplan, E. H. 1989. What are the risks of risky sex? *Oper. Res.* 37:198–209
34. Kempton, W., 1987. Variation in folk models and consequent behavior. *Am. Behav. Sci.* 31:203–18
35. Kintsch, W. 1986. Learning from text. *Cogn. Instr.*3:87–108
36. Krimsky, S., Plough, A. 1988. *Environmental Hazards*. Dover, Mass: Auburn
37. Lau, R., Kaine, R., Berry, S., Ware, J., Roy, D. 1980. Channeling health: a review of the evaluation of televised health campaigns. *Health Educ. Q.* 7:56–89
38. Lichtenstein, S., Fischhoff, B., Phillips, L. D. 1982. Calibration of probabilities: state of the art to 1980. See Ref. 32
39. Lichtenstein, S., Newman, J. R. 1967. Empirical scaling of common verbal phrases associated with numerical probabilities. *Psychon. Sci.* 9:563–64
40. Lichtenstein, S., Slovic, P., Fischhoff, B., Layman, M., Combs, B. 1978. Judged frequency of lethal events. *J. Exp. Psychol. Hum. Learn. Mem.* 4: 551–78
41. Linville, P. W., Fischer, G. W., Fischhoff, B. Perceived risk and decision making involving AIDS. 1993. In *The Social Psychology of HIV Infection,* ed. J. B. Pryor, G. D. Reeder. Hillsdale, NJ: Erlbaum. In press
42. Maharik, M., Fischhoff, B. 1992. The risks of nuclear energy sources in space: Some activists' perceptions. *Risk Anal.* 12:383–92
43. Means, M. L., Voss, J. F., 1985. Star wars: a developmental study of expert and novice knowledge studies. *J. Mem. Lang.* 24:746–57
44. Merton, R. F. 1987. The focussed interview and focus groups. *Public Opin. Q.* 51:550–66
45. Merz, J. F. 1991. *Toward a standard of disclosure for medical informed consent: development and demonstration of a decision—analytic methodology*. Ph.D. diss. Carnegie Mellon Univ.
46. Merz, J. F., Fischhoff, B., 1990. Informed consent does not mean rational consent: cognitive limitations on decision-making. *J. Legal Med.* 11: 321–50
47. Morgan, M. G., Florig, H. K., Nair, I., Cortes, C., Marsh, K., Pavlosky, K. 1990. Lay understanding of power-frequency fields. *Bioelectromagnetics* 11:313–35
48. Morrison, D. M. 1985. Adolescent contraceptive behavior: a review. *Psychol. Bull.* 98:538–68
49. Natl. Res. Counc. 1989. *Improving Risk Communication*. Washington, DC: Natl. Acad. Press
50. Oden, G. C. 1987. Concept, knowledge, and thought. *Annu. Rev. Psychol.* 38:203–27
51. Poulton, E. C. 1989. *Bias in Quantifying Judgment*. Hillsdale, NJ: Erlbaum
52. Quadrel, M. J. 1990. *Elicitation of adolescents' perceptions: qualitative and quantitative dimensions*. Ph.D. diss. Carnegie Mellon Univ.
53. Quadrel, M. J., Fischhoff, B., Davis, W. 1993. Adolescent invulnerability. *Am. Psychol.* In press
54. Reder, L. M. 1985. Techniques available to author, teacher, and reader to improve retention of main ideas of a chapter. In *Thinking and Learning Skills: Vol. 2. Research and Open Questions,* ed. S. F. Chipman, J. W. Segal, R. Glaser, pp. 37–64. Hillsdale, NJ: Erlbaum
55. Rohrmann, B., 1990. *Analyzing and evaluating the effectiveness of risk communication programs*. Unpubl. Univ. of Mannheim
56. Roth, E., Morgan, G., Fischhoff, B., Lave, L., Bostrom, A. 1990. What do we know about making risk comparisons? *Risk Anal.* 10:375–87
57. Rouse, W. B., Morris, N. M. 1986. On looking into the black box: prospects and limits in the search for mental models. *Psychol. Bull.* 100:349–63
58. Schriver, K. A. 1989. *Plain language for expert or lay audiences: designing text using protocol aided revision*. Pittsburgh: Commun. Design Cent., Carnegie Mellon Univ.
59. Shaklee, H., Fischhoff, B. 1990. The psychology of contraceptive surprises: judging the cumulative risk of contraceptive failure. *J. Appl. Psychol.* 20: 385–403
60. Slovic, P. 1987. Perceptions of risk. *Science* 236:280–85
61. Slovic, P., Fischhoff, B., Lichtenstein, S. 1984. Modeling the societal impact of fatal accidents. *Manage Sci.* 30:464–74
62. Slovic, P., Fischhoff, B., Lichtenstein, S. 1979. Rating the risks. *Environment* 21:14–20, 36–39
63. Svenson, O. 1981. Are we all less risky and more skillful than our fellow drivers? *Acta Psychol.* 47:143–48
64. Svenson, O., Fischhoff, B. 1985. Lev-

els of environmental decisions. *J. Environ. Psychol.* 5:55–68

65. Tversky, A., Kahneman, D. 1973. Availability: a heuristic for judging frequency and probability. *Cogn. Psychol.* 4:207–32

65a. US Environ. Prot. Agency Off. of Air and Radiat., US Dep. of Health and Hum. Serv., Cent. for Dis. Control. 1986. *A Citizen's Guide to Radon: What It Is and What to Do About It,* OPA-86-004

66. von Winterfeldt, D., Edwards, W., 1986. *Decision Analysis and Behavioral Research.* New York: Cambridge Univ. Press

67. Wallsten, T. S., Budescu, D. V., Rapoport, A., Zwick, R., Forsyth, B. 1986. Measuring the vague meanings of probability terms. *J. Exp. Psychol. Gen.* 115:348–65

68. Weinstein, N. 1987. *Taking Care: Understanding and Encouraging Self-Protective Behavior.* New York: Cambridge Univ. Press

69. Weinstein, N. D. 1980. Unrealistic optimism about future life events. *J. Pers. Soc. Psychol.* 39:806–20

70. Wilson, R. W., Thornberry, O. T. 1987. Knowledge and attitudes about AIDS: provisional data from the National Health Interview Survey, August 10–30, 1987. *Adv. Data,* No. 146

71. Yates, J. F., ed. 1992. *Risk Taking.* Chichester: Wiley

72. Yates, J. F. 1989. *Judgment and Decision Making.* Englewood Cliffs, NJ: Prentice Hall

Annu. Rev. Publ. Health 1993. 14:205–17

SENTINEL EVENT STRATEGIES IN ENVIRONMENTAL HEALTH

Tim E. Aldrich

Department of Epidemiology, School of Public Health, University of North Carolina, Chapel Hill, North Carolina 27599–7400

Paul E. Leaverton

Department of Epidemiology and Biostatistics, College of Public Health, University of South Florida, Tampa, Florida 33612–3899

KEY WORDS: surveillance, epidemiology, disease control, space-time clusters, decision rules

---

INTRODUCTION

In 1979, 1980, and 1981, the three Yves Biraud Seminars in Talloires, France, explored developments in the relatively new field of environmental epidemiology. Since those early conclaves, the field has advanced considerably, yet the evolution of new technologies, specific to the purpose, have been slow (5, 25). Many of the research methods used for environmental epidemiology have been borrowed from infectious disease investigations or from occupational studies. This chapter describes the application of a specific public health monitoring technique, borrowed from occupational epidemiology—surveillance for sentinel health events (53).

Disease surveillance has been defined as a "state of continuing watchfulness" (60). The salient characteristic here is **watchfulness**, which is the objective of detecting a meaningful change of state, i.e. disease incidence. A surveillance system has been defined as the systematic collection, analysis, and dissemination of data. Many industries began to develop company-based surveillance systems in the 1970s as a response to the Occupational Safety and Health Administration (OSHA) legislation and the need for more data to study potential health effects from occupational exposures.

0163-7525/93/0510-0205$02.00

A similar process is now occurring for environmental exposures with the implementation of federal legislation under "Superfund" (55). The emergence of exposure registries has prompted the search for innovative techniques for analyzing the available data to detect evidence of increased disease risk as soon as possible (5, 50). From occupational data applications and the earlier Yves Biraud deliberations, the objective has been clear, early recognition of emerging health risks—the sentinel event strategy arises directly from these objectives.

SENTINEL EVENT STRATEGIES

One case of a disease may have different implications than another. For example, one additional case of lung cancer in a community with 30 cases may not be significant, particularly if that individual is a smoker. By contrast, one case of pediatric osteogenic sarcoma near a nuclear power plant can be a cause for substantive concern. In the *Case of the Redheaded League,* Sherlock Holmes quipped to Dr. Watson: "The more bizarre a thing is the less mysterious it is likely to prove." This adage is a prelude to what is called sentinel event reasoning. Simply stated, some events mean more than others; that is, they are important because of recognized characteristics that are known or suspected about the disease etiology (6, 50, 53). Selective surveillance for these health events can be very productive; because these events tend to be rare (i.e. "bizarre"), there is reason to hope that their causation may also be more simple to study (i.e. "less mysterious") (6).

Defining Sentinel Events

As proposed by Rutstein et al (53), sentinel events are occurrences of single cases of disease. In subsequent years, other meanings have been given to sentinel events, e.g. the event may be statistical. This sort of expansion of the concept has led to three different applications of the sentinel event strategy and to two examples of innovative variations.

SINGLE EVENTS Focal to Rutstein's strategy for sentinel events were their singularity and their preventability (53). Rutstein often cited cervical cancer deaths as an example. The North Carolina State Center for Health and Environmental Statistics prepares a sentinel event list that features such causes of death as "death during child birth" and "oral cancer in a person less than 30 years of age." A death (or case, for cancer) of either of these types provides evidence that a prevention action could be warranted. These sentinel events could guide a county health director to implement specific interventions, such as targeting of natality care, public education regarding smokeless tobacco, and screening. These applications of sentinel events are directly in-line with

Rutstein's admonition to search for singularity of occurrence and the ability for prevention (53).

LOCALIZED CLUSTERING OF RARE EVENTS Another approach to the study of sentinel events borrows more from Holmes than Rutstein and does not rely on single events (6, 7). Rare health events can be bizarre when they occur in a small aggregate or in unusual populations. Such an intent accepts that some events are expected, e.g. pediatric osteogenic sarcoma—a rare but nonzero occurrence in a state's population. When the occasional, rare osteogenic sarcoma case occurs, it is still more rare from a population distribution perspective. Two such cases within a single residential, subdivision would certainly be bizarre. This localization of occurrence is the key to this variation on a sentinel event strategy. Although these (sentinel) rare events may not be preventable in any way that we currently understand, epidemiologists can examine the risk factors for their occurrence. The logical linkage of occurrence and risk was also intrinsic to Rutstein's thinking (53). In this example, if the two pediatric osteogenic sarcomas occurred in a setting with no known risk factors, they might be disregarded as sentinels and considered random occurrences. However, if the two cases occurred near a nuclear waste disposal facility, they would command greater attention. In this same sense, the occurrence of a third case in the same vicinity would mandate closer evaluation. In this particular sentinel event approach, a single case may not serve as a sentinel, yet it may pose a warning. Later discussions in this chapter elaborate these principles and discuss their application (6, 30).

CHANGES IN A "LOGICAL" PATTERN An extension of the previous application of sentinel event reasoning is the recognition of incidence patterns on a population scale and not necessarily on a cause and effect level. For example, cerebrovascular deaths (strokes) are relatively common in older persons, especially in older blacks. Further, the high frequency of the event obscures potentially significant occurrences, or sentinels. Thus, an analysis of stroke mortality could be focused on deaths of persons less than 30 years of age. Finding a curious aggregate of these, a further examination of the pattern of persons over 30 might also indicate an increased occurrence. The incidence in persons over 30 probably would have been disregarded as a random fluctuation without the corroborating increase among younger persons (21). In North Carolina, this strategy has been applied to late-stage cervical cancer diagnoses as a means of targeting screening programs. The distribution of late-stage cervical cancers was first studied for women under the age of 50; this was compared with late-stage diagnoses for women of older ages. Concordant high proportions for late-stage diagnoses targeted geographic areas for concern regarding access to screening services and to public health education about screening efficacy.

SURROGATE EVENTS One of the most innovative applications of the sentinel event philosophy is its extension beyond the subject event. Two examples are provided.

Increased occurrences along a spectrum of biologic effects For many years, carcinogenesis has been associated with mutational events, hence the application of in vitro tests (8). A logical extension of this reasoning for sentinel event applications is along the logic of the biologic spectrum leading to cancer. That is to say, other adverse health events might have related etiologies, but their occurrence might precede neoplasia. Congenital anomalies (birth defects) are the foremost candidate for this logic. Finding a small cluster of rare cancers might lead to marginal statistical significance for it being a random event. However, a concordant increase in birth defects could provide the added, bizarre ingredient to the study for justifying further research. Other applications of this approach include strategic dermatologic manifestations (e.g. chloracne due to suspected chlorinated hydrocarbon exposures and increased respiratory illnesses associated with a suspected airborne contaminant).

Sentinel species A particularly splendid extension of this logic for sentinel event research relates to the same reasoning that was applied to arrive at the use of in vivo test systems for bioassays of potential carcinogens (36). Simply stated, animals experience accelerated life spans compared with humans. Where similar hazardous exposure occurs in the ambient environment, they may manifest adverse disease more quickly than humans (47). In fact, there is evidence that animals may develop tumors as a result of carcinogenic exposures in common with their owners (24, 32, 48).

EXAMPLES OF SENTINEL EVENTS

In the Honan province of China, two communities were identified as having dramatically different esophageal cancer rates. A regional pattern of gullet cancer among local poultry in one of the provinces (40, 41) led to the community with the higher esophageal cancer rate being systematically relocated; their poultry was not permitted to be taken along. However, the esophageal cancer rates in the migrants were not diminished. Eventually, the practice of eating strongly pickled vegetables was identified as the causal association; the similar pattern among the chickens had been the result of shared foods (41).

Recognition of spatial patterns and unusual case occurrences are consistent with sentinel reasoning. This approach of seeking sentinel cancers associated with occupational exposures was raised to a new level by the mapping of cancer mortality by the National Cancer Institute (42). One excellent example of studies directed to rare diseases involves a pediatric liver cancer case that was linked to a paternal work place exposure (18).

IMPLEMENTING SENTINEL EVENT STRATEGIES

Sentinel strategies can be used for environmental health practice. We now discuss routine and ad hoc approaches, simple inspections and complex data bases, reasoning on single events, and sophisticated statistical methods.

Routine, Periodic Inspection

In North Carolina, a biennial review process is applied to each county. This review, called "community diagnosis," is based on the statistical information available from vital records for each county. In this approach, sentinel events are inspected for occurrences of single cases that would represent bases for public health intervention (e.g. a maternal death). Similarly, trends and demographic patterns are inspected for targeting programs and resources (e.g. oral cancer in youths and late-stage cervical cancer). In the future, geographic patterns of disease occurrence may also be studied in a community diagnosis process by using Geographic Information Systems (GIS) technology to evaluate environmental evidence for sentinel patterns.

Disease Registries

Disease registries are one of the preeminent approaches to studying environmental health risk and to resolving reports of disease clusters (34, 51). Registries are an ideal setting for the application of sentinel strategies that employ the diseases registered. Cancer databases provide many states with incidence information that may be applied for sentinel event assessments; 41 states now have some level of population-based cancer surveillance, and there are several birth defect registries, as well (6, 14, 61). Another source of secondary surveillance data is death certificates, a nation-wide resource. Also, there are databases in place for pursuit of the animal sentinel event strategy (33).

Directed Analyses

In addition to these programmatic approaches, others may be employed that simply use a particular perspective within research methods. For example, **surveillance studies** involve systematic assessment of selected sentinel events along a line of common exposures (e.g. gradients along a water shed, or distances of air pollution migration up a valley). The concomitant variation of disease having potentially common biologic mechanisms offers another example of a surveillance study (Mill's Canons listed in Ref. 49).

Another such directed strategy would employ **"time-series analyses"** for evidence of systematic trends that may signal a subtle shifting in disease risk that cannot be explained as a secular trend or geographic correlate. Finally, following-up of disease **cluster reports** offers a particularly heuristic challenge for sentinel event evaluations. Each of these methods for directed analyses is discussed in turn and in somewhat more detail in the later sections of this chapter.

OTHER PRACTICAL CONSIDERATIONS

Which events should be considered sentinel? Returning to the Holmes quote, the event should be bizarre, such that one case alone is noticed. Miller notes that "virtually every known carcinogen and teratogen has first been recognized by an alert clinician" (44). The alert clinician in each case was knowledgeable about disease occurrence, so that when an unusual (bizarre) case occurred, the clinician noticed it (9). Thus, rare diseases and diseases occurring in unusual population groups are at the forefront of a list of sentinel health events (see Table 1) (21).

Further, the sentinel events should have temporal validity. Most cancers are not useful sentinels, because their latency is too long, in the range of 15–30 years. Rutstein et al's (53) original list included several cancers, but also many other acute and subchronic conditions. Monitoring adverse reproductive outcomes, neurologic conditions, and acute diagnoses is also needed (Table 1) (6, 12, 52). Further, as our understanding of genetic factors associated with susceptibility to hazardous exposures grows, there is the potential for monitoring specific biologic markers and individuals with genetic predisposition (12, 31, 35, 37, 45).

From the original intent of sentinel event reasoning, the objective was to know enough about the suspect exposures to anticipate what events might be expected as a sequela from them, so that the first case of one of those diseases would signal intervention. Practically speaking, however, there are two necessary antecedent circumstances:

1. There needs to be a system in place for monitoring communities around hazardous point sources, so that one case of an unusual health event will be noticed, or so that a pattern of unusual health events (if the occurrence is not too rare) will be detected.
2. A means is needed for detecting unusual disease aggregates so that valid clusters can be identified, as they may occur near a point source that has not previously been identified or classified as hazardous.

Table 1 Sample listing of sentinel health events and conditions[a]

Health events
Liver carcinoma (specifically in nonsmokers and nondrinkers)
Glioblastoma
Amelanotic melanoma
Pediatric solid tumors
Genitourinary cancers in children
Exotic lymphoma cell types
Exotic leukemias (or occurring in uncharacteristic age groups)
Bladder, lung, or upper respiratory cancers (specifically in nonsmokers)
Midline or septal birth defects
Health conditions
Unusual allergies
Unusual neurologic symptoms
Idiopathic hematuria
Persistent, unresolved rashes
Persistent, idiopathic nasopharyngitis
Extreme liver enzyme functions in a nonsmoker
Extreme renal function values in a nonsmoker

[a] From Ref. 6.

Both of these objectives are consistent with surveillance systems. Currently, the approach is being driven by an inefficient process of disease cluster reports (16, 51, 54). Prospective identification of impending increases in disease rates on a small scale and at as early a time as possible is best. However, imaginative use of disease surveillance systems is needed to accomplish these ends.

THE CURRENT STATUS OF DISEASE SURVEILLANCE

The required elements for a sentinel event surveillance system are a reportable list, a reporting system, and statistical methods for discerning an increase (6). The sentinel event approach has been used with occupational mortality for a national analysis (62). The *Future of Public Health* report from the Institute of Medicine Committee encouraged states to develop capabilities for environmental health research of populations exposed to hazardous materials, especially for exposures that cross state lines (37). Also, many larger industries are developing surveillance medical systems (38). The National Institute of Occupational Safety and Health operates a medical surveillance system based on this design—Sentinel Events Notification System for Occupational Risks (SENSOR) (15).

To this end, the opportunity exists for linkage of disease registry data with environmental databases (20). One such approach was recently used with cancer mortality and hazardous waste sites on the National Priority List; that study used county of residence/location as the basis of analysis (27). In addition, the Agency for Toxic Substances and Disease Registry is developing national exposure and disease registries (1, 2).

Surveillance Strategies

Today, much of what we call "risk assessment" for environmental hazards does not use much or any human data for determining risks (31, 58). What is needed in environmental epidemiology is a research method based on prospectively identifying meaningful rare event aggregates (4). Such a research method is, by definition, the operation of a surveillance system; yet, this system will be most productive if it is strategically designed to operate with sentinel events (6, 60). However, disease surveillance systems are expensive in comparison to mathematical modeling means for evaluating potential carcinogenicity of specific agents, despite the improvement in certainty and the avoidance of interspecies extrapolation. The wisdom to see long-term benefit for epidemiologic surveillance systems like these is slow in coming and the morass of politics and science is not helping bring such system designs about (11, 26).

Analytic Issues

Central to the process of environmental health surveillance is establishing what disease incidence is expected in a population. When national data are applied to a small geographic area to approximate an expected disease rate, several potential errors can occur. A fraction of a case may be expected; thus, even one case will indicate an increased rate. This circumstance leads to the use of the Poisson distribution for rare event studies. Also, the potential exists for committing the "ecologic fallacy" when an increase disease rate is found and assigned to a particular factor (e.g. a hazardous, local industry) when another factor actually explains the increase (e.g. an age artifact) (19).

Time-Series Analysis

Identifying a "meaningful" increase in disease occurrence is both a sophisticated problem and a subtle one. One of the best established methods for conducting disease surveillance is a comparison over time (56, 59). The process of disease surveillance has become increasingly complicated in recent years because of rapid, localized population growth (e.g. "boom towns") and shifting demographic characteristics (e.g. the aging of the population). These changing population parameters are called secular trends (literally, belonging to the world). Consequently, the selection of an appropriate comparison population is a critical consideration. Further, the decision that an observed increase in disease occurrence is a "real" one and not simply random "noise" makes decision-making all the more uncertain.

Because surveillance analyses can be so complicated, it is a sound strategy to develop models of the expected disease rates and to determine in advance the thresholds of observed cases/rates that will represent statistical significance (30). Table 2, taken from a rare event surveillance system developed in Texas, shows the small number of cases that may be needed to declare an increased rate for mortality around a specific hazardous waste site (see also Ref. 29). The approaches use Poisson distributions for solutions and Standardized Mortality Ratio (SMR) tests, so that age, race, sex, and population change over time can be controlled.

In addition to the problem of declaring an increase, there is the issue of false findings (an increase that is a random swing). A statistical solution can be built into the decision threshold to limit the possibility of one false positive per series of tests (13). Also, a sequential approach may be used so that an increase will first trigger an "ALERT" that a threshold has been passed; then,

Table 2 Sample statistical decision table for use with a public health surveillance system applied to sentinel events—numbers of deaths and (magnitude of SMR value required)[a]

Expected number of deaths	Observed number of deaths: For an ALERT[b]	Observed number of deaths: For an ACTION[b]
0.05	1 (20)[c]	3 (60)
0.1	2 (20)	3 (30)
0.2	2 (10)	4 (20)
0.4	2 (5)	4 (10)
0.5	2 (4)	5 (10)
1	3 (3)	6 (6)
2	5 (2.5)	9 (4.5)
4	8 (2)	12 (3)
5	9 (1.8)	14 (2.8)
10	15 (1.5)	22 (2.2)
15	21 (1.4)	29 (1.93)
20	26 (1.3)	36 (1.8)
25	33 (1.32)	43 (1.72)
30	38 (1.27)	49 (1.63)

[a] From Ref. 22.
[b] ACTION and ALERT levels correspond to $p_2 = 0.001$ and $p_1 + p_2 = 0.09$ for a two-year error level of 0.01.
[c] ( ) Corresponding SMR associated with the specific expected number of deaths and the observed number of deaths.

if the elevated occurrence continues for a second interval, "ACTION" can be taken (22). This same approach permits a single, very high increase to signal "ACTION" based on one time period alone (22, 30).

Spatial Analyses

It is also possible to monitor disease occurrence for evidence of geographic patterns. With these methods, the research question is, Are geographic areas with similar (usually elevated) rates adjacent to each other? Interpreting these analyses can be complicated. Today, there is a new technology to assist with geographic analyses; the advent of GIS technology has been a boon to many large geographic area applications (3, 13, 57). This technology will facilitate cluster investigations and studies of exposure from hazardous point sources (10, 23, 28, 46).

Clustering in Time and Space

In addition to studying a pattern of disease occurrence over time and in space, there is also the approach using space and time (3), e.g. the REMSA technique (which also uses demographic traits) (7). REMSA aims to answer the question, What part of all the available population "space" is being occupied by a subset of cases? This method searches for a small cell, within the available population space, to see how unlikely is a certain aggregation of cases (7). With this technique, individual population characteristics are treated as independent probabilities (e.g. age, race, sex). Consequently, epidemiologists can detect a cluster of cases that occur within a small population strata, as well as one that occurs in a short period of time or in a small geographic area—all with the unifying characteristic that the aggregate is unlikely to occur because of chance. This test uses a negative binomial solution to evaluate the probability of unusual cases clustering (7).

The Surveillance Mandate

Active collection of surveillance data is similar to a cohort study or epidemiologic surveillance, which means it can be costly (60). Through the fiat of state law, many states require reporting of cancer or other chronic diseases of public health significance. This approach compels institutions and professionals to report cases to a central agency. As a compromise, the data set is usually small to encourage compliance. In this latter approach, the emphasis is on case identification; for special research purposes (as discussed under analytic issues above), a more detailed data set may be collected for the subset of cases of interest.

One critical characteristic of a surveillance system is the reporting of the data to appropriate health officials. These reports may be extensive or brief. Many disease registries now publish a concise report annually and make available their database for interested researchers; periodically (every 3–5 years), these registries publish a detailed report with extensive analyses and narratives. The Centers for Disease Control has provided a discussion of surveillance systems and a description of their structure (39).

CONCLUSION

Public health practice needs to evolve toward more efficient and systematic methods (37). Surveillance for sentinel health events signaling potentially important emerging environmental health problems is one effort directed to that end. It is not an easy task, because of the statistical and epidemiological difficulties involved in sorting out real signals from the background noise of random disease occurrences. Few real successes have been obtained to date, yet prototype strategies are identified (17, 43, 51). Further, the public demand for disease cluster investigation will not go away. Nor should it. Computer and biological (including biological markers) technology exists to improve present efforts (52). And, these technologies are becoming more useful (31, 35). This important public health issue requires more attention by environmental epidemiologists and statisticians (6, 12, 25, 52). We need to harness efficiently all the tools becoming available to create systematic methods for identifying and detecting sentinel health events as we deal with the growing environmental health concerns of today and tomorrow.

Literature Cited

1. Agency Toxic Subst. Dis. Regist. 1988. *Establishment of the National Exposure Registries*. Atlanta: Public Health Serv.
2. Agency Toxic Subst. Dis. Regist. 1990. *Final Report of the Panel on the National Disease Registry*. Atlanta: Public Health Serv.
3. Aldrich, T. E., Drane, J. W. 1992. *CLUSTER: User's Manual for Software to Assist with the Investigation of Rare Health Events*. Atlanta: Agency Toxic Subst. Dis. Regist. 114 pp.
4. Aldrich, T. E., Garcia, N., Zeichner, S., Berger, S. 1959. Cancer clusters: a myth or a method. *Med. Hypothesis* 12:41–52.
5. Aldrich, T. E., Griffith, J. D. 1991. A sobering start to the cluster busters' conference and Counterpoint from a Cluster Buster (letter). *Am. J. Epidemiol.* 133(5):512–13
6. Aldrich, T. E., Meyer, R. E., Qualters, J., Atkinson, D. A. 1989. Rare health events as sentinels of environmental contamination. *Proc. 1989 Public Health Conf. Rec. Stat.*, DHHS Publ. No. (PHS) 90–124:323–26
7. Aldrich, T. E., Wilson, C. C., Easterly, C. E. 1986. Population-surveillance for rare health events. *Proc. 1985 Public Health Conf. Rec. and Stat.*, DHHS Publ. No. (PHS) 86-1214:215–20
8. Ames, B. N., McCann, J., Yamasaki, E. 1975. Methods for detecting carcinogens and mutagens with the Salmonella/mammalian microsome mutagenicity test. *Mutat. Res.* 31:347–64
9. Armenian, H. K. 1991. Case investigation in epidemiology. *Am. J. Epidemiol.* 134(10):1067–72
10. Beral, V. 1990. Childhood leukemia near nuclear power plants in the United Kingdom: the evolution of a systematic approach to studying rare disease in small geographic areas. *Am. J. Epidemiol.* 132(Suppl.):S63–S68
11. Brownlea, A. 1981. From public health

to political epidemiology. *Soc. Sci. Med.* 15D:57–67

12. Buffler, P. A., Aase, J. M. 1982. Genetic risk and environmental surveillance: epidemiologic aspects of monitoring industrial populations for environmental mutagens. *J. Occup. Med.* 24(4):305–14
13. Chen, R. 1978. A surveillance system for congenital malformations. *J. Am. Stat. Assoc.* 73:323–27
14. Edmonds, L. D., Layde, P. M., James, L. M., Oakley, G. 1987. Congenital malformation surveillance: two American systems. Int. J. Epidemiol. 10: 247–51
15. Ehrenberg, R. 1988. Sentinel events notification system for occupational risks (SENSOR): 1987. In *Proc. Workshop Needs Resourc. Occup. Mortal. Data.* CDC DHHS Publ. No. (PHS) 88–1463:448–49
16. Enterline, P. E. 1985. Evaluating cancer clusters. *Am. Ind. Hyg. Assoc. J.* 46:10–13
17. Falk, H., Baxter, P. J. 1981. Hepatic angiosarcoma registries: implications for rare tumor studies. *Banbury Rep. No. 9: Quantification of Occupational Cancer,* pp. 543–51. Cold Spring Harbor, NY: Cold Spring Harbor Lab. 691 pp.
18. Falk, H., Herbert, J. T., Edmonds, L., Heath, C. W., Thomas, L. B., Popper, H. 1981. Review of four cases of childhood hepatic angiocarcinoma—elevated environmental arsenic exposure in one case. *Cancer* 47:382–91
19. Feinleib, M., and Leaverton, P. E. 1984. Ecologic fallacies in epidemiology. In *Health Information Systems,* eds. P. E. Leaverton, L. Masse, 4:33–62. New York: Praeger. 195 pp.
20. Frisch, J. D., Shaw, G. M., Harris, J. A. 1990. Epidemiologic research using existing databases of environmental measures. *Arch. Environ. Health* 45(5):303–7
21. Garfinkel, L. 1987. Cancer clusters. *J. Clinic.* 37(1):20–25
22. Glasser, J. H. 1986. Health statistics surveillance systems for hazardous waste disposal. *Proc. 1985 Public Health Conf. Rec. Stat.* DHHS Publ. No. (PHS) 86–1214:221–24
23. Glick, B. 1979. The spatial autocorrelation of cancer mortality. *Soc. Sci. Med.* 13D:123–30
24. Glickman, L. T., Domanski, L. M., Maguire, T. G., et al., 1983. Mesothelioma in pet dogs associated with exposure of their owners to asbestos. *Environ. Res.* 32:305–13
25. Goldsmith, J. R. 1988. Keynote address: improving the prospects for environmental epidemiology. *Arch. Environ. Health* 43(2):69–74
26. Gough, M. 1987. Environmental epidemiology: separating politics and science. *Issues Sci. Technol.* Summer:20–31
27. Griffith, J. D., Duncan, R. C., Riggan, W. B., Pellom, A. C. 1989. Cancer mortality in US counties with hazardous waste sites and ground water pollution. *Arch. Environ. Health* 44:69–74
28. Grimson, R. C., Wang, K. C., Johnson, P. W. C. 1981. Searching for hierarchial clusters of disease: spatial patterns of sudden infant death syndrome. *Soc. Sci. Med.* 15:287–93
29. Hanrahan, L. A., Mirkin, I., Olson, J., Anderson, H., Fiore, B. 1990. SMRFIT: a statistical analysis system (SAS) program for standardized mortality ratio analysis and poisson regression model fits in community disease cluster investigation. *Am. J. Epidemiol.* 132 (Suppl):S116–22
30. Hardy, R. J., Schroeder, G. D., Cooper, S. P., Buffler, P. A., Prichard, H. M., Crane, M. 1990. A surveillance system for assessing health effects from hazardous exposures. *Am. J. Epidemiol.* 132:S32–S42
31. Hatis, D. B. 1986. The promise of molecular epidemiology for quantitative risk assessment. *Risk Anal.* 6(2):181–93
32. Hayes, H. M. Jr., Hoover, R., Tyrone, R. E. 1981. Bladder cancer in pet dogs: a sentinel for environmental cancer? *Am. J. Epidemiol.* 104:673–77
33. Hayes, H. M. Jr., Wison, G. P., Moraff, H. 1979. The veterinary medical data program (VMDP): past, present, and future. In *Proc. Int. Symp. Animal Health Dis. Data Banks.* APHIS Misc. Publ. No. 1381, pp. 127–32. Washington, DC: USDA
34. Houk, V. N., Thacker, S. B. 1987. Registries: one way to assess environmental hazards. *Health Environ. Digest* 1:5–6
35. Hulka, B. S., Wilcosky, T. C., Griffith, J. D. 1990. *Biological Markers in Epidemiology.* New York: Oxford Univ. Press. 236 pp.
36. Innes, J. R. M., Ulland, B. M., Valerio, M. G., et al. 1969. Bioassay of pesticides and industrial chemicals for tumorigenicity in mice. A preliminary note. *J. Natl. Cancer Inst.* 42: 1101–14
37. Inst. Med. 1988. *The Future of Public Health.* New York: Natl. Acad. Sci.

38. Joiner, R. L. 1982. Occupational health and environmental information systems: basic considerations. *J. Occup. Med.* 24(10):863–66
39. Klauke, D. N., Buehler, J. W., Thacker, S. B. 1988. Guidelines for evaluating surveillance systems. *Morbid. Mortal. Wkly. Rep.* 37(S-5):1–18
40. Li, F. P., Shiang, E. L. 1980. Cancer mortality in China. *J. Natl. Cancer Inst.* 65:217–21
41. Mason, T. J., Hayes, H. M. Jr. 1982. Disease among animals as sentinels of environmental exposures. In *Environmental Epidemiology,* ed. Leaverton, P. E., Masse, L., Simches, S. O., 7:67–72. New York: Praeger. 176 pp.
42. Mason, T. J., McKay, F. W. 1973. *U.S. Cancer Mortality by County: 1950–1969*. Washington, DC: GPO. 150 pp.
43. Mason, T. J., Vogler, W. J. 1990. Bladder cancer screening at the Dupont chambers works: a new initiative. *J. Occup. Med.* 32(9):874–77
44. Miller, R. W. 1981. Area wide chemical contamination: lessons from case histories. *J. Am. Med. Assoc.* 245: 1548–51
45. Nicholson, W. J. 1984. Research issues in occupational and environmental cancer. *Arch. Environ. Health* 39(3):190–202
46. Ohno, Y, Aoki, K., Aoki, N. 1979. A test of significance for geographic clusters of disease. *Int. J. Epidemiol.* 8:273–81
47. Priester, W. A., McKay, F. W. 1980. The occurrence of tumors in domestic animals. *Natl. Cancer Inst. Monogr.* 54:1–210.
48. Reif, J. S., Dunn, K., Oglive, G. K., Harris, C. K. 1992. Passive smoking and canine lung cancer risk. *Am. J. Epidemiol.* 135(3):234–39
49. Roht, L. H., Selwyn, B. J., Holguin, A. H., Christensen, B. L. 1982. *Principles of Epidemiology: A Self Teaching Guide* (Reference to Mill's Canons). New York: Academic. 261 pp.
50. Rothman, K. J. 1987. Clustering of disease. *Am. J. Public Health* 77(1):14–16
51. Rothman, K. J. 1990. A sobering start for the cluster busters' conference. *Am. J. Epidemiol.* 132(Suppl.):S6–S13
52. Rothwell, C. J., Hamilton, C. B., Leaverton, P. E. 1991. Identification of sentinel health events as indicators of environmental contamination. *Environ. Health Perspect.* 94:261–63
53. Rutstein, D. D., Mullan, R. J., Frazier, T. M., Halperin, W. E., Melius, J. M., Sestito, J. P. 1984. Sentinel health events (occupational): a basis for physician recognition and public health surveillance. *Am. J. Public Health* 39(3):1054–62
54. Schulte, P. A., Ehernburg, R. L., Singal, M. 1987. Investigation of occupational cancer clusters. *Am. J. Public Health* 77(1):52–56
55. Schulte, P. A., Kaye, W. E. 1988. Exposure registries. *Arch. Environ. Health* 43(2):155–61
56. Serfling, R. E. 1963. Methods for current statistical analysis of excess pneumonia-influenza deaths. *Public Health Rep.* 78:494–506
57. Shulman, J., Slevin, S., Merrill, D. W. 1988. Density equalized map projections: a method for analyzing clustering around a fixed point. *Stat. Med.* 7:491–506
58. Stallones, R. 1983. Assessment of risks to public health. In *Risk Assessment in the Federal Government: Managing the Process,* Chair. R. Stallones. Washington, DC: Natl. Acad. Press
59. Stroup, D. F., Williamson, G. D., Hearndon, J. L. 1989. Detection of aberrations in the occurrence of notifiable disease surveillance data. *Stat. Med.* 8:323–39
60. Thacker, S. B., Berkelman, R. L. 1988. Public health surveillance in the United States. *Epidemiol. Rev.* 10:164–90
61. Utility of cancer registries varies. 1990. *Public Health Macroview* 3(5):2–3
62. Wagener, D. K., Buffler, P. A. 1989. Geographic distribution of deaths due to sentinel health event (occupational) causes. *Am. J. Ind. Med.* 16:355–72

Annu. Rev. Publ. Health. 1993. 14:219–41

CONTAINING COSTS WHILE IMPROVING QUALITY OF CARE: The Role of Profiling and Practice Guidelines*†

D. W. Shapiro and R. D. Lasker
Physician Payment Review Commission, Washington, DC 20037

A. B. Bindman[1,2] *and P. R. Lee*[1]
[1]Institute for Health Policy Studies, University of California, San Francisco, California 94109; [2]Division of General Internal Medicine, San Francisco General Hospital, San Francisco, California 94110

KEY WORDS: cost containment, quality improvement, utilization review, economic incentives, practice patterns

INTRODUCTION

The rapidly rising cost of medical care is the driving force behind US health policy today. Health care is claiming an increasing share of our society's human, financial, and physical resources. In addition, rising costs are a critical barrier to improving the availability and quality of health care for the population as a whole. The need to control costs has stimulated numerous proposals for private and public reforms, ranging from managed competition to all-payer rate setting, national expenditure caps, and regional budgeting.

Slowing the rise in costs while maintaining or improving quality of care is challenging, because attempts to control expenditures risk curtailing necessary, as well as unnecessary, services. Meeting this challenge requires strategies that address both cost and quality. Initiatives aimed solely at cost-cutting risk harming patients by eliminating necessary and appropriate

*This chapter presents solely the view of the authors and not necessarily those of their institutions.

care, and efforts to improve the quality of care need to consider the accompanying costs. Profiling and practice guidelines are tools that can be used in conjunction with economic incentives to help practitioners, patients, and payers reduce the rate of increase in costs while not sacrificing quality.

This chapter briefly reviews the factors that contribute to rising costs and analyzes what is needed to preserve quality while controlling costs. We then discuss the roles that profiling and practice guidelines can play in this effort, including the infrastructure and incentives that can make them more effective in improving practice.

THE PROBLEM OF RISING EXPENDITURES FOR HEALTH CARE

It is well known that health care is expensive, but the aggregate numbers are nonetheless stunning. Expenditures for health care in the United States are projected to total $809 billion in 1992, more than 13% of the gross national product (GNP) (43). Spending for physician services alone is estimated to exceed $165 billion in 1992 (43).

Recent analyses bring home the impact of these expenditures on employers and the public. Health-care spending by business now exceeds corporate profits (23). The average household spends $8000 per year for health care—one-third paid directly by members of the household and the remainder indirectly through taxes and reduced wages (insurance premiums paid by employers) (45). Even with Medicare, out-of-pocket expenses are increasing for the elderly. In 1972, the elderly spent 10.6% of their income on health care; this rose to 17.1% in 1991 (12).

What has raised the problem of health-care costs to crisis proportions is the rate at which these expenditures are increasing. During the past 20 years, health-care spending in the United States rose at an annual rate of 11.6%, while GNP rose at an average annual rate of 8.8% (46). As a result, the share of GNP devoted to health care rose from 7.3% in 1970 to 12.2% in 1990 (22). By the year 2020, health-care expenditures will reach 36% of GNP if real per capita health-care expenditures continue to rise at the rate they have over the past decade (1).

As health care claims an increasing portion of the federal budget, resources are being diverted from other important needs. Total federal health expenditures rose from $17.7 billion in 1970 to $195.4 billion in 1990 and are expected to reach $325 billion by 1995 (22). Federal health expenditures are projected to rise by 7.0% annually, social security expenditures are expected to rise by 2.2%, and net interest on the debt by 1.4%; all other federal expenditures are expected to decline in real dollars (33b).

Spending for physicians' services has paralleled that for health care in general, rising from $13.6 billion in 1970 to $125.7 billion in 1990 (22). Spending for physicians' services in the Medicare program has increased at an average annual rate of 13% since the program's inception in 1966 (33b).

The public might readily support devoting 13% of GNP—or even more—to health care if it was convinced that good value was being obtained for the money. There is no evidence that this is the case, however. There are few standardized ways to measure quality, but reported health outcomes (such as infant mortality and life expectancy) are not better in the United States than in other industrialized nations that spend only about 6–9% of GNP on health care (39). The public attributes the high cost of care in the United States to wasteful practices and unnecessarily high prices (34b).

Given the size and complexity of the US health-care system and the many factors contributing to the rise in health-care costs, reducing the rate of cost increases will require a significant amount of resources and time. A substantial, coordinated effort must be begun now so that it can have effect before the adverse consequences of high health-care costs become truly intolerable to the nation.

The Role of Price and Volume in Cost Increases

Four factors account for the increases in spending on health care: the growing number of persons in the population and the growing proportion of the elderly, general inflation, medical care price inflation above general inflation, and the greater volume and intensity (type) of services being delivered per patient. Medical care price inflation and greater volume and intensity of services are particularly important because they are responsible for almost half of the increase in health-care expenditures (22) and are potentially amenable to control within the health-care system.

Prices and volume of services have gone up for a variety of reasons. Price increases are likely due to the lack of a competitive market for health services and rising costs of administration, supplies, and liability (16). The increases in volume and intensity of services are being driven by many factors, including technological advances (of proven and unproven benefit), reimbursement policies, unbundling (billing separately for individual components of care that could be billed for collectively), "defensive medicine" inspired by the threat of malpractice suits, excess capacity in the health-care system, the number and specialty distribution of physicians, the training of physicians in tertiary-care environments that foster the use of expensive technologies, and patient demand (particularly because patients are usually buffered from the true costs of services by health insurance, which itself is often purchased by their employers). These factors need to be addressed by initiatives in many different areas.

Increased volume and intensity of services are stimulated in part by relative payment levels for services that disproportionately reward procedural and surgical services compared with evaluation and management services. The new resource-based Medicare Fee Schedule was intended to ameliorate these payment-based incentives. It will have its strongest impact when it is fully implemented in 1996, particularly if the fee schedule is modified so that practice costs also become resource based. Other payers will likely alter their payments over time toward a similar pattern of reimbursements (33a).

Purely financial approaches to health-care cost control run the risk of decreasing spending on appropriate, as well as inappropriate, services. For example, the RAND Health Insurance Experiment demonstrated that economic incentives, such as copayments and deductibles, reduce utilization. However, patients could not discriminate between appropriate and inappropriate care and reduced both alike when these economic incentives were applied (42). Often, neither patients nor physicians know which care is appropriate.

Efforts to Control Price Increases

Some public and private payers have been able to moderate the increases in the prices they pay for services. Preferred provider organizations (PPOs) have used their ability to supply patients to physicians as a lever to obtain discounts in fees. Such price cuts have put a notch in the trend toward increased prices, but they do not appear to have affected the underlying rate of increase in expenditures (3). Health maintenance organizations (HMOs) have instituted payments based on capitation; for some HMOs (group and staff model), the savings have been substantial when compared with fee-for-service payments (25). Much of these savings come from the substitution of ambulatory care for more expensive hospital care. For more loosely organized HMOs, which consist largely of physicians in independent practice, the savings have not been as substantial.

The quality of care in group and staff model HMOs has compared favorably over the years with fee-for-service practice (26, 27, 31). In the RAND Health Insurance Experiment, outcomes were similar among HMO and fee-for-service plans, except that low-income persons who were sick at the beginning of the experiment had somewhat worse outcomes in the HMO (47).

The Medicare program has addressed both hospital and physician prices through regulation. In recent years, Congress has periodically reduced payments for certain procedures and services in the Medicare program. The Medicare Fee Schedule now sets all Medicare physician fees nationwide by formula.

Medicare hospital payment levels have been set by formula since 1983 under the prospective payment system. Between 1983 and 1986, real hospital cost increases slowed to about 2% per year (33b). This slowing has been attributed to reductions in length of stay and admissions that were observed during this time (41). A recent comprehensive study did not find any reduction in the quality of care that elderly patients received while they were in the hospital after prospective payment was begun. However, patients were discharged earlier and more often in "unstable" condition (35). In recent years, hospital costs have again been rising at their historical rate of 6% per year, although Medicare expenditures have increased at a lower rate because only small yearly updates in payment have been granted (34a).

The success of some payers in holding down price increases has led to concern about increased cost shifting to other payers. Such cost shifting creates greater disparities among payers and cushions for providers the reduction in overall health-care expenditures that might have otherwise occurred as a result of successful price moderation by some payers. All-payer rate setting (for example, the application to all payers of the same fee schedule for physician services) has been suggested to prevent these adverse effects.

Although price controls have produced some reductions in health-care expenditures for some payers, relying on this strategy alone has not been successful in constraining rising overall costs. For instance, the volume of Medicare services continued to increase at an average of 7% per year from 1981 through 1991, even though the average annual price increases of 6% before 1986 were cut by Congress to 2% after 1986 (33b). Furthermore, reductions in unit prices may stimulate increased volume and intensity of services. Although the results of studies are mixed, some opposite volume effect can be anticipated from price changes (11, 33a). Clearly, both price and volume must be addressed to control total costs successfully.

Controlling Volume Without Reducing Quality

The challenge in controlling volume is to reduce only those services that are of little or no benefit to patients, while permitting and encouraging the delivery of necessary care. This is not an easy task, and most efforts to control volume have not accomplished it well.

Theoretically, there are three ways to control costs without compromising quality: identifying and eliminating unnecessary services; choosing the less costly of alternative effective approaches to care, such as the delivery of some services in an outpatient rather than inpatient setting or the use of a lower priced generic equivalent of a prescription drug; and providing preventive services that can save money in the long term.

Two types of studies suggest that curtailing the increases in volume and intensity of services without compromising the quality of care should be possible. The first type, small-area analyses, has identified large variations in the utilization of health services among similar populations of patients. The second, appropriateness studies, which assess whether services are indicated for specific clinical presentations, have identified substantial amounts of unnecessary care.

Small-area studies by Wennberg and others have documented variation in the utilization of many health services among different geographic areas (8, 44, 49, 51). Variation seems to be greatest for conditions in which there is uncertainty about the best approaches to care (48). For example, the appropriate indications for performing prostatectomy, tonsillectomy, and hysterectomy are not clearly delineated, and their utilization rates vary greatly across regions (29, 36).

Some variation is legitimately due to differences among areas in their need for a service, as measured by the prevalence of a condition in a population (32b, 51). However, some variation represents inappropriate under- or overuse of the service. Utilization rates have been related to income, gender, race, and health insurance status—often without clear differences in patient outcomes. Variation has also been correlated with the availability of services or equipment. Physicians' practice patterns and patients' choices may have important effects on utilization (15, 50).

Variations unrelated to the prevalence of disease or patient outcomes present opportunities for intervention and savings, e.g. the rate of cesarean section deliveries varies among practitioners for reasons not necessarily related to outcomes, such as type of insurance (14, 15). One hospital, for example, reduced its cesarean section rate from 17.5% to 11.5% without compromising maternal or fetal outcomes (30). The Maine Medical Assessment Foundation has organized groups of physicians to study practice variations. Providing educational feedback on rates of service use that substantially exceeded what seemed necessary to the groups has resulted in decreases in those rates toward the median, with significant savings in costs (20).

Appropriateness studies define clinical indications for which a service is appropriate, inappropriate, or equivocal. These ratings are determined by the degree of consensus of a group of experts who interact in a structured manner and use a carefully prepared literature synthesis. Such studies have found that one third of carotid endarterectomies and 17% of coronary angiograms and endoscopies were performed for what were judged to be inappropriate indications (10).

In these types of studies, inappropriate use has been found in all areas, including those with high and low utilization rates (9, 21). This implies that some procedures in both high- and low-use areas could be foregone without hurting patients' health. These studies have not measured the extent to which the procedures are underutilized.

STRATEGIES TO CONTROL VOLUME Two types of strategies have been employed to control volume: utilization review and financial incentives. Utilization review has primarily focused on individual cases for preauthorization approval of procedures or hospitalizations, concurrent review of care for hospitalized patients, or postservice review. Medicare, which has taken this approach, contracts with Peer Review Organizations (PROs) for review of individual cases to detect inappropriate utilization.

This case-by-case approach has been criticized as being ineffective, inefficient, and antagonistic (17). Without efficient ways of identifying which cases to review, utilization review of individual cases is so expensive that it is sensible only for more costly procedures. Because it focuses on outliers (by definition a small proportion of physicians), the total volume of services provided is not likely to change much, and most physicians' practices remain unaffected. Physicians who are targeted for review are frustrated by the intrusiveness ("hassle") of the review process and by the lack of a sound, consistent basis for deciding which services are approved (13, 37, 38). Unsound decisions can be deleterious to patients by restricting or discouraging practitioners from providing them with necessary care.

A variety of financial incentives, such as capitation, withholds, expenditure caps, global budgeting for hospitals, and the Medicare Volume Performance Standard, have been implemented to counteract the strong incentive to provide more services that is inherent in fee-for-service payment. Capitation sets a fixed amount of payment per enrollee over a period of time (typically one year), no matter which services are delivered. Expenditure caps are the equivalent of capitation applied to an entire population. Global budgets, which allocate a fixed, predetermined amount of resources to an organization to provide care, have usually been applied to hospital payments (e.g. Maryland, Canadian provinces). Withholds are mechanisms by which a portion of payment is reserved and adjusted to varying degrees according to the overall performance—usually financial performance—of one or more physicians.

In the Medicare physician payment reforms enacted in 1989, Congress linked physician payments to an expenditure target (the Volume Performance Standard) designed to slow the rate of increase in Medicare expenditures. Discrepancies between the Volume Performance Standard and actual Medicare expenditures form the basis each year for adjustments of future levels of physician payments (33a). It remains to be seen how well the Volume Performance Standard system achieves its goal, particularly as it applies only to Medicare payments.

These types of financial incentives attempt to control volume by rewarding individual or group practitioners who provide fewer services or who provide them more efficiently. Incentives targeted to an individual physician affect individual patient care decisions more strongly than incentives conditioned on group performance. However, the latter is less strongly tied to the care of any individual patient than the former and may stimulate collective action to reduce costs. Unlike utilization review, financial incentives aimed at controlling volume permit physicians and patients to decide on their own which services are, or are not, needed. No external standards are applied.

REQUIREMENTS FOR CONTROLLING VOLUME WITHOUT IMPAIRING QUALITY For utilization review and financial incentives to control costs without compromising the quality of care, three requirements must be met. First, physicians, institutions, payers, and the public need accurate and reliable information about practice: its costs, service use, and outcomes. Such information can be used to focus utilization review so that it can be more efficient and less intrusive; can help identify where efforts should be targeted to evaluate and improve patterns of practice; and can be used to monitor the quality of care by determining whether appropriate care is being given and whether that care is, in fact, effective.

Second, physicians, patients, and payers need information that enables them to distinguish appropriate from inappropriate approaches to care. Payers need this information to develop explicit standards for utilization review. If these standards are not sound, review decisions may be deleterious to patients' health. Practitioners and patients need this information to respond appropriately to financial incentives. Otherwise, wrong decisions may be made, and the quality of care may be seriously compromised. The fact that rates of inappropriate use of services are similar in high- and low-utilization areas (9, 21) suggests that, without guidance as to when a service is appropriate, financial incentives will decrease both inappropriate and appropriate uses of services.

Finally, a proper infrastructure and incentives are required to facilitate these efforts. An organization is needed to convene physicians and to catalyze and monitor changes in practice. A data infrastructure is needed to collect and analyze data on the cost, process, and outcomes of care. Payment policies, such as relative prices and the services covered by insurance, should be supportive of the goal of constraining inappropriate services while encouraging the delivery of necessary services. Other incentives, such as professionalism, peer pressure, external review, malpractice litigation, and credentialing, need to be applied appropriately. All financial incentives need to be calibrated to realistic levels of performance.

None of these three requirements is well satisfied now, but new methods are becoming available. Profiling of physician practice patterns has the potential to be an unintrusive source of valid, relevant information about the process, outcomes, and cost of care that is being provided in practice. Profiling of institutions (e.g. hospitals, groups practices, HMOs) and communities will be increasingly possible with uniform datasets, as will profiling of the full care received by individual patients. Practice guidelines and outcomes research offer a way of determining and describing the best care in a particular situation, i.e. ways to distinguish appropriate and effective care from inappropriate or ineffective care in practice. In the remainder of this chapter, we analyze how these tools can help efforts to address both the cost and quality of care.

USING PROFILING TO OBTAIN INFORMATION ABOUT PRACTICE

Profiling of physician practice patterns can potentially supply information about costs, service use, and quality of care (process and outcome) in actual practice. Rather than focusing on individual occurrences of care, profiling uses epidemiologic methods to compare the patterns of practice of different providers. The provider being profiled can be an individual, a group, or a health-care organization, such as a hospital or HMO. The provider's pattern of practice is expressed as a rate: some measure of utilization (costs or services) or outcome (e.g. functional status, patient satisfaction, morbidity, or mortality) aggregated over time for a defined population of patients under the provider's care. Examples of profiling rates include the number of sigmoidoscopy claims an internist submits to the Medicare program per 100 Medicare patients seen and the percentage of a hospital's patients undergoing coronary artery bypass graft operations who die within the subsequent 30 days.

Three features of profiles make them advantageous in conveying useful information about medical practice. Profiles focus on patterns of practice, rather than individual instances of care. Profiling is efficient and unintrusive, because of its use of available administrative and claims databases. Finally, a provider's practice pattern is given a context by comparing it with another pattern, or norm. This enables the profile to be evaluated and acted upon if necessary.

The norm used for comparison in a profile can be either a rate derived from the practice patterns of other similar providers, called a practice-based norm, or a rate that would be expected if providers followed an accepted practice guideline, called a standards-based norm. Practice-based norms do not necessarily reflect appropriate care. For example, the mean rate at which internists currently perform sigmoidoscopies for eligible patients may be too high or too low. Standards-based norms should reflect patterns that would be expected from care consistent with valid practice guidelines for similar populations in practice. For example, the vast majority of a family practitioner's elderly patients should receive flu vaccination.

For profiling comparisons to be valid, the providers being compared need to be similar in important respects, or the relevant differences between them need to be adequately considered. For example, it would not be reasonable to compare the rate at which cardiologists perform electrocardiograms (EKGs) per 100 office visits with the rate of family practitioners. The patients and medical problems treated by the two types of physicians are not likely to require similar numbers of EKGs. The profiling rates could be adjusted for relevant differences in patients, such as relative proportions of patients with medical problems requiring EKGs. Alternatively, physician specialty could serve as a proxy for the mix of patients and problems, so that EKG rates could be compared separately among cardiologists and among family practitioners.

Ultimately, profiles are designed to generate some type of action, which is usually taken if the utilization or outcome rate for a particular physician differs from the norm by a certain amount. For example, a pulmonologist might be notified by the Medicare program if his or her bronchoscopy rate is greater than two standard deviations above the mean for other pulmonologists practicing in the same community. Alternatively, if a standards-based norm is available for performing bronchoscopy in the Medicare population, all pulmonologists might benefit from learning the extent to which their rates are high or low in relation to the norm.

Uses of Profiling

Profiling has applications in three areas: quality improvement, assessment of physician performance, and utilization review. In all three areas, profiling can be used to help ensure that volume control does not compromise quality of care.

QUALITY IMPROVEMENT Profiling can play a role in several aspects of quality improvement. It can be used to target potential problem areas by identifying conditions or procedures where there are large variations in outcome. An example of this might be substantial differences among hospitals in 30-day mortality following coronary artery bypass graft surgery.

It can also be helpful in determining how and by whom performance should be changed to improve outcome. Through feedback and discussion of the results of an outcomes profile, physicians may be able to identify specific differences in the process of care (not necessarily attributable to them) that are likely to underlie differences in outcome (40). It will often be necessary to develop additional profiles or to investigate the actual process of care in greater detail (32a).

ASSESSMENT OF PROVIDER PERFORMANCE Profiling can be used to identify physicians or other providers who do, or do not, meet a certain standard of care. This can be useful in ensuring that physicians do not reduce their delivery of needed services. A particular physician's outcome of care or rate of performing a service could be compared with the rate that would be expected for physicians who followed a practice guideline. Performance would be "acceptable" if the physician's rate does not deviate substantially from this norm. When there is a significant deviation, further inquiry could be undertaken to understand the reasons for the discrepancy.

UTILIZATION REVIEW Profiling can be used in two complementary modes for utilization review: focusing on outliers or improving median performance (40). In the outlier approach, physicians whose service use deviates substantially from the norm are identified. Feedback or case-by-case review is initially used to change these physicians' patterns of practice.

Profiling also has the potential to improve the frequency with which services are provided by the average physician. For example, in cases where a standards-based norm is available for a particular service, all profiled physicians could be notified of the extent to which their utilization rates differ from the norm. Practice guidelines could be distributed at the same time to inform physicians how they might change their behavior so as to use the service more appropriately. When standards-based norms and practice guidelines are not available, it may be possible to bring a community's physicians together to review the profiling results. In some cases, they may be able to identify a utilization rate, or range of rates, that they believe is appropriate and to suggest ways that physicians could achieve this rate without compromising patient outcome.

Improving the Quality of Profiling

The availability of large claims databases and advances in the technology with which to analyze them have led to rapid increases in the use of profiling. As profiling has become more widespread, however, diverse groups have raised concerns about the quality of the profiles and the data on which they are based, the uses to which they have been put, and access to the information contained in them.

For example, the following types of questions have been raised about profiles comparing hospitals' mortality rates 30 days after coronary artery bypass graft (CABG) operations:

1. Which databases were used in the analysis? How were they linked, and how accurate and reliable is the information in them?
2. How many CABG operations were performed at each hospital per year? How likely is it that the differences across hospitals are due to chance alone?
3. Does the profile account for differences in the mix of different CABG operations each hospital performs? (Higher mortality rates might be

expected for hospitals performing higher proportions of, for example, emergency or repeat CABGs.)

4. Does the profile account for differences in the patients undergoing CABG operations in each hospital that could account for differences in mortality?
5. Does the profile compare similar hospitals (e.g. tertiary-care teaching hospitals) or all hospitals in the state?
6. What time frame was used in the analysis? How likely is it that death during that period was related to the CABG rather than to other causes?

Many of these concerns relate to the data used to develop and evaluate profiles (6). Current databases are not ideal for profiling, because they were developed for other purposes. Profiling would be improved if databases were available that provided the following: information to identify similar providers or to account for important differences across providers, such as differences in patient case mix; adequate numbers of observations; clinically meaningful indicators of the process or outcome of care and its costs; and utilization and outcome rates that reflect appropriate, cost-effective care. In addition, profiles need to be constructed to provide physicians with information that they can act on to improve the process and outcomes of care.

COMPARABILITY ADJUSTMENTS Because provider and patient factors can have a substantial effect on utilization and outcome rates, profile results are most meaningful if they compare the practice patterns of similar types of providers who care for similar patient populations. To make these comparability adjustments, data are required that can be used to characterize, accurately and reliably, relevant aspects of both the provider and the patient.

For example, physicians participating in a PPO might be profiled on the rate at which they bill for chest x-rays per 100 visits of PPO enrollees to that physician. Physicians might question the results on several grounds:

1. Their specialty designation is wrong or they are a member of a specialty that the PPO does not distinctly recognize.
2. They provide chest x-rays in their office, whereas most of the other physicians in the PPO refer patients who need chest x-rays to a radiologist.
3. They are referred more patients with cardiac or pulmonary conditions than other PPO physicians in their specialty.

To account for these possibilities, data are needed to control for physician specialty and patient condition/diagnosis and to distinguish the referring or ordering physician from the physician who actually provides each service. Medicare claims files currently include these data elements, but the codes that are used to describe physician specialty and patient condition/diagnosis are not interpreted or used uniformly. Administrative databases of other payers frequently do not include all of this information. Improvements in coding and modifications in claim forms that would facilitate making these comparability adjustments would not be particularly difficult to achieve, yet they would make claims data much more supportive of profiling.

Interpretation of other types of profiles may require more sophisticated comparability adjustments than are necessary for utilization review (28). For example, comparisons of morbidity and mortality rates are challenging because many provider and patient variables—some known and some unknown—contribute to complications following a particular procedure. New computerized databases of clinical care may make such information easier and cheaper to collect.

NUMBER OF OBSERVATIONS PER PROVIDER Unless a service is provided frequently or an outcome occurs often, the number of observations in a profile may be insufficient to ensure that differences in rates across providers are not due to chance alone. Although currently available databases contain information on thousands, sometimes millions, of patients, the frequency with which an individual physician performs a procedure over the course of a year or the frequency with which an adverse outcome occurs following this procedure may not be high enough to detect statistically significant differences (28). To some extent, this reflects the fact that each claims file covers only a portion of a physician's practice. Comprehensive databases covering all patients that a physician cares for are more likely to provide an adequate number of observations. This could be achieved by linking data sets with uniform formats across payers (33b). Even so, observations for a particular service or condition may be insufficient, requiring profilers to aggregate utilization or outcome rates across groups of physicians, rather than to profile rates of individual physicians.

INDICATORS FOR ASSESSING QUALITY Profiling for assessment of performance and quality improvement depends on having data about clinically meaningful aspects of the process and outcome of care. The choice of indicators is critical to avoid being misled by profiles. For example, several process measures could potentially assess quality of care for diabetes. One that is commonly used is whether a minimum number of random blood sugar levels were ordered. However, this test is rarely useful in managing diabetes. A better process indicator would be the ordering of glycosylated hemoglobin levels, which is a more integral component of good quality care.

It would be ideal if relevant process and outcome indicators were accurately and reliably recorded in available databases. This is generally not the case

(6). Claims files do not contain information about many pertinent aspects of the process of care, such as medications and preventive services, both of which are often uncovered; postoperative visits, which are included in global fees; aspects of the history and physical examination, which are included in visits; and laboratory and imaging results. Many of the most meaningful patient outcomes, such as functional status or condition-specific indicators of morbidity, are also poorly documented. Medical records should be an excellent source of relevant information for profiling. But, some of these data may be unreliable, because physicians may fail to document all of their findings or all of the services they provide. Moreover, because data must be abstracted, obtaining information from medical records is often costly.

Accurate, reliable, and relevant information about the process of care may be best obtained from condition-specific encounter forms (5). Such forms could be developed to monitor compliance with integral components of the process of care embodied in specific diagnostic or management guidelines.

RATES FOR ASSESSING QUALITY Physicians' performance can be compared with rates that would be expected from appropriate, cost-effective care. Such rates cannot be derived from current practice patterns of physicians, because practice-based norms do not necessarily reflect appropriate care. These comparison rates can be generated in the future by profiling physicians who care for patients with particular conditions according to valid practice guidelines. It may be possible to design a process that generates the information required to track compliance. If guidelines were presented in a real-time computer format, physicians could supply the relevant information in the course of using the guideline. The computer record could then serve as the basis for reviewing the physicians' compliance with the guidelines.

USING PRACTICE GUIDELINES TO IDENTIFY APPROPRIATE, COST-EFFECTIVE CARE

Practice guidelines are statements of approaches to care for particular clinical situations. Based on evidence and expert judgment, they identify—to the extent possible—effective approaches to care. It follows that guidelines should only be developed when there is evidence that care is effective.

Guidelines can be used in different ways to help ensure that appropriate, cost-effective care is provided. Their most fundamental use is to help clinicians and patients choose the best approaches to care based on its benefits, risks, and cost. Guidelines can also form the basis of utilization review decisions concerning the appropriateness of care. Implementing practice guidelines in community practice can generate rates of service use and outcomes that are associated with care in accordance with the guidelines. These rates can be used as the standards-based norms in profiling.

Constructing Guidelines to Address Both the Costs and Benefits of Care

Guidelines can help control volume without sacrificing quality if cost and quality are considered together when guidelines are constructed. Guidelines constructed in this manner can identify three kinds of treatment: ineffective treatment that can be withheld; the most cost-effective among equally effective treatment alternatives; and alternatives that are more effective, yet also more expensive.

Guidelines can address cost and quality without foreclosing treatment options—in other words, without making value-laden decisions involving trade-offs between the costs and benefits of effective services. In its 1992 report to Congress, the Physician Payment Review Commission suggested this could be achieved by the following: incorporating elements that enable guidelines to be used in different ways to promote the delivery of appropriate, cost-effective care; developing guidelines organized around the indications for particular services, as well as around particular conditions; and developing guidelines on topics for which changes in practice have the greatest potential to reduce the amount of resources being spent on unnecessary services (33b).

ELEMENTS OF GUIDELINES Practice guidelines have three basic elements: a desired patient outcome, short-term clinical measures and target values that correlate with this desired outcome, and specific approaches for achieving both the target and the outcome. The desired patient outcome—the ultimate goal of a practice guideline—is the improvement in functional status, patient satisfaction, morbidity, or mortality expected from following the course of action described in a guideline. A guideline for treating high blood pressure, for example, would express these benefits in terms of decreased morbidity and mortality from coronary artery disease, renal disease, stroke, and other diseases, which can be achieved by lowering the blood pressure. The clinical measure that correlates with achieving this outcome is blood pressure, for which a target range is established. The specific approaches to care to achieve the target range of blood pressure might include diet, exercise, and various medications.

The overall cost of care can largely be influenced by whether a guideline's clinical measures and target values are chosen on the basis of both cost and effectiveness. Short-term goals that are more rigorous than necessary to achieve the desired patient outcome may entail undue risk and cost. For example, blood pressure targets that are too low might not yield better long-term outcomes than higher targets, but may incur greater morbidity and costs.

Guidelines can provide physicians, patients, and payers with explicit information that allows them to compare different approaches to care. The criteria for evaluation should include effectiveness in achieving the clinical target and desired patient outcome, the adverse outcomes that may be expected from following the proposed courses of action (such as side-effects of medications), and expected costs.

In many instances, the most appropriate approach to care may vary according to characteristics of the patient or the physician's practice environment. Guidelines are best targeted to the types of patients that practitioners typically see. For example, guidelines focusing on the evaluation of symptoms in primary care settings should be tailored to a typical primary care patient population, rather than to patients referred to specialists (even though most medical literature focuses on the latter). Primary care patient populations generally have a lower prevalence and severity of disease than patients referred to specialists, so they require, as a group, less expensive and less invasive diagnostic testing.

Guidelines should attempt to account for common differences in the local availability and quality of health-care resources. Suggested approaches to care in practice guidelines presume certain effectiveness rates for diagnostic or therapeutic procedures, certain levels of sensitivity and specificity for laboratory tests, and the availability of particular services. In some localities, however, expertise may not meet these standards. In addition, access to technology, specialist care, and ancillary services may vary in different types of practices and in different regions of the country. For this reason, a guideline's suggested approach to care may not be achievable in some locations and may not be the most effective or efficient course to follow in others. Guidelines can address this problem by making explicit their assumptions about the quality and availability of care and by identifying, whenever possible, alternative approaches to care that are applicable to different types of practice environments.

SERVICE GUIDELINES An effective way for guidelines to help control volume is to identify and reduce the delivery of services that are of little or no benefit to patients. Guidelines that are organized around the appropriate and inappropriate indications for a particular procedure are best suited for this task. Guidelines in this form, called "service guidelines," may be particularly useful in helping patients avoid unnecessary procedures and in conducting utilization review (which is often targeted at procedures). They can also help physicians respond appropriately to generalized financial incentives.

GUIDELINE TOPICS Many factors should be considered in choosing topics on which to formulate practice guidelines, including costs. Guidelines can affect costs by identifying appropriate care—especially care that could lower future expenditures—that is currently being underdelivered. Cost control can also be enhanced by developing guidelines that focus on common conditions now being treated inappropriately or in an unduly expensive fashion. Such conditions often include those for which practitioners and patients find the benefits, risks, and costs of alternative approaches to care difficult to weigh. Service guidelines can be most useful if they are targeted at commonly provided diagnostic and therapeutic procedures that are likely to be used inappropriately or that entail substantial risk or cost.

Realizing the Potential of Practice Guidelines

To date, guidelines have not played a major role in cost containment and quality improvement efforts. Several steps could make them more effective. Efforts could be focused on developing service guidelines, as described above. Methods of evaluating guidelines could be developed to identify existing guidelines that are the most promising, which could then be put into the hands of practitioners, patients, and payers.

The ability of guideline developers to formulate the needed elements of practice guidelines depends on the availability of the right types of data and scientific evidence. Outcomes research should be directed to topics on which guidelines need to be formulated, but the evidence to do so is lacking. The outcomes studies would be most helpful if they were explicitly designed to provide the information needed by guideline developers, such as short-term measures that are closely correlated with patient outcomes and the least rigorous target values that achieve these outcomes, and when outcomes, clinical targets, and approaches to care differ for different types of patients. The results from randomized, clinical trials may not be generalizable from the patients in the studies to the types of patients typically seen in community practice. Outcomes research needs to be conducted on more general populations, so that the effectiveness of treatment in actual practice can be determined.

The most efficient and meaningful way to test the effectiveness and costs of treatment approaches may be to study whether guidelines incorporating them improve patient outcomes and control costs in actual practice (33b). Guideline developers can facilitate this process by identifying relevant process and outcome indicators that can be used to monitor compliance with guidelines. For many conditions, it may be possible (by combining data from a variety of sources) to follow short- and long-term outcomes and incurred costs for patient populations managed according to promising guidelines. Similar studies can also be used to compare the effectiveness and cost of different approaches to care embodied in "competing" guidelines, particularly if they control for compliance and relevant patient factors. For example, different approaches to testing for the presence of coronary artery disease could be used over a period of time by different physicians in separate defined patient populations, and the short- and long-term results could be compared.

More research is needed on the best ways to produce guidelines. Because the availability, quality, and applicability of scientific evidence may vary, all guidelines ultimately require a process involving expert judgment to synthesize a coherent approach from fragmentary knowledge. It is important that existing practices and biases are not simply codified, and that guideline developers consider diverse perspectives. Little is known about the quality and reliability of processes being used to develop guidelines (18), but guideline development can likely be made more efficient.

USING PROFILING AND PRACTICE GUIDELINES TO CHANGE PRACTICE

The ultimate objective of developing practice guidelines and profiling is to change medical practice for the better. Ways must be found for the information from profiling and practice guidelines to affect clinical practice. This requires developing valid, actionable profiles; establishing an infrastructure to support these activities; and creating supportive environments and incentives to encourage efforts to improve the appropriateness and cost-effectiveness of care.

The Convener Function

Effective change based on practice guidelines and profiling can be encouraged through proper supporting structures. Publication of practice guidelines alone has not in itself produced substantial changes in practice (24). By contrast, feedback of profiling of physicians' practice patterns has been successful in improving physician performance (40). This is particularly true when the profiling entity acts as a convener that brings physicians together to interact as a group in interpreting profiling results. This setting also facilitates discussing practice guidelines, relating them to profiling data, and using them to help decide the next steps in gathering data and changing practice patterns.

In situations where a convener has been used, physicians have been able to compensate somewhat for the limitations of profiles or the lack of practice guidelines and still identify effective courses of action. By using the convener function, physicians can try to understand the patterns of care and plan how to change those patterns when desired. They may be able to make comparability adjustments based on their knowledge of physicians' practices, to identify reasonable target rates, and to devise ways to achieve their target rates without compromising patient outcome (40). Profiles can thus be useful, even if they are not perfect.

Although the convener function has been used most often in the context of quality improvement, it also has important applications to utilization review. For many services, inappropriate utilization is likely to be common, yet appropriate utilization rates are not known, and practice guidelines that identify appropriate and inappropriate indications for using the service are not yet available. In these cases, identifying outliers on the basis of practice-based norms may overlook many providers who over- or underutilize the service. Providing feedback alone will not give providers the information they need to take corrective action. Convening physicians in a community to review the profiling results may, in some cases, make up for these limitations. By using the utilization rates as a starting point for discussion, they may be able to identify reasonable, if not well-documented, target rates and courses of action to follow (20). They can then use or derive practice guidelines to help achieve target values or determine prospectively what approaches to care are best in practice.

Infrastructure

The convener function requires not only effective educational and feedback techniques, but also an organizational structure and personnel that can encourage and enable independent physicians in a community to work together as a group. First, there must be a mechanism for collecting the necessary data, developing valid and relevant profiles from these data, and disseminating profiling results to appropriate parties. There is broad interest in improving data systems so that they are standardized and can be linked across payers. New proposals envision centralized claims processing for different payers, which would enable comprehensive databases to be assembled efficiently (2, 19, 33b). Coding systems need to be refined and necessary data elements included.

Second, some entity needs to act as a convener by bringing physicians in a community together in the context of a structured group process to examine and understand profiling results and to help plan effective action and monitor its success. It may be important for these activities to occur in a setting protected from public disclosure (4). Effective models for accomplishing these tasks need to be identified, improved, and implemented.

Incentives

The best incentive for improving practice is the professional interest of physicians in delivering the most appropriate and cost-effective care possible. Profiling and practice guidelines offer avenues for physicians to play a central role in improving quality and moderating costs.

Other incentives need to be harmonized with this professional objective. Direct financial incentives applied to individual patients may too strongly influence care; broader financial incentives are less vulnerable to this problem, but need to be strong enough to have an effect. Financial incentives need to be based on levels of performance that can be realistically attained without harming the quality of care. Payment policies can help support the use of guidelines: For example, the most cost-effective approaches could be fully covered, less-efficient approaches could be partially covered, and inappropriate care could be excluded from coverage. Relative levels of payment that do not stimulate the delivery of more intensive services are important to encourage appropriate and cost-effective care. The malpractice system can provide an incentive to the extent that it recognizes guidelines as establishing the standard of care (7). Public release of individual-specific quality of care information may serve some needs, but could jeopardize the willing participation of physicians in the quality improvement process.

CONCLUSION

The rapidly rising cost of health care is a major factor driving health-care policies in both the public and private sectors. Too often, policies have been instituted to slow rising costs that do not give due consideration to the impact of the policies on the quality of care. Cost containment that is blind to quality is a risk to the health of the public. But, we can no longer afford continued increases in the volume of care without ensuring its effectiveness. The only rational course is to consider cost and quality together. Profiling and practice guidelines can facilitate this integration. Physicians, payers, and patients need to have access to profiles to know what care is being delivered and access to practice guidelines to know what care is appropriate. These tools can be used now to help control volume responsibly, and they could be much more useful in the future if the needed infrastructure and incentives are created to support them.

Profiling and practice guidelines can be most effective if they are used by practitioners to review and improve their patterns of practice. The alternative to self-management is increasing external controls over the practice of medicine. These controls are likely to be less effective, more costly, and more troublesome for physicians, patients, and payers. External regulation is also likely to result in worsening cycles of resistance and evasion countered by more regulation. This course is as untenable for the health-care system as is continuing unchecked the current rate of increase in expenditures.

Containing health care costs in the United States will be a difficult task at best. Success will require addressing simultaneously many factors, including the supply and specialty distribution of physicians, uncontrolled development and use of medical technology, the excess supply of hospital beds, the fragmented system of financing, lack of incentives for efficient care, market failure, high administrative costs, and defensive medicine. It is also important to address obstacles to changing behavior. In the present circumstances, profiling and practice guidelines are likely to have only a modest impact. Within a context of health-care reform that includes an overall strategy for cost containment, such as a cap on expenditures, all-payer rate regulation with universal coverage, and incentives for managing care that promote quality as well as efficiency, profiling and practice guidelines would have a significant, indeed essential, role. With their help, costs can be controlled in a manner that is consonant with Americans' desire for the highest quality of care.

Literature Cited

1. Adv. Counc. on Soc. Secur. 1991. *Economic Security and Health Care: Economic Implications 1991–2020,* pp. 3–9. Expert panel rep. to Adv. Counc. on Soc. Secur. Washington, DC: Adv. Counc. on Soc. Secur.
2. Am. Med. Peer Rev. Assoc. Task Force. 1992. *A National Quality Improvement Program*. Washington, DC: Am. Med. Peer Rev. Assoc.
3. Berenson, R. A. 1991. A physician's view of managed care. *Health Aff.* 10(4):106–19
4. Berwick, D. M. 1991. The double edge of knowledge. *J. Am. Med. Assoc.* 266(6):841–42
5. Brand, D. A., Acampora, D., Gottlieb, L. D., Glancy, K. E., Frazier, W. H. 1983. Adequacy of tetanus prophylaxis in six hospital emergency rooms. *N. Engl. J. Med.* 309(11):636–40
6. Brand, D. A., Quam, L., Leatherman, S. 1992. Data needs of profiling systems. In *Conference on Profiling,* No. 92-2, pp. 20–45. Washington, DC: Physician Payment Rev. Comm.
7. Brennan, T. A. 1991. Practice guidelines and malpractice litigation: collision or cohesion? *J. Health Polit. Policy Law* 16(1):67–85
8. Brewer, W. R., Freedman, M. A. 1982. Causes and implications of variation in hospital utilization. *J. Public Health Policy* 3(4):445–54
9. Chassin, M. R., Kosecoff, J., Park, R. E., Winslow, C. M., Kahn, K. L., et al. 1987. Does inappropriate use explain geographic variations in the use of health care services? A study of three procedures. *J. Am. Med. Assoc.* 258(18):2533–37
10. Chassin, M. R., Kosecoff, J., Park, R. E., Winslow, C. M., Kahn, K. L., et al. 1989. *The Appropriateness of Selected Medical and Surgical Procedures: Relationship to Geographic Variations*. Ann Arbor, Mich: Health Adm. Press
11. Christensen, S. 1992. Volume responses to exogenous changes in Medicare's payment policies. *Health Serv. Res.* 27(1):65–79
12. Families USA Found. 1992. *The Health Cost Squeeze on Older Americans*. Washington, DC: Families USA Found.
13. Goldman, R. 1992. The reliability of peer assessments of quality of care. *J. Am. Med. Assoc.* 167(7):958–60
14. Gould, J. B., Davey, B., Stafford, R. S. 1989. Socioeconomic differences in rates of cesarean section. *N. Engl. J. Med.* 321(4):233–39
15. Goyert, G. L., Bottoms, S. F., Treadwell, M. C., Nehra, P. C. 1989. The physician factor in cesarian birth rates. *N. Engl. J. Med.* 320(11):706–9
16. Harvard Community Health Plan. 1991. *Who Will Cure America's Health Care Crisis? Harvard Community Health Plan Annual Report 1991*. Brookline, Mass: Harvard Community Health Plan
17. Inst. of Med. 1991. *Medicare: a Strategy for Quality Assurance,* ed. K. N. Lohr, Vol. 1. Washington, DC: Natl. Acad. Press
18. Inst. of Med. 1992. *Guidelines for Clinical Practice: From Development to Use*. ed. M. J. Field, K. N. Lohr. Washington, DC: Natl. Acad. Press
19. John A. Hartford Found. 1991. *Community Health Management Information*

System: CHMIS Overview. New York: Hartford Found.
20. Keller, R. B., Chapin, A. M., Soule, D. N. 1990. Informed inquiry into practice variations: the Maine Medical Assessment Foundation. *Qual. Assur. Health Care* 2(1):69–75
21. Leape, L. L., Park, R. E., Solomon, D. H., Chassin, M. R., Kosecoff, J., et al. 1990. Does inappropriate use explain small-area variations in the use of health care services? *J. Am. Med. Assoc.* 263(5):669–72
22. Levit, K. R., Lazenby, H. C., Cowan, C. A., Letsch, S. W. 1991. National health expenditures, 1990. *Health Care Financ. Rev.* 13(1):29–54
23. Levit, K. R., Lazenby, H. C., Letsch, S. W., Cowan, C. A. 1991. National health care spending, 1989. *Health Aff.* 10(1):117–30
24. Lomas, J., Anderson, G. M., Domnick-Pierre, K., Vayda, E., Enkin, M. W., et al. 1989. Do practice guidelines guide practice? The effect of a consensus statement on the practice of physicians. *N. Engl. J. Med.* 321(19): 1306–11
25. Luft, H. S. 1978. How do health maintenance organizations achieve their "savings"? Rhetoric and evidence. *N. Engl. J. Med.* 298(24):1336–43
26. Luft, H. S. 1981. *Health Maintenance Organizations: Dimensions of Performance*. New York: Wiley-Intersc.
27. Luft, H. S. 1988. HMOs and quality of care. *Inquiry* 25(1):147–56
28. McNeil, B. J., Pedersen, S. H., Gatsonis, C. 1992. Current issues in profiles: potentials and limitations. In *Conference on Profiling*, No. 92-2, pp. 46–70. Washington, DC: Physician Payment Rev. Comm.
29. McPherson, K., Wennberg, J. E., Hovind, O. B., Clifford, P. 1982. Small-area variations in the use of common surgical procedures: within and between England and Wales, Canada and the United States of America. *Soc. Sci. Med.* 15A:273–88
30. Myers, S. A., Gleicher, N. 1988. A successful program to lower cesarean-section rates. *N. Engl. J. Med.* 319(23): 1511–16
31. Natl. Adv. Comm. on Health Manpower. 1967. *Report of the National Advisory Commission on Health Manpower*. Washington, DC: GPO
32a. O'Connor, G. T., Plume, S. K., Olmstead, E. M., Coffin, L. H., Morton, J. R., et al. 1991. A regional prospective study of in-hospital mortality associated with coronary artery bypass grafting. *J. Am. Med. Assoc.* 266(6): 803–9
32b. Pasley, B., Vernon, P., Gibson, G., McCauley, M., Andoh, J. 1987. Geographic variations in elderly hospital and surgical discharge rates, New York State. *Am. J. Public Health* 77(6):679–84
33a. Physician Payment Rev. Comm. 1991. *Annual Report to Congress 1991*. Washington, DC: Physician Payment Rev. Comm.
33b. Physician Payment Rev. Comm. 1992. *Annual Report to Congress 1992*. Washington, DC: Physician Payment Rev. Comm.
34a. Prospect. Payment Assess. Comm. 1992. *Report and Recommendations to the Congress*. Washington, DC: Prospect. Payment Assess. Comm.
34b. Public Agenda Found. 1992. *Faulty Diagnosis: Public Misconceptions about Health Care Reform*. New York: Public Agenda Found.
35. Rogers, W. H., Draper, D., Kahn, K. L., Keeler, E. B., Rubenstein, L. V., et al. 1990. Quality of care before and after implementation of the DRG-based prospective payment system: a summary of effects. *J. Am. Med. Assoc.* 264(15): 1989–94
36. Roos, N. P., Roos, L. L., Henteleff, P. D. 1977. Elective surgical rates—do high rates mean lower standards? *N. Engl. J. Med.* 299(7):360–65
37. Rubin, H. R., Rogers, W. H., Kahn, K. L., Rubenstein, L. V., Brook, R. H. 1992. Watching the doctor-watchers: how well do peer review organization methods detect hospital care quality problems? *J. Am. Med. Assoc.* 267(17): 2349–54
38. Sanazaro, P. J., Mills, D. H. 1991. A critique of the use of generic screening in quality assessment. *J. Am. Med. Assoc.* 265(15):1977–81
39. Schieber, G., Poullier, J.-P., Greenwald, L. M. 1991. Health care systems in twenty-four countries. *Health Aff.* 10(3):22–38
40. Schoenbaum, S. C., Murrey, K. O. 1992. Impact of profiles on medical practice. In *Conference on Profiling*, No. 92-2, pp. 71–125. Washington, DC: Physician Payment Rev. Comm.
41. Schwartz, W. B., Mendelson, D. N. 1991. Hospital cost containment in the 1980s: hard lessons learned and prospects for the 1990s. *N. Engl. J. Med.* 324(15):1037–42

42. Siu, A. L., Sonnenberg, F. A., Manning, W. G., Goldberg, G. A., Bloomfield, E. S., et al. 1986. Inappropriate use of hospitals in a randomized trial of health insurance plans. *N. Engl. J. Med.* 315(20):1259–66
43. Sonnefeld, S. T., Waldo, D. R., Lemieux, J. A., McKusick, D. R. 1991. Projections of national health expenditures through the year 2000. *Health Care Financ. Rev.* 13(1):1–27
44. Stano, M. 1986. A further analysis of the "variations in practice style" phenomenon. *Inquiry* 23(2):176–82
45. Steuerle, C. E. 1992. The search for adaptable health policy through finance-based reform. In *American Health Policy: Critical Issues for Reform,* ed. R. B. Helms. Washington, DC: Am. Enterprise Inst. In press
46. US Gen. Account. Off. 1991. *Health Care Spending Control: The Experience of France, Germany, and Japan,* GAO/HRD-92-9. Washington, DC: GAO
47. Ware, J. E., Brook, R. H., Rogers, W. H., Keeler, E. B., Davies, A., et al. 1986. Comparison of health outcomes at a health maintenance organization with those of fee-for-service care. *Lancet* 1:1017–22
48. Wennberg, J. E., Barnes, B. A., Zubkoff, M. 1982. Professional uncertainty and the problem of supplier-induced demand. *Soc. Sci. Med.* 16(7): 811–24
49. Wennberg, J. E., Gittelsohn, A. M. 1973. Small area variations in health care delivery. *Science* 182:1102–8
50. Wennberg, J. E., Gittelsohn, A. M. 1982. Variations in medical care among small areas. *Sci. Am.* 246(4): 120–34
51. Wilson, P., Tedeschi, P. 1984. Community correlates of hospital use. *Health Serv. Res.* 19(3):333–55

Annu. Rev. Publ. Health. 1993. 14:243–70

THE INSURANCE GAP: Does It Make a Difference?

Joel S. Weissman[1,2] *and Arnold M. Epstein*[1–3]

[1]Division of General Medicine (Section on Health Services Research), Department of Medicine, Brigham and Women's Hospital; [2]Department of Health Care Policy, Harvard Medical School; [3]Department of Health Policy and Management, Harvard School of Public Health, Boston, Massachusetts 02115

KEY WORDS: health insurance access, uninsured, Medicaid, underutilization

---

For the first time in more than 20 years, the United States Congress is seriously debating the merits of universal health insurance. National anxiety about health insurance reform stems largely from perceptions that one's insurance status, especially the lack of insurance, affects the amount and type of care that one receives. This article reviews the evidence on the association between insurance status and access to health care. The focus is on comparisons of health care utilization among persons who are uninsured, receive Medicaid, or are privately insured.[1] We begin the review by presenting a theoretical framework for the study of access. Next, we describe the populations of interest. The article examines the literature of the last ten years that addresses differences in patients' utilization of care vis-a-vis the source of payment. We end with a brief discussion of the implications for health outcomes, the need for further research, and the existing policy debate.

[1]All statistics cited in the text are for populations less than 65 years of age unless noted. Persons over age 65 are almost universally insured by Medicare, so comparisons between insured and uninsured elderly are virtually impossible. Moreover, the health status of those over 65 is vastly different, which makes it difficult to compare them with younger persons. Hence, they are often excluded from most of the relevant analyses.

0163-7525/93/0510-0243$02.00

A CONCEPTUAL FRAMEWORK FOR THE STUDY OF INSURANCE AND ACCESS TO HEALTH CARE

How Might Health Insurance Affect Use of Health Services?

Economic theory argues that lacking health insurance, or having inadequate health insurance, has clear implications for individuals' use of health services. Health insurance reduces the price of care to individuals at the time of demand and moves them along the demand curve, thus enabling them to purchase more services at a subsidized price. Health insurance may encourage persons to consume more of an insured good than they would have if they had to pay the full cost, a tendency known as moral hazard (66). Furthermore, better payment, which is often linked to source of payment, may stimulate providers to render more or better services.

Health insurance has obvious benefits. Consumers benefit by trading a fixed premium (in advance) for uncertain and potentially devastating expenditures on huge medical bills; providers benefit by gaining higher and more stable incomes; and society benefits if workers are more productive or if communicable disease is better controlled because of the availability of health insurance. To counterbalance the social cost of inadequate insurance, the United States health care system has developed several programs and policies, including free clinics, public hospitals, and charity care, that form the fabric of the health care safety net. An important question is whether these policies are sufficient to make health care accessible to persons regardless of their payment source.

Defining and Measuring Access

Access cannot be defined absolutely. There is no set of specified services or characteristics, and no single index can completely summarize the overall access to health care for a particular group. Andersen et al (7) define access as "those dimensions which describe potential and actual entry of a given population to the health care delivery system." They further define "equity of access" as "services [that] are distributed on the basis of people's need for them. Inequity exists when one's race, income . . . or insurance coverage . . . are important predictors of realized access." We prefer a definition that specifies some of the criteria or concepts of access and reflects recent interest in health outcomes. Thus, we define access to be the attainment of timely, sufficient, and appropriate health care of adequate quality such that health outcomes are maximized.

We present a framework in Figure 1 that builds upon the conceptual approach for the study of access pioneered by Aday, Andersen, and coworkers (1, 6, 7). Several points follow from the framework illustrated in the figure:

HEALTH POLICY CHARACTERISTICS	
	Insurance coverage System characteristics[a] Utilization controls
PATIENT (CONTROL) CHARACTERISTICS	
Predisposing	Age Sex Education Occupation Ethnicity Income Residency (urban/rural) Health behaviors
Need	Perceived health Restricted activity Chronic conditions Other health status measures
ACCESS INDICATORS	
Intermediate indicators	Regular source of care Location of care Convenience/acceptability
Process indicators (Quantity and quality of utilization)	Number and intensity of visits, procedures, drugs, etc. Expenditures Appropriateness/sufficiency (e.g. timeliness, preventive care, care for serious problems) Technical quality Negligent adverse events Patient-doctor communication
Outcome indicators	Satisfaction Mortality/health status Preventable disease conditions

Figure 1 A framework for studying access to care.

The top half of the figure refers to characteristics of the health care system or of individuals. The bottom half of the figure lists indicators for measuring access. The health policy variables are limited to characteristics of patients or providers that are directly affected by policies of the health care system. Insurance coverage falls into this category. The patient variables include those "predisposing" and "need" characteristics that might influence demand for utilization and outcomes. Good studies usually control for one or more of these variables. Intermediate access indicators are those attributes that may be desirable in terms of how patients interact with the system, yet would not be considered definitive indicators of access. Indicators of ultimate access to care include the quantity, and outcomes of health care. In a research context, they constitute the dependent variables.

[a] System characteristics refer primarily to organizational factors, such as the availability or supply characteristics of the system or region in which individuals reside. Examples include supplies of physicians, nurses, and beds; or capitation versus fee-for-service.

1. The purpose is to study access problems within the context of health system policies, not other social policies, such as housing or income support, even though the latter may possess equal or greater potential for health enhancement than changes to the health care system.
2. Health status appears twice in the model, first as a measure of need and again as an outcome indicator.
3. Both process and outcome may be necessary to characterize access fully.
4. Access barriers are not limited to financial ones. Race, ethnicity, social class, geographic isolation, culture, education, and psychosocial and organizational factors have all been linked to health and health care (see Refs. 20, 60). Many of the studies reviewed for this article do not control for these potentially confounding variables.
5. Finally, persons in different insurance groups may differ from each other in ways that are directly related to their need and demand for services and their health status. This state of affairs arises from a phenomenon known as biased selection, which describes what happens when people are allowed to choose among insurance options, including the choice of having no insurance. Persons who expect to consume substantial amounts of services are more likely to buy extensive insurance, thereby creating adverse selection. Of course, some adverse selection is intentional—the Medicaid program was designed to care for the poorest, sickest citizens. The effect of biased selection on research is apparent. Medicaid recipients may have poorer health status not because of access to care, but because they are sicker to begin with. And, at least some of the uninsured may have lower utilization of medical care not because they face access barriers, but because they are a self-selected group with a lower preference for health-care consumption. Therefore, underutilization is a relative term, and it may be complicated by the tendency of insured groups to overutilize care.

CHARACTERISTICS OF PATIENTS WHO ARE UNINSURED OR ARE COVERED BY MEDICAID

In 1989, about 160 million Americans under age 65 had some private insurance, more than 18 million had coverage by Medicaid, and 34.4 million were uninsured[2] (33). Figures from the Current Population Survey (CPS) for 1987 and 1988 demonstrate that slightly fewer than one third of the uninsured were poor, and more than three-quarters were poor or near-poor[3] (23, 64).

[2]Estimates of the uninsured population are controversial. Changes in the wording of questionnaires and contrasting interpretations of their meaning have led to different figures. For more information, see Ref. 63.

[3]Federal poverty status considers both the size of a family and the total family income. The poverty threshold for a family of four in 1986 was $11,203 (23). Most authors refer to the poor as at or below the poverty threshold. "Near-poor" usually refers to persons whose income is between the poverty level and 150–200% of poverty.

Medicaid eligibility is based on a variety of financial and demographic (categorical) factors. There is considerable variation by state in the income cut-off, in the make-up of eligible families (e.g. single parents versus married with unemployed spouse), and in coverage of the medically needy. Most states set their income cut-off well below the federal poverty level. As a result of this and other restrictions in categorical eligibility, only 41% of all persons below the poverty level were covered by Medicaid in 1986 (24).

The health status of persons varies by insurance class. Higher proportions of persons with Medicaid report themselves to be in fair or poor health or to have limitations in activities than any other insurance class (49, 55, 73). This is most likely because of the adverse selection that occurs as a result of categorical eligibility for the disabled or medically needy programs. The data comparing the health status of uninsured and privately insured groups are inconsistent. Unadjusted figures suggest that uninsured persons are close in health status to the privately insured, because they are only slightly more likely to report fair or poor health (15, 23, 55, 73). After adjustments for age, however, the uninsured are less healthy, whereas adjustments for income provide mixed results (23, 64, 73). We are unaware of any analyses of general health status measures that controlled for age and income simultaneously. Research comparing insured and uninsured persons in terms of activity limitations also yields inconsistent results (6, 15, 49, 64).

INTERMEDIATE INDICATORS OF ACCESS

There are two principal concerns over source of care: whether persons have a usual (or regular) source of care and the site or location of their care. Persons without a usual source of medical care may lack an entry point to the health-care system when an acute problem strikes and, therefore, may be less likely to receive necessary treatment in a timely manner.[4] The location of care is important, because persons whose usual source is a hospital outpatient department or emergency room may lack continuity of care with a particular provider. In addition, care may not be comprehensive in approach and may be more expensive than care received from other sources. The literature on intermediate indicators also includes several studies that examine the convenience of care and the use of municipal hospitals. These issues are also addressed below.

Having a Usual Source of Care

Uninsured persons are more likely than either the privately or the publicly insured to lack a usual source of care, as highlighted by figures from numerous

[4]The direction of causality is debatable. Persons who are high utilizers of care may be more likely to obtain a regular source of care.

surveys (Table 1). Uninsured children may be less likely to lack a usual source of care than uninsured adults (Table 1) (16, 71). Repeated surveys in 1982 and 1986 by the Robert Wood Johnson Foundation (RWJF) suggest that over the four-year period, the proportion of uninsured persons not having a usual source of care increased by approximately 50% (64, 69).

The variation by payer groups in having a usual source of care does not appear to be an artifact of differences in patients' socioeconomic characteristics (not shown in Table). At least three studies include a multivariate analysis of the probability of having a usual source, two of them using data from the RWJF Access Surveys (2, 35, 69). In an analysis of the 1982 survey that controlled for age, sex, income, health status, race/ethnicity, and urban/rural residence, the uninsured were 1.6 times as likely as the insured not to have a regular source of care (47). Similar results were found in a 1986 survey (46) and in a study of low-income persons in California (51). In the 1986 RWJF survey, 61% of those without a regular source did not want one (46). For patients with these preferences, lacking a regular source may not be indicative of an access problem. More worrisome reasons for lacking a regular

Table 1 Persons without a usual source of care, various studies, various years

	Uninsured	Public/Medicaid	Private
1980 NMCUES			
Howell (49)	25	15	13
Rosenbach (71)[e]	18	16	13
1982 RWJF Survey			
Needleman (64)[a]	22	11	10
1986 RWJF Survey			
Robert Wood Johnson (69)[b]	31		16
1987–1988 Orange County Survey			
Hubbell (51)	39	13[c]	
1987 NMES			
Cornelius et al (26)	35	13	18
1988 NHIS			
Bloom (16)[d]	21		8

The figures reported by Rosenbach (1985) and by Bloom (1990) refer only to children, which may explain the lower percentages of uninsured without a usual source of care in those studies.
[a] Lewin/ICF tabulations from the 1982 Robert Wood Johnson Foundation Access Survey.
[b] Includes person aged 65 and older.
[c] All insured low-income adults (below 200% of poverty).
[d] Children 17 years of age or under.
[e] Low-income children (below 150% of poverty).

source of care include prohibitive cost and difficulty getting appointments. Uninsured respondents were significantly more likely than the insured to report no regular source because of financial problems ($p < .05$), but not because of local resource inaccessibility, in analyses that controlled for age, sex, health status, income, race, urban/rural residence, and education (46).

Whether having a regular physician is a matter of patient preference, as suggested above, or of financial necessity, the impact of insurance coverage may be especially important to poor persons who lose their insurance involuntarily. In a study of loss of Medicaid status among medically indigent adults in California, Lurie et al (58, 59) found a considerable drop in the proportion of persons who reported having a regular physician—from a baseline figure of 96% down to 40% after six months, and then only back up to 50% after one year. The proportion of persons having a regular physician among the control group (who kept their Medicaid status) remained the same as at baseline (94%). It is very unlikely that patients who lost their insurance suddenly changed their preference for a regular source of care. These results suggest that persons who are poor may be strongly affected in terms of having a regular source of care when insurance is lost.

Location of Care

Most of the surveys listed in Table 1 also examined the site of the usual source of care and found differences by insurance class.[5] The most recent findings are available from the 1987 National Medical Expenditure Survey (NMES). Of those with a usual source, uninsured and publicly insured patients were less likely than privately insured to have a private physician as their usual source of care and more likely to rely on hospital-based or other sources (26).

Convenience

Convenience of care (measured by travel and waiting times) may be associated with rates of service, especially for minor problems or visits for preventive care. Most national surveys have queried patients on travel and waiting times. Uninsured and publicly insured patients are more likely to have longer travel times and longer waiting times once they arrive at a physician's office (Table 2). The longer travel times may reflect the rural residences of some patients or the more frequent use of public transportation by others, rather than restricted access to near-by care. Nevertheless, the inconvenience associated with longer travel time has potential implications for obtaining medical services in a timely manner.

[5]One exception is Rosenbach (71) who, using NMCUES, found only small differences by payer in the proportions of low-income children whose regular source was a private physician.

Table 2 Travel time and waiting time for persons with a usual source of care, 1977, 1987

	Percentage of population with indicated health insurance status		
	Uninsured	Public/Medicaid	Private
Davis & Rowland (28) (1977 NMCES)			
Traveling ≥30 minutes	25		18[a]
Leicher et al (55) (1980 NMCUES)			
Traveling ≥60 minutes	5.5	4.5	2.5
Waiting ≥60 minutes	24.0	29.4	18.0
Cornellus et al (26) (1987 NMES)			
Traveling ≥60 minutes[b]	3.9	4.9	1.7
Waiting ≥60 minutes[b]	15.5	19.8	8.5

[a] Includes all insured.
[b] All differences $p < .05$.

Use of Public Hospitals

Public hospitals have long been characterized as the provider of last resort for the poor and uninsured. When municipal hospitals are absent or closed, access to care by those who rely on them may suffer because of the inability or unwillingness of other area facilities to serve the needy population. A national study of metropolitan areas found 33–40% more uncompensated admissions per 100 uninsured poor persons in cities with public hospitals than in cities without public hospitals (85). When the public hospital in Shasta County, California, shut down, Bindman et al (12) surveyed its patients. One year later, they found that the percentages of persons who had no regular provider were denied medical care, had to wait seven or more days for an appointment, or missed medications before refill had all increased; a similar group in another county reported decreases in all of those categories ($p < .05$ for all comparisons).

ULTIMATE INDICATORS OF ACCESS

Ambulatory Visits

The introduction of Medicaid in 1966 had an enormous effect on the ability of the very poor to obtain physician care (70). Until that time, the poor routinely utilized physicians less often than the nonpoor in spite of having more health problems. By 1974, the trend had reversed itself. Persons with low incomes had 13% more physician visits than persons with higher incomes (these figures were not adjusted for health status) (27, 29). Low-income children still saw physicians less often than children in families of higher income in 1974, but the differential compared with 1964 was substantially reduced (27, 29). And, low-income persons in states with strong Medicaid programs had substantially more physician visits than low-income persons in Arizona (which did not have a Medicaid program at the time of the study) or in states with limited Medicaid programs (13).

As evidenced by numerous surveys (Tables 3 and 4), uninsured persons are more likely to go without seeing a physician and have fewer physician visits than the privately insured, whereas Medicaid recipients have higher utilization patterns than these two groups. The percentage of persons who do not see a physician at all during a year is a gross indicator of initial access to the system—a physician cannot prescribe medicines or refer to specialists if there is no initial contact. The mean number of visits per person and/or the mean number of visits per user (of at least one visit) reflect the intensity of use for those who do enter the system. Findings of less use by uninsured relative to insured groups have been replicated in studies that stratify their samples by age and sex (23, 64), by race and geographic region (28), and by income (73).

Perhaps the most important concerns for access are for those who are ill. Among those in poor or fair health, insured patients saw physicians almost 70% more often than uninsured persons in 1977 (28), and nearly twice as often as the uninsured in 1980 (55). Similarly, among the poor/near-poor[6] with poor or fair health status, those on Medicaid saw a physician 7.1 times per year, compared with 5.7 for other insured and 3.9 for uninsured (7, 92). The use-disability ratio, a measure of physician visits per 100 days of restricted activity, provides another approach to controlling for health status. Using this ratio, Howell (49) and Andersen et al (6) found lower use of physicians by the uninsured than by persons with private or Medicaid coverage. Insured persons in the 1987 RWJF survey reporting fair or poor health were more than twice as likely as uninsured persons to visit a doctor ($p < .05$); for those having chronic or serious illnesses, the ratio was 1.5 ($p < .05$) (34).

Studies controlling for multiple factors confirm these differences. Assuming that the uninsured would use services at the same rate as the insured after adjustment for age, sex, income, and health status, Lewin/ICF (64) used the 1980 National Medical Care Utilization and Expenditure Survey (NMCUES) to estimate the expected level of utilization and the utilization shortfall for

[6]Within 150% of poverty.

Table 3 Percentage reporting no physician visits during one year, various studies, various years

	Uninsured	Medicaid	Private/Other
1977 NMCES			
Wilensky & Berk (93)[e]	50	30	36
1980 NMCUES			
Kasper (53)[d]	43.7	21.2	24.4
Rosenbach (71)[a]	36.3	24.8	31.0
1982 RWJF			
Andersen et al (6)	30	15	18
1984 NHIS			
Rowland & Lyons (73)	40.8	17.2	25.9
1986 RWJF			
Freeman et al (34)[b]	44		35.7
1987–1988 Orange County Survey			
Hubbell et al (51)[c]	32		11

[a] Low-income children.
[b] Adults, only.
[c] Low-income, below 200% of poverty levels.
[d] Calculated from age-specific rates.
[e] Poor/near poor (under 150% of poverty), all ages, figure given is 1 minus the probability of a visit.

the uninsured. The authors estimated a 36.9% shortfall for physician visits for the uninsured. In an analysis of low-income children, Rosenbach (72) found that Medicaid beneficiaries were significantly more likely ($p < .05$) to have, at least once, visited a physician in an office setting than either the uninsured or the privately insured. The analysis controlled for age, race, education, income, health status, and physician supply variables.

In a study based on over 92,000 persons from the 1982 National Health Interview Survey (NHIS), Newacheck and colleagues (65) assessed the effect of Medicaid on health care utilization by constructing a multivariate model with control for age, sex, race, and family size (predisposing characteristics); perceived health status and restricted activity (variables indicating need); and region and urban/nonurban location. After statistical adjustment, poor persons with Medicaid had about the same or slightly more physican contacts than persons (without Medicaid) above poverty, whereas poor persons without Medicaid had significantly fewer mean annual visits. The impact of Medicaid may be understated in these models, because the non-Medicaid group included both the insured and the uninsured.

Although the studies cited above suggest that differences in physician visits

Table 4 Physician visits by the uninsured as a percentage of Medicaid use and insured use, various studies, various years[a]

Survey	Percentage of Medicaid	Percentage of private insured
1977 NMCES		
Davis & Rowland (28)		65
Wilensky & Berk (93)[b]	53	68
1980 NMCUES		
Leicher et al (55)	40	53
Long & Settle (57), low-income adults and children		68
1984 Survey of Income & Program Participation		
Long & Rodgers (56)		63
1984 NHIS		
Rowland & Lyons (73)	46	79
1986 NHIS		
Congressional Research Service (24)		64
Congressional Research Service, <$15,000 income		53
Long & Rodgers (56)		75
1986 Robert Wood Johnson Survey		
Freeman et al (35)		72

[a] Lower figure with respect to Medicaid; high figure with respect to private insured.
[b] All ages; poor/near poor (under 150% of poverty).
Source: Adapted and expanded from Garrison (38, Table 1).

by insurance coverage persist even with control for many other characteristics, we know of two studies that did not find significant associations or found associations that were inconsistent. Yelin et al (95) examined patients with specific symptoms and discrete diagnoses (e.g. back pain, emphysema, diabetes) in the 1976 NHIS. The authors found no consistent differences in the use of physicians by payment source. Cornelius (25) estimated the likelihood of any ambulatory utilization and the number of visits for over 1000 patients, controlling for demographic variables, health status, residence, and the usual source of care. The findings pointed toward lower use for uninsured patients, but the coefficients were not statistically significant. The studies by both Yelin et al and Cornelius had small numbers of subjects for stratified or multivariate analysis. Because of this limitation and the lack of other contradicting studies, we conclude that the weight of the evidence demonstrates less ambulatory care use by the uninsured and a clear impact from Medicaid coverage.

Timeliness Indicators: Foregone or Delayed Care

Poor access to care is directly implicated when patients forego or delay receiving care as a consequence of their insurance status. As a result, patients could develop unnecessary morbidity or greater severity of illness. The RWJF surveys provide some of the richest information on the subject derived from patient reports (Table 5). In 1982, for example, 15% of uninsured persons reported not receiving needed care, compared with 5% of insured persons, a ratio of 3 to 1; 4% of those having no insurance or public insurance had been refused care for financial reasons, compared with 1% of the privately insured (2). Multivariate analysis of the 1986 survey (47), as well as several studies summarized in Table 5 using other patient samples, provides complementary results.

Involuntary loss of insurance, especially among the poor, also has a deleterious effect on access. One natural experiment occurred as a result of the 1981 Omnibus Budget Reconciliation Act (OBRA), which instituted changes that effectively denied Aid to Families with Dependent Children (AFDC) and its associated Medicaid coverage to many families on welfare who had jobs (74). In a study of Medicaid patients in Hennepin County, Minnesota, who lost their AFDC eligibility and, hence, their Medicaid coverage as a result of this legislation, 15% reported that their new private policies did not cover prescription medications, 6% did not cover physician services, and 1% did not cover inpatient admissions.[7] Compared with their responses before they lost Medicaid, roughly three times as many persons reported not having enough money to pay their doctors; therefore, they delayed seeking medical care or went without it (62).

Another natural experiment took place in California in 1982, when the state transferred responsibility for the medically indigent adult (MIA) population to the counties and reduced the state subsidy. This plan effectively eliminated Medicaid insurance for this group of patients. At the UCLA Medical Center, Lurie et al (58) compared MIAs with other Medicaid patients who did not lose their eligibility and found two- to threefold differences in the proportion who could identify a usual source of care, were satisfied with their care, or agreed with the statement, "I can get medical care whenever I need it." In a second study of MIAs in Orange County, Akin et al (5) followed persons who applied for Medicaid, but were found ineligible, and assessed the clinical importance of the patients' conditions according to a 5-point scale (where 1 represented the least severe conditions and 5 represented conditions that would most likely lead to long-term disability). Of the patients with more serious

[7]About 70% of respondents had some private coverage two years after the implementation of OBRA, compared with about 50% before OBRA.

Table 5 Problems with getting care, various studies, various years

Study	Type of problem	Percentage of subjects with indicated problem		
		Uninsured	Public	Insured
1977 Michigan				
Gortmaker (40)	Unmet dental needs reported by parents (for children ages 3–17)		18	8
1980 NMCUES				
Needleman et al (64)	Health care condition during the year for which care was desired but not received;	8.9		5.0
	Among those who did not obtain care, those who did not for economic reasons	66		33
1982 RWJF Survey				
Aday & Andersen (2); all ages	Needed help but did not get it;	15	8	5
	Were refused care for financial reasons;	4	4	1
	Found it more difficult to get care now than in previous years	11	4	0
1986 RWJF Survey				
Freeman et al (35)	Needed care but did not get it for economic reasons;	13		6[a]
	Had serious symptoms but did not get care	67		41[a]
Hayward et al (46)	Relative risk of needing supportive medical care but not getting it;	1.9[b]		
	Relative risk of not seeing a physician in past year for respondents with one or more chronic conditions	1.3[b]		

Table 5 (*Continued*)

Study	Type of problem	Percentage of subjects with indicated problem		
		Uninsured	Public	Insured
1988 DCHA Uninsured Patient Survey, Washington, DC	Unable to get care thought needed	21.4		
Billings & Teicholz (11)	Unable to fill prescription;	17.7		
	Unable to get diagnostic test recommended by MD;	9.4		
	Unable to get advice of specialist	15.6		
1989 Massachusetts Survey	Unable to get care for financial reasons;	10		1
Blendon et al (15)	Failed to receive care for a serious or chronic condition;	48		19
	Failed to receive care for a serious symptom	51	28	

Public includes Medicaid; Insured refers to private insurance, but includes Medicaid if a separate figure is not provided.
[a] All US, insured and uninsured.
[b] Adjusted relative risk compared with the insured, controlling for age, sex, income, health status, race.

problems (levels 3 to 5), 76% had not received treatment four weeks later. A third study by Brown & Cousineau (18) indicated that loss of Medicaid coverage led to approximately 19% fewer inpatient discharges and 78% fewer visits than expected.

The studies reviewed in the preceding paragraphs focus on care that was not obtained. Because the uninsured and underinsured face financial and other barriers to care, even when they eventually receive care they may have delayed seeking or receiving treatment when symptoms first appeared. Billings & Teicholz (11) interviewed 955 uninsured hospital patients in Washington, DC, in 1988, and found that almost 20% reported delays in treatment of the medical problem that ultimately resulted in admission. Weissman et al (89) interviewed more than 17,000 patients in the Boston area and found that those who were poor, black, or uninsured or who did not have a regular doctor were 40–80% more likely to report delay than others ($p < .01$); persons who were both poor and uninsured were 12 times as likely as other patients ($p < .01$) to report delays because of the cost of care.

Preventive Care

The use of preventive care may be particularly sensitive to insurance status, because the need for it is less immediate and the benefits are more obscure. Woolhandler & Himmelstein (94) used multiple logistic regression to control for overall health status and demographic variables and found that uninsured women were 64% more likely than insured women to lack adequate blood pressure screening. The 1986 RWJF survey focused just on persons (both sexes) with hypertensive disease and found only a 10% differential (35).

Other studies have focused on preventive health care services targeted at women. In the 1982 RWJF access survey, women with private insurance were about 40% more likely to have a Papanicolaou smear or a breast examination by a physician than the uninsured or publicly insured (2). Insured women in the 1986 RWJF survey were 2½–3 times as likely as uninsured women to receive a Papanicolaou smear, a breast examination, or a mammography, controlling for age, income, education, having a usual site of care, and health status (45). In the 1982 NHIS, uninsured women were 28–38% less likely than insured women to receive a Papanicolaou smear, a breast examination, or a glaucoma test (94). The authors, who found consistent results after controlling for education, race, health status, and income, noted that uninsured women are more likely to be poor and, therefore, to be at elevated risk for contracting the diseases that these tests discover.

Although most children are insured, they are often not covered for preventive services. The notable exceptions are children who are beneficiaries of Medicaid, because they are eligible for the Early and Periodic Screening, Diagnosis, and Treatment program (EPSDT). The services provided under the aegis of EPSDT may include physical examinations, vision and dental checkups, and follow-up care, although availability of screening and follow-up services varies considerably by state. Results from the program's evaluations are mixed, however (2, 65, 77).

Prenatal Care

Prenatal care can be a highly cost-effective service for poor women (75), yet one third of pregnant women do not get adequate prenatal care (86). The adequacy of prenatal care is clearly associated with private insurance, as demonstrated by several studies (Table 6). In 1986, 20% of uninsured pregnant women failed to get prenatal care during their first trimester, compared with 15% for the US as a whole (35). In the study by the US General Accounting Office (87), Medicaid recipients and the uninsured began their care later and made fewer visits than the comparison group. Lack of money to pay for care, lack of transportation, and lack of awareness about the pregnancy were cited as the principal barriers to care among those interviewed.

Prescription Drug Use

Very little information is available about differences in prescription drug use by payment source, particularly for the uninsured. We know that the poor who have Medicaid use more prescription medications, presumably because prescription medications are a covered benefit. Overall, the uninsured poor and near poor use 2.0 prescription drugs per year, those with Medicaid part of the year (uninsured otherwise) used 3.0, and those on Medicaid all year used 6.0 (7, 92).[8] The figures for a subset of the same populations who perceived their health to be fair or poor were 5.6, 6.8, and 12.1, respectively.

Some states have tried to control the use of expensive and perhaps nonessential drugs by Medicaid recipients by imposing such controls as utilization review, formularies, limits on number of prescriptions, and copayments (52). These strategies, especially the last three, may cause access problems. In a study of over 10,000 Medicaid recipients (all ages) in New Hampshire, Soumerai et al (80) found that the imposition of a limit of three drugs per month caused a meaningful drop of 30% in the number of prescriptions filled, with no change observed in a comparison state. The reduction in use was greatest for "ineffective" drugs (58%). However, surprisingly large reductions in utilization were observed for medications normally considered to be essential, including insulin (28%), thiazides (28%), and furosemide (30%). A change to a $1 copayment returned drug use to just below pre-cap levels.

[8]Wilensky & Berk examined all age groups.

Table 6 Use of prenatal care, by insurance status, various studies

	Uninsured	Public/Medicaid	Insured/national average
St. Clair et al (83)			
Percent of under-utilizers among low-income women (n = 185)[a]	43	64	42
Freeman et al (35)			
Percent who failed to get care during first trimester	20		15[b]
Adler & Emmerich (4)			
Mean estimated gestational age at first prenatal visit (n = 98)[a]	18 weeks	13 weeks	8 weeks
Norris & Williams (67)			
Percent with prenatal care in first trimester (white/hispanic/black)		65/56/67	82/60/70
Buescher et al (19)			
Percent with inadequate prenatal care	44[d]	38	14[e]
Piper et al (68)			
Effects of Medicaid expansion on prenatal care		No significant effects noted.	
Howell et al (50)			
Percent began care in first trimester	70[f]	69[g]	92[h]
Schwethelm et al (76)			
Percent began care in first trimester	84	76	91
Percent began care in third trimester	1.8	3.1	0.8
Freund et al (36)			
Percent of deliveries with prenatal care in first trimester (four Medicaid Competition Demonstration sites)		32–36	76[c]
US GAO (87)			
Percent with inadequate prenatal care for noncomplicated pregnancy	24	16	2

[a] $P < .05$ for differences across groups.
[b] Figure is for US as a whole.
[c] National average.
[d] Received care in public health department.
[e] All other live births in county.
[f] Non-Medicaid residents of low-income areas.
[g] Enrolled for four or more months of pregnancy.
[h] Non-Medicaid residents of high-income areas.

Hospital Care

The use of hospital care is important for at least two reasons. First, hospital care is usually provided for diseases or conditions that are considered much more serious than those treated on an outpatient basis and, therefore, may have greater implications for health status. Second, because hospital care is so expensive, differential utilization has a large financial impact.

The results of numerous surveys examining differences in hospital use by payer are generally consistent (Table 7). In every study, hospital use is substantially lower by the uninsured than by the privately insured. Medicaid patients are hospitalized more often than either of the other two groups, and

Table 7 Hospital service use by the uninsured as a percentage of privately insured and Medicaid use, various studies, various years

Survey	Of privately insured	Of Medicaid recipients
1977 NMCES		
Davis & Rowland (28)	52	
Wilensky & Berk (7,92)[a]	50	39
1980 NMCUES		
Kasper (53)	50	30
Long & Settle (57), low-income adults and children	33	
1982 Robert Wood Johnson Survey		
Aday et al (2)	86	42
Aday & Andersen (3)	66	35
Freeman et al (35)	61	
1984 Survey of Income & Program Participation		
Long & Rodgers (56)	31	
1984 NHIS		
Rowland & Lyons (73)	72	36
1986 NHIS		
Congressional Research Service (24)	76	
Congressional Research Service, <$15,000 income	60	
Long & Rodgers (56)	63	
1986 Robert Wood Johnson Survey		
Freeman et al (35)	81	72

Hospital service use is measured by hospital days, mean admissions, or percent hospitalized. Therefore, figures may vary within the same data source.

Private insured may include public insured (Medicaid) if separate figure not provided.

[a] Wilensky & Berk included all ages.

Source: Adapted from Garrison (38, Table 1).

so the percentage figures comparing the uninsured with Medicaid patients are even lower where statistics for each group were available.

Discrepancies in access to hospital care for the uninsured may have narrowed over time. Freeman et al (35) report a 39% hospitalization gap in 1982, compared with a 19% gap in 1986. This finding is consistent with other research that shows increases in the number and proportion of self-pay patients in US hospitals between 1980 and 1985 (78). In recent years, managed care programs may also have led to reduced hospital utilization for privately insured persons.

As with the analyses of physician use, a number of other factors influence hospitalizations. Studies that used multivariate approaches to compare hospital use among persons with different insurance coverage have all found lower usage by uninsured persons. Chen & Lyttle (22) found that the uninsured had significantly fewer hospitalizations and total hospital days than either Medicaid or privately insured persons, after adjusting for demographic and supply characteristics, as well as perceived health status. In a study of the Community Hospital Program in 11 sites nationally, Cornelius (25) examined hospital utilization for 1150 persons who had an episode of illness that forced them to curtail their usual activities for three or more consecutive days. With control for age, sex, race, income, health status, usual source of care, and use of ambulatory services, uninsured persons were significantly less likely ($p < .05$) to have any inpatient use from 1978 to 1981 than the privately insured. Finally, using the same simulation methods described previously, Needleman et al (64) estimated shortfalls for the uninsured of 46% in inpatient admissions and 38% in hospital outpatient visits, with adjustment for age, sex, income, and health status.

Although overall rates of hospital use are lower for the uninsured, their rates of hospitalization may be higher for certain illnesses. Weissman et al (90) examined rates of admission for cellulitis, asthma, bleeding ulcers, and ten other conditions for which admission was thought to be more likely if ambulatory care was less than optimal. These results showed generally higher rates for the uninsured, as well as Medicaid, patients. Billings & Teicholz (11) also found a high proportion of "preventable" admissions by the uninsured and those insured by Medicaid compared with the privately insured.

Intensity—Resource Use in the Hospital

Until recently, many thought that once initial entry to the health care system was achieved, all patients received uniform care appropriate to their medical condition. This belief was reinforced by the 1977 National Medical Care and Expenditure Survey (NMCES), which showed that, for people who used the hospital at least once, the average number of stays was nearly equivalent across insurance groups (7, 92).[9] Growing evidence to the contrary suggests that differences in fact exist.

The weight of the evidence on length of stay for hospital patients indicates that self-pay or free-care patients stay fewer days in the hospital than the privately insured and that Medicaid patients stay longer (9, 30, 31, 43, 54, 61, 79, 88, 96). The results in these studies held after controlling for hospital type, patient demographic characteristics, case mix, and other factors. Two studies, however, found longer lengths of stay among self-pay patients—a 1970 study of New England hospitals by Hornbrook & Goldfarb (48) and a more recent study of New York patients [cited in Needleman et al (64)]. Customary patterns in lengths of stay by payer may be changing. The spread of managed care may have resulted in shorter lengths of stay for insured populations, and recent unpublished data from the Commission on Professional Hospital Activities suggest that the gap between insured and uninsured has narrowed considerably or even disappeared (32).

Disparities in length of stay between uninsured and insured patients are mirrored by findings of studies that focused on overall use of hospital services. In multivariate analyses controlling for case mix, hospital type, and other factors, uninsured patients underwent fewer procedures than Blue Cross patients but about the same number as Medicaid recipients (88), and incurred costs about 10% less than those incurred by Medicaid or Blue Cross patients (61). Wenneker et al (92) found that privately insured patients admitted with circulatory disorders or chest pain were 28–80% more likely to undergo angiography, angioplasty, or bypass grafting than either uninsured or Medicaid patients. Hadley and colleagues (43) demonstrated that rates of five high-cost or high-discretion procedures were 29–75% lower for uninsured patients than for those privately insured.

Finally, there is evidence that the uninsured may receive fewer life-saving therapies from hospitals. On the basis of an examination of 1808 hospital charts of cancer patients in New Hampshire and Vermont, Greenberg et al (41) found that insured patients were more likely than uninsured to be treated by surgery (odds ratio 1.52, $p < .05$) rather than radiation therapy or chemotherapy. Hadley et al (43) also suggest that treatment for the privately insured is more aggressive. In five of seven selected procedures, the insured were about twice as likely as the uninsured to have "not abnormal" (i.e. normal) biopsy results.

Not all of the extra resource use by the insured is necessarily beneficial. We are unaware of any studies to date that compare the appropriateness of procedure use in relation to payment status. However, a study of obstetrical care provides relevant information. Stafford (81) examined the records of

[9]Wilensky & Berk examined all age groups.

nearly one-half million deliveries in California in 1986, of which nearly one-quarter were by cesarean section. The privately insured were about 50% more likely than self-pay or indigent[10] patients to undergo this procedure. The similarity in rates between uninsured patients and patients of the Kaiser HMO suggests that some portion of the gap between privately insured and uninsured use may be related to unnecessary care for the insured groups. In a subsequent study, Stafford (82) also noted similar trends for vaginal births after cesarean.

Quality of Care in Hospitals

Above we noted the absence of research on variations in the appropriateness of specific procedures by payment status. Two groups of researchers have, however, examined the process of care using other techniques to gauge its quality. Burstin et al (21) explored the distribution of adverse events (injuries suffered as a result of medical management) and negligent adverse events among more than 30,000 patients hospitalized in New York State in 1984. The mean rate for adverse events was 4.2%; about 27% of the adverse events were determined to be negligent. Furthermore, the likelihood that an adverse event was caused by negligence was significantly associated with payer. Self-pay patients suffered a 40.3% neligent adverse events rate, compared with 29.1% for Medicaid and 20.3% for private patients (p=.017). Self-pay patients were also more likely than others to suffer disability leading to death as a result of their injuries. A second recent study, by Hand and colleagues (44), examined hospital predictors of quality of care for nearly 6000 women diagnosed with breast cancer in nearly 100 Illinois hospitals. Hospitals that cared for a large proportion of uninsured or Medicaid patients had lower quality of care as evidenced by a higher proportion of women diagnosed with a late stage tumor and a lower proportion of women receiving an appropriate test of hormone receptor status. Actions by individual hosptials are only partly responsible for delays in diagnosis, but the omission of hormone receptor tests is more clearly an institutional responsibility.

OUTCOMES OF CARE

Although numerous studies document lack of access to health care services for the poor and uninsured, many fewer have examined whether barriers to care have been sufficiently large to affect health outcomes. We do know, for example, that uninsured patients are less satisfied with their care than privately

[10]Indigent services are presumably for medically indigent adults, not eligible for Medicaid, who are seen primarily in municipal hospitals.

insured groups, whereas Medicaid patients do not differ significantly from the privately insured (22, 69).

The bulk of the literature on health care outcomes primarily considers clinical consequences. For example, as part of the study discussed above, Lurie et al (58) found that hypertensive patients who lost Medicaid coverage were more likely at follow-up six months later to have worsening blood pressure control and lower perceived health status. The health of the comparison group improved or stayed the same.

Delays in ambulatory care may result in diagnosis or treatment later in the course of disease. Three studies—two about 20 years old and one very recent—found that uninsured patients were more likey to present at later stages of cancer or with more advanced tumors compared with privately insured patients (8, 10, 37). Two studies disagree about the chances for survival from cancer. Greenberg et al (41) found no significant differences in survival from lung cancer by payer, whereas Ayanian et al (8) found that uninsured and Medicaid women had shorter median survival times from breast cancer after controlling for age, stage, race, and income. Other studies have examined patients in general, rather than those with cancer, and found that uninsured patients are likely to be admitted to the hospital with more advanced disease stage (39) and other characteristics that suggest greater severity (43).

Once in the hospital, uninsured patients may also have higher in-hospital mortality rates than patients with other payment sources (43, 96, 97). None of these studies, however, could identify specific clinical causes of the poor outcomes.

The evidence on variation in birth outcomes is inconsistent. Some research shows that babies born to uninsured mothers have poorer outcomes (17, 87). However, research by Howell et al (50) suggests that patient income has at least as strong an effect as payer on birth outcomes, and work by Piper et al (68) and Haas et al (42) report no significant changes in birth outcomes when insurance coverage is provided to populations of uninsured women.

SUMMARY AND IMPLICATIONS

Research on the association of insurance status with access to care should be an important component of the political debate over health insurance reform. The voluminous literature on health-care process indicates clearly that the source of payment has a substantial effect on the amount, location, and even quality of care received in the US health care system. This form of inequity appears to be important to most Americans, as evidenced by public opinion polls that indicate strong support for options that make insurance coverage more available for those currently uninsured (14).

Uninsured patients are less likely to have a regular doctor and more likely to receive care from emergency departments or hosptial outpatient clinics.

Data on waiting times suggest that their care is also less convenient. Perhaps as a result, the uninsured delay important care more than others and tend to receive fewer preventive health services. There are also marked disparities in the total number of ambulatory visits, with the uninsured making many fewer on average than either Medicaid or privately insured groups.

Recipients of Medicaid are a heterogeneous group, comprising poor women and their children and the sick poor. The evidence on utilization of care suggests that provision of Medicaid coverage has led to increased numbers of physician visits for beneficiaries, although other problems in access persist. For example, Medicaid beneficiaries closely resemble uninsured groups in their reduced access to private physicians as a usual source of care. There are still many gaps in our understanding of the behavioral aspects of supply and demand for Medicaid services. We know little, for example, about whether evidence of lower access for Medicaid beneficiaries is due more to care-seeking behavior associated with their socioeconomic position, to the tendency of physicians to locate their practices in affluent neighborhoods, or to Medicaid's poor reimbursement rates. These issues are important, because an often-mentioned solution to the problem of the uninsured is to expand the Medicaid program.

Although measuring the process of care is important, there is a recent trend among policy-makers and researchers to ask more about the quality and outcomes of care. As a result, mere calculation of such indices as visit rates is insufficient; we also need to learn what happened during the visit and what the outcome was. The dramatic differences in process of care do not appear to result in similarly dramatic differences in outcome, although several studies affirm that such variation does occur. The relatively small number of studies contrasting outcomes by payer status should not be surprising. The focus on outcomes is a relatively recent phenomenon; outcome data are generally more difficult to obtain than utilization data, and the impacts of discrepancies in use on eventual outcomes are likely to be confounded by a large number of other social and economic factors.

Assessing the evidence on insurance status and access to care can be like using a metal detector to search for coins and jewelry on the beach. One must scan through a great deal of raw material to locate a few valuable items. For example, differences among and within insurance groups make suspect conclusions from analyses that fail to adjust for health status, as well as age and income. The heterogeneity of patients within payer groups raises concerns that comparisons of payment groups in their entirety, rather than subgroups defined by health or other characteristics, will fail to illuminate factors other than payer that may be important. Perhaps one of the greatest deficits in the access literature is the lack of studies that distinguish underservice in one group from overservice in another. For example, as we discussed above, newer evidence suggests that gaps among payer groups in hospital lengths of stay are shrinking, largely because of aggressive utilization review programs aimed at privately insured patients (32). Future research should address differences in levels of appropriate and important care, as well as the function of patient preferences in explaining dissimilarities in access indicators.

Medical care can alleviate pain and discomfort, prevent unnecessary morbidity and mortality, and relieve anxiety. Yet, factors other than medical need, including the source of payment, seem to play a large role in allocating services and, in some instances, in determining health outcomes, including satisfaction. Our knowledge of how variations by payer are mediated is still incomplete. Although recent public opinion polls demonstrate broad societal tension over problems with access, there is still no consensus on the appropriate policy solution. Clearly, we have a long way to go before inequities in the provision of health care are substantially reduced.

ACKNOWLEDGMENTS

We wish to acknowledge the valuable contributions of Denise Dougherty, Julie Goldman, Wendy Landman, and Kimberly Levin to the work reported here. We appreciate the work of Ann Seymour in preparing the manuscript.

Literature Cited

1. Aday, L. A., Anderson, R. M. 1975. *Development of Indices of Access to Medical Care*. Ann Arbor, Mich: Health Adm. Press
2. Aday, L. A., Andersen, R. M. 1984. The national profile of access to medical care: Where do we stand? *Am. J. Public Health* 74(12):1331–39
3. Aday, L. A., Fleming, G. V., Andersen, R. 1984. *Access to Medical Care in the US: Who Has it, Who Doesn't*. Chicago: Univ. Chicago Press
4. Adler, K., Emmerich, M. 1990. Late prenatal care for the uninsured in Eau Clair. *Wisc. Med. J.* Jan.
5. Akin, B. V., Rucker, L., Hubbell, F. A., Cygan, R. W., Waitzkin, H. 1989. Access to medical care in a medically indigent population. *J. Gen. Intern. Med.* 4:216–20
6. Andersen, R. M., Aday, L. A., Lyttle, C. S., Cornelius, L. J., Chen, M. S. 1987. *Ambulatory Care and Insurance Coverage in an Era of Constraint*. Cent. Health Adm. Stud. Cont. CHAS Res. Ser. No. 35. Pluribus Press
7. Andersen, R. M., McCutcheon, A., Aday, L. A., Chiu, G. Y., Bell, R. 1983. Exploring dimensions of access to medical care. *Health Serv. Res.* 18(1):50–74
8. Ayanian, J. Z., Kohler, B. A., Abe, T., Epstein, A. M., 1992. Outcomes of breast cancer for women on Medicaid and uninsured women. Chicago, Ill:AHSR
9. Becker, E. R., Sloan, F. A. 1983. Utilization of hospital services: the roles of teaching, case mix, and reimbursement. *Inquiry* 20:248–57
10. Berg, J. W., Ross, R., Latourette, H. B. 1977. Economic status and survival of cancer patients. *Cancer* 39:467–77
11. Billings, J., Teicholz, N. 1990. Uninsured patients in District of Columbia hospitals. *Health Aff.* Winter: 158–65
12. Bindman, A. B., Keane, D., Lurie, N. 1990. A public hospital closes. *J. Am. Med. Assoc.* 264(22):2899–2904
13. Blendon, R. J., Aiken, L. H., Freeman, H. E., Kirkman-Liff, B. L., Murphy, J. W. 1986. Uncompensated care by hospitals or public insurance for the poor. Does it make a difference? *N. Engl. J. Med.* 31(18):1160–63
14. Blendon, R. J., Donelan, K. 1990. The public and the emerging debate

over national health insurance. *N. Engl. J. Med.* 323(3):208–12

15. Blendon, R. J., Donelan, K., Lukas, C. V., Thorpe, K. E., Frankel, M., et al. 1992. Caring for the uninsured and underinsured. The uninsured and the debate over the repeal of the Massachusetts universal health care law. *J. Am. Med. Assoc.* 267(8):1113–17
16. Bloom, B. 1990. Health insurance and medical care: health of our nation's children, United States, 1988. *Advance Data from Vital and Health Statistics,* No. 188. Hyattsville, Md: Natl. Cent. Health Stat.
17. Braveman, P., Oliva, G., Grisham Miller, M., Reiter, R., Egerter, S. 1989. Adverse outcomes and lack of health insurance among newborns in an eight-county area of California, 1982–1986. *N. Engl. J. Med.* 321(8): 508–12
18. Brown, E. R., Cousineau, M. R. 1991. Loss of Medicaid and access to health services. *Health Care Financ. Rev.* 12(4):17–26
19. Buescher, P. A., Smith, C., Holliday, J. L., Levine, R. H. 1987. Source of prenatal care and infant birth weight: the case of a North Carolina county. *Am. J. Obstet. Gynecol.* 156(1):204–10
20. Bunker, J. P., Gomby, D. S., Kehrer, B. H., eds. 1989. *Pathways to Health: The Role of Social Factors.* Menlo Park, Calif: Kaiser Family Found.
21. Burstin, H. R., Lipsitz, S. R., Brennan, T. A. 1992. Socioeconomic status and risk for substandard medical care. *J. Am. Med. Assoc.* Nov. 3, 1992.
22. Chen, M., Lyttle, C. S. 1987. Multivariate analysis of access to care. In *Ambulatory Care and Insurance Coverage in an Era of Constraint,* ed. F. M. Anderson, L. A. Aday, C. S. Lyttle, L. J. Cornelius, M. S. Chen. Cont. CHAS Res. Ser., No. 35. Cent. Health Adm. Stud.
23. Congr. Res. Serv. Library of Congress. 1988. *Health Insurance and the Uninsured: Background Data and Analysis.* Washington, DC: GPO
24. Congr. Res. Serv. Library of Congress. 1988. *Medicaid Source Book: Background Data and Analysis.* Prep. Subcomm. Health Environ. Comm. Energy Commer. Washington, DC: US House of Representatives
25. Cornelius, L. J. 1991. Access to medical care for black Americans with an episode of illness. *J. Natl. Med. Assoc.* 83(7):617–26
26. Cornelius, L. J., Beauregard, K., Cohen, J. 1991. *Usual Sources of Medical Care and Their Characteristics.* Rockville, Md: Public Health Serv. Agency Health Care Policy Res., AHCPR Publ. No. 91-0042. NMES Res. Find. 11
27. Davis, K. 1976. Achievements and problems of medicaid. *Public Health Rep.* 91(4):309–16
28. Davis, K., Rowland, D. 1983. Uninsured and underserved: inequities in health care in the United States. *Milbank Mem. Fund Q.* 61(2):149–76
29. Donabedian, A. 1976. Effects of Medicare and Medicaid on access to and quality of health care. *Public Health Rep.* 91:322
30. Dowd, B. E., Johnson, A., Madson, R. 1986. Inpatient length of stay in twin cities health plans. *Med. Care* 24(8):694
31. Duncan, R. P., Kilpatrick, K. E. 1987. Unresolved hospital charges in Florida. *Health Aff.* Spring:157–66
32. Firshein, J., ed. 1992. Briefly this week. In *Faulkner and Gray's Medicine and Health.* 46(16)
33. Foley, J. D. 1991. *Uninsured in the United States: The nonelderly population without health insurance.* Anal. March 1990 Curr. Populat. Surv. Washington, DC: Employee Benefit Res. Inst.
34. Freeman, H. E., Aiken, L. H., Blendon, R. J., Corey, C. R. 1990. Uninsured working-age adults: characteristics and consequences. *Health Serv. Res.* 24(6):811–23
35. Freeman, H. E., Blendon, R. J., Aiken, L. H., Subman, S., Mullinix, C. F., et al. 1987. Americans report on their access to health care. *Health Aff.* Spring: 6–18
36. Freund, D. A., Hurley, R. E., Paul, J., Grubb, C., Rossitter, L. F., Adamache, K. W. 1989. Interim findings from the Medicaid competition demonstrations. *Adv. Health Econ. Health Serv. Res.* 10:153–81
37. Friedman, B., Parker, P., Lipworth, L. 1973. The influence of medicaid and private health insurance on the eaely diagnosis of breast cancer. *Med. Care* 11(6):485–90
38. Garrison, L. P. 1990. Medicaid, the uninsured, and national health spending: Federal policy implications. *Health Care Financ. Rev.* Ann. Suppl. 167–70
39. Gonnella, J., Hornbrook, M., Louis, D. 1984. Staging of disease: a case mix measurement. *J. Am. Med. Assoc.* 251:637
40. Gortmacher, S. L. 1981. Medicaid and the health care of children in poverty

and near poverty: some successes and failures. *Med. Care* 19(6):567–82
41. Greenberg, E. R., Chute, C. G., Stukel, T., Baron, J. A., Freeman, D. H., et al. 1988. Social and economic factors in the choice of lung cancer treatment: a population based study in two rural states. *N. Engl. J. Med.* 318:612–17
42. Haas, J., Udvarhelyi, I. S., Morris, C., Epstein, A. M. 1992. The impact of providing health coverage to poor, uninsured pregnant women in Massachusetts. *J. Am. Med. Assoc.* In press
43. Hadley, J., Steinberg, E. P., Feder, J. 1991. Comparison of uninsured and privately insured hospital patients: condition on admission, resource use and outcome. *J. Am. Med. Assoc.* 265(3): 374–79
44. Hand, R., Sener, S., Imperato, J., Chmiel, J. S., Sylvester, J., Fremgen, A. 1991. Hospital variables associated with quality of care for breast cancer patients. *J. Am. Med. Assoc.* 266(24): 3429–32
45. Hayward, R. A., Shapiro, M. F., Freeman, H. E., Corey, C. R. 1988. Who gets screened for cervical and breast cancer? Results from a new national survey. *Arch. Intern. Med.* 148:1177–81
46. Hayward, R. A., Bernard, A. M., Freeman, H. E., Corey, C. R. 1991. Regular source of ambulatory care and access to health services. *Am. J. Public Health* 81(4):434–38
47. Hayward, R. A., Shapiro, M. R., Freeman, H. E., Corey, C. R. 1988. Inequities in health services among insured Americans: do working-age adults have less access to medical care than the elderly? *N. Engl. J. Med.* 318(23):1507–12
48. Hornbrook, M. C., Goldfarb, M. G. 1983. A partial test of a hospital behavioral model. *Soc. Sci. Med.* 17:667–80
49. Howell, E. M. 1988. Low-income persons' access to health care: NMCUES Medicaid data. *Public Health Rep.* 103 (5):507–14
50. Howell, E. M., Herz, E. J., Wang, R., Hirsch, M. B. 1991. A comparison of Medicaid and non-Medicaid obstetrical care in California. *Health Care Financ. Rev.* 12(4):1–16
51. Hubbell, F. A., Waitzkin, H., Mishra, S. I., Dombrink, J. 1989. Evaluating health-care needs of the poor: a community oriented approach. *Am. J. Med.* 87(2):127–31
52. Jencks, S. F., Benedict, M. B. 1990. Accessibility and effectiveness of care under Medicaid. *Health Care Financ. Rev.* Annu. Suppl. 47–56
53. Kasper, J. D. 1986. Perspectives on health care: United States, 1980. *National Medical Care Utilization and Expenditure Survey,* Ser. B, Descript. Rep. 14, DHHS Publ. No. 86-20214. Washington, DC: Off. Res. Demonstr. Health Care Financ. Adm.
54. Kelly, J. V. 1985. Provision of charity care by urban voluntary hospitals. In *Hospitals and the Uninsured Poor: Measuring and Paying for Uncompensated Care*. New York: United Hosp. Fund NY
55. Leicher, E. S., Howell, E. M., Corder, L., LaVange, L. M. 1985. Access to medical care in 1980. *National Medical Care Utilization and Expenditure Survey*. Health Care Financ. Adm. Office Res. Demonstr. Public Health Serv. Natl. Cent. Health Stat. Ser. B, Descr. Rep. No. 12
56. Long, S. H., Rogers, J. 1989. *The Effects of Being Uninsured on Health Care Service Use: Estimates from the Survey of Income and Program Participation*. Presented at Annu. Meet. Allied Soc. Sci. Assoc., Atlanta.
57. Long, S. H., Settle, R. F. 1985. *Cutbacks in Medicaid eligibility under the omnibus budget reconciliation act of 1981: Implications for access to health care services among the newly eligible*. Prep. Health Care Financ. Adm. Contract No. 500-83-0058
58. Lurie, N., Ward, N. B., Shapiro, M. F., Brook, R. 1984. Termination from Medi-Cal-does it affect health? *N. Engl. J. Med.* 311(7):480–84
59. Lurie, N., Ward, N. B., Shapiro, M. F., Gallego, C., Vaghaiwalla, R., Brook, R. H. 1986. Termination of Medi-Cal benefits. A follow-up study one year later. *N. Engl. J. Med.* 314 (19):1266–68
60. Mechanic, D. 1979. Correlates of physician utilization: why do major multivariate studies of physician utilization find trivial psychosocial and organizational effects? *J. Health Soc. Behav.* 20:387–96
61. Melnick, G. A., Mann, J. M. 1989. Are Medicaid patients more expensive? A review and analysis. *Med. Care Rev.* 46(3):229–53
62. Moscovice, I., Davidson, G. 1987. Health care and insurance loss of working AFDC recipients. *Med. Care* 25(5): 413–25
63. Moyer, M. E. (1989). A revised look at the number of uninsured Americans. *Health Aff.* 8(2):102–10

64. Needleman, J., Arnold, J., Sheila, J., Lewin, L. S. 1990. *The Health Care Financing System and the Uninsured*. Washington, DC: Lewin/ICF, Final rep. HCFA Contract No. 500-89-0023
65. Newacheck, P. W. 1988. Access to ambulatory care for poor persons. *Health Serv. Res*. 23(3):401–19
66. Newhouse, J. P. 1978. *The Economics of Medical Care*. Reading, Mass: Addision-Wesley
67. Norris, F. D., Williams, R. L. 1984. Perinatal outcomes among Medicaid recipients in California. *Am. J. Public Health* 74(10):1112–17
68. Piper, J. M., Ray, W. A., Griffin, M. R. 1990. Effects of Medicaid eligibility expansion on prenatal care and pregnancy outcome in Tennessee. *J. Am. Med. Assoc*. 264(17):2219–23
69. Robert Wood Johnson Found. 1987. *Access to Health Care in the United States: Results of a 1986 Survey*. Special rep. No. 2. RWJF
70. Rogers, D. E., Blendon, R. J. 1977. The changing American health scene. Sometimes things get better. *J. Am. Med. Assoc*. 237(16):1710–14
71. Rosenbach, M. L. 1985. *Insurance Coverage and Ambulatory Medical Care of Low-Income Children: United States, 1980*, Ser. C, Anal. Rep. No. 1 DHHS Publ. No. 85-20401. Natl. Cent. Health Stat. Public Health Serv. Washington, DC: GPO
72. Rosenbach, M. 1986. The impact of Medicaid on physician use by low-income children. *Am. J. Public Health* 79(9):1220–26
73. Rowland, D., Lyons, B. 1989. Triple jeopardy: rural, poor, and uninsured. *Health Serv. Res*. 23(6):975–1004
74. Rowland, D., Lyons, B., Edwards, J. 1988. Medicaid: health care for the poor in the Reagan era. *Annu. Rev. Public Health* 9:427–50
75. Schramm, W. F. 1985. WIC prenatal participation and its relationship to newborn Medicaid costs in Missouri: a cost/benefit analysis. *Am. J. Public Health* 75(8):851–57
76. Schwethelm, B., Margolis, L. H., Miller, C., 1989. Risk status and pregnancy outcome among Medicaid recipients. *Am. J. Prev. Med*. 5(3): 157–63
77. Short, P. F., Lefkowitz, D. 1991. *Encouraging preventive services for low-income children: the effect of expanding Medicaid*. Annu. Meet. Assoc. Health Serv. Res. San Diego, Calif
78. Slaon, F. A., Morrisey, M. A., Valvona, J. 1988. Hospital care for the "self-pay" patient. *J. Health Polit. Policy Law* 13(1):83–103
79. Sloan, F. A., Valvona, J., Mullner, R. 1986. Identifying the issues: a statistical profile. In *Uncompensated Hospital Care: Rights and Responsibilities*, ed. F. Sloan, J. Blumstein, J. Perrin. Baltimore: Johns Hopkins Univ. Press
80. Soumerai, S. B., Avorn, J., Ross-Degan, Gortmaker, S. 1987. Payment restrictions for prescription drugs under Medicaid: effects on therapy, cost, and equity. *N. Engl. J. Med*. 317(9):550–56
81. Stafford, R. S. 1990. Cesarean section use and source of payment: an analysis of California hospital discharge abstracts. *Am. J. Public Health* 80(3): 313–15
82. Stafford, R. S. 1991. The impact of nonclinical factors on repeat cesarean section. *J. Am. Med. Assoc*. 265(1):59–63
83. St.Clair, P. A., Smeriglio, V. L., Alexander, C. S., Connel, F. A., Niebyl, J. R. 1990. Situational and financial barriers to prenatal care in a sample of low-income inner-city women. *Public Health Rep*. 105(3): 264–66
84. Sulvetta, M. B., Swartz, K. 1986. *The Uninsured and Uncompensated Care: A Chartbook*. Washington, DC: Natl. Health Policy Forum, George Washington Univ.
85. Thorpe, K. E., Brecher, C. 1987. Improved access to care for the uninsured poor in large cities: do public hospitals make a difference? *J. Health Polit. Policy Law* 12(2):313–24
86. Torres, A., Kenney, A. M. 1989. Expanding Medicaid coverage for pregnant women: estimates of the impact and cost. *Family Plan. Perspect*. 21(1): 19–24
87. US Gen. Account. Off. 1987. *Prenatal Care: Medicaid Recipients and Uninsured Women Obtain Insufficient Care*. Rep. to Chairman, Subcomm. Hum. Resourc. Intergovern. Relat. Comm. Govern. Operat. House of Representatives. Publ. No. GAO/HRD-87-137. Washington, DC
88. Weissman, J. S., Epstein, A. M. 1989. Case mix and resource utilization by uninsured hospital patients in the Boston metropolitan area. *J. Am. Med. Assoc*. 261(24):3572–76
89. Weissman, J. S., Fielding, S. L., Stern, R. S., Epstein, A. M. 1991. Delayed access to health care: risk factors, reasons, and consequences. *Ann. Int. Med*. 114(4):325–31
90. Weissman, J. S., Gatsonis, C., Epstein,

A. M. 1992. Rates of avoidable hospitalization by insurance status in Massachusetts and Maryland. *J. Am. Med. Assoc.* 268(17):2388–94

91. Weissman, J. S., Van Deusen Lukas, C., Epstein,A. M. 1992. Bad debt and free care in Masschusetts hospitals: the role of uninsured and underinsured patients. *Health Aff.* Summer: 148–61
92. Wenneker, M. B., Weissman, J. S., Epstein, A. M. 1990. The association of payer with utilization of cardiac procedures in Massachusetts. *J. Am. Med. Assoc.* 264(10):1255–60
93. Wilensky, G., Berk, M. 1985. The poor, sick, uninsured and the role of Medicaid. In *Hospitals and the Uninsured Poor: Measuring and Paying for Uncompensated Care,* ed. S. J. Rogers, A. M. Rousseau, S. W. Nesbitt. New York: United Hosp. Fund NY
94. Woolhandler, S., Himmelstein, D. U. 1988. Reverse targeting of preventive care due to lack of health insurance. *J. Am. Med. Assoc.* 259(19):2872–74
95. Yelin, E. H., Kramer, J. S., Epstein, W. 1983. Is health care use equivalent across social groups? A diagnosis-based study. *Am. J. Public Health* 73(5):563–71
96. Yergan, J., Flood, A. B., Diehr, P., LoGerfo, J. P. 1988. Relationship between patient source of payment and the intensity of hospital services. *Med. Care* 26(11):1111–14
97. Young, G. J., Cohen, B. B. 1991. Inequities in hospital care, the Massachusetts experience. *Inquiry* 28:255–62

Annu. Rev. Publ. Health. 1993. 14:271–92

RETIREE HEALTH BENEFITS

M. A. Morrisey
Lister Hill Center for Health Policy and Department of Health Care Organization and Policy, University of Alabama at Birmingham, Birmingham, Alabama 35294

KEY WORDS: elderly, health insurance, Medicare, medigap, employers

---

INTRODUCTION

In this paper, we review what is known about the private health insurance held by the elderly in the United States. Virtually all persons over age 65 are covered by the Medicare program. However, nearly 80% of the elderly also have some form of private coverage. This coverage falls into two broad categories: individually purchased and employer sponsored. The former includes the well-known "medigap" policies, as well as "extra cash," indemnity, specific disease, and nursing home policies. Employer-sponsored coverage is generally of two types: active worker coverage provided to those persons, and their dependents, who are over age 65 and still employed, and post-retirement coverage for those workers, and their dependents, who have retired.

A host of public policy issues are associated with retiree health insurance. The ill-fated Medicare Catastrophic Coverage Act, for example, sought to extend Medicare for extended acute care services and prescription drugs. Yet, many of the elderly already had coverage for these services and saw the program as requiring additional taxes with no additional benefits. Further, there is growing evidence that the Medicare program effectively subsidizes the cost of retiree health benefits. There have been calls for taxes on supplemental plans to eliminate this subsidy.

Some have been concerned that the elderly are unable to choose intelligently among the array of medigap and individually available retiree health insurance policies. Allegedly, the elderly have needlessly purchased multiple duplicative policies. As a result, some states have restricted the range of options available and provided consumers with guides to the purchase of insurance. The federal government enacted the Baucus amendment in 1982 to encourage states to

0163-7525/93/0510-0271$02.00

bring some uniformity to the offerings in the medigap market. The Omnibus Budget Reconciliation Act (OBRA) of 1990 required the medigap policies to conform to one of ten models developed by the National Association of Insurance Commissioners (NAIC).

With respect to employer-sponsored coverage, serious concerns exist among employers that the costs of retiree benefits will be unacceptably high. New accounting standards now require firms to report the future costs of retiree health benefits as a liability on their financial reports. This has led to an appreciation of the magnitude of the potential costs. Current workers are now concerned that the promise of health insurance will not honored after retirement. Federal legislation provides a guarantee of pension benefits. No federal guarantee exists for retiree health benefits. Further, there are concerns that changes in Medicare will lead to increases in the private cost of employer sponsored benefits.

This paper provides an empirical background to these and related issues. We do not systematically deal with questions of long-term care insurance or with the Medicaid program. These topics deserve more extensive treatment than can be provided in the space available. After a brief discussion of the coverage under the Medicare program, we review the literature on individually purchased retiree coverage. We then discuss employer-sponsored coverage. The fourth section deals with the effects of retiree benefits on the use of health-care services and, particularly, on the costs to the Medicare program. The final section speculates about the future.

THE MEDICARE PROGRAM

In 1987, some 29.8 million persons in the United States were aged 65 or older, and 28.8 million (96.6%) had coverage under Medicare (39). By 2030, an estimated 66.5 million persons will be elderly by this definition, some 19% of the US population (6).

Medicare provides coverage for inpatient and ambulatory care. Inpatient coverage is provided through the Hospital Insurance Trust Fund and is designated Part-A coverage. It includes 90 days of hospital care per episode of illness with a 60-day lifetime reserve. An episode begins when a beneficiary enters a hospital and ends when he or she has been out of a hospital or skilled nursing home for 60 consecutive days. All services, except those provided by a physician in-hospital, are covered. Care in a skilled nursing facility (SNF) is covered up to 100 days, if medically necessary and subsequent to a hospitalization. Unlimited medically necessary home health visits are also covered. An initial hospital deductible of $652 is not paid by Medicare. The beneficiary is also responsible for a copayment of one fourth the deductible for each day of hospitalization between 61 and 90. The first 20 days of SNF care involves a copayment of one eighth of the deductible per day. For terminally ill beneficiaries with life expectancy of six months or less, Part-A covers hospice care, but special limits and a copayment apply. The cost of Part-A coverage is paid by current workers through payroll deductions from their earnings.

Supplemental Medical Insurance, or Part-B, covers physician and outpatient services. An annual deductible of $100 applies, as does a 20% coinsurance applied to the amount of the bill deemed reasonable by Medicare. Historically, "reasonable" was based upon a determination of the provider's usual, customary, and reasonable charge. The provider was generally free to collect the balance of the bill from the beneficiary. The new Medicare Fee Schedule now being phased-in replaces the reasonable determination and puts further limits on the provider's ability to "balance bill." Three fourths of the cost of Part-B coverage is paid from general federal tax revenues. The remainder is paid by a monthly premium from the beneficiary. The premium was $31.80 in 1992.

MEDIGAP AND OTHER INDIVIDUALLY PURCHASED COVERAGE

Privately purchased insurance coverage designed to supplement Medicare has been available since the inception of Medicare. Mueller (26) reported that by 1967, some 46% of the Medicare elderly had some form of private supplemental coverage. By 1972, the percentage had risen to 53.2% (27). Although the data sources and the assumptions used to develop the estimates have varied by study (2, 15, 26, 27, 34), Figure 1 presents the trend in private insurance supplements. By 1987, 79% of elderly Medicare recipients had a private supplement of some kind. An additional 7.1–8.2% had Medicaid as a supplement (15, 34).

Types of Coverage

Rice & McCall (29) provide the most extensive information on the types of coverage held by the elderly. Their findings are based upon a 1982 survey of 1657 Medicare beneficiaries in six states. They identified seven types of supplemental insurance: medigap, hospital indemnity, specific disease, nursing home, health maintenance organization (HMO), major medical, and other. Medigap coverage is generally designed to cover the deductibles and copayments that the beneficiary is faced with under Medicare. Hospital indemnity plans generally pay a cash amount per hospital admission or per day of hospitalization. Specific disease policies pay a cash amount or cover medical expenses associated with a particular disease, such as cancer. Major

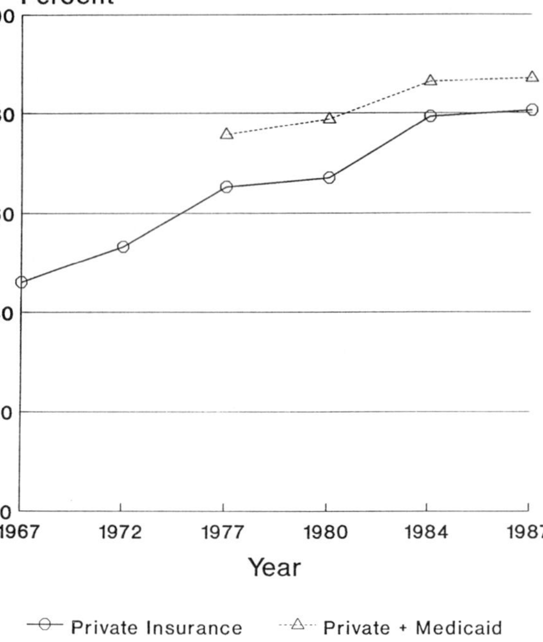

Figure 1 Percent of the Medicare elderly population with additional health insurance.

medical policies usually cover health-care expenses after a deductible is met. Major medical is generally provided by employer-sponsored plans.

The extent of coverage under these plan types is summarized in Table 1. Approximately 70% of this sample had some form of private supplement. The choice of plan varied significantly by state, however. Fifty to seventy percent

Table 1 Percent of Medicare elderly with private coverage, 1982[a]

	Calif.	Fla.	Miss.	NJ	Wash.	Wisc.
Medigap	53.5%	57.2%	53.5%	71.7%	63.7%	52.4%
Hospital indemnity	14.7	23.3	18.3	9.4	3.9	17.3
Specified disease	1.4	1.8	12.4	0.0	2.5	9.8
Nursing home	3.6	3.7	0.6	1.0	5.1	1.9
HMO	9.3	1.4	0.0	0.0	7.6	2.0
Major medical	15.7	7.6	8.6	9.5	14.1	10.8
Other	1.8	5.0	6.5	8.4	3.0	5.8
One or more	76.9	82.3	69.2	76.1	81.4	80.3

[a] Adapted from Rice & McCall (29).

of the elderly had a medigap policy. Seven to nearly sixteen percent reported having major medical coverage, depending upon state.

Another way to categorize health insurance is by the source of coverage. Jensen & Morrisey (15) provide the cleanest typology. Using data from all four waves of the 1984 Survey of Income and Program Participation, they found that 86.4% of the Medicare elderly had some form of supplement. Nearly 46% had a medigap or other individually purchased policy; 19% had employer-sponsored post-retirement coverage. Another 7% had both post-retirement and medigap coverage. Less than 5% had active worker coverage; 7% had Medicaid coverage.

Short & Vistnes (35) used the 1987 National Medical Expenditure Survey (NMES) to examine coverage under multiple plans. They found that 78.6% of the Medicare elderly had private supplements. Almost 59% had only one policy, 16% had two, and 4% had three or more. Among those elderly with Medicaid coverage, nearly 2% also had a private supplement.

Characteristics of the Privately Insured Elderly

Several studies have examined the characteristics of the elderly with private Medicare supplements (2, 9, 15, 17, 35, 36). The data used in these studies range from 1976 through 1987. Most use multivariate techniques to estimate the probability of owning some form of private supplemental coverage. The results are broadly consistent. The young-old, generally those aged 65–69 or 65–74, were more likely to have supplemental coverage, as were those with more years of schooling. Whites were more likely than minorities to own a private supplement, as were those in good to excellent health. The results are somewhat mixed with respect to sex. Taylor et al (36) found that women were more likely to own a nongroup supplement. Nongroup supplements are most likely to be medigap policies. On the other hand, Short & Vistnes (35) found that elderly women were more likely to have Medicaid coverage. This may simply be an indication that women were less likely to have employer-sponsored post-retirement benefits.

Although somewhat dated, the Long et al study (17) suggested that the effect of income largely washes out when Medicaid coverage was considered along with private supplements. They found that among low-income groups, the probability of owning a private supplement increased rapidly with income. However, the probability of Medicaid coverage declined. The net effect was that the presence of public or private supplements was approximately uniform across income groups.

A determination of who has which form of supplemental coverage is complex and depends upon the type of supplement and the treatment of duplicate coverages. Jensen & Morrisey (15) provide a useful summary (see Table 2). Medigap-only coverage was somewhat less common among the young-old, men, the highest income groups, and nonwhites. In contrast, the young-old, men, and higher income groups were more likely to have employer-sponsored post-retirement benefits. Not surprisingly, active worker coverage for the elderly was most common among higher income groups, men, and the young-old. These individuals were more likely to still be in the labor force.

Combined retiree-medigap coverage was most common among women and higher income groups. This suggests that many of those with multiple coverage are the spouses of men with retiree benefits. In fact, Jensen & Morrisey (15) report that 68.5% of those with both retiree and medigap coverage are a dependent on another's employer-sponsored post-retirement policy. Morrisey et al (25) indicated that most employer summary plan booklets were silent on how long spouses were covered under the retiree benefit. One explanation for the double coverage is that many women were hedging their bets, as it were, given the uncertainty of their post-retirement benefits.

Table 2 also demonstrates that those with Medicaid coverage tended to be older and unmarried (including widows) women. Also, nonwhites and low-income elderly were more likely to have Medicaid as a supplement to Medicare. Clearly, Medicaid plays an important role in filling the gap in coverage for the low income. However, these data also indicated that the low-income elderly were more likely to be without any form of Medicare supplement, even after allowance is made for Medicaid coverage.

Covered Services

Medigap policies, as their name implies, tend to cover the gaps in the coverage provided through Medicare. The gaps that are filled tend to be on the front end. Extended nursing home care, long hospital stays, and the portion of a physicians charge over the Medicare limit are generally not paid. More than 97% of the plans in the Rice & McCall (29) study of six states covered the Medicare hospital deductible and the daily copayment required of hospital days 61 through 90. The copayment on lifetime reserve days was almost always covered as well. However, there was considerable variance in the coverage of hospital days in excess of 150. Only 26% of medigap policies in New Jersey offered such coverage, compared with 92% of the plans in Washington state. The copayments associated with Medicare stays in SNFs were generally covered by the medigap plans; however, plans seldom covered additional nursing home days and generally did not cover stays in non-Medicare certified facilities.

Physician office visit coverage also varied across the states. Cafferata (2) found that 53% of those with nongroup coverage in 1977 had coverage for office visits, whereas Rice & McCall (29) reported that only 14% did in Florida and 78% did in New Jersey. Virtually all of the medigap plans covered

Table 2 Extent of non-Medicare health insurance among the Medicare elderly, 1984[a]

	Percentage within category with:						
Category	Medigap cov. only	Retiree cov. only	Retiree & medigap only	Act. worker cov. only	Medicaid only	Other categories	No supplements
Total Medicare elderly	45.6%	19.0%	7.1%	4.2%	7.1%	3.5%	13.6%
By age group:							
ages 65–69	41.3	22.3	7.9	8.1	5.3	3.8	11.4
ages 70–74	48.0	19.5	7.0	3.5	6.8	3.0	12.3
ages 75+	47.6	15.6	6.5	1.3	8.9	3.5	16.6
By sex and marital status:							
men, married	40.4	27.3	5.5	7.4	3.8	2.4	13.4
women, married	50.7	17.0	11.7	3.4	3.0	3.8	10.5
men, unmarried	41.0	19.7	3.3	2.3	8.0	3.6	22.1
women, unmarried	48.0	12.9	6.7	2.5	12.1	4.1	13.6
By age and sex:							
men aged 65–74	38.9	26.9	4.9	8.0	4.0	2.9	14.3
women aged 65–74	48.4	16.5	9.5	4.4	7.4	3.8	9.9
men aged 75+	43.6	22.7	5.0	2.7	6.1	2.2	17.6
women aged 75+	50.0	11.5	7.3	0.5	10.5	4.2	16.0
By race:							
white	47.5	19.7	7.5	4.3	5.5	3.1	12.5
minority	26.7	11.7	2.9	3.6	22.8	6.9	25.5
By family income:							
less than $10,000	44.6	6.6	6.0	0.9	15.9	5.0	21.0
$10,000–$19,999	48.8	23.8	6.8	3.5	3.0	2.1	12.1
$20,000–$29,999	44.6	25.6	8.6	6.9	2.3	3.6	8.4
$30,000+	41.7	26.1	8.5	9.5	3.4	3.0	7.8

[a] Adapted from Jensen & Morrisey (15).

the 20% coinsurance rate required by Medicare. However, the majority did not cover any amount over that judged reasonable by Medicare. Balance billing, therefore, was not typically covered. In general, only about one quarter of the plans covered nonhospital prescription drugs.

Rice & Gabel (28) argue that these medigap supplements become much less important as the use of health-care services increases. Using 1980 data, they found that above about $7500 in annual health care expenditures, the medigap type plans offered little additional insurance protection, because much of this expense is related to nursing home care.

Given the theory of decision making under uncertainty (8a), one would generally expect people to buy insurance against large loss, moderate probability events. These are not the events covered by medigap policies. Nonetheless, people buy medigap coverage for two principal reasons: First, consumers may be misinformed. Second, and more importantly, Medicare effectively subsidizes the claims cost of private insurance supplements. The resultant lower premiums have arguably encouraged the purchase of medigap plans. The empirical evidence on this second reason also relates to employer-sponsored coverage and is discussed later.

Consumer Information and Federal Legislation

A commonly held view has been that Medicare beneficiaries are unable to wade through the various coverages and provisions offered in the Medicare supplement market and, as a result, buy unnecessary and duplicative coverages. The data reported earlier suggest that duplicate coverage was relatively infrequent and tended to be concentrated among women and those with higher incomes. In this section, we review the literature on the extent to which the elderly are aware of the coverage they have and the effects of legislation designed to standardize the range of policies offered.

Cafferata (3) used 1977 data to compare perceptions of the elderly concerning Medicare coverage with actual coverage provisions. Generally, the elderly were more likely to be correct for services that were more routinely used. Further, the most common error was a false negative. That is, the respondent believed that a service was not covered by Medicare when, in fact, it was. For example, 82.7% knew that a semi-private hospital room was covered, but only 21% knew about coverage of inpatient mental-health services. In regression analysis, the younger elderly, whites, the more highly educated and those with higher medical expenses were more often correct.

In 1986, McCall and colleagues (21) revisited their 1982 survey of Medicare beneficiaries to compare perceptions of the coverage offered by Medicare and by their medigap policy (if they had one) with the actual policy provisions. The results with respect to Medicare were similar to Cafferata's, but suggested a slightly lower level of knowledge. In addition, their regression analysis suggested that those who were widowed or unmarried were less knowledgeable, and those who had purchased a supplemental policy were more knowledgeable of the extent of Medicare coverage.

With respect to supplemental coverage, depending upon the state, 21–41% of those with a medigap policy knew if the policy covered SNF care. Only 26–46% knew if custodial nursing home care was covered. However, 51–84% knew whether the Part-A deductible was covered, and 42–84% knew whether the Part-B coinsurance was covered. And, 66–88% knew if prescription drugs were covered. Some caution must be exercised with these data, because there were only 558 responses. In regression work, those with more than a high school education were more likely to know their coverage correctly. The old-old and unmarried were less knowledgeable. There was no statistically significant difference in knowledge by race.

Because of a perception of confusion among the elderly, Congress has passed two pieces of legislation to simplify the medigap insurance market: Public Law 96-265, commonly referred to as the Baucus Amendment, and provisions of OBRA 1990. The Baucus Amendment essentially called for a review of state laws and regulations on medigap policies for consistency with model regulations developed by the NAIC.

McCall et al (20) used their survey of Medicare beneficiaries to determine whether state regulations increased the loss ratio of policies held in the state. Higher ratios imply that more premium dollars go to paying claims. They also examined whether abusive practices of insurance agents were reduced. Using regression techniques, they concluded that the specification of minimum loss ratios and the promulgation of consumer guides to coverage appeared to promote higher quality insurance products. Consumer guides and press announcements by the insurance commissioner on abusive practices appeared to reduce the perception of abusive behavior.

Scheffler (31) analyzed the effect of the 1982–1983 introduction of the Baucus amendment on the share of the Medicare supplement market held by Blue Cross. He found that the Blue Cross share of the over age 65 market increased as a result. He offered two explanations. First, other plans might have been forced to expand their coverage and raise their premiums to meet the minimums specified by the law. If Blue Cross coverage was initially broader, then its relative price was now lower, and some people would switch to Blue Cross. Alternatively, or additionally, the overall market for supplements may have expanded because of increased confidence in the product.

The General Accounting Office (GAO) (11) interviewed insurance commissioners in 12 states. They concluded that abusive sales practices had probably declined. In 1988, about 38% of the companies offering medigap policies had loss ratios below .6 and .75 for individual and group policies. However, 88% of premium dollars were collected from companies that met these minimums. More recently, GAO (12) reports that for 1988, aggregate loss ratios for mature and credible plans were .79 and .95 for individual and group plans, respectively, and .82 for each category of plan in 1989. A mature and credible plan is three or more years old and has at least $150,000 in premiums in the state. These ratios were well above the required minimums, although a few companies did have ratios that were too low. Unfortunately, the GAO did not have a control group on which to base it conclusions.

OBRA 1990 raised the loss ratio minimum on individual policies and required all medigap policies to conform to one of ten policies that were to be developed by the NAIC. It prevents the sale of duplicate coverage and provides for a six-month open enrollment period when a person turns 65. The ten plan options were released in 1991 and are to be used with plans sold after July 30, 1992. Rice & Thomas (30) provide a summary.

EMPLOYER-SPONSORED POST-RETIREMENT BENEFITS

Retiree health insurance benefits are held by about one third of the Medicare elderly, or by perhaps 43% of those with a private insurance supplement (22, 35). This magnitude makes it important. The issues surrounding employer-sponsored benefits are more complex than medigap policies. Medigap coverage is simply purchased by the elderly sometime after they become eligible for Medicare. Economic theory suggests that employer-sponsored coverage is purchased by current workers, in the form of lower money wages and other fringe benefits, throughout their working years. [See Morrisey (24) for a summary of the empirical literature.] Thus, the issues concern not only who currently has retiree coverage, but who has been promised coverage, the nature of that promise, and the risk of default. The benefits do not tend to be directly related to Medicare. This raises questions about how employer-sponsored benefits relate to Medicare. The answers have important implications for the out-of-pocket payments made by the elderly and the claims experienced by the employer-sponsored plan. Finally, because the benefits involve a future promise to pay, they raise issues of how firms deal with this liability.

Who Has Coverage and Who Provides It?

In 1977, only 19.7% of the population over age 65 had employer-sponsored health insurance (34). Jensen & Morrisey (15) report that, in 1984, 19% of the Medicare elderly had employer-sponsored post-retirement health benefits. Another 7.1% had both medigap and post-retiree benefits. This totals approximately 6.5 million elderly. Another 4.2% of the Medicare elderly (1.1 million persons) had active worker coverage provided by an employer. These persons strictly had not retired, although they were covered by Medicare because of their age. By 1987, some 8.4 million persons aged 65 and over had some form of health insurance provided through an employer (22).

These numbers underestimate the likely number of true retirees with employer-sponsored health insurance. Schultz (33) reports that nearly one half of men are out of the labor force before age 65. The proportion of the early retirees with employer-sponsored health benefits is unknown. However, Morrisey et al (25) report that among those receiving employer-sponsored post-retirement health benefits in 1988, 37.2% were early retirees. Thus, many early retirees are receiving employer-sponsored benefits, and they may be early retirees because they can take advantage of employer-sponsored health insurance.

Current recipients of post-retirement benefits have retired from large firms. Morrisey et al (25) report that over 94% of current retirees were employed by a firm with more than 1000 workers. These retirees overwhelmingly worked for manufacturing firms (71%), although 12% had worked in the service industry. Their former employers tended to be located in the northeast (49%) or the south (31%). Those firms located in the west were least likely to have retirees receiving health insurance benefits. Over 52% had worked for a firm that had a retiree health plan that had existed for more than ten years.

Those Promised Coverage

The story for those promised retiree benefits is much different. Using 1986 Bureau of Labor Statistics (BLS) data on medium- and large-size firms, Jensen & Morrisey (14) report that 68% of current workers in these firms have been promised post-retirement benefits beyond age 65. The benefits are to continue indefinitely in almost every case. Approximately 85% of these workers do not expect premium sharing upon retirement. The data are roughly similar for workers in state and local governments. A larger proportion have been promised continuous benefits after age 65 (75%); however, only about 60% percent of these avoid premium sharing after retirement.

Morrisey et al (25) used Health Insurance Association of America (HIAA) data from 1988 to examine the proportion of workers promised coverage. The advantage of this data set is that it included representation of smaller firms. However, whereas the BLS data relied on its own coding of employer summary plan booklets, the HIAA relied on a telephone survey of benefits managers. Overall, these data suggest that nearly 58% of workers are promised benefits. Many more medium and small employers are promising coverage than currently offering it, presumably because the newer plans do not yet have eligible retirees. Further, a much wider range of industries are promising post-retirement health benefits.

Nature of Coverage

The BLS data for 1986 indicate that 79% of workers promised retiree benefits in private-sector medium- and large-size firms would get benefits that are the "same as active workers" (14). Approximately 18% would get less extensive coverage. This was an increase from 1981, when only 47.5% of workers had benefits the same as those of active workers. For state and local government workers in 1987, the BLS data indicated that 92.4% were promised benefits identical to those extended to active workers. These findings are consistent with 1977 data reported by Cafferata (2) and with 1988 results from Morrisey et al (25).

Less than half of private-sector workers and only 18.8% of government workers in the BLS sampling frames faced deductibles or coinsurance for hospital care. Extended care, i.e. nursing home care, was promised to nearly three quarters of the private-sector retirees and over 80% of government retirees. The criteria for eligibility for extended care is unclear. Because the plans mimic active worker coverage, it is unlikely that residence in a Medicare-certified SNF is required. Prior hospitalization may be required, and few plans cover intermediate or custodial care, so the plans are not a substitute for long-term care coverage. In the private sector, 94% of retirees and over 99% of government workers who were promised retiree insurance have coverage for physician visits. Seven to eight percent face a deductible that is lower than Medicare's, and most have the same 20% coinsurance feature. Most of the plans would pay at least some portion of a physician's bill above the Medicare reasonable rate.

Nonhospital prescription drug coverage is included for 98% of private and 91% of government workers promised coverage. Stop-loss features are common and included in the packages of 75% of private-sector retirees and 65% of government retirees. A stop-loss limits the amount an individual must pay out-of-pocket for covered services. The plan's liability often has a maximum expenditure limit over the life of the subscriber. Over three quarters of those promised retiree health benefits have a limit that exceeds $250,000.

In addition, retirees generally face the same utilization review programs as active workers. The 1988 HIAA survey indicated that 76% of those promised retiree coverage would face preadmission certification, 78% would have concurrent review, and 74% would have large-claim case management.

One important aspect of coverage that is unclear is the effect of a retiree's death on health benefits for a surviving spouse. For 1986, BLS data indicated that in approximately 2% of cases, the coverage is immediately canceled. Coverage continued for a limited period for 17% of workers promised retiree coverage. It continued indefinitely for one third of retirees. However, nearly half (48%) were in plans in which the summary plan booklet was silent on the continuation of coverage for the spouse. This may explain why elderly women are more likely to have both employer-sponsored retiree coverage and medigap coverage.

Coordination Between Employer Plans and Medicare

With medigap coverage, the coordination between the private plan and Medicare is reasonably clear. The medigap plan essentially pays for the deductibles, copayments, and coinsurance associated with Medicare covered services. Coordination is much more complex between an employer-sponsored retiree plan and Medicare. Three approaches to coordination are commonly used: coordination of benefits, carve-out, and exclusion.

Consider the following example: Suppose a retiree has $600 in covered physician services in one year and a $2000 hospitalization. For simplicity, suppose these bills are considered reasonable under the Medicare definition. Medicare would pay 80% of the amount over the $100 annual deductible for the physician services and all of the hospital bill after the $652 Medicare hospital deductible. Thus, it would pay $1748. Suppose the employer's retiree plan has a $150 deductible and an 20% coinsurance provision. Under the coordination of benefits (COB) approach, the firm calculates the amount payable in the absence of Medicare, which is $1960 (80% of $2450). With COB, Medicare's payment of $1748 is available to first satisfy the deductible and coinsurance provisions of the private plan. Thus, the retiree ends up paying nothing out-of-pocket. Medicare pays $1748, and the firm pays the remainding $852. Morrisey et al (25) report that 15.3% of firms used the COB method in 1988.

Under the carve-out method, the firm again calculates the amount payable absent Medicare, which again is $1960. In this case, however, the Medicare payment is first applied to the amount the firm would pay. Thus, Medicare pays $1748, as always, the firm's liability is $212, and the retiree pays $640. This approach is used by an estimated 66% of firms.

The exclusion approach is less common, used by only 5.4% of firms. It generally yields an out-of-pocket liability for the retiree somewhere between the COB and carve-out approaches. The firm applies its deductible and coinsurance rate to the amount left after Medicare has paid. Thus, $1748 of the $2600 total bill is paid by Medicare. Of the remaining $852, the firm applies its $150 deductible and 20% coinsurance. The firm pays $561.60, and the retiree pays $290.40.

Under the most common method of coordination, the carve-out, the Medicare retiree may still face significant out-of-pocket payments. In practice, the effect of the coordination method depends upon the size of the deductible and coinsurance of the firm. A private plan with no copayments, for example, has identical payments for Medicare, the firm, and the retiree, regardless of the coordination method. If a firm were interested in minimizing its payments, it could impose a large deductible and use the carve-out method. Morrisey et al (25) related a firm's deductible with its type of coordination method. Workers with carve-out methods are least likely to face an employer deductible, and their deductibles are lower. This suggests that employers are not using the carve-out method as a purely cost-saving device. A plausible explanation for the common use of the carve-out method is that it retains some of the beneficiary cost sharing, thereby reducing the incentive to overuse medical services.

Vesting and Changes in Coverage

It is not clear how many current workers will actually receive post-retirement benefits. The issue is called "vesting," that is, the conditions under which a worker becomes eligible for retiree health benefits. There is little empirical evidence on this point. The only published work appears to be that of DiCarlo & Gabel (7) and Morrisey et al (25). Both groups report results of an HIAA survey. Virtually all plans require the worker to retire from the firm that provides the coverage; portability, therefore, appears to be rare. They also found that 74% of plans require early retirees to have worked for the firm for a specified number of years. (There does not appear to be any evidence of the time in service necessary for "regular" retirees.) Just over half of the plans use the same minimum number of years as was required by the firm's pension plan. Andrews (1) notes that most firms have a ten-year vesting period for their pension plan.

There has been considerable concern over the extent to which a firm can modify or terminate a retiree health plan. Vogel (38) and Schmidt (32) have suggested that employers initially did not give much consideration to retiree health benefits and believed that they could change or terminate the plans largely at will. The laws governing pension plans (essentially the Employee Retirement Income Security Act of 1974) apparently do not apply to retiree health benefit plans. However, the courts have applied contract law to retiree health benefits and ruled that the benefits could be changed after retirement only if the employer explicitly states this in writing. Thus, except for certain conditions relating to bankruptcy (see Ref. 10), employers can make changes only if their plan documentation explicitly reserves the right to do so. The impression from the literature is that most companies have revised the language of their promise to current workers to allow for such changes.

In addition to legal contract protections, there are economic reasons to believe that the labor market would impose some constraints on the freedom of employers to change or eliminate benefits. Labor theory implies that workers are basically paid what they are worth. The payment could take many forms: money wages, current fringe benefits, pensions, and, of course, a promise of retiree health insurance. In a reasonably competitive labor market, higher retiree benefits would imply that workers receive lower current wages. If a firm were to renege on its promise of payment or reduce the benefit package substantially, wages to current workers would have to rise to make them whole. Failure to do so would lead to increased resignations, as the better workers obtained employment elsewhere. Current retirees would clearly lose. However, unless the firm were to cease operations, it would pay a price for restricting or eliminating coverage to its retirees.

There is some evidence that wages and pensions do behave in a manner suggested by this theory. The basic argument is that firms that offer wages and pensions provide lower wages than firms that only pay money wages. Ippolito (13) argues that the appropriate comparison is between the present value of money wages on the one hand and the present value of money wages plus the pension on the other. One must compare the income streams over the life cycle of the workers. If a worker has a zero chance of dying, if the firm has zero chance of failing or otherwise terminating the pension, and if the worker has zero chance of being terminated, then the present value of the pension should be equal to the present value of the reductions in wages over the entire working life. Montgomery et al (23) offer a test of this lifetime model by using 1983 Survey of Consumer Finances data from the Internal Revenue Service. When lifetime wages were imputed and used in the model, they found a coefficient of –.8 on pension value. This implies that 80% of the pension was offset by reductions in lifetime wages. Because workers do die before retirement, pension plans do occasionally fail, and termination does occur before retirement, the 80% compensating differential is plausible. Indeed, it is dramatic evidence of wage adjustments. For a more detailed discussion of compensating differentials in health care, see Morrisey (24).

Prefunding

Currently, most employers use a pay-as-you-go approach to pay for retiree health benefits. This is consistent with the practices used for active workers. Current medical claims are paid from currently paid premiums or from monies set aside this year to pay for medical costs. This is very different from the approach used to pay for pensions, which are typically prefunded, i.e. the employer invests money today to have cash available in the future to pay pension benefits.

Doran et al (8) argue that there are three reasons for the different treatment: lack of appreciation of the actual future costs of retiree health benefits, perhaps spurred by the early belief that benefits could always be changed; general accounting standards that allowed pay-as-you-go accounting; and a tax code that allows prefunding of health benefits, but greatly limits the tax subsidy from doing so. As a result, other uses of capital appear to provide the firm with a greater return on its investment.

Accurately computing likely retiree medical claims costs is no simple task. One must first estimate the number of workers likely to be vested each year and then calculate their expected average medical expenditure. This implies making assumptions about life expectancy, future use rates, and rates of increase in health-care costs. These in turn imply a series of assumptions about government policy with respect to Medicare.

Doran et al (8) provide an example: Suppose one considers a stable work force of 10,000 active workers plus 1600 current retirees covered by a plan that has a $500 deductible and 75% coinsurance with a $7500 annual out-of-pocket stop-loss. Assuming that the medical care component of the GNP ultimately rises to 17%, the present value would be $24 million for current retirees and an additional $70 million for future retirees. These are the dollars one would set aside today to pay for the post-retirement health-care costs of current retirees and workers. (Of course, one can compute the amount the firm would have to invest every year to be consistent with this amount.)

If the proportion of benefits paid by Medicare were to decline by three tenths of 1% per year for 20 years, there would be a 15% increase in the present value of retiree health benefits. If Medicare were to become the secondary payer, costs would increase by an estimated 235%. If life expectancy increased by one year, the present value of the liability would increase by 6%.

The Financial Accounting Standards Board (FASB) has ruled that firms must begin reporting the present value of their unfunded retiree health benefits on their financial statements effective for fiscal years beginning after December 15, 1992. Several authors have estimated the aggregate magnitude of this unfunded liability. Chollet (4) estimates total liability of $279.4 billion (in 1988 dollars). The GAO (37) estimates that the total liability was $335 billion (in 1991 dollars).

Some have asserted that the FASB ruling would cause employers to cut future retiree benefit costs. However, DiCarlo & Gabel (7) report that less than 5% of employers in the HIAA survey planned to phase out retiree coverage. Only 4% planned to drop spousal coverage; 30% planned to tighten eligibility and 15% said they would cut benefits. Forty percent planned to expand the use of managed care. Although plans are not necessarily actions, they suggest some tightening of benefits but no wholesale elimination of coverage.

Others have argued that the FASB rule would lead to a decline in the value of firms. The argument is that the reporting of these unfunded liabilities would reveal to investors that the future profits of firms were smaller than they had thought. As a result, stock prices would decline. H. F. Mittelstaedt and M.

Warshawsky (1991, personal communication) test this hypothesis with data on 2005 firms, some with unfunded health benefit liabilities and some without. They conclude that the market valuation of corporate equity over the period 1986–1988 did reflect the future retiree benefit liability (even in advance of the FASB rule). However, the coefficient estimates are less than the value that would indicate full adjustment by the market. They offer two explanations: First, the market may indeed lack knowledge on the full extent of liability, so the adjustments were not yet complete. Second, the market may expect that changes will occur in the environment to reduce corporate liability.

EFFECTS OF SUPPLEMENTAL COVERAGE ON USE OF SERVICES

It is now well established in the health services literature that when people have to pay less out-of-pocket for medical services, they use more (18). Thus, one should expect that, other things equal, those persons with insurance coverage that supplements Medicare use more health services. Also, supplementary coverage increases Medicare's expenditures. Stated somewhat differently, it can be argued that Medicare subsidizes the cost the supplemental coverage.

Link et al (16) were the first to examine the effects of supplements on the use of health services. Using the 1976 Health Interview Survey and controlling for other factors, they found that there was a 33% increase in the predicted hospital use because of the presence of a supplement. There was an estimated 42% increase in physician visits. Christiansen et al (5) updated the study using 1984 data. They found a 27% increase in the probability of a hospitalization and a 24.3% increase in physician visits. Neither of these studies could differentiate between medigap-type policies and employer-sponsored plans. Both relied on the elderly's recall of insurance coverage. Further, the studies could not control for the presence of adverse selection. That is, those most likely to use services are also those most likely to either purchase a supplemental plan or work for a firm that provides retiree benefits. Adverse selection results in an overstatement of the use effects of supplemental coverage.

Taylor et al (36) used the 1977 National Medical Care Expenditure Survey (NMCES) data, which yielded better measures of actual insurance coverage and allowed a separation of nongroup and group coverage. This is a reasonable first approximation of medigap-type and employer-sponsored plans. They also experimented with a two-stage regression procedure to adjust for the adverse selection problem, but concluded that there was no meaningful problem. With respect to hospital care, they found no statistically significant effects on the probability of admission. However, group coverage increased hospital expenditures by an estimated 30%. Physician expenditures increased by 26% for those with group coverage and 39% among those with nongroup coverage.

The study also found that those with nongroup supplemental coverage increased Medicare expenditures by about $30 per individual per year. Group coverage increased Medicare expenditures by approximately $8 per year, although this result was not statistically significant.

It is important to sketch the effect of supplemental coverage on Medicare expenditures. Suppose I use 12 physician visits per year when I only have Medicare coverage. At $50 per physician visit, this implies a total cost of $600. Medicare would pay 80% of this amount after the $100 deductible is paid, in this instance, $400. However, if I have a medigap policy that covers the deductible and the coinsurance, I pay nothing out-of-pocket when I visit the doctor. As a result, I may choose to have 16 visits instead of 12. The total cost is $800 (16 × $50). Medicare now pays $560. The medigap policy lowered the out-of-pocket price of a physician visit. As a result, the beneficiary obtained more visits. Medicare paid 80% of the cost of each additional visit. This chain of events leads to the conclusion that Medicare expenditures rise when supplemental coverage is present. It also suggests that Medicare is subsidizing the claims experience of the supplemental plan. My extra four visits were the result of the medigap plan; however, the plan only had to pay 20% of the extra claims cost.

More recent data continue to support empirically the effect of supplemental coverage on Medicare expenditures. Scheffler (31), using 1981 and 1984 Blue Cross data, concluded that Medicare expenditures increased by two tenths of 1% for each 1% increase in the Blue Cross supplemental market share.

McCall et al (19) use their 1982 survey of Medicare beneficiaries from six states. These data are combined with Medicare claims data on the individuals. Three innovations are considered: differential effects for self-reported healthy (excellent or good health) and nonhealthy (fair or poor health) elderly; differential use by those with basic, nonbasic, and no supplemental coverage; and differential use by those with first dollar coverage, without first dollar coverage, and with no supplemental coverage. Basic coverage refers generally to medigap- and employer-type major medical coverage that covered both hospital and physician office services. The results are summarized in Table 3.

Several findings are noteworthy. First, nonhealthy Medicare beneficiaries with supplemental coverage used more hospital days and more Part-B services. Use of Part-B services was 42% higher than that of nonhealthy beneficiaries without supplemental coverage. These differences were statistically significant. Second, although self-described healthy Medicare beneficiaries with supplemental insurance coverage did have generally higher use rates than those without extra coverage, the differences were not statistically significant

Table 3 Effect of supplemental coverage on the use of services[a]

	Hospital days		Part-B services		Medicare charges	
	Healthy	Nonhealthy	Healthy	Nonhealthy	Healthy	Nonhealthy
Owns policy	−4.8%	31.1%[b]	15.2%	42.4%[d]	11.7%	35.8%
Owns basic	−2.0	36.1[b]	17.3	42.2[c]	14.2	40.4
Owns nonbasic	−10.7	24.0	10.7	44.0[c]	7.5	28.5
First dollar	2.3	44.7[c]	12.8	61.7[d]	3.3	72.0[c]
Nonfirst dollar	−16.4	−3.2	22.1	2.1	40.0	−25.6

[a] Adapted from McCall et al (19).
[b,c,d] Significant at the 90%, 95%, and 99% confidence level, respectively.

at the usual levels. Third, those who owned a basic plan, one that covered both hospital and physician services, did use more services generally than those with nonbasic coverage and both tended to use more than those without supplemental coverage. However, the statistically significant results were limited to nonhealthy beneficiaries. Fourth, it appears that a principal motivating factor in the use of both hospital and Part-B services was the presence of first dollar coverage. Such coverage eliminated financial barriers to initial visits. Although the healthy had small and statistically insignificant increases in use, the nonhealthy had large increases. Hospital days were 44.7% higher, and Part-B services were nearly 62% higher.

Finally, the study revealed that total allowed Medicare charges were 72% higher for the nonhealthy with first dollar coverage. Medicare charges were higher for most categories of beneficiaries with supplemental coverage; however, these results lacked statistical significance. One might suppose that this result is contaminated because of adverse selection. The nonhealthy beneficiaries with supplemental coverage are more disposed to acquire the coverage because they intend to use it. However, the authors indicate that in more sophisticated analysis that uses a two-stage regression process to correct for choice of coverage, the results were similar. One might also challenge the use of charges rather than actual payments by Medicare, which biases the coefficients upward. Nonetheless, there is strong and consistent evidence that supplemental coverage increases Medicare program costs, particularly when first dollar coverage is added.

SUMMARY AND CONCLUSIONS

Some 80% of elderly Medicare beneficiaries have private supplemental insurance. Approximately 50% of these have some form of medigap of privately purchased coverage. Those holding private coverage tend to be younger, more highly educated, and white. Women are more likely to hold medigap type plans, and men are more likely to have employment related coverage. The extent of multiple coverage is relatively rare. One estimate puts multiple coverage at about 20% of those with private supplemental coverage.

Contrary to conventional wisdom, those with multiple coverage are not the very old and poorly educated. Rather, they tend to be younger and more highly educated. Also, women are more likely to have both employer-sponsored and medigap coverage, maybe because of the uncertainty about whether a wife will continue to have employer-sponsored post-retirement coverage after her husband has died. Medigap-type health insurance is heavy on first dollar coverage; the Medicare deductibles and copayments are covered. Provisions of OBRA 1990 will homogenize this coverage even more.

Employer-sponsored health benefits are common. Some 8.4 million elderly Medicare beneficiaries have employer-sponsored coverage. A large but undetermined number of early retirees also have coverage. These recipients have generally been the workers in very large firms. However, the future will not look like the past. Two thirds of current workers are promised health benefits upon retirement. The benefits provided under these plans are both broad and deep.

The nature of benefit coordination between these plans and Medicare can reduce the size of the apparent benefits. The carve-out method of coordination is the most common and can result in sizable out-of-pocket payments by the beneficiary. However, it is not obvious that employer-sponsored plans have been designed to exploit this opportunity. There is little information on the conditions under which a worker is vested for health benefits. The sketchy evidence that does exist suggests that a worker must retire from the firm and have had time in service about equal to that required for the firm's pension plan. Firms apparently can change their retiree benefit plans if they have explicitly retained the right to do so. There are sound economic reasons to suggest that many firms would honor their commitments, even in the absence of legal requirements.

Supplemental retiree coverage leads to additional use of health services, particularly by those in poorer health and particularly by those with plans that feature first-dollar coverage. The increased use of services as a result of supplemental coverage also increases Medicare's costs. In fact, Medicare effectively subsidizes the claims costs of supplemental plans for Medicare covered services.

Over the next decade, the nature of retiree health benefits will change significantly. Employers are likely to continue to honor the bulk of their promises for retiree benefits. As a result, the importance of medigap coverage will decline as current workers retire with employer-sponsored coverage. The benefits offered will also change, but not dramatically. Utilization review and managed care will become more important factors. However, in the absence of income tax law changes, health insurance benefits of all types will continue to be actively used as a form of untaxed compensation. Promised retiree benefits are simply another way of providing untaxed compensation to current workers and should be expected to be both continued and honored.

Literature Cited

1. Andrews, E. S. 1985. *The Changing Profile of Pensions in America*. Washington, DC: Empl. Benefit Res. Inst.
2. Cafferata, G. L. 1984. Private health insurance of the Medicare population. *Data Preview* 18. Washington, DC: Natl. Cent. Health Serv. Res.
3. Cafferata, G. L. 1984. Knowledge of their health insurance coverage by the elderly. *Med. Care* 22(9):835–47
4. Chollet, D. J. 1989. Retiree health insurance benefits: trends and issues. In *Retiree Health Benefits: What is the Promise?*, pp: 19–36. Washington, DC: Empl. Benefit Res. Inst.
5. Christiansen, S., Long, S. H., Rogers, J. 1987. Acute health care costs for the aged Medicare population: overview and policy options. *Milbank Q*. 65(3): 397–425
6. Davis, K., Rowland, D. 1986. *Medicare Policy*. Baltimore: Johns Hopkins Univ. Press
7. DiCarlo, S., Gabel, J. 1989. Facing up to postretirement health benefits. *Res. Bull.*, Sept. Washington, DC: Health Insur. Assoc. Am.
8. Doran, P. A., MacBain, K. D., Reimert, W. A. 1987. *Measuring and Funding Corporate Liabilities for Retiree Health Benefits*. Washington, DC: Empl. Benefits Res. Inst.

8a. Feldstein, P. J. 1988. *Health Care Economics*. New York: Wiley. 3rd ed.

9. Garfinkel, S., Corder, L. 1985. Supplemental health insurance coverage among aged Medicare beneficiaries. *Natl. Med. Care Util. Expend. Surv.*, Ser. B, Rep. 5, DHHS no. 85-20205. Washington, DC: Health Care Financ. Admin.
10. Gen. Acc. Off. 1991. *Employee Benefits: Effect of Bankruptcy on Retiree Health Benefits*, Rep. no. GAO/HRD-91-115. Washington, DC
11. Gen. Acc. Off. 1991. *Medigap Insurance: Better Consumer Protection Should Result from 1990 Changes to Baucus Amendment*. Rep. no. GAO/HRD-91-49. Washington, DC
12. Gen. Acc. Off. 1992. *Medigap Insurance: Insurers Whose Loss Ratios Did Not Meet Federal Minimum Standards in 1988–89*, Rep. no. GAO/HRD-92–54. Washington, DC
13. Ippolito, R. A. 1987. The implicit pension contract: developments and new directions. *J. Hum. Resourc*. 22: 441–67
14. Jensen, G. A., Morrisey, M. A. 1992. Employer-sponsored post-retirement health benefits: not your mother's Medigap plan. *Gerontologist*. 32(5): 693–703
15. Jensen, G. A., Morrisey, M. A. 1992. Health insurance coverage of the Medicare elderly. In *Trends in Health Benefits*, ed. J. A. Turner, W. Wiatroski. Washington, DC: Pension Welf. Benefits Admin. In press
16. Link, C. R., Long, S. H., Settle, R. 1980. Cost sharing, supplementary insurance, and health services utilization among the Medicare elderly. *Health Care Financ. Rev*. 2(2):25–31
17. Long, S. H., Settle, R. F., Link, C. R. 1982. Who bears the burden of Medicare cost sharing? *Inquiry* 19(3): 222–34
18. Manning, W. G., Newhouse, J. P., Duan, N., Keeler, E. B., Leibowitz, A., et al. 1987. Health insurance and the demand for medical care: evidence from a randomized experiment. *Am. Econ. Rev*. 77:895–903
19. McCall, N., Rice, T., Boismier, J., West, R. 1991. Private health insurance and medical care utilization: evidence from the Medicare population. *Inquiry* 28(3):276–87
20. McCall, N., Rice, T., Hall A. 1987. The effect of state regulations on the quality and sale of insurance policies to Medicare beneficiaries. *J. Health Polit. Policy Law* 12(1):53–76
21. McCall, N., Rice, T., Sangl, J. 1986.

Consumer knowledge of Medicare and supplemental health insurance benefits. *Health Serv. Res.* 20(6, pt. 1):633–58

22. Monheit, A. C., Schur, C. 1989. Health insurance coverage of retired persons. *Natl. Med. Care Expend. Surv. Res. Find.* 2, DHHS Publ. no. PHS-89-3444. Washington, DC: Natl. Cent. Health Serv. Res.
23. Montgomery, E., Shaw, K., Benedict, M. E. 1990. *Pensions and Wages: An Hedonic Price Theory Approach,* Rep. 3458. New York: Natl. Bur. Econ. Res.
24. Morrisey, M. A. 1992. Compensating differentials: taxing the uninsured. In *American Health Policy: Critical Issues for Reform,* ed. R. Helms. Washington, DC: Am. Enterp. Inst. In press
25. Morrisey, M. A., Jensen, G. A., Henderlite, S. E. 1990. Employer-sponsored health insurance for retired Americans. *Health Aff.* 9(1):57–73
26. Mueller, M. 1972. Private health insurance in 1970. *Soc. Sec. Bull.* 35:3–19
27. Mueller, M. 1974. Private health insurance in 1972. *Soc. Sec. Bull.* 37:20–40
28. Rice, T., Gabel, J. 1986. Protecting the elderly against high health care costs. *Health Aff.* 5(3):5–21
29. Rice, T., McCall, N. 1985. The extent of ownership and the characteristics of Medicare supplemental policies. *Inquiry* 22(2):188–200
30. Rice, T., Thomas, K. 1992. Evaluating the new Medigap standardization regulations. *Health Aff.* 11(1):195–207
31. Scheffler, R. M. 1988. An analysis of "Medigap" enrollment: assessment of current status and policy initiatives. In *Lessons From the First Twenty Years of Medicare,* ed. M. V. Pauly, W. L. Kissick, pp. 181–208. Philadelphia: Univ. Penn. Press
32. Schmidt, P. K. 1989. Retiree health benefits: an illusory promise? In *Retiree Health Benefits: What Is the Promise?* Washington, DC: Empl. Benefit Res. Inst.
33. Schultz, J. H. 1988. *The Economics of Aging.* Dover, Mass: Auburn House
34. Short, P. F., Monheit, A. 1988. Employers and Medicare as partners in financing health care for the elderly. In *Lessons From the First Twenty Years of Medicare,* ed. M. V. Pauly, W. L. Kissick, pp. 301–320. Philadelphia: Univ. Penn. Press
35. Short, P. F., Vistnes, J. P. 1992. Multiple sources of Medicare supplementary insurance. *Inquiry* 29(1):33–43
36. Taylor, A. K., Short, P. F., Horgan, C. M. 1988. Medigap insurance: friend or foe in reducing Medicare deficits? In *Health Care in America,* ed. H. E. Frech III, pp. 145–78. San Francisco: Pacific Res. Inst. Public Policy
37. Thompson, L. H. 1991. *Significant Reductions in Corporate Retiree Health Liabilities Projected If Medicare Eligibility Age Lowered to 60.* Testimony before the House Subcomm. on Health, Comm. on Ways and Means, Nov. 5
38. Vogel, J. 1987. Until death do us part: vesting of retiree insurance. *Ind. Relat. Law J.* 9(2):18341
39. Waldo, D. R., Sonnefeld, S. T., McKusick, D. R., Arnett, R. H. 1989. Health expenditures by age group, 1977 and 1987. *Health Care Financ. Rev.* 10(4):111–20

Annu. Rev. Publ. Health 1993. 14:293–312

THE RELATIONSHIP BETWEEN HEALTH AND LABOR MARKET STATUS

Thomas N. Chirikos
Department of Health Policy and Management, College of Public Health, University of South Florida, Tampa, Florida 33612

KEY WORDS: work disability, population health trends, social security, health status measurement, costs of chronic disease

---

INTRODUCTION

Few relationships seem more self-evident than the impact of poor health on labor market behavior. Chronic health conditions that diminish basic physical and mental capabilities are typically expected to disrupt normal work functioning, not only by preventing the performance of some job-related tasks altogether, but also by raising the difficulty or cost of discharging these role responsibilities beyond levels that a reasonable person would judge tolerable. As a result, individuals with impaired health are expected to reduce the amount of time spent in the labor force, the date or age of their complete withdrawal from the job market, and/or the kind of work performed. Because the onset of chronic health problems is not uncommon at any age, and incidence rises steeply with age, health-related work adjustments are likely to be required of most persons at some stage of the life course. In fact, an extensive set of institutional arrangements for retirement and disability insurance benefits has developed over time to cushion the expected losses in market income brought about by these health-induced changes in work effort. Yet, the impact of poor health on labor market status (and the corresponding magnitude of the economic toll exacted by various health problems) is at present neither fully understood nor measured with any precision. Uncertainty about the relationship arises from the difficulty of gauging the extent to which the severity of physical and mental conditions varies across the population in poor health and the degree to which institutional arrangements, such as disability program

0163-7525/93/0510-0293$02.00

benefits themselves, induce members of this population to withdraw from the market. Among other things, judgments about the effectiveness and efficiency of public sector income support and medical insurance programs hinge on our ability to narrow the range of this uncertainty.

This article reviews the empirical evidence that has accumulated over the past two decades on the net effect of health conditions on labor market status. This research effort was mainly developed in response to early retirement trends and the public policy controversies they created, and was shaped by the analytic constructs and data available to investigators, mostly economists, working on those controversies. The next section sketches this background to provide both a framework and evaluative criteria for the review. This discussion is intentionally nontechnical in nature, and some issues of econometric estimation are suppressed altogether. The third section then summarizes the findings of recent empirical studies that primarily focus on the role of impaired health in reducing work effort either in amount or kind. Because virtually every analysis shows that health matters to some degree, the discussion focuses on the causes and consequences of variations in the magnitude of measured health effects across studies. Conclusions drawn from the review of the literature are presented in the final section.

CONCEPTUAL OVERVIEW

Policy Questions

Research on the relationship between impaired health and labor market status is most conveniently understood as a response to various public policy issues and prescriptions. At one level, empirical estimates of this relationship are used to calculate the indirect toll that chronic disease exacts from the national economy (29, 57, 95). The extent to which health conditions either prevent individuals (with or without employer accommodation) from engaging in market work or impose burdens that can be relieved only by cutting back on work effort will be reflected in reductions in the amount of time spent in labor force activities. Individuals with impaired health may also earn less for each hour spent working, because they are not as productive, they cannot devote sufficient time or talent to higher paying jobs, or they encounter discriminatory practices by employers. By a line of reasoning long familiar to economists, the value of these morbidity costs of health-related losses in economic output (i.e. the hours reduction multiplied by the lower hourly wage rate of persons with health conditions) can be used to gauge the value of social benefits that accrue to interventions that lower incidence or prevalence rates of chronic health problems.

At a somewhat different level, empirical research on the relationship between poor health and labor market status has been impelled by the impact of recent trends in the American labor force on the financing of public sector programs, particularly the Social Security system. The main issue has been the dramatic decline over the past four decades in the labor force participation rates of older American men. (This rate is defined as the proportion of age- and sex-specific population groups that is either working or looking for work during a given reference period). For example, Bureau of Labor Statistics data show that about one half of all men over 65 years of age were in the labor force in 1950, whereas only about one sixth of men this age are either working or looking for market work at present. Similarly, the participation rate of men aged 55–64 years has declined from about 87% in 1950 to only 68% at present; even the rate for men aged 45–54 has declined from about 96% to only 90% over the same period.

These trends are commonly explained either in terms of the poor health of aged persons or the increased availability of public and private pensions and social insurance benefits (5, 73, 96). In recent years, the health explanation of nonparticipation has generally been discounted, in part because it often relies on post hoc justification of labor market withdrawal by retired persons themselves, and in part because the period in question was marked by significant increases in life expectancy at older ages and the corresponding assumption that average health levels were rising (46). More significance has accordingly been attached to the explanation based on the growth and generosity of pension programs, particularly the rising number of workers covered by Social Security and the expanding asset value of retirement income and medical care insurance benefits provided by this program.

Pension programs not only accommodated the conventional retirement goals of increasingly larger cohorts of men reaching their seventh decade, they also underwent design changes that permitted even earlier retirement, e.g. after 1961, men eligible for Social Security were allowed to retire with actuarially reduced benefits at age 62; more than one in ten retired worker beneficiaries is now 62–64 years of age. The relative importance of health factors and pension inducements is a pivotal question in recent policy changes designed to shore up Social Security financing. In 1983, for instance, the eligibility age for full retirement benefits was raised from 65 to 67 years, with gradual implementation expected to be completed by the year 2027. This change raised concerns that workers in poor health or in physically demanding jobs will be disadvantaged (100). Similar proposals for raising the age of Medicare coverage, and concern that it will disadvantage workers who must stay longer in the work force to keep their medical insurance coverage, have also been set forth (37). Clearly, if poor health causes involuntary withdrawals from market work, these policy changes might impose higher costs on individuals with health problems.

The health-labor market relationship plays an even more crucial role in accounting for the rapid growth of disability transfer programs, especially the Social Security Disability Insurance (SSDI) program. Social Security Administration statistics show that SSDI beneficiary rolls have grown at more than 7% per year since the inception of the program. In 1990, there were approximately 3 million SSDI beneficiaries. (The number of disabled recipients of working age in the Supplemental Security Income program has also grown rapidly, with about 3 million persons on the rolls in 1990). Because the correlation between the temporal decline in labor force participation and the growth in the disability rolls is high, several investigators conclude that these programs induce individuals with impaired health to leave the labor market (22, 70, 88). If poor health causes only involuntary reductions in work effort, trends in nonparticipation and disability program rolls would not necessarily be correlated, because health-impaired persons who are incapable of market work would not be enumerated as members of the labor force in the first place. However, if health problems do not just cause involuntary withdrawals from the labor market, incentive effects may be inferred from the correlation between these trends. Economic inducements of disability programs, incidentally, also have important health programming implications. For instance, economic incentives built into these programs may influence the effectiveness of medical/vocational rehabilitation efforts (14, 17). Medical care insurance benefits available through these programs may also keep disabled beneficiaries from returning to market work (2, 27). Such incentives will be the subject of renewed interest because of the recently enacted Americans With Disabilities Act (ADA), which extends the mandate of the Rehabilitation Act of 1973 that employers make reasonable accommodation to facilitate the employment of individuals with chronic health impairments (30, 105).

Analytic Approach

Despite their diversity, the policy issues sketched above have been approached analytically in a remarkably similar fashion, viz. the estimation of multivariate regression models in which, among others, poor health is a predictor variable and work effort is the outcome of interest. Given the importance economic factors play in the controversies about the inducement of program benefits, as well as labor market decision making generally, most analysts now also typically incorporate a variable or variables characterizing the economic incentives facing the individual. In highly simplified terms, the general approach used in analyzing the health-labor market status relationship may be represented as:

$$W_i = \alpha - \beta_h H_i + \Sigma_j \beta_j Y_{ij} + \Sigma_k \beta_k X_{ik} + \epsilon_i, \qquad 1.$$

where W represents the work effort of individual i as measured, say, by the number of hours or weeks worked during some reference period; H represents a measure of impaired health; Y_j represents the set of economic inducements for continued work and leisure, such as wage earnings, pension income, and health insurance coverage; and X_k is a vector of other exogenous factors, such as age and gender, that influence labor market status. The α, β_h, β_j, and β_k are parameters to be estimated by means of ordinary least-squares regression (or more appropriate techniques, such as probit or Tobit regression when the dependent variable is dichotomous or truncated). And, ϵ is a normally distributed error term with the standard properties. The analytic approach boils down to testing the estimated β_h under the null hypothesis and, assuming that the coefficient is indeed significantly less than zero, evaluating the magnitude of the coefficient as a means of gauging how much poor health really matters.

This approach was adopted because it is easily derived from the well-established microeconomic theory of household labor-leisure choices. Its implementation was further facilitated when several microlevel data sets pertaining to the labor market behavior of older American men became available in the late 1960s, most notably the National Longitudinal Surveys of Labor Market Experience (86) and the Longitudinal Retirement History Survey (63). However, this analytic approach only yields usable results relative to the policy questions described above if certain conditions are met. Several of the most crucial of these conditions are summarized below to provide some criteria for the review of the empirical literature.

First, impaired health must be suitably measured (13, 31, 42). The variable(s) used to characterize health status must be valid, at least in the sense of what is usually referred to as construct validity; they must be reliable in the sense of providing a comparable yardstick of health differences at a point in time, as well as any differences that may occur over time; and they must be exogenous to the labor market behavior that they are supposed to explain. In each case, a plausible mechanism linking the health variable to permanent (as opposed to transitory) changes in labor market status must be identified. Of special significance here is whether poor health influences the willingness, as well as the capacity or ability, to perform job requirements. Chronic health conditions may lower earnings potential (wages) and, thus, lower the value of the time spent by individuals with impaired health in market work. They may also raise the value of nonmarket time to the impaired individual, perhaps by imposing self-care requirements that reduce the amount of usable time available for either market or nonmarket pursuits. Furthermore, by affecting life expectancy, impaired health may also influence the time horizon over which economic decisions are made and/or the rate of time preference (discount rate) that is applied to the calculation of the individual's assets (48, 85, 111, 112). Such factors may make departure from the work force relatively attractive, even if the impaired individual can still perform job requirements. However, any one of these explanations is consistent with a statistically significant β_h coefficient in Equation 1. In the absence of other tests, the standard approach cannot discriminate between involuntary and voluntary health-related exits from the work force on the basis of the measured health effect alone.

Second, the specification of the regression model must account for factors likely to confound the relationship of interest. One such confounding factor is whether health status itself is treated simply as an exogenous determinant of labor market status or as an endogenous or dependent variable as well. The large literature on occupational exposures to chronic disease and other work-induced health problems implies that health is not necessarily exogenous to work effort. Consequently, the following equation might also be estimated either as a complement to Equation 1 or as a constituent element of a larger, multi-equation model in which it and Equation 1 are estimated jointly:

$$H_i = \alpha - \beta_w W(t)_i + \Sigma_j \beta_j Y_{ij} + \Sigma_k \beta_k X_{ik} + \epsilon_i. \qquad 2.$$

The variables in Equation 2 are defined as before, except that $W(t)$ may index work effort at different time points (t) to allow for the cumulative effects of work on health to play themselves out. Although this type of extended model is of increasing interest to researchers, the direction of causality in many of the studies under review has been limited to the estimation of Equation 1 alone on the assumption that health status is completely exogenous.

A variant of Equation 2, which has been the focus of active interest in the current literature, hypothesizes that individual evaluations or self-reports of health status are systematically linked to the economic and sociodemographic variables on the right-hand side of Equation 2, as well as to underlying health or physical/mental conditions. A particularly relevant version (referred to below as the disability model) posits that the self-report of a work-limiting health problem is influenced by these predictor variables, i.e.

$$D_i = \alpha + \beta_h H_i + \Sigma_j \beta_j Y_{ij} + \Sigma_k \beta_k X_{ik} + \epsilon_i. \qquad 2a.$$

In this case, D_i represents reported work disablement (i.e. the responses of the ith individual to survey questions about whether a health or physical condition limits the amount or kind of work done or prevents market work altogether); H reflects the underlying physical or mental capabilities of that individual; and the Y_j and X_k are the previously defined vectors of economic and sociodemographic variables. Among others, this formulation implies that economic incentives facing individuals are significant determinants of self-appraised health status. Indeed, Equation 2a may be interpreted straightforwardly from the perspective of the work-disability literature as an outcome that is responsive to economic and job-related factors, as well as to underlying physical and mental capabilities (84, 109). In this connection, if D is used as a proxy measure of H in Equation 1, the measured effects of health on work status will be biased upwards. (This can be seen by replacing H with D in Equation 1 and then substituting 2a for D in that equation). As described below, adjustment for this potential bias to ensure that the precision of the estimated magnitude of β_h will not be compromised is possible.

Third, however the health variable is measured or modeled, it must also be tracked over time—an especially relevant consideration if the statistical modeling is cross-sectional in nature, but the policy question is interpreted from the viewpoint of trends over time. Put differently, cross-sectional models convey something about the chances that an average person in poor health will be working, but they cannot indicate whether the number of such persons is increasing or decreasing over time. The issue may be conceptualized as writing the total differential of temporal change in work effort, and then estimating the relative contributions of each term in that differential. In the simple linear case, for instance, the differential of work effort ΔW is approximated as

$$\Delta W = \beta_h \Delta H + \Sigma_j \beta_j \Delta Y_j + \Sigma_k \beta_k \Delta X_k, \qquad 3.$$

and the relative contribution of health is simply $\beta_h \Delta H / \Delta W$. This is a nontrivial matter in the present context, because the question of whether average health levels are increasing or decreasing (i.e. ΔH) is subject to active, but as yet unresolved, debate (28, 36, 46, 103, 108). Mortality rates have been declining, so a mortality-related measure of health would imply a declining health effect over time, all other things equal. Disability-based measures of health, which have been rising over time, clearly lead to the opposite inference, even if the measured cross-sectional effect of each type of health measure is roughly equal.

EMPIRICAL EVIDENCE

Scope and Classification

The pool of empirical findings on the labor market effects of poor health is potentially extensive, given its linkage to labor supply issues in the economics literature, as well as to behavioral and epidemiologic research in the health literature. To keep the review manageable, the papers selected for inclusion were delimited in several respects. Only research results pertaining to the United States published since the early 1970s are considered. This excludes not only relevant analyses in other countries, but much of the early literature on the health-retirement relationship that attributed virtually all withdrawals from the work force to the onset of chronic health conditions (83). In addition, only studies treating health as a determinant of labor market outcomes are considered. This excludes investigations conducted on adjacent topics, such as the healthy worker effect (106), return to work as an epidemiologic endpoint of highly detailed or specific disease processes (74), disease-specific cost-of-illness studies based simply on descriptive data (82), the impact of retirement on health (76), and the reciprocal impact of socioeconomic status on health (102). The vast literature on occupational disease is also excluded. Finally, within the narrower limits of research on health and labor market behavior, only those labor supply studies judged to treat health status in more than a perfunctory fashion as a control variable are included.

Even within this comparatively narrow focus, there is a sizable literature that is not always easy to classify or synthesize. A major dividing line suggested by the preceding methodological discussion is whether health is treated in a given study simply as an exogenous predictor variable, typically in the framework of single-equation models of labor supply, or whether there is a more extensive modeling strategy in which some health attribute is treated as a dependent (endogenous) variable or object of individual choice. Most of the studies reviewed in this article fall into this first category. Typically, these investigations were carried out earlier in the time period encompassed by the review and, perhaps as a result, with less appreciation for the conceptual and methodological pitfalls of this line of inquiry. These studies represent the first generation of analytic results on the health-labor market status relationship. Fewer and generally more recent studies fall into the second category. These analyses tend to be more methodologically oriented and use considerably more sophisticated statistical techniques. They are sketched briefly in the subsection below devoted to second-generation results.

First-Generation Results

Representative studies in this category use information obtained in household surveys of generalizable samples of American adults to predict the effects of health status on labor market outcomes. Many, although not all, are cross-sectional in nature, as they investigate the influence of some health measure on a contemporaneous measure of labor supply, such as the probability of being in the work force or the annual number of hours worked during a defined reference period, cf. Equation 1. Many of these studies use responses to disability or work-limitation questions as the health variable (3, 4, 43, 45, 49, 52–55, 61, 67, 72, 93, 94, 97). Other sets of studies investigate similar labor market outcomes, but they use different measures to represent health status: indicators or summary indexes of functional impairments, such as the difficulty in walking, seeing, and stooping, or the complete inability to perform these functions (13, 15, 16, 31, 32, 47, 71); reported onset, presence, symptoms, or severity level of specific diseases or physical/mental conditions (7, 8, 10, 40, 50, 62, 77, 79, 80, 95, 115); self-ratings of health (health excellent, good, fair, poor) and/or combinations of self-ratings and one or more of the other types of health reports (35, 58, 59); and, in longitudinal data sets, the mortality experience (date of death) of respondents (1, 88). Several studies investigate not only the direct effects of health on labor supply, but the indirect effects via changes in the wage rate (15, 79) or just the wage rate (12, 65); others use the health variable to split the sample and investigate interaction effects (72, 94). Still others appraise the impact of health conditions of one member of a household (e.g. the spouse) on the labor market outcomes of another member of that household (11, 33, 61, 87). Some studies go beyond the cross-sectional relationship to probe whether disease conditions early in life significantly lower market earning later in life (7, 8), or whether a history of continuously or intermittently poor health over time lowers the chances of working regular hours or earning the same per hour at present (35).

Broadly considered, two inferences can be drawn from these studies. The first, as anticipated, is that health matters. In virtually every case, impaired health exacts some toll by either restricting the ability of individuals to engage in market work or shifting their preferences for time spent in the labor market, reducing the wages of workers in poor health, and/or changing the labor market behavior of other persons in the household of the health-impaired individual. This conclusion is generally invariant to sociodemographic characteristics, occupational or industrial attachment, or the type of physical or mental health condition. Although most studies concentrate only on samples of older white men, interaction studies that look at other gender and race groups find that health problems compound even further the well-known labor market disadvantages of women and minorities.

There are predictably a few exceptions that perhaps prove the general rule that health matters. Haveman et al (59) failed to detect significant health effects on decisions by men in their early sixties either to continue working, apply for SSDI benefits, or take early Social Security benefits. However, the health variable in this study was not well measured, thereby biasing its regression coefficient toward zero. Several studies find significant health effects on work effort, but not necessarily on wages, particularly the wages of women and blacks (32, 80). This may result from the lesser overall attachment of these groups to the labor force, although it is also sensitive to the modeling techniques utilized to incorporate wages into the statistical analysis. Mixed results of the effects of job requirement-health status interactions are also in evidence (16, 31, 71). Finally, the estimated effects of health conditions of one household member (usually the spouse) on the labor market behavior of another household member also differ, with only some analyses detecting statistically significant effects of male health problems on female work effort (11, 33, 87).

Despite the near universal finding that health is a significant determinant of work effort, the second major inference drawn from the review is that the magnitude of measured health effects varies substantially across studies. One reason for this may actually be how economic variables are measured and the overall labor supply equation is specified. This possibility is suggested by the continuing controversy about the role of economic inducements in the historical rise in disability program rolls, much of it sparked by Parsons' (88) influential work on this issue. Parsons showed that the replacement rate (the proportion of market earnings replaced by SSDI and state disability program benefits) accounted for more of the observed trends in the labor force participation of older men than health factors, indexed in this study by a mortality experience measure constructed from longitudinal data. This study has been criticized by, among others, Haveman & Wolfe (56), who conducted a replication study indicating that Parsons' replacement rate variable and model specification overstate the importance of economic incentives (also see Refs. 19, 20, 90–92, 99.) Regrettably, Haveman & Wolfe deploy a different health measure than the one used by Parsons, so their replication analysis does not yield an altogether convincing comparison of results. Nonetheless, if the replacement rate explains too much, it will bias the effects of other determinants downward, most prominently poor health. Subsequent research not only tends to confirm that Parsons' replacement rate measure overstates the effects of economic variables, but also points to the likelihood that his mortality measure understates the impact of poor health (1, 21, 70, 96).

The more likely reason for variations in measured health effects is the fact that a variety of different health variables have been employed in estimating labor supply equations. These differences are clearly nontrivial, but precise estimates of their magnitude are not easily quantified, because of differences in the health scales themselves and because of variations in model specification. A few studies, however, have attempted to gauge the effects of incorporating different health measures in comparable regression models (1, 9, 21, 34). One of these studies (34) estimates otherwise identical models of the labor market behavior of various gender and race subgroups of older persons with either a work-limiting health (disability) report or a summary index of physical/mental impairments as the relevant health variable. The results show that the measured health effect on the probability of being in the labor force, and the direct and indirect effects on annual hours worked for those in the labor force, is between one-quarter and one-third lower for men and one-quarter and almost one-half less for women when the impairment measure is compared with the disability report. Bound's (21) recent study suggests that the differential effects of using disability, self-rated health, or mortality measures in a labor force participation model are perhaps even an order of magnitude greater still. Whatever the true effect of health status on labor market status, these comparison studies predict that the measured effect is higher when disability and self-rated health indexes are used and lower when impairment, functional limitations, or mortality experience indexes are used. Generally speaking, that prediction is borne out in the first-generation literature.

Several recent studies attempt to account for variations in measured health effects by examining the extent to which self-reported poor health may be misrepresented by survey respondents in order to rationalize labor market choices decided on other grounds (1, 9, 18, 21, 26, 104). At one level, Butler et al (26) infer from a (tetrachoric) correlation analysis of survey responses of individuals with arthritis that self-reported symptoms of the disease differ significantly by the respondent's work status. This inference, however, hinges on several strong assumptions that the investigators cannot test directly with the data at hand. At another level, studies have been carried out to appraise the potential bias in using work-limiting health reports by comparing longitudinally the date of these reports and the date at which market work ceased.

To illustrate, Bazzoli (9) examined the effects of reported work limitations before retirement and those reported immediately after retirement on the marginal probability of retiring, and then interpreted discrepancies as the source of potential measurement error. Because she finds a statistically significant effect of the post-retirement disability report, but fails to find a significant effect on the pre-retirement report, she concludes that the importance of health is overstated in early retirement studies. Boaz & Muller (18) dispute this finding. Using a similar strategy, they investigate not only retirement, but death and medical care utilization, of those reporting work-limiting health problems at different time points. Not unlike earlier studies (6, 67), they find significant differences in mortality experience of men who report health limitations after retirement; they also find significantly different medical care utilization patterns. Boaz & Muller thus conclude that early retirees are, indeed, in poorer health and that the use of work limitation reports does not exaggerate the impact of health on work withdrawal. But, it is unclear that such pre- and post-retirement comparisons provide a decisive test of potential measurement error in self-reported health indexes. One reason is that the investigators have no independent way of controlling for the physical/mental conditions of survey respondents at the time they actually left the labor force. A more compelling reason is that the assumption that the health limitation measures in these analyses are simply an exogenous variable has been seriously questioned in second-generation studies.

Second-Generation Results

Although recent articles have tended to attribute variations in measured health effects to the impact of using self-reported versus objective measures of health, what is really at issue is the degree to which there are choice elements, especially economic choices, in health status evaluation. Some disability specialists worry that this formulation casts individuals with impaired health who withdraw from the work force as malingerers (113, 114). Yet, only the most extreme version of the medical model can account for work disablement without any reference to economic choice mechanisms. Similarly, only an extreme version of the economic model of labor supply that assumes completely unchanging preferences over the course of the life cycle can account for work withdrawals induced by the onset of disease, functional limitations, or other decrements to physical and mental capacities by economic motivations alone. The second-generation literature now taking shape maneuvers between these two extreme views by treating economic and health decision-making as being interrelated or jointly determined. Second-generation research is characterized by efforts, typically in a multi-equation framework, to explain the determinants of self-appraised health levels and labor market behavior simultaneously.

Impetus for this line of research stems in part from another study by Parsons (89) that uses a multi-equation model to test first the likelihood that an individual is out of the labor force, and then that the declaration of health status (disability report) varies systematically with this probability of nonparticipation. He finds a significant effect of (predicted) nonparticipation on self-reported work limitations and interprets this as the misrepresentation of true health status attributable to economic motivations. There are, however, other ways to interpret this finding. One way is simply to acknowledge the tautological character of responses to work-limiting health questions in labor force participation equations (64, 68; also see 107). The other is to revise the implied sequence or direction of causality. In contrast to Parsons' supposition that individuals decide first whether to participate in the work force and then report a health status rationalizing that choice, individuals might first judge the seriousness and burden of their health impairments and then formulate a strategy for modifying their work activities that accommodates those judgments. Earnings and other economic benefits of market work may compensate for the added burden of chronic conditions, so persons with higher potential market income may be more likely to sustain work when in poor health than individuals with lower opportunity costs. Responses to work-limiting health questions may gauge ex post the willingness of persons with health problems to cut back their market work, based on an interrelated appraisal of their economic circumstances and the burden that their health conditions place on work effort. On this interpretation, work-limiting health reports can be treated as endogenous variables in disability models (Equation 2a) that include both economic and impairment variables as predictors (31, 34, 69, 110). Models of this sort should be expected to show that work-limited (disabled) persons have lower opportunity costs than the nondisabled, controlling for the level of impairment, job requirements, and other work determinants. One study (34) tested this hypothesis rigorously and provided compelling evidence in its favor.

The advantages of treating reported health status as an endogenous variable in a multi-equation framework have been recognized for some time (51, 75). Recent analyses draw on both self-reported work disability or self-rated health status and use relatively sophisticated statistical techniques to test the joint determination of health and labor market status (1, 21, 25, 78, 81, 98, 101). Space limitations preclude a description of these studies, but several interesting characteristics may be briefly noted. First, although some analyses model the reciprocal effects of health and work activity itself (Equations 1 and 2), most focus on the joint determination of health and work effort in response to economic and other common determinants (Equations 1 and 2a). In this latter category, some studies specify equations for health status and for labor market participation, by estimating them separately (recursively) in sequential fashion; in others, the equations are jointly estimated, e.g. by using the predicted values of one outcome from an estimating equation that includes all of the exogenous variables in the model as a predictor variable in the estimating equation of the other dependent variable.

Many of these studies find that economic choice factors play a crucial role in determining health levels. Sickles & Taubman (98) show that changes in Social Security benefits and eligibility for transfer income affects both self-rated healthiness and withdrawal from the work force. Burtless (25) finds that occupational factors, sociodemographic characteristics, and economic incentives affect self-rated health status, which in turn determines work effort. His analysis also suggests that economic sectors in which health risks are greater are more likely to develop institutional arrangements (pension and disability insurance programs) that facilitate earlier retirement, i.e. health factors shift economic inducements, which then lead to higher probabilities of labor market withdrawal. Although these studies are quite promising, data constraints in terms of disease prevalence and the underlying presence of functional impairments force them to treat health status as a black box. When new population surveys fill these data gaps, the application of these second-generation models should yield considerably more fruit.

If choice elements of the health-work relationship are important, they should be evident not only in decisions to withdraw from market work, but also in the duration of work disability episodes. Drawing on longitudinal data and new techniques for modeling survival functions that overcome problems of incomplete spells and sample losses (right-side censoring), several studies have examined the durations of periods of sustained work activity and, correspondingly, of disability episodes. Chirikos & Nestel (38, 39) model the capacity for continuing work and the length of work disability spells by means of a competing risks model of retirement, disability, and death. They show that older men generally have the health capacity to continue working for several years beyond the current normal retirement age, and those who do not are not necessarily concentrated in physically demanding jobs. They also show that disability episodes have finite durations, the lengths of which are mediated by various health and economic determinants. Equivalent studies focusing on populations of disabled beneficiaries find similar effects (44, 60, 66). These analyses also suggest that the demand for workers with impaired health generally, and the impacts of employer discrimination and accommodation in particular, play critical roles in reducing the length of time these workers remain out of the labor market (41, 50, 65, 115). Given the provisions of the recently enacted ADA, the willingness of employers to facilitate the continuing employment of chronically impaired individuals is an especially crucial aspect (24).

CONCLUSIONS

In their pioneering book on participation in the American labor force, Bowen & Finegan (23, 62) observed that "the labor force status of an individual will be affected by his health is an unassailable proposition [because] a priori reasoning and casual observation tell us it must be so, not because there is a mass of supporting evidence." In the quarter-century since this observation was made, a large literature has grown up aimed at providing just such supporting evidence. As the preceding review of that literature shows, there is now unambiguous empirical proof of Bowen & Finegan's main contention that health affects work effort. However, this literature leaves the magnitude of the health effect, either absolutely or relative to other determinants of work behavior, still very much in doubt. Consequently, major issues of public sector policy that hinge on the measured impact of poor health have not yet been resolved very well; moreover, estimates of morbidity losses in cost-of-illness studies are probably quite imprecise. On both grounds, additional research is called for.

To begin with, the conceptual framework for health status measurement must be refined and built into new data collection efforts. The bundle of health capacities that influence the ability to perform market work must be distinguished from the bundle that affect the preferences for market work. More detailed data on measurable pathology, residual impairment, and medical/vocational rehabilitation coupled to the physical and mental capabilities needed to perform particular job assignments must be available to model work ability; more penetrating probes of the economic circumstances of the households of health-impaired individuals and the temporal sequence of work-related decisions after the onset of a chronic condition are needed to model health-constrained work preferences. Better data of this sort may eliminate two pitfalls: One is the absence of strictly comparable empirical evidence in this literature and, thereby, cumulative additions to the knowledge base. Too many studies have been discrete (albeit often ingenious) efforts that introduce a health proxy variable into the analysis without any serious consideration of how health status is expected to shape labor market activity or why. The other pitfall has been the essentially nonproductive debate about whether preferences and financial incentives play any role in health-related decision making. There is convincing evidence that they do; but this neither implies that impaired individuals who withdraw from market work are malingerers nor guarantees that pension and disability benefits can be cut back without imposing serious hardships on current program recipients because of their poor health. More disaggregate data may improve our ability to gauge the costs of health-induced reductions in market work and, correspondingly, the benefits attributable to interventions that reduce the likelihood of such episodes.

New research should pay more attention to health differences across the mix of sociodemographic groups in the work force, the future occupational composition of employment, and the role of employer demand in accommodating impaired workers. More is known at the moment about older white men than about any other group, and much of this knowledge is bounded by the structural features of the economy in the 1970s and early 1980s. The growing proportion of the adult female population that is working, the rapid growth in the number of younger workers with sufficiently impaired health conditions to qualify for disability insurance benefits, and the growing fraction of total employment in the service sector argues for revising research priorities. Stratified analyses of health effects on the demand for, and supply of, these groups should be accorded especially high priority. Stratified analyses of the labor market effects of specific diseases are also needed, although the long list of diseases that can be potentially studied and the significant interaction effects attributable to comorbidities argue for according this strategy lower priority. The need to cut across demographic, socioeconomic, and disease groupings implies that requisite labor supply data must be generated from general population surveys. To be sure, surveys of special population groups will continue to provide valuable data, including the start up of a new National Institute on Aging-funded longitudinal study of retirement and health that will draw a nationally representative sample of older individuals. Yet, these special data collection efforts will fail to provide much insight about health and work in other relevant population subgroups. Regularly administered population surveys, such as the National Health Interview Survey and the Current Population Survey, should be asked to provide more relevant data for research in this area.

ACKNOWLEDGMENTS

With the usual disclaimers, I thank Gilbert Nestel for valuable comments on a preliminary draft of the paper and Linda Chirikos for help with the bibliography.

Literature Cited

1. Anderson, K., Burkhauser, R. V. 1985. The retirement-health nexus: a new measure of an old puzzle. *J. Human Resour*. 20:315–30
2. Andrews, R. A., Ruther, M., Baugh, D. K., Pine, P. L., Rymer, M. P. 1988. Medicaid expenditures for the disabled under a work incentive program. *Health Care Financ. Rev*. 9(3):1–8
3. Andrisani, P. J. 1977. Effects of health problems on the work experience of middle-aged men. *Ind. Gerontol*. Spring:97–111
4. Angel, R. 1984. The costs of disability for hispanic males. *Soc. Sci. Q* 65(2): 426–43
5. Baily, M. N. 1987. Aging and the ability to work: policy issues and recent trends. In *Work, Health, and Income Among the Elderly,* ed. G. Burtless, pp. 59–102. Washington, DC: Brookings Inst.
6. Baker, D., Packard, M., Rader, A. D., Reno, V., Upp, M. 1982. Mortality and early retirement. *Soc. Secur. Bull*. 45(12):3–10
7. Bartel, A., Taubman, P. 1979. Health and labor market success: the role of various diseases. *Rev. Econ. Stat*. 61(1):1–8
8. Bartel, A., Taubman, P. 1986. Some economic and demographic consequences of mental illness. *J. Labor Econ*. 4(2):243–56
9. Bazzoli, G. J. 1985. The early retirement decision: new empirical evidence on the influence of health. *J. Human Resour*. 20(2):214–34
10. Benham, L., Benham, A. 1982. Employment, earnings, and psychiatric diagnosis. In *Economic Aspects of Health,* ed. V. R. Fuchs, pp. 203–20. Chicago: Univ. Chicago Press.
11. Berger, M. C. 1982. Family allocation of time: the effects of health on labor supply. *Atlantic Econ. J*. 10(4):14–24
12. Berger, M. C., Leigh, J. P. 1988. The effect of alcohol use on wages. *Appl. Econ*. 20:1343–51
13. Berkowitz, M. 1978. The search for a health variable. In *Policy Analysis with Social Security Research Files,* pp. 411–32. Washington, DC: HEW Publ. no.(SSA)79–11808
14. Berkowitz, M. 1981. Disincentives and the rehabilitation of disabled persons. In *Annu. Rev. Rehab.,* ed. E. Pan, T. Backer, C. Lash, 2:40–57. New York: Springer
15. Berkowitz, M., Fenn, P., Lambrinos, J. 1983. The optimal stock of health with endogenous wages. *J. Health Econ*. 2(2):139–47
16. Berkowitz, M., Johnson, W. G. 1974. Health and labor force participation. *J. Human Resour*. 9:117–28
17. Better, S. R., Fine, P. R., Simison, D., Doss, G. H., Walls, R. T., et al. 1979. Disability benefits as disincentives to rehabilitation. *Milbank Mem. Fund Q./Health Soc*. 57(3):412–27
18. Boaz, R. F., Muller, C. F. 1990. The validity of health limitations as a reason for deciding to retire. *Health Serv. Res*. 25(2):361–86
19. Bound, J. 1989. The health and earnings of rejected disability insurance applicants. *Am. Econ. Rev*. 79(3):482–503
20. Bound, J. 1991. The health and earnings of rejected disability insurance applicants: reply. *Am. Econ. Rev*. 81(5):1427–34
21. Bound, J. 1991. Self-reported versus objective measures of health in retire-

ment models. *J. Human Resour.* 26(1): 106–38

22. Bound, J, Waidmann, T. 1990. Disability transfers and the labor force attachment of older men: evidence from the historical record. *NBER Working Paper No. 3437*. Cambridge, Mass: Nat. Bur. Econ. Res. 56 pp.
23. Bowen, W., Finegan, T. 1969. *The Economics of Labor Force Participation*. Princeton, NJ: Princeton Univ. Press
24. Burkhauser, R. V., Kim, Y. W. 1991. *The Importance of Employer Accommodation on the Job Duration of Disabled Workers: A Hazard Model Approach*. Working paper. Syracuse Univ. 35 pp.
25. Burtless, G. 1987. Occupational effects on the health and work capacity of older men. See Ref. 5, pp. 103–50
26. Butler, J. S., Burkhauser, R. V., Mitchell, J. M., Pincus, T. P. 1987. Measurement error in self-reported health variables. *Rev. Econ. Stat.* 69(4):644–50
27. Bye, B. V., Riley, G. F. 1989. Eliminating the Medicare waiting period for Social Security disabled-worker beneficiaries. *Soc. Secur. Bull.* 52(May)2–15
28. Chirikos, T. N. 1986. Accounting for the historical rise in work-disability prevalence. *Milbank Q.* 64(2):271–301
29. Chirikos, T. N. 1989. Aggregate economic losses from disability in the United States: a preliminary assay. *Milbank Q.* 67(Suppl. 2, Pt. 1):59–91
30. Chirikos, T. N. 1991. The economics of employment. *Milbank Q. Suppl. The Americans With Disabilities Act* 69(1/2):150–79
31. Chirikos, T. N., Nestel, G. 1981. Impairment and labor market outcomes: a cross sectional and longitudinal analysis. In *Work and Retirement: A Longitudinal Study of Men*, ed. H. S. Parnes, pp. 93–131. Cambridge, Mass: MIT Press
32. Chirikos, T. N., Nestel, G. 1982. The economic consequences of poor health, by race and sex. *Proc. Am. Stat. Assoc. Soc. Stat. Sect.*, pp. 473–78
33. Chirikos, T. N., Nestel, G. 1983. Economic consequences of poor health in mature women. In *Unplanned Careers: the Working Lives of Middle-Aged Women*, ed. L. Shaw, pp. 93–108. Lexington, Mass: Lexington Books
34. Chirikos, T. N., Nestel, G. 1984. Economic determinants and consequences of self-reported work disability. *J. Health Econ.* 3:117–36
35. Chirikos, T. N., Nestel, G. 1985. Further evidence on the economic effects of poor health. *Rev. Econ. Stat.* 67(1):61–9
36. Chirikos, T. N., Nestel, G. 1985. Longitudinal analysis of functional disabilities in older men. *J. Gerontol.* 40(4):426–33
37. Chirikos, T. N., Nestel, G. 1988. Work capacity of older men and age-eligibility for Medicare benefits. *Med. Care* 26(9):867–81
38. Chirikos, T. N., Nestel, G. 1989. Occupation, impaired health and the functional capacity of men to continue working. *Res. Aging* 11(2):174–205
39. Chirikos, T. N., Nestel, G. 1991. Occupational differences in the ability of men to delay retirement. *J. Human Resour.* 26(1):1–26
40. Chirikos, T. N., Nickel, J. L. 1984. Work disability from coronary heart disease in women. *Women Health* 9(1): 55–74
41. Craft, J. A., Benecki, T. J., Shkop, Y. M. 1980. Who hires the seriously handicapped? *Ind. Relat.* 19(1):94–9
42. Dean, D. H., Milberg, W. 1988. Using better measures of disability status. In *Measuring the Efficiency of Public Programs*, ed. M. Berkowitz, pp. 199–231. Philadelphia: Temple Univ. Press
43. Diamond, P. A., Hausman, J. A. 1984. The retirement and unemployment behavior of older men. In *Retirement and Economic Behavior*, ed. H. Aaron, G. Burtless, pp. 97–134. Washington, DC: Brookings Inst.
44. Dykacz, J., Hennessey, J. 1989. Postrecovery experience of disabled-worker beneficiaries. *Soc. Secur. Bull.* 9(Sept.):42–66
45. Elesh, D., Lefcowitz, M. J. 1977. The effects of health on the supply of and returns to labor. In *The New Jersey Income-Maintenance Experiment: Vol. 2. Labor Supply Responses*, ed. H. W. Watts, A. Rees, pp. 289–319. New York: Academic
46. Feldman, J. J. 1983. Work ability of the aged under conditions of improving mortality. *Milbank Mem. Fund Q./Health Soc.* 61(3):430–44
47. Fechter, A. 1978. Health conditions and earnings capacity: a human captial model. See Ref. 13, pp. 385–410
48. Fuchs, V. R. 1982. Time preference and health: an exploratory study. See Ref. 10, pp. 93–120
49. Gordon, R. H., Blinder, A. S. 1980. Market wages, reservation wages, and retirement decisions. *J. Public Econ.* 14(2):277–308

50. Greenwald, H. P., Dirks, S. J., Borgatta, E. F., McCorkle, R., Nevitt, M. C., et al. 1989. Work disability among cancer patients. *Soc. Sci. Med.* 29(11):1253 59
51. Grossman, M., Benham, L. 1974. Health, hours and wages. In *The Economics of Health and Medical Care,* ed. M. Perlman, pp. 205–33. New York: Halsted
52. Gustman, A. L., Steinmeier, T. L. 1986. A disaggregated, structural analysis of retirement by race, difficulty of work and health. *Rev. Econ. Stat.* 68(3):509–13
53. Hanoch, G., Honig, M. 1983. Retirement, wages, and labor supply of the elderly. *J. Labor Econ.* 1(2):131–51
54. Hardy, M. A. 1982. Job characteristics and health: differential impact on benefit entitlement. *Res. Aging* 44:457–78
55. Hausman, J. A., Wise, D. A. 1985. Social security, health status, and retirement. In *Pensions, Labor, and Individual Choice,* ed. D. A. Wise, pp. 159–91. Chicago: Univ. Chicago Press
56. Haveman, R. H., Wolfe, B. L. 1984. The decline in male labor force participation: comment. *J. Polit. Econ.* 92(3):532–41
57. Haveman, R., Wolfe, B., Buron, L., Hill, S. 1992. *Productivity Losses from Health/Disability in the United States from 1973 to 1983: An Earnings Capacity Approach.* Presented to Annu. Meet. Am. Econ. Assoc., New Orleans. 36 pp.
58. Haveman, R. H., Wolfe, B. L., Warlick, J. L. 1984. Disability transfers, early retirement, and retrenchment. See Ref. 43, pp. 65–96
59. Haveman, R. H., Wolfe, B. L., Warlick, J. L. 1988. Labor market behavior of older men, estimates from a trichotomous choice model. *J. Public. Econ.* 36:153–75
60. Hennessey, J., Dykacz, J. 1989. Projected outcomes and length of time in the disability insurance program. *Soc. Secur. Bull.* 52(Sept.):2–41
61. Hurd, M. D. 1990. The joint retirement decision of husbands and wives. In *Issues in the Economics of Aging,* ed. D. A. Wise, pp. 231–58. Chicago: Univ. Chicago Press
62. Inman, R. P. 1987. The economic consequences of debilitating illness: the case of multiple sclerosis. *Rev. Econ. Stat.* 69(4):651–60
63. Ireland, L. M. 1972. Retirement history study: introduction. *Soc. Secur. Bull.* 35(Nov.):3–8
64. Johnson, W. G. 1977. The effect of disability on labor supply, comment. *Ind. Labor Relat. Rev.* 30(3):380–81
65. Johnson, W. G., Lambrinos, J. 1985. Wage discrimination against handicapped men and women. *J. Human Resour.* 20(2):264–77
66. Johnson, W. G., Ondrich, J. 1990. The duration of post-injury absences from work. *Rev. Econ. Stat.* 72:578–86
67. Kingson, E. R. 1982. The health of very early retirees. *Soc. Secur. Bull.* 45(9):3–9
68. Lambrinos, J. 1981. Health: a source of bias in labor supply models. *Rev. Econ. Stat.* 63(2):206–12
69. Leigh, J. P. 1985. An empirical analysis of self-reported, work-limiting disability. *Med. Care* 23(4):310–19
70. Leonard, J. S. 1986. Labor supply incentives and disincentives for disabled persons. In *Disability and the Labor Market,* ed. M. Berkowitz, M. A. Hill, pp. 64–94. Ithaca, NY: ILR Press
71. Levy, J., McManus, L. 1978. Functional limitations and job requirements: effects on labor force choices. See Ref. 13, pp. 447–60
72. Luft, H. S. 1975. The impact of poor health on earnings. *Rev. Econ. Stat.* 57(1):43–57
73. Lumsdaine, R. L., Wise, D. A. 1990. Aging and labor force participation: a review of trends and explanations. *NBER Working Paper No. 3420*. Cambridge, Mass: Nat. Bur. Econ. Res. 69 pp.
74. MacKenzie, E. J., Shapiro, S., Smith, R. T., Siegel, J. H., Moody, M., et al. 1987. Factors influencing return to work following hospitalization for traumatic injury. *Am. J. Public Health* 77(3):329–34
75. Menefee, J. A. 1980. The demand for health and retirement. In *Retirement Policy in an Aging Society,* ed. R. L. Clark, pp. 18–51. Durham, NC: Duke Univ. Press
76. Minkler, M. 1981. Research on the health effects of retirement: an uncertain legacy. *J. Health Soc. Behav.* 22(June): 117–30
77. Mitchell, J. M. 1991. Work behavior after the onset of arthritis. *Med. Care* 29(4):362–76
78. Mitchell, J. M., Anderson, K. H. 1989. Mental health and the labor force participation of older workers. *Inquiry* 26(Summer):262–71
79. Mitchell, J. M., Burkhauser, R. V. 1990. Disentangling the effect of arthritis on earnings: a simultaneous estimate of wage rates and hours worked. *Appl. Econ.* 22:1291–1309

80. Mitchell, J. M., Butler, J. S. 1986. Arthritis and the earnings of men: an analysis incorporating selection bias. *J. Health Econ.* 5(1):81–98
81. Mullahy, J., Sindelar, J. 1989. Life-cycle effects of alcoholism on education, earnings, and occupation. *Inquiry* 26:272–82
82. Murt, H. A., Parsons, P. E., Harlan, W. R., Thomas, J. W., Lepkowski, J. M., et al. 1986. Disability, utilization and costs associated with musculoskeletal conditions, United States, 1980. *Nat. Med. Care Utilization and Expenditure Survey, Ser. C, No. 5.* Washington, DC: NCHS
83. Myers, R. J. 1982. Why do people retire from work early? *Soc. Secur. Bull.* 45(9):10–14
84. Nagi, S. 1976. An epidemiology of disability among adults in the United States. *Milbank Mem. Fund Q./Health Soc.* 54(4):739–67
85. Oi, W. Y., Andrews, E. S. 1991. *The ADA in a Labor Market for People with Disabilities.* Presented at Am. Econ. Assoc. Meet., New Orleans, 29 pp.
86. Parnes, H. S. 1975. The national longitudinal surveys: new vistas for labor market research. *Am. Econ. Rev.* 65: 244–49
87. Parsons, D. O. 1977. Health, family structure, and labor supply. *Am. Econ. Rev.* 67(Sept.):703–12
88. Parsons, D. O. 1980. The decline in male labor force participation. *J. Polit. Econ.* 88(1):117–34
89. Parsons, D. O. 1982. The male labour force participation decision: health, reported health, and economic incentives. *Economica* 49:81–91
90. Parsons, D. O. 1984. Disability insurance and male labor force participation: a response to Haveman and Wolfe. *J. Polit. Econ.* 92(3):542–49
91. Parsons, D. O. 1991. The health and earnings of rejected disability insurance applicants, comment. *Am. Econ. Rev.* 81(5):1419–26
92. Parsons, D. O. 1991. Self-screening in targeted public transfer programs. *J. Polit. Economy* 99(4):859–76
93. Passmore, D. L., Ay, U., Rockel, S., Wade, B., Wise, J. 1983. Health and youth employment. *Appl. Econ.* 15: 715–29
94. Quinn, J. 1977. Microeconomic determinants of early retirement: a cross-sectional view of white married men. *J. Human Resour.* 12(3):329–46
95. Salkever, D. S. 1984. *Morbidity Costs: National Estimates and Economic Determinants.* Final rep. submitted to the US Nat. Cent. Health Serv. Res. Washington, DC: Nat. Tech. Inf. Serv.
96. Sammartino, F. J. 1987. The effect of health on retirement. *Soc. Secur. Bull.* 50(2):31–47
97. Scheffler, R. M., Iden, G. 1974. The effect of disability on labor supply. *Ind. Labor Relat. Rev.* 28(Oct.):122–32
98. Sickles, R. C., Taubman, P. 1986. An analysis of the health and retirement status of the elderly. *Econometrica* 54(6):1339–56
99. Slade, F. P. 1984. Older men: disability insurance and the incentive to work. *Ind. Relat.* 23(2):260–69
100. Soc. Sec. Adm. 1986. Increasing the Social Security retirement age: older workers in physically demanding occupations or ill health. *Soc. Sec. Bull.* 49:5–23
101. Stern, S. 1989. Measuring the effect of disability on labor force participation. *J. Human Resour.* 24(3):361–95
102. Syme, S. L., Berkman, L. F. 1976. Social class, susceptibility and sickness. *Am. J. Epidemiol.* 104(1):1–8
103. Verbrugge, L. M. 1989. Recent, present, and future health of American adults. *Annu. Rev. Public Health* 10: 333–61
104. Waldron, I., Herold, J., Dunn, D. 1982. How valid are self-report measures for evaluating relationships between women's health and labor force participation? *Women Health* 7(2):53–66
105. Weaver, C. L. 1991. *Disability and Work: Incentives, Rights, and Opportunities,* ed. C. L. Weaver. Washington, DC: AEI Press
106. Wen, C. P., Tsai, S. P., Gibson, R. L. 1983. Anatomy of the healthy worker effect: a critical review. *J. Occup. Med.* 25(4):283–88
107. Wilson, R. W., Drury, T. F. 1981. Factors affecting the use of limitation of activity as a health status measure. In *Silver Anniversary of the National Health Survey Act,* pp. 9–14. Hyattsville, Md: Nat. Cent. Health Stat.
108. Wilson, R. W., Drury, T. F. 1984. Interpreting trends in illness and disability: health statistics and health status. *Annu. Rev. Public Health* 5: 83–106
109. Wolfe, B. L. 1984. Measuring disability and health (editorial). *J. Health Econ.* 3:187–93
110. Wolfe, B. L., Haveman, R. 1990. Trends in the prevalence of work disability from 1962 to 1984, and their correlates. *Milbank Q.* 68(1):53–80
111. Wolfe, J. R. 1983. Perceived longevity

and early retirement. *Rev. Econ. Stat.* 65:544–51

112. Wolfe, J. R. 1985. A model of declining health and retirement. *J. Polit. Econ.* 93(6):1258–67
113. Yelin, E. H. 1986. The myth of malingering: why individuals withdraw from work in the presence of illness. *Milbank Q.* 64(4):622–49
114. Yelin, E. H. 1989. Displaced concern: the social context of the work-disability problem. *Milbank Q.* 67 (Suppl. 2, Pt. 1):114–65
115. Yelin, E. H., Greenblatt, R. M., Hollander, H., McMaster, J. R. 1991. The impact of HIV-related illness on employment. *Am. J. Public Health* 81(1):79–84

Annu. Rev. Publ. Health. 1993. 14:313–33

EMERGENCY MEDICAL SERVICES AND SUDDEN CARDIAC ARREST: The "Chain of Survival" Concept

Richard O. Cummins
Department of Medicine, University of Washington, Seattle, Washington 98195

KEY WORDS: sudden cardiac death, emergency medicine

OVERVIEW

This article reviews the problem of out-of-hospital cardiac arrest and decribes the structure and processes of the emergency medical services (EMS) systems that treat cardiac arrest outside the hospital. People are more likely to survive out-of-hospital cardiac arrest when the following sequence of events occurs as rapidly as possible: recognition of early warning signs, activation of the emergency medical system, basic cardiopulmonary resuscitation (CPR), defibrillation, intubation, and intravenous medications. The descriptive device of a "chain of survival" communicates this understanding usefully (33). Although separate specialized programs are necessary to develop strength in each link, all of the links must be interconnected. Weakness in any link lessens the chances of survival and condemns a community to poor results. The chain of survival concept has been confirmed by several decades of research about sudden cardiac arrest. This research has identified effective system interventions that will increase the number of neurologically intact survivors. Although a few urban systems may have approached the current practical limit for survivability from sudden cardiac arrest, most EMS systems, both in the United States and in other countries, operate with defects in their EMS chain and with poor resuscitation rates.

The Problem of Unexpected Out-of-Hospital Cardiac Arrest

Out-of-hospital cardiac arrest is an important public health problem for several reasons. First, ischemic heart disease is the leading cause of death in the

0163-7525/93/0510-0313$02.00

United States and in all major developed nations. In the United States, an estimated 1.6 million persons each year have a heart attack because of coronary artery disease; 600,000 of them die. For men and women aged 40–69, the mortality rate is 320 per 100,000 and 90 per 100,000, respectively. Heart attack deaths comprise 55% of the 1 million deaths from cardiovascular disease. Other causes include stroke (16%), hypertensive disease (3%), rheumatic heart disease (1%), and other cardiovascular diseases (26%) (2). In 1989, an estimated 350,000–400,000 of the 600,000 persons who died prematurely from acute heart attack died out-of-hospital. More out-of-hospital deaths from cardiac arrest due to ischemic heart disease occur than from all causes of cancer (450,000–500,000 per year). Among persons over age 65, an estimated 1.1 million have clinically recognized coronary heart disease; yet, more than 250,000 persons die each year from acute heart attack, 150,000 of whom die out-of-hospital (37).

Second, the expense of ischemic heart disease is enormous (2). The total estimated economic cost of cardiovascular diseases is $85 billion: physician and nursing services, $13 billion; hospital and nursing home services, $53 billion; medications, $6 billion; lost output due to disability, $14 billion; lost output due to death, $38–57 billion.

Third, unexpected out-of-hospital cardiac arrest is an important public health problem because the current "standard treatment" is both expensive and futile. Most communities in the United States have created some form of EMS system (6, 12, 33, 57). Virtually every urban area has paramedic care, and most rural areas are serviced by emergency medical technicians (57). The US Department of Transportation guidelines dictate that in a given EMS system, emergency care should be provided within ten minutes for over 90% of the EMS responses. By this definition, over 90% of the US population is now considered "served" by an EMS system. The standard of care in the United States dictates that a resuscitative effort be made for persons with sudden cardiac arrest once the EMS system is called (6). Although exact figures are not available, at least 90% of the 350,000–400,000 persons who die from sudden cardiac arrest are thought to be treated by their local EMS system. Unfortunately, only 3–5% of persons on whom an out-of-hospital resuscitation is attempted live to be discharged from the hospital. One can argue, therefore, that 95–97 times out of 100, the resuscitation efforts are wasted. These figures come close to what some experts define as a "futile" medical intervention that should be abandoned (93).

The Structure and Process of Emergency Cardiac Care

Patient outcomes from unexpected cardiac arrest depend on the process of care, primarily the time intervals from collapse to delivery of four major EMS interventions: CPR, defibrillation, intubation, and intravenous medications.

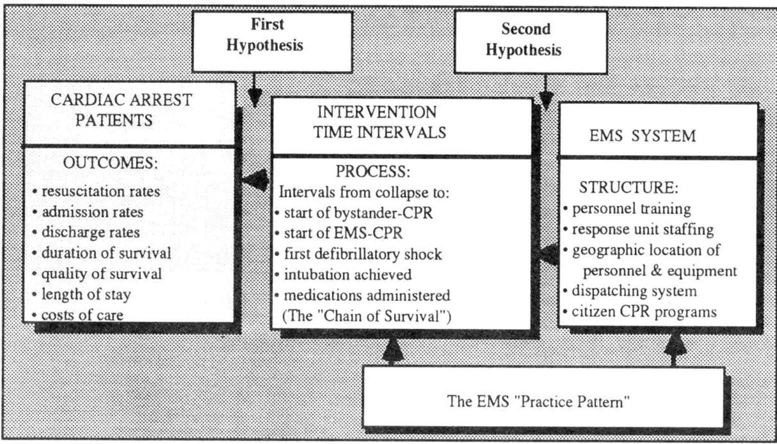

Figure 1 How patient outcomes depend on the process of care, primarily the time intervals from collapse to delivery of care (first hypothesis). Time intervals, in turn, are associated with the structure of the EMS system (second hypothesis). This structure and process comprises the EMS "practice pattern" related to sudden cardiac arrest.

These intervention time intervals, in turn, are associated with the structure of the EMS system, which consists primarily of personnel and equipment and their respective locations. This overview is best conceptualized in Figure 1.

THE PRACTICE PATTERN OF EMS SYSTEMS AND THE IMPORTANCE OF TIME From the perspective of individual patients, the treatment of cardiac arrest involves the rapid initiation of basic CPR, electrical defibrillation, endotracheal intubation, and intravenous medications (37, 40). Timing is critically important. One widely accepted hypothesis in emergency cardiac care is that patient outcomes are determined by the speed with which the four major interventions are delivered by the EMS system (18, 20, 33, 37, 40, 78, 90, 97, 107).

The magnitude of the contribution of timing, however, once adjusted for other factors, as well as the relative contribution of each of the interventions, remains unclear. The key intervention time intervals are determined by the structure of the EMS system. EMS practice patterns can best be understood in terms of the ways they are structured to deliver the four major interventions.

Personnel training In regard to cardiac arrest, the key to understanding EMS structure is that different types of personnel have different levels of skills and authorization to provide each of the different interventions. This leads to numerous structural mixes. Paramedics are the most familiar emergency

Table 1 How different levels of EMS personnel are distinquished by the interventions that they are trained and permitted to perform

	CPR	Defibrillation	Intubation	Start IVs	Give medicines
First responder	yes	no	no	no	no
First responder-D	yes	yes	no	no	no
EMTS	yes	no	no	maybe	no
EMT-Ds	yes	yes	maybe	maybe	no
Paramedics	yes	yes	yes	maybe	maybe

personnel. In general, they receive 1200–2000 hours of training. They can deliver the three main interventions of Advanced Cardiac Life Support (ACLS): endotracheal intubation, intravenous medications, and defibrillation. Emergency medical technicians (EMTs) are emergency personnel who have received 110 hours of training in a certification-granting curriculum. They always can deliver the intervention of CPR and, in some locations, defibrillation. Extra training in defibrillation requires 4–12 hours. Some systems use emergency personnel known as first responders, who have received 40–50 hours of training in a certification-granting curriculum. Although they always can perform CPR, they may or may not be trained and equipped to defibrillate and they never administer medications.

The structural picture is more complicated, however, because many variations in these personnel definitions exist. Some paramedics, for example, may be allowed to start an intravenous infusion, but are not allowed to administer medications. This is also true for some EMTs. Some systems limit the number of defibrillations or medications that can be administered. Some systems train EMTs to use advanced airway techniques similar to endotracheal intubation, but they are not permitted to defibrillate or administer medications. The most significant variation, however, is whether the first responding personnel, either EMTs or first responders, are allowed to defibrillate. Table 1, a personnel/intervention matrix, displays some of this structural complexity.

Response unit staffing and geographic location of personnel and equipment
In the United States, 60% of the EMS services are combined with fire-fighting services. This means an EMS response comes from a fire station in either a specific medical response vehicle (ambulance) or a fire-fighting vehicle (fire truck). These vehicles are staffed by cross-training fire fighters who have the skills of first responders or EMTs. As noted above, they may or may not be trained to defibrillate. Other EMS systems may have ambulances respond from hospitals or from free-standing base stations (quarters) devoted solely to emergency medical services. Again, these personnel may range from first

responders to paramedics. In King County, Washington, for example, EMTs trained to defibrillate respond from 56 different fire department stations. Two-person paramedic response teams respond from nine different paramedic stations. Because the geographic area covered is constant, the paramedic response intervals average longer than the more densely located EMT-Ds. the time intervals, therefore, to EMS-CPR and first defibrillatory shock are generally shorter than the time intervals to intubation and intravenous medications, because only paramedics can perform intubation and start intravenous lines.

An obvious variation on this two-tiered pattern, however, has been to place paramedics in each individual fire station. Thus, a person skilled in all three interventions (defibrillation, intubation, and intravenous medications) would respond as part of the first tier from the 56 different fire stations. An additional variation is that one-paramedic response teams are used, as opposed to the more traditional two-paramedic teams. Again, these one-paramedic/one-EMT response teams can be either widely disbursed geographically in separate fire stations, or located in a few specific paramedic locations. Finally, personnel who are trained to a specific skill level and then geographically dispersed to minimize response intervals may not be equipped in a manner consistent with their skills. For example, paramedics who are placed in stations that do not have an Advanced Life Support (ALS) vehicle, lack the advanced equipment (defibrillators, intubation kit) to apply their advanced skills.

THE CHAIN OF SURVIVAL METAPHOR The chain of survival metaphor captures the complexity of EMS structure (33, 79, 80). The concept is straightforward: An EMS system must be organized with multiple divisions; each division requires separate attention; and weaknesses in any one link will

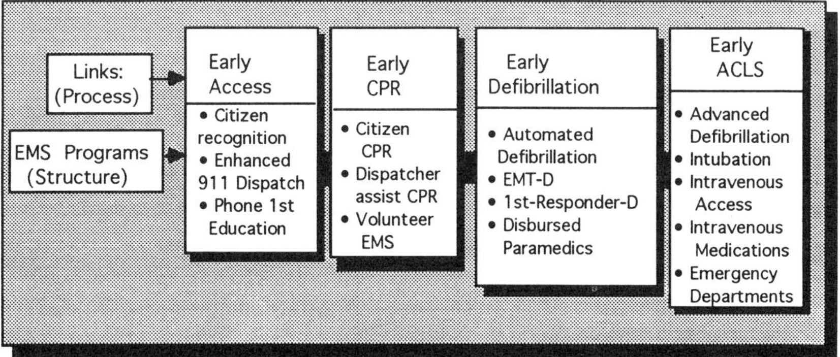

Figure 2 The "chain of survival. Separate EMS program components (structure) are required to produce strong links (process) in the chain.

condemn a system to poorer survival rates. Figure 2 summarizes these interactions among the elements of the chain of survival and EMS structure.

THE LINKS IN THE CHAIN OF SURVIVAL

The Early Access Link

Early access begins the chain of survival and gets trained help to the patient as quickly as possible. To start the resuscitation chain, someone must recognize a medical emergency and gain access to and activate the emergency medical system. Time is required to recognize the emergency, decide to make the call, and locate the telephone and the proper number. Then, the dispatcher must interrogate the caller and decide to send the emergency vehicles. Dispatchers may require additional time to route the call to the proper response station or vehicle. Ambulance response time is the interval from receipt of the call by the emergency dispatcher to arrival of the unit at the scene by the emergency personnel. Additional time may be required after arrival at the scene before responders actually make contact with the patient. Recognition, call processing, and ambulance response time add seconds, usually minutes, to that critical interval between the arrest and the initiation of emergency treatment.

The most common approach to shorten this interval between collapse and arrival of emergency personnel has been to add more ambulances. However, this is expensive and inefficient. Studies have demonstrated that, after a certain point, an increase in the number of ambulances fails to decrease response time significantly (54, 55). In one model, response time varied inversely as the square root of the number of vehicles per square miles; an 80% increase in the number of vehicles reduced average response time only by one minute (54). This same one-minute reduction in average response time could be achieved by greater public awareness and more efficient dispatching systems, and at far less cost.

Strength can be gained in the early access link by education of the public, specifically those individuals most likely to witness a cardiac arrest, and by installation of an efficient emergency communication system. Educational and public service programs, such as those developed by the American Heart Association (AHA) (72) and the American Red Cross (4), attempt to inform the public of what to do in the event of a cardiac arrest. In CPR classes and in AHA-sponsored schoolsite and worksite training, people learn to recognize the warning signs of a heart attack and a person in cardiac arrest, and to quickly call the EMS system whenever a person collapses. Persons uninformed about chest pain and respiratory distress may fail to comprehend the signs of an impending cardiac arrest. When a person collapses, such witnesses may take an excessively long time to call the emergency dispatch center. Witnesses may call neighbors, relatives, or even their local doctor before calling the emergency dispatch number.

Lack of a three-digit "911" (or its equivalent in other countries) emergency dispatch system can produce confusion and delays because witnesses call the wrong number or multiple numbers, or spend time searching for the number. In one community in North Carolina, the telephone book lists 85 different emergency numbers (56, 57). In contrast, in Seattle, Washington, which has an enhanced 911 system, 90% of 1271 persons interviewed could identify 911 as their EMS notification number (67). Investigators from Minneapolis performed a before-and-after evaluation of implementation of a 911 emergency number system (68). They noted that the percentage of emergency callers who could activate the EMS system in less than one minute went from 63% before to 82% after the system was implemented. The percentage of callers who needed only one telephone call to activate the system went from 40% before the 911 system was started to 74% after the system began. Another study demonstrated that imprecise knowledge of how to notify the emergency system can cause confusion and delays (42). Persons living in 911 communities knew the correct number to call 85% of the time; persons residing in regional systems in which several fire districts operate under one dispatching center knew the correct number to call only 47% of the time; and in systems where a local seven-digit number for a particular fire district must be called, only 36% of the people could give the correct number. Many persons who lived adjacent to a 911 area thought 911 was their emergency number; when they mistakenly called 911, delays of 30 seconds to two minutes resulted. Given the transient and mobile nature of today's populations, a standard, universal access number must be adopted.

The Early CPR Link

The next link in the chain of survival is for people at the scene of the cardiac arrest to start basic CPR immediately (25, 72). This action should occur immediately after witnesses recognize a cardiac arrest, and simultaneously with their efforts to gain access to and activate the EMS system. EMS systems must depend on citizens, rather than emergency responders, to initiate CPR. Otherwise, the CPR is simply started too late.

For almost three decades, the chest compressions and positive pressure ventilations of standard CPR have helped return pulseless, nonbreathing patients to a state of spontaneous respiration and cardiac perfusion (62, 92).

The current perspective on the value of early CPR is that it buys time for the primary cardiac arrest patient (10, 25, 31, 62, 71, 72, 91, 92) by producing enough low blood flow to the central nervous system and the myocardium to maintain temporary viability. To make this contribution to survival, however, basic CPR must be started early, and the earlier the better. This initial CPR must be followed quickly by defibrillation, intubation, and cardiovascular medications. If the emergency personnel who carry the defibrillator arrive late, at about 8–12 minutes after the person's collapse, then early bystander CPR is less effective in preventing death (38). Recent data from the Belgian Cardiopulmonary-Cerebral Resuscitation Registry suggest some prolonged benefit from bystander-CPR, even with late arrival of advanced life support personnel (10, 11). The combination of late CPR (more than four minutes) and late advanced life support (more than 12 minutes) is particularly lethal and has been referred to as the resuscitation "failure zone" (74).

Many reports provide data to compare the survival rates of cardiac arrest victims who receive "early" CPR (defined here as CPR initiated by citizens or bystanders) with the survival rates of those who receive "late" CPR (that CPR initiated by emergency responders) (22, 25, 27, 38, 46, 52, 53, 64, 66, 89, 90, 95, 97, 101–103, 112). "Early" usually differs from "late" CPR by about four minutes. In all but one system, comparisons between early and late CPR reveal a positive benefit of early CPR. The magnitude of this contribution may be considerable, and odds ratios for improved survival with early CPR can range as high as 11.5.

The association between early CPR and improved survival is related to the presence of ventricular fibrillation (VF) (10, 27, 59, 106). Researchers have observed that when CPR is started early, victims are more likely to be in VF when a monitoring unit arrives at the patient's side (106). In a study from King County, Washington, 80% of cardiac arrest victims were in VF/VT (ventricular tachycardia) if they had received early bystander CPR, compared with 68% if they had received delayed CPR (27). In Stockholm, Sweden, 67% of persons in cardiac arrest who had CPR started by bystanders were in VF/VT, whereas only 45% of persons without bystander CPR were in VF/VT (59). The Belgian Cardiopulmonary-Cerebral Resuscitation Registry has reported a 42% prevalence of VF in cardiac arrest patients who received bystander-CPR, compared with 29% in arrest patients who received delayed CPR (10). These three studies suggest that CPR prolongs the duration of VF and that the presence of VF should be considered a dependent, rather than an independent, variable in analyses of survival data. In addition, victims who receive early CPR are more likely after electrical shock to convert to a cardiac rhythm associated with restoration of spontaneous circulation (27, 87). In King County, Washington, persons who were in VF at the time of EMS arrival had a 37% rate of long-term survival if they had received bystander CPR, compared with 29% if they had not (statistically significant, $P<0.05$) (27). In Houston, 40% of the patients with VF/VT survived to discharge if they had received bystander CPR, versus 19% for VF/VT patient without bystander CPR (87).

There are several approaches to insure that basic CPR is performed by a bystander before the emergency responders arrive. The most widely advocated is citizen CPR training. Endorsed and conducted by the AHA and the American Red Cross, such programs have trained millions of laypersons in CPR (71). The AHA has suggested that a 20% prevalence of CPR training among adults might significantly reduce morbidity and mortality from out-of-hospital cardiac arrest (94). Some communities have achieved this level of adult training, despite physician reluctance to "prescribe" CPR training for the family members and friends of high risk patients (48, 67, 96). In the Seattle area, for example, Leonard Cobb and coworkers have trained more than 2 million people (19). In Minneapolis, a survey of 2310 adults noted that 23% had been trained in CPR (77).

There are problems, however, with the concept that a threshold level of citizen training can be "protective." The Minneapolis survey observed that despite having an estimated 23% of the population trained in CPR, only 10% of these trained adults had ever witnessed a cardiac arrest (77). At only 30% of cardiac arrests was a CPR-trained witness present. Of the persons trained in Minneapolis, just 19% maintained certification by retraining every year; similarly, only 21% of trainees in Los Angeles returned for their one-year recertification (50). In Seattle and King County, data suggest that some knowledge of CPR techniques is so prevalent that many citizens attempt to perform CPR even without formal training (43), and despite a high prevalence of disagreeable physical characteristics (saliva, blood, emesis) encountered during the performance of bystander CPR (69). Cobb has observed that the outcome for CPR performed by these untrained citizens is similar to the outcomes for trained laypersons (18, 19).

Another approach to achieve early CPR is "targeted CPR" training (18, 19, 49, 67, 77, 84, 85). Targeted CPR programs teach CPR to middle-aged people, residents and staff of senior centers, survivors of a myocardial infarction, and the family members of persons who have been identified as having cardiac arrest risk factors. These programs are slowly becoming more widespread and represent an important change in the focus of CPR training. Much CPR training in the United States focuses on the young, especially school-age children and young adults. These people are easy to train and they show energetic interest. They are not, however, the group most likely to witness a cardiac arrest. Cardiac arrest victims are typically aging men who live at home (10, 65, 105) and are usuallly nonprofessional and poorly educated (63). In one location, the average age of persons who experience cardiac arrest is 65. Of this group, 75% are men, and 77% of the cardic arrests happen at home (37, 65). Therefore, the individuals with the highest likelihood of witnessing a cardiac arrest and being called upon to perform CPR are those persons living with or closely associated with middle-aged men. There is an excellent prognosis even for the elderly (over age 70) resuscitated from cardiac arrest (9, 91). Unfortunately, few middle-aged women in the United States have received formal CPR training (67, 68).

A final method to achieve early CPR is "dispatcher-assisted" CPR instruction. This refers to programs in which emergency telephone dispatchers offer CPR instructions to people at the time they call to report a cardiac arrest (13, 17, 43, 60). Panicked bystanders can be focused by the dispatchers and encouraged to perform CPR when they "draw a blank" at the sudden sight of a cyanotic and breathless loved one.

The Early Defibrillation Link

The purpose of early defibrillation is to reestablish a normal spontaneous rhythm in the heart. There are several new approaches to help achieve early defibrillation: automated defibrillators used by the first responding emergency personnel; automated defibrillators used by "community" responders, i.e. people whose usual occupation or training would not require responding to emergencies; and "home defibrillation" programs for high risk patients.

The rationale for early defibrillation emerges from data that demonstrate that almost 85% of persons with ambulatory, out-of-hospital, primary cardiac arrest experience ventricular tachyarrhythmias during the early minutes after their collapse (36). In one report, 157 ambulatory (not hospitalized) patients experienced fatal arrhythmias while continuous cardiac monitoring was in place (36). The very first initial dysrhythmia in 62% was ventricular tachycardia that evolved to VF. Although this study involved a select population of patients who had some indication for ambulatory cardiac monitoring, the rhythms they experienced are probably representative of the usual initial rhythms of the sudden cardiac arrest victim.

Prehospital studies, in which the rhythm of arrest cannot be identified until the emergency personnel arrive with a defibrillator/monitor four to eight minutes later, have observed the percentage of persons in ventricular tachyarrhythmias to be 60% or less (44, 87). Nearly all eventual survivors emerge from the group of people who remain in VF when emergency personnel arrive. For example, in King County, Washington, over 92% of the cardiac arrest survivors are from this group (44), as are over 80% in Houston, Texas (87).

In England, where general practitioners are the most frequent responders to patients with chest pain and cardiac arrest, early defibrillation alone has produced successful resuscitations (21). Many patients in Britain call for their general practitioner during the early stages of a myocardial infarction, and some studies have noted that about 5% of these patients experience a cardiac arrest after the arrival of the general practitioner (83, 88). The British Heart Foundation donated 78 defibrillators to 25 general practices and reported on the experiences after one year (21). A total of 19 patients suffered cardiac arrest in the vicinity of a general practitioner with a defibrillator: 13 (68%) of these people were in VF; nine were successfully resuscitated outside the hospitals; and six were discharged alive (21).

Research in the early 1980s demonstrated the ability of personnel less well-trained than paramedics, namely EMTs, to use defibrillators successfully (39, 41, 99, 108). Implementation of early defibrillation programs for other levels of personnel, such as firefighters and minimally trained first responders, spread slowly. This was, however, more often because of implementation barriers and administrative inertia than from any doubt of clinical efficacy (24, 111).

The proposals to allow less well-trained emergency personnel to operate defibrillators initially attracted controversy, but most concerns have disappeared. Conceptually, early defibrillation programs represented the transfer of what was a medical act—diagnosis of the rhythm and operation of a defibrillator—into the hands of nonphysicians. Although this transfer of skills to paramedics had been accepted for years, authorities in many locations hesitated to extend acceptance to emergency personnel with less training than paramedics. Rational reasons for this hesitancy vanished by the late 1980s, however, with the widespread acceptance of the principle of early defibrillation and the successful development of the new technology of automated external defibrillators (23, 29).

The principle of early defibrillation holds that the professional rescuer who arrives first at the scene of a cardiac arrest should carry and be trained to operate a defibrillator. With few exceptions, the defibrillator used should be an automated external defibrillator (24, 26, 28–30, 86, 98, 107). Automated external defibrillators perform with high accuracy (5, 28, 35, 98, 109) and eliminate the need to train the operator in the complex skills of rhythm recognition. Their simplicity of operation decreases the time and expense of initial training and continuing education and markedly expands the range of people who can operate the devices. Clinical studies also show that systems using automated defibrillators can deliver the first shock up to one minute faster than with conventional defibrillators (28, 98).

With each passing year, more communities in the United States have allowed the use of both automated and conventional defibrillators by EMTs and even first responders. Although the term "first responders" refers specifically to individuals who have completed an official 40-hour course, it can refer generically to a large group of public safety employees, such as firefighters, ambulance personnel, part-time emergency volunteers, members of police forces, highway patrol personnel, security guards, and crew members of public transportation vehicles. Programs that permit first responder (usually firefighter) defibrillation, have been started in many locations (75, 76, 80, 81). The International Association of Fire Chiefs has now endorsed this concept for its members and has started an initiative called "RapidZap." RapidZap plans to equip all fire department emergency response vehicles with automated defibrillators by the year 2000 (75, 76, 80, 81).

Just how effective are programs to give defibrillators to EMTs and first responders? Clinical studies have thus far observed variable degrees of success. The published survival rates for systems whose prehospital response teams consist only of EMTs trained to defibrillate range from 6% to 26% for patients in VF (41, 44, 47, 51, 59, 104). The most important comparison, however, is between the survival rate in communities before and after they instituted an early defibrillation program. In suburban communities in King County, Washington, for example, the survival rate for patients in VF increased from 7% to 26% (41). Similarly, in communities in Iowa, it increased from 3% to 19% (99). In southeastern Minnesota, the survival rate was 4% without EMT-defibrillation and 17% with such a program (104), whereas in northeastern Minnesota, the survival rate was 2.5% without and 10% with EMT-defibrillation (7). When an early defibrillation program was started in certain communities in Wisconsin, the survival rate rose from 3.6% to 6.4% for all cardiac arrests and was 11% for patients initially noted to be in VF (82). These initial improvements in survival rates should be maintained and increased as experience and competency continue to improve over time.

Two other techniques that have been advocated as training approaches to help achieve early defibrillation are home defibrillation programs for high-risk patients and early defibrillation programs for community responders, such as public safety workers, security personnel, stadia ushers, and other laypersons who may have a perceived duty to respond to an emergency. Although these approaches have been under evaluation for several years, their specific effects on community-wide survival rates from cardiac arrest have not been determined (58). Moore et al (73) observed that of 95 VF survivors, only 63 (66%) were eligible for placement of a home defibrillator, and only 38 of 47 (81%) persons approached agreed to participate. This suggests that approximately half (.66 × .81) of VF survivors would receive the device and appropriate training. McDaniel et al (70) experienced recruitment problems in a similar home defibrillation study, in which only 8% of survivors of acute myocardial infarction participated in their study. The reasons for such low participation in both of these projects included the following: Patients lived alone or outside the study area, they had no telephone, or they had religious objections. Physicians considered resuscitation medically inappropriate, discharged the patient to a nursing home, implanted automatic internal defibrillators, or eliminated the patient from the study (70, 73).

Nevertheless, enough experience has accumulated to establish the feasibility of training family members of high-risk patients and community responders to use automated defibrillators (14, 15, 34, 45, 70, 73). Despite some decline in skill retention and performance, family members and lay responders can remember most of their training and retain the skill for up to one year. They can also apply and operate the device at that dramatic moment of the cardiac arrest of a family member or coworkers (34, 45).

So far, clinical experience to demonstrate the practicality and effectiveness of these home and community responder defibrillation programs has been limited. In a case series of 30 patients with witnessed cardiac arrest in which laypersons used automated defibrillators before the arrival of trained emergency personnel, eight of 15 patients were resuscitated to an organized rhythm associated with spontaneous circulation, and five were discharged from the hospital (14). In a series of 48 high-risk patients whose family members were trained to operate automated defibrillators, five cardiac arrests occurred, the automated defibrillator was used four times, and three patients had successful restoration of circulation (100).

Researchers from King County, Washington, however, have experienced less positive results with home (45) and community responder defibrillation (34). Eisenberg et al (45) placed automated defibrillators in the homes of 59 people who had survived prehospital cardiac arrest. Ten cardiac arrests occurred in this group; the device was used in six. Only two patients were in VF; one of them was resuscitated, but survived only a few months with residual neurological deficits. In another King County study, 14 automated defibrillators were placed in a variety of community settings, and 146 laypersons working in those settings were trained to operate the device (34). Only three cardiac arrests occurred in these settings; recognition and operating errors prevented proper attachment and use of the defibrillator in each of these patients. However, simpler, lighter, and more sophisticated automated defibrillators, with more user-friendly protocols and simpler electrode pad placement, have recently been developed. Better results may be achieved with currently available devices.

Better results have already been achieved in other studies of community responder placement of automated defibrillators. At the 1986 World's Exposition in Vancouver, British Columbia, 160 security personnel were trained to operate an automated defibrillator in the event of a cardiac arrest (110). Five cardiac arrests occurred among Expo's 22.1 million visitors. An automated external defibrillator was attached to each of these victims. Two were in VF, and both were successfully shocked and returned to a spontaneous circulation. Both of these patients were moving and semiconscious by the time emergency personnel arrived. In England, automated external defibrillators have been placed on long-distance aircraft of one international air carrier (16). This pilot study had to cease when the air carrier was purchased by another company, but the training had been accepted with full enthusiasm by the senior cabin attendants. High-risk or isolated industrial settings represent another interesting target group for implementation of early defibrillation programs. Automated defibrillators have, for example, been placed and used successfully by safety personnel at oil platforms in the North Sea, at electricity plants, and onboard passenger boats (1990, personal communications).

The Early Advanced Cardiac Life Support Link

In many instances, CPR and defibrillation alone do not achieve or sustain resuscitation. The unique interventions of the early ACLS link—endotracheal intubation and intravenous medications—are necessary to improve the chances of survival further. In the United States, ACLS for prehospital cardiac arrest is generally provided by paramedics (6). These individuals receive 1000–3000 hours of classroom training and field instruction, and generally can provide intubation, defibrillation, and intravenous medications.

In other locations, ACLS is provided by either nurses or emergency physicians (referred to as "ambulance doctors"). They respond in specially equipped vehicles, known as "doctor-manned ambulances." In the United States, however, such programs were abandoned years ago, because physician-staffed ambulances were considered to be an inefficient use of physician resources and paramedics could perform the same functions with comparable effectiveness (6). Physician-staffed ambulances in Europe, however, may well be more cost-effective than they are in the United States, depending on relative operating costs, professional salaries, the population density, and combinations with air-rescue services. In Norway, for example, nine combined doctor ambulances with helicopters are popular and respond to about 4500 patients a year in a population service area of 4 million people.

Although defibrillation has classically been considered part of ACLS care, early defibrillation has now achieved such importance that it stands by itself as a separate link in the chain of survival. EMTs and other early responders now share this skill with paramedics, physicians, and nurses. Still, in view of the sequential nature of ACLS therapy during a resuscitation attempt, it is difficult to separate precisely the value of defibrillation from other interventions, such as intubation and intravenous medications, which have usually been almost simultaneously performed.

Although early defibrillation alone achieves a considerable portion of all survivors, intubation and intravenous medications are also important. These interventions are thought to not only promote the return of a spontaneous rhythm and circulation, but also stabilize and maintain patients during the immediate post-resuscitation period.

THE MAXIMUM PRACTICAL SURVIVAL RATE?

We do not know the number of people who have been resuscitated from sudden cardiac death. Nor do we know how many people, with a reasonable chance of intact neurologic survival, can be resuscitated. One could argue that the highest survival rates currently reported for out-of-hospital cardiac arrest are a reasonable target for all locations. Although achievement of such survival rates is not practical in every community, this approach does expose the gap between what a community does achieve and what is achieved elsewhere. The highest published rates come from sophisticated urban/suburban systems in communities like King County, Washington (37), and Seattle (107). Their EMS systems can be termed "mature." Over the past 10–15 years, these locations established strong links in the chain of survival. The annual survival rates for King County from 1976 through 1987 fluctuate 15–20% for all cardiac arrests and 25–30% for all patients presenting in VF. These overall survival rates, however, have remained moderately stable despite a several system interventions, such as EMT-defibrillation with manual defibrillators (41), EMT-defibrillation with automated defibrillators (28), dispatcher-assisted-CPR (43), and transcutaneous pacing (32). Therefore, this level of VF survival rate may represent the practical limits for prehospital emergency care.

How many people would be saved if all emergency medical systems in the United States approached the hypothesized maximum survival rate of 20%, which occurs in these mature EMS systems? If an estimated 3% survival rate (40) is applied to the presumed annual 400,000 cardiac arrests, approximately 12,000 people per year now survive out-of-hospital cardiac arrest (3). If this population of nontraumatic cardiac arrest patients had a survival rate of 20%, then 80,000 survivors, or an additional 68,000 people, would be saved. The AHA estimates that a full nationwide implementation of all life-saving emergency cardiac care mechanisms in each community may save up to 100,000 lives annually in the United States (72). Without proper implementation of such prehospital care systems, such save rates will not be achieved, as those not resuscitated before hospital arrival rarely survive (8, 61).

SUMMARY

Early access to the EMS system helps insure early CPR, defibrillation, and advanced care. Early access is easiest to achieve with 911 systems and widespread community education and publicity. It may also be taught during citizen-CPR classes. Early CPR helps patients by slowing the process of dying, but its effectiveness disappears within minutes, and defibrillation must soon follow. A citizenry well-informed about cardiac emergencies and well-trained in CPR appears to be the best method to achieve early recognition and early CPR. The earliest possible delivery of defibrillation is critical and, almost by itself, sufficient for many sudden death cases. It has, therefore, emerged as the single most effective intervention for patients in nontraumatic cardiac arrest. Automated external defibrillators help accomplish this goal and now permit widespread implementation of a variety of early defibrillation programs. Early advanced care helps those who do not immediately convert to an organized cardiac activity or who do not achieve a spontaneous circulation following early defibrillation. Advanced care allows a system to approach its highest possible survival rate by respiratory and anti-arrhythmic stabilization and monitoring of patients in the post-resuscitation period.

At present, early CPR and rapid defibrillation, combined with early advanced care, can result in long-term survival rates as high as 30% for witnessed VF. Because neurological and psychological recovery from cardiac arrest are tied to the time within which these critical interdependent treatment modalities are delivered (1, 87), high resuscitation rates will also lead to a high percentage of patients who recover to their pre-arrest neurologic level.

The public health challenge is to develop programs that will allow recognition, access, bystander-CPR, defibrillation, and advanced care to be delivered as quickly as possible, ideally within moments of the collapse of a sudden death victim. Achievement of such a goal requires the deployment of multiple properly directed programs within an EMS system; each program lends strength to the chain of survival, thereby enhancing successful recovery and long-term survival.

What benefits would occur if a majority of EMS systems in the United States could establish cost-effective programs with respectable survival rates? The AHA estimates that full implementation of potential life-saving mechanisms in the community may save 10,000–100,000 lives each year in the US (2). If the maximum survival rate for all nontraumatic cardiac arrests in mature EMS systems is about 20% (33) among the annual 400,000 out-of-hospital cardiac arrests, 80,000 persons would be saved (33). It is difficult to envision other public health measures that have the potential to save so many lives. There is a mistaken impression by the general public that EMS systems are highly effective in resuscitation of out-of-hospital cardiac arrest victims. This is clearly not the case. Implementation of the things we already know work, combined with innovative research, should help this field of medicine live up to community expectations.

Literature Cited

1. Abramson, N., Safar, P., Detre, K., Group BIS. 1989. Factors influencing neurologic recovery after cardiac arrest. *Ann. Emerg. Med.* 18:477–78 (abstr.)
2. Am. Heart Assoc. 1989. *Heart and Stroke Facts,* p. 44. Dallas: Am. Heart Assoc. 1990 ed.
3. Am. Heart Assoc. 1986. *1987 Heart Facts,* p. 31. Dallas: Am. Heart Assoc.
4. Anon. 1987. *American Red Cross: Adult CPR.* Boston: Am. Nat. Red Cross
5. Atkins, J., Streigler, H., Burstain, T., Foster, G. 1989. Improved survival rates with automatic defibrillators. *Prehosp. Disat. Med.* 1:69(abstr.)
6. Atkins, J. M. 1986. Emergency medical service systems in acute cardiac care: state of the art. *Circulation* 74:iv-4
7. Bachman, J. W., McDonald, G. S., O'Brien, P. C. 1986. A study of out-of-hospital cardiac arrests in Northeastern Minnesota. *J. Am. Med. Assoc.* 256:477–83
8. Bonnin, M., Pepe, P. E. 1990. Key role of prehospital resuscitation in survival from out-of-hospital cardiac arrest. *Ann. Emerg. Med.* 19:466(abstr.)
9. Bonnin, M., Pepe, P., Clack, P. 1989. Survival prognosis for the elderly after out-of-hospital cardiac arrest. *Ann. Emerg. Med.* 18:469(abstr.)
10. Bossaert, L., Vanhoeyweghen, R., Group CRS. 1989. Bystanders Cardiopulmonary Resuscitation (CPR) in out-of-hospital cardiac arrest. *Resuscitation* 17(Suppl.):S55–S69
11. Bossaert, L., Vanhoeyweghen, R., Group CRS. 1989. Evaluation of cardiopulmonary resuscitation techniques. *Resuscitation* 17:S99–S109
12. Braun, O., McCallion, R., Fazackerley, J. 1990. Characteristics of midsized urban EMS systems. *Ann. Emerg. Med.* 19:536–46
13. Carter, W. B., Eisenberg, M. S., Hallstrom, A. P., Schaeffer, S. 1984. Development and implementation of emergency CPR instructions via telephone. Part 1. *Ann. Emerg. Med.* 13: 695–700
14. Chadda, K., Kammerer, R., Kuphal, J., Miller, K. 1987. Successful defibrillation in the industrial, recreational and corporate settings by laypersons. *Circulation* 76:iv-12(abstr.)
15. Chadda, K. D., Kammerer, R. 1987. Early experiences with the portable automatic external defibrillator in the home and public places. *Am. J. Cardiol.* 60:732–33
16. Chapman, P. J. C., Chamberlain, D. 1987. Death in the clouds. *Br. Med. J.* 294:181
17. Clawson, J. J. 1989. Emergency medical dispatching. In *Principles of EMS Systems: A Comprehensive Text for Physicians,* ed. W. R. Roush, R. D. Aranosian, T. M. H. Blair, K. A. Handal, R. D. Kellow, R. D. Stewart, Dallas: Am. Coll. Emerg. Physicians
18. Cobb, L. A., Hallstrom, A. P. 1982. Community-based cardiopulmonary resuscitation: what have we learned? *Ann. NY Acad. Sci.* 382:330–42
19. Cobb, L. A., Hallstrom, A. P., Thompson, R. G., Mandel, L. P. 1980. Community cardiopulmonary resuscitation. *Annu. Rev. Med.* 31:453–62
20. Cobb, L. A., Werner, J. A., Trobaugh, G. B. 1980. Sudden cardiac death: I. A decade's experience with out-of-hospital resuscitation. *Mod. Concepts. Cardiovasc. Dis.* 49:31–36
21. Colquhoun, M. 1988. Use of defibrillators by general practitioners. *Br. Med. J.* 297:336–37
22. Copley, D. P., John, A. M., Rogers, W. J., Russell, R. O. J. 1977. Improved outcome for prehospital cardiopulmonary collapse with resuscitation by bystanders. *Circulation* 56:901–5
23. Cummins, R. O. 1989. From concept to standard-of-care? Review of the clinical experience with automated external defibrillators. *Ann. Emerg. Med.* 18: 1269–75
24. Cummins, R. O. 1987. EMT defibrillation: national guidelines for implementation. *Am. J. Emerg. Med.* 5(3): 254–57
25. Cummins, R. O., Eisenberg, M. S. 1985. Prehospital cardiopulmonary resuscitation: is it effective? *J. Am. Med. Assoc.* 253:2408–12
26. Cummins, R. O., Eisenberg, M. S., Bergner, L., Hallstrom, A. P., Hearne, T., Murray, J. A. 1984. Automatic external defibrillation: evaluation of its role in the home and in emergency medical services. Part 1. *Ann. Emerg. Med.* 13(9):789–801
27. Cummins, R. O., Eisenberg, M. S., Hallstrom, A. P., Litwin, P. E. 1985. Survival of out-of-hospital cardiac arrest with early initiation of cardiopulmonary resuscitation. *Am. J. Emerg. Med.* 3:114–18
28. Cummins, R. O., Eisenberg, M. S.,

Litwin, P. E., Graves, J. R., Hearne, T. R., Hallstrom, A. P. 1987. Automatic external defibrillators used by emergency medical technicians. A controlled clinical trial. *J. Am. Med. Assoc.* 257(12):1605–10

29. Cummins, R. O., Eisenberg, M. S., Moore, J. D., Hearne, T. R., Andresen, E., et al. 1985. Automatic external defibrillators: clinical, training, psychological and public health issues. *Ann. Emerg. Med.* 14(8):755–60
30. Cummins, R. O., Eisenberg, M. S., Stultz, K. R. 1986. Automatic external defibrillators: clinical issues for cardiology. *Circulation* 73:381
31. Cummins, R. O., Graves, J. 1989. Clinical results of standard CPR: prehospital and inhospital. In *Clinics in Critical Care Medicine: Cardiopulmonary Resuscitation,* ed. W. Kaye, N. Bircher, pp. 87–102. New York: Churchill-Livingstone
32. Cummins, R. O., Graves J. 1989. Prehospital transcutaneous pacing by paramedics and emergency medical technicians: clinical and system effectiveness. *Prehosp. Disast. Med.* 4(2): 196
33. Cummins, R. O., Ornato, J. P., Thies, W., Pepe, P., et al. 1991. Improving survival from cardiac arrest: the chain of survival concept. *Circulation* 83: 1832–47
34. Cummins, R. O., Schubach, J. A., Litwin, P. E., Hearne, T. R. 1989. Training lay persons to use automatic external defibrillators: success of initial training and one-year retention of skills. *Am. J. Emerg. Med.* 7:143–49
35. Cummins, R. O., Stults, K, R., Haggar, B., Kerber, R. E., Schaeffer, S., Brown, D. D. 1988. A new rhythm library for testing automatic external defibrillators: performance of three devices. *J. Am. Coll. Cardiol.* 11:597–602
36. de Luna, A. B., Coumel, P., Leclercq, J. F. 1989. Ambulatory sudden cardiac death: mechanism of production of fatal arrhythmia on the basis of data from 157 cases. *Am. Heart J.* 117:151–59
37. Eisenberg, M. S. 1984. Who shall live? Who shall die? In *Sudden Cardiac Death in the Community,* ed. M. S. Eisenberg, L. Bergner, H. P. Hallstrom, pp. 44–58. Philadelphia: Praeger Sci. 44–58
38. Eisenberg, M. S., Bergner, L., Hallstrom, A. 1979. Paramedic programs and out-of-hospital cardiac arrest: I. Factors associated with successful resuscitation. *Am. J. Public Health* 69:30–38
39. Eisenberg, M. S., Bergner, L., Hallstrom, A. 1980. Out-of-hospital cardiac arrest: improved survival with paramedic services. Lancet 8172:812–15
40. Eisenberg, M. S., Bergner, L., Hallstrom, A. P., Cummins, R. O. 1986. Sudden cardiac death. *Sci. Am.* 254:37–43
41. Eisenberg, M. S., Copass, M. K., Hallstorm, A. P., Blake, B., Bergner, L., et al. 1980. Treatment of out-of-hospital cardiac arrest with rapid defibrillation by emergency medical technicians. *N. Engl. J. Med.* 302: 1379–83
42. Eisenberg, M. S., Hallstrom, A., Becker, L. 1981. Community awareness of emergency phone numbers. *Am. J. Public Health* 71:1058–60
43. Eisenberg, M. S., Hallstrom, A. P., Carter, W. B., Cummins, R. O., Bergner, L., Pierce, J. 1985. Emergency CPR via telephone. *Am. J. Public Health* 75:47–50
44. Eisenberg, M. S., Hallstrom, A. P., Copass, M. K., Bergner, L., Short, F., Pierce, J. 1984. Treatment of ventricular fibrillation: emergency medical technician defibrillation and paramedic services. *J. Am. Med. Assoc.* 251(13):1723–26
45. Eisenberg, M. S., Moore, J., Cummins, R. O., Andresen, E., Litwin, P. E., et al. 1989. Use of the automatic external defibrillator in home of survivors of out-of-hospital ventricular fibrillation. *Am. J. Cardiol.* 63:443–46
46. Eitel, D. R., Walton, S. L., Guerci, A. D., Hess, D. R., Sabulsky, N. K. 1988. Out-of-hospital cardiac arrest: a six-year experience in a suburban-rural system. *Ann. Emerg. Med.* 17:808–12
47. Gentile, D., Auerbach, P., Gaffron, J., Foon, G., Phillips, J. 1988. Prehospital defibrillation by emergency medical technicians: results of a pilot study in Tennessee. *J. Tenn. Med. Assoc.* 999:144–48
48. Goldberg, R. J. 1987. Physicians and CPR training in high risk family members. *Am. J. Public Health* 77: 671–72
49. Goldberg, R. J., Gore, J. M., Love, D. G., et al. 1984. Layperson CPR: are we training the right people? *Ann. Emerg. Med.* 13:701–4
50. Gombeski, W., Effron, D., Ramirez, A., Moore, T. 1982. Impact on retention: comparison of two CPR training

programs. *Am. J. Public Health* 72: 849–52
51. Gray, A. J., Redmond, A. D., Martin, M. A. 1987. Use of the automatic external defibrillator-pacemaker by ambulance personnel: the Stockport experience. *Br. Med. J.* 294:1133–35
52. Gudjonsson, H., Baldvinsson, E., Oddsson, G., Asgeirsson, E. 1982. Results of attempted cardiopulmonary resuscitation of patients dying suddenly outside the hospital in Reykjavik and the surrounding area, 1976–1979. *Acta Med. Scand.*212:247–51
53. Guzy, P. M., Pearce, M. L., Greenfield, S. 1983. The survival benefit of bystander cardiopulmonary resuscitation in a paramedic-served metropolitan area. *Am. J. Public Health* 73:766–69
54. Hallstrom, A. P. 1984. Improving the EMS system. See Red. 37, pp. 126–39
55. Hallstrom, A. P., Eisenberg, M. S., Bergner, L. 1984. The potential use of automatic defibrillators in the home for management of cardiac arrest. *Med. Care* 22(12):1083–87
56. Hunt, R. C., Allison, E. J., Yates, J. G. 1986. The need for improved emergency medical servies in Pitt County. *NC Med. J.* 47:39–42
57. Hunt, R. C., McCabe, J. B., Hamilton, G. C., Krohmer, J. R. 1989. Influence of emergency medical services systems and prehospital defibrillation on survival of sudden cardiac death victims. *Am. J. Emerg. Med.* 7:68–82
58. Jacobs, L. 1986. Medical, legal and social implications of automatic external defibrillators. *Ann. Emerg. Med.* 15: 863–64
59. Jakobsson, J., Nyquist, O., Rehnqvist, N. 1987. Cardiac arrest in Stockholm with special reference to the ambulance organization. *Acta Med. Scand.* 222: 117–22
60. Kellerman, A. L., Hackman, B. B., Somes, G. 1989. Dispatcher-assisted cardiopulmonary resuscitation: validation of efficacy. *Circulation* 80:1231–39
61. Kellermann, A. L., Staves, D., Hackman, B. 1988. In-hospital resuscitation following unsuccessful prehospital advanced cardiac life support: "heroic efforts" of an exercise in futility? *Ann. Emerg. Med.* 17:589–94
62. Kouwenhoven, W. B., Jude, J. R., Knickerbocker, G. G. 1960. Closed-chest cardiac massage. *J. Am. Med. Assoc.* 173:1064–67
63. Kraus, J., Borhani, N., Franti, C. 1980. Socioeconomic status, ethnicity and risk of heart disease. *Am. J. Epidemiol.* 111:404–17
64. Lewi, P. J., Mullie, A., Quets, A. 1989. Relevance and significance of pre-CPR conditions in cardio-pulmonary-cerebral resuscitation: a grapic analysis by means of spectramap. *Resuscitation* 17(Suppl.):S35–S44
65. Litwin, P. E., Eisenberg, M. S., Hallstrom, A. P., Cummins, R. O. 1987. Location of cardiac arrest and its effect on survival from cardiac arrest. *Ann. Emerg. Med.* 16:787–91
66. Lund, I., Skulberg, A. 1976. Cardiopulmonary resuscitation by lay people. *Lancet* 2:702–4
67. Mandel, L. P., Cobb, L. A. 1985. CPR training in the community. *Ann. Emerg. Med.* 14:669–71
68. Mayron, R., Long, R. S., Ruiz, E. 1984. The 911 emergency telephone number: impact on emergency medical systems access in a metropolitan area. *Am. J. Emerg. Med.* 2:491–93
69. McCormack, A. P., Damon, S. K., Eisenberg, M. S. 1989. Disagreeable physical characteristics affected bystander CPR. *Ann. Emerg. Med.* 18(3):283–85
70. McDaniel, C. M., Berry, V. A., Haines, D. E., Dimarco, J. 1988. Automatic external defibrillation of patients after myocardial infarction by family members: practical aspects and psychological impact of training. *PACE* 11:2029–34
71. Montgomery, W., et al. 1987. Advanced cardiac life support in perspective. In Jaffe A, ed. *Textbook of Advanced Cardiac Life Support,* ed. A. Jaffe, pp. 1–10. Dallas: Am. Heart Assoc. 2nd ed.
72. Montgomery, W., Donegan, J., McIntyre, K. 1986. Standards and guidelines for cardiopulmonary resuscitation and emergency cardiac care. Part I: Introduction. *J. Am. Med. Assoc.* 255 (21):2905–14
73. Moore, J. E., Eisenberg, M. S., Cummins, R. O., Hallstrom, A., Litwin, P., Carter, W. 1987. Lay Person Use of Automatic External Defibrillation. *Ann. Emerg. Med.* 16(6): 669–72
74. Mullie, A., Vanhoeyweghen, R., Quets, A. 1989. Influence of time intervals on outcome of CPR. *Resuscitation* 17(Suppl.):S23–S33
75. Murphy, D. M. 1987. Rapid defibrillation: fire service to lead the way. *J. Emerg. Med. Serv.* 12:67–71
76. Murphy, D. M. 1989. RapidZap. In

RapidZap: Automatic Defibrillation, ed. J. R. Graves, D. J. Austin, R. O. Cummins. Englewood Cliffs, NJ: Brady Co.

77. Murphy, R. J., Luepker, R. V., Jacobs, D. R., Gillum, R. F., Folsom, A. R., Blackburn, H. 1984. Citizen cardiopulmonary resuscitation training and use in a metropolitan area: the Minnesota Heart survey. *Am. J. Public Health* 74:513–15
78. Myerburg, R. J., Zaman, L., Luceri, R. M. 1985. Clinical characteristics of sudden death: implications for survival. *Cardiovasc. Clin.* 15:107–17
79. Newman, M. 1988. Early access, early CPR and early defibrillation: cry of the 1988 Conference on Citizen CPR. *J. Emerg. Med. Serv.* 13:30–35
80. Newman, M. 1989. Chain of survival concept takes hold. *J. Emerg. Med. Serv.* 14:11–13
81. Newman, M. 1989. Defibrillation shakes the nation: results of the JEMS 1988 National Early Defibrillation Study. *J. Emerg. Med. Serv.* 14:50–59
82. Olson, D. W., Larochelle, J., Fark, D., Milbrath, M., Hendlet, G., Aufderheide, T. 1989. EMT-D: the Wisconsin experience. *Ann. Emerg. Med.* 18:806–11
83. Pai, G., Haites, N., Rawles, J. 1987. One thousand heart attacks in Grampian: the place of cardiopulmonary resuscitation in general practice. *Br. Med. J.* 294:352–54
84. Pane, G., Salness, K. 1987. A survey of participants in a mass CPR training course. *Ann. Emerg. Med.* 16:1112–16
85. Pane, G., Salness, K. 1989. Targeted recruitment of senior citizens and cardiac patients to a mass CPR training course. *Ann. Emerg. Med.* 18:152–54
86. Paris, P. M. 1988. EMT-Defibrillation: a recipe for saving lives. *Am. J. Emerg. Med.* 6:282–87
87. Pepe, P. 1990. Advanced cardiac life support: state of the art. In *Emergency and Intensive Care,* ed. J. Vincent, pp. 565–85. Berlin: Springer-Verlag
88. Rawlins, D. 1981. Study of the management of suspected cardiac infarction by British immediate care doctors. *Br. Med. J.* 282:1677–79
89. Ritter, G., Wolfe, R. A., Goldstein, S., Landis, J. R., Vasu, C. M., Acheson, A. 1985. The effect of bystander CPR on survival of out-of-hospital cardiac arrest victims. *Am. Heart J.* 110: 932–37
90. Roth, R., Stewart, R. D., Rogers, K., Cannon, G. M. 1984. Out-of-hospital cardiac arrest: factors associated with survival. *Ann. Emerg. Med.* 13:237–43
91. Safar, P. 1989. History of cardiopulmonary-cerebral resuscitation. See Ref. 31, pp. 1–54
92. Safar, P., Torrey, C. B., Hopltey, W. J., Wilder, R. J. 1961. Ventilation and circulation with closed-chest cardiac massage in man. *J. Am. Med. Assoc.* 176:574–76
93. Schneiderman, L., Jecker, N., Jonsen, A. 1990. Medical futility: its meaning and ethical implications. *Ann. Int. Med.* 112:949–54
94. Selby, M., Kautz, J., Moore, T., Gombeski, W., Ramirez, A., et al. 1982. Indicators of response to a mass media CPR recruitment campaign. *Am. J. Public Health* 72:1039–42
95. Spaite, D. W., Hanlon, T., Criss, E. A., Valenzuela, T. D., Wright, A. L., et al. 1989. Prehospital cardiac arrest: the impact of witnessed collapse and bystander CPR in an EMS system with short response times. *Prehosp. Disast. Med.* 4(1):69(abstr.)
96. St. Louis, P., Carter, W. B., Eisenberg, M. S. 1982. Prescribing CPR: survey of physicians. *Am. J. Public Health* 72:1158–60
97. Stueven, H., Troiano, P., Thompson, B., Mateer, J. R., Kastenson, E. H. 1986. Bystander/first responder CPR: ten years experience in a paramedic system. *Ann. Emerg. Med.* 15:707–10
98. Stults, K., Brown, D., Kerber, R. 1986. Efficacy of an automated exeternal defibrillator in the management of out-of-hospital cardiac arrest: validations of the diagnostic algorithm and initial experience in a rural environment. *Circulation* 73:701–9
99. Stults, K. R., Brown, D. D., Schug, V. L., Bean, J. A. 1984. Prehospital defibrillation performed by emergency medical technicians in rural communities. *N. Engl. J. Med.* 310:219–23
100. Swenson, R. D., Hill, D. L., Martin, J. S., Wirkus, M., Weaver, W. D. 1987. Automatic external defibrillators used by family members to treat cardiac arrest. *Circulatin* 76:iv–463(abstr.)
101. Thompson, R. G., Hallstrom, A. P., Cobb, L. A. 1979. Bystander-initiated cardiopulmonary resuscitation in the management of ventricular fibrillation. *Ann. Int. Med.* 90:737–40
102. Tweed, W. A., Bristow, G., Donen, N. 1980. Resuscitation from cardiac arrest: assessment of a system providing only basic life support outside of hos-

pital. *Can. Med. Assoc. J.* 122: 297–300

103. Vertesi, L., Wilson, L., Glick, N. 1983. Cardiac arrest: comparison of paramedic and conventional ambulance services. *Can. Med. Assoc. J.* 128:809–13
104. Vukov, L. F., White, R. D., Bachman, J. W., O'Brien, P. C. 1988. New perspetives on rural EMT defibrillation. *Ann. Emerg. Med.* 17:318–21
105. Walters, G., Glucksman, E. 1989. Planning a pre-hospital cardiac resuscitation programme: an analysis of community and system factors in London. *J. R. Coll. Physicians* 23:107–10
106. Weaver, W. D., Cobb, L., Dennis, D., et al. 1985. Amplitude of ventricular waveform and outcome after cardiac arrest. *Ann. Int. Med.* 102:53–55
107. Weaver, W. D., Cobb, L. A., Hallstrom, A. P. 1986. Considerations for impriving survival from out-of-hospital cardiac arrest. *Ann. Emerg. Med.* 15:1181–86
108. Weaver, W. D., Copass, M. K., Cobb, L. A. 1984. Improved neurologic recovery and survival after early defibrillation. *Circulation* 69(5):948–48
109. Weaver, W. D., Hill, D., Fahrenbruch, C. E., Copass, M. K., Martin, J. S., et al. 1988. Use of the automatic external defibrillator in the management of out-of-hospital cardiac arrest. *N. Engl. J. Med.* 319:661–66
110. Weaver, W. D., Sutherland, K., Wirkus, M. J., Bachman, R. 1989. Emergency medical care requirements for large public assemblies and a new strategy for managing cardiac arrest in this setting. *Ann. Emerg. Med.* 18:155–60
111. White, R. D. 1986. EMT-Defibrillation: time for controlled implementation of effective treatment. *AHA Emerg. Cardiac Care Newslett.* 8:1–3
112. Wright, D., James, C., Marsden, A. K., Mackintosh, A. F. 1989. Defibrillation by ambulance staff who have had extended training. *Br. Med. J.* 299:96–97

Annu. Rev. Publ. Health 1993. 14:335–53

NATIONAL HEALTH SYSTEMS THROUGHOUT THE WORLD

Milton I. Roemer
Department of Public Health, University of California, Los Angeles, California 90024

KEY WORDS: health system, market intervention, resource development, management, delivery of service

---

Every country has a national health system, which reflects its history, its economic development, and its dominant political ideology. Because of these diverse circumstances, there are several types of health systems. In this article, we examine the highlights of these systems in both industrialized and developing countries. The type of health system in a country depends on the characteristics of each of the system's component parts.

COMPOSITION OF HEALTH SYSTEMS

Any national health system in a country at any stage of economic development may be analyzed according to five principal component parts: resources, organization, management, economic support, and delivery of services.

The resources of a health system consist of human resources (personnel), facilities (hospitals, health centers, etc.), commodities (drugs, equipment, supplies, etc.), and knowledge. Each of these may be produced or acquired in different ways and to various extents.

Health programs may be organized under diverse sponsorships. In virtually all health systems, there is one principal authority of government (at several levels), other governmental agencies with health functions, voluntary health agencies, enterprises, and a private health-care market. The proportions among these five major forms of organization vary greatly in different countries.

The management of health systems entails several processes: health planning, administration (supervision, consultation, coordination, etc.), reg-

0163-7525/93/0510-0335$02.00

ulation, and legislation. The methods of carrying out each managerial process tend to vary mainly with a country's dominant political ideology.

The economic support of the various parts of a health system usually depends on one or more financial mechanisms. These may be governmental tax revenues (at different levels), social insurance (statutory), voluntary insurance, charity, and personal households. In economically less developed countries, foreign aid may play a role. The relative proportions among these different forms of support influence many features of a health system.

Finally, these four component parts of a health system lead to the crucial fifth part: the delivery of health services. These services may be analyzed according to several main subdivisions: primary health care (preventive and curative), secondary care, and tertiary care. In most health systems, furthermore, there are special modes of delivery of health services to certain populations and for certain disorders.

The combined characteristics of these five component parts permit the designation of each national health system according to certain types. Although history, economic level, and political ideology determine these types, their attributes may be classified according to the degree of market intervention by government. The organization of every health system, it was noted, includes a private health-care market. The proportions and characteristics of this market depend on the extent of intervention in the market process—supply, demand, competition, and price—by government. This may be measured, as we shall see, in different ways, appropriate to each component.

By such analysis, the national health systems in the world's approximately 165 sovereign countries may be scaled into four main types. Going from the least market intervention to the most, these health system types are: entrepreneurial, welfare-oriented, comprehensive, and socialist. This scaling may be applied, furthermore, to countries at high, middle, and low levels of economic development. In this chapter, we examine health systems in illustrative industrialized countries, as well as in selected developing countries of both middle and low economic levels. Health systems, of course, change over time, and this article describes the situation in the late 1980s to 1990.

ENTREPRENEURIAL HEALTH SYSTEMS

An entrepreneurial health system in a highly industrialized country is best illustrated by that in the United States. Indeed, in 1990, probably no other country belongs in this category, although Australia may have fitted into it 20 years ago.

Health resources of all sorts are relatively abundant in the United States. Physicians are plentiful (about 220 per 100,000 population), and for each physician there are 15–20 associated health personnel—nurses, pharmacists, dentists, technicians, physical therapists, administrators, etc. These personnel are prepared by universities, hospitals, and other training centers that are sponsored about half by units of government and half by nongovernment agencies. Within medicine, there is a high degree of specialization, so that only about 15% of doctors are generalists. Of all doctors serving ambulatory patients, about half are in group practice clinics (three or more working together). About two thirds of hospital beds are in nongovernmental institutions, and 10% of the total are operated for profit.

The major health authority of the US federal government is the Department of Health and Human Services, which promotes disease prevention and gives medical care to selected population groups. In the 50 US states and 3100 counties, there are local public health authorities engaged in environmental sanitation, communicable disease control, preventive service for mothers and infants, and certain other functions. Voluntary health agencies, which focus on certain persons, diseases, or services, are especially numerous. The largest channel for providing health care, however, is the private market of thousands of independent medical practitioners, pharmacies, laboratories, and so on.

Economic support for the US health system comes predominantly from private sources—for about 60% of the vast expenditures in 1987 of $2200 per capita. Of these health funds spent in the private sector, about half are derived from voluntary insurance, sold by hundreds of commercial or nonprofit companies. The public sector of 40% is derived partly from social insurance (social security legislation) and partly from federal, state, and local tax revenues. Charity and industrial management contribute only a small fraction (under 5%) of health system costs. As a share of gross national product (GNP), US health expenditures consume 11.5 percent—the largest percentage of any country. Still, some 15% of the population are without adequate economic protection for health care costs.

Because the US health system is so pluralistic in structure and function, primary health care is not delivered in a uniform way. Most is provided by private practitioners who are paid fees for each service rendered, whether the source of payment is private or public. The largest governmentally sponsored programs of medical care are Medicare for the elderly and totally disabled and Medicaid for the poor; under both of these programs, doctors and other practitioners are paid by the fee-for-service method, administered with much elasticity. This applies to services in hospitals, which usually have "open" medical staffs, as well as to care for the ambulatory patient.

In spite of these highly entrepreneurial characteristics, the US health system has been undergoing rapid changes. The long-term trend of economic support has been toward increased financing through collectivized mechanisms. The delivery of health service has also been subjected to various patterns of organization, so that teams of health personnel working in clinics and community health centers, as well as hospitals, are becoming increasingly common. Various legislative strategies are being actively debated to achieve universal population coverage for health services in the United States.

An entrepreneurial type of health system in a middle-income developing country is found in the Philippine Republic. Despite the general poverty of the national population (GNP per capita in 1986 was $590), of all health-related expenditures in 1980, 75% came from private sources. There are 76 provinces with locally elected governors, but the central Ministry of Health (MoH), like other ministries, has its own representatives in each province. The Provincial Health Officers, and below them District Health Officers, theoretically supervise MoH hospitals, but most of their work concerns conventional preventive public health services.

Major responsibility for financing medical care is vested in the Philippine Medical Care Commission, which is independent of the MoH. It administers a social insurance program, which covered about 28% of the population in 1980. Unlike policies in welfare-oriented health systems, these constitute higher paid employees in both public and private employment. The services are rendered, furthermore, by private physicians and private hospitals that are paid on a fee-for-service basis. When costs rose steeply in the late 1970s, the solution was not to reduce private fees but to increase cost-sharing required from patients.

The output of physicians and nurses in the Philippines is quite high, but more than half of the new graduates leave the country. In 1984, therefore, there were only 14.3 physicians per 100,000 people; more than half of these were settled in and around the national capital, with 22% of the population. There are 23 medical schools, but only three are governmental; the other 20 are small private schools run by private doctors as profit-making enterprises. Likewise, 87% of 132 nursing shcools are privately owned and operated.

In 1981, 59% of all Philippine physicians were engaged entirely in private practice. Nearly all of the 41% in government employment also did private work part-time. Among dentists, 84% were wholly private. Hospitals are relatively abundant, with 1.8 beds per 1000 people in 1981. Of the 1600 facilities, however, 74% are private, with 55% of the total beds. Only affluent patients and some covered by the social insurance (who can afford the copayments) can use the private hospitals. Even the public hospitals, moreover, charge for drugs and diagnostic procedures, except to totally indigent patients. The 45% of beds in public hospitals are typically overcrowded, with frequent occupancy of one bed by two patients.

The Philippine health system had some 2000 health centers for ambulatory service in 1982. Although theoretically staffed by a doctor, nurse, and midwife, the health centers actually have many vacancies. The services offered are limited essentially to prevention, and patients coming for treatment (except for first-aid) are usually sent to a private physician or a hospital outpatient department. The rate of health center utilization, therefore, is very low.

The high percentage of private spending in the total Philippine health expenditures has been noted. Considering personal household spending, a 1975 survey found that drugs and medical supplies accounted for 45%; private physicians and healers, 25%; and fees paid to hospitals and other facilities, 30%.

Kenya is a low-income, developing country of Africa, with entrepreneurial health system policies. Its GNP per capita in 1986 was only $324, but its ruling Kenya African National Union party has been committed to a policy of free private enterprise.

The seven provinces and, within these, 41 districts are each headed by a medical officer who is appointed by the central government. Below the district level, planning in 1972 called for 254 rural health units (staffed entirely by auxiliary personnel), but by 1984 only 120 of these were in operation. The Kenyan government estimated that primary health care had been brought within reach of about 30% of the rural population. The Ministry of Local Government also has responsibilities for health in the country's four main cities.

Loosely linked to the MoH is a National Hospital Insurance Fund, which insures about 12% of the population. As in the Philippines, it is the higher paid employed or self-employed persons who must pay premiums, and there is no contribution from employers. The insurance fund is explicitly intended to increase the use of private hospitals or private beds in public hospitals.

There are many nongovernmental health agencies in Kenya, the most important of which are religious missions from Europe and America. In 1981, these missions controlled about 25% of the hospital beds, whereas 46% were in government facilities and 29% were purely private. The mission hospitals got 24% of their operating costs from government grants, but 60% came from private patient fees (sometimes through insurance).

Kenya's physicians numbered 10.5 per 100,000 people in 1981; of these, 53% were in the national capital, Nairobi, with 6% of the population, and 94% of the people had to depend on the remaining 47% of doctors. In 1982, at least 70% of all Kenyan physicians were entirely in private practice, and the 30% in government also practiced privately part-time.

Not surprisingly, a 1983–1984 British study of health expenditures in Kenya found 49% to come from public sources and 51% from private. Household interviews revealed, furthermore, that 56% of the private expenditures came from a small proportion of families with high incomes. Also, 83% of the private spending came from the 15% of people who were city residents. The outcome of all these entrepreneurial policies is a life expectancy at birth, as of 1986, of only 57 years, compared with 61 years in other countries of comparable income level (GNPs of $400 per capita or less).

WELFARE-ORIENTED HEALTH SYSTEMS

Many health systems of Western Europe are welfare oriented, as are the systems of Canada, Japan, and Australia. The health system of the Federal Republic of Germany has mobilized economic support, to make health service available to practically all its people, for the longest period of time; thus, it may well illustrate this type of system in an industrialized country.

After many years of voluntary health care insurance organizations among low-income workers, Germany enacted mandatory legislation for such insurance in 1883. The kinds of workers covered and the scope of health services provided were gradually broadened. The insurance is now carried by several hundred relatively small "sickness funds," which are regulated by government as to their costs, benefits, and methods of administration. The principal governmental responsibility for this social insurance is the Ministry of Labor and Social Affairs in the central government, and also in each of the nine "lander," or provinces. Preventive public health work is done by the Ministry of Youth, Family Affairs, and Health, working in local communities.

Physicians and other health personnel are trained in universities and schools sponsored entirely by units of government. Hospitals are also sponsored mainly (52.3% of beds in 1980) by units of government; of the nongovernmental hospital beds, two-thirds are under voluntary nonprofit agencies and one-third are proprietary. The medical staffs of the proprietary hospitals are open to any qualified local physician, but in government and voluntary nonprofit facilities there are "closed" medical staffs of salaried physicians.

The payment of nonsalaried physicians for their services is a complex process, resulting from long historical developments. The sickness funds enter into contracts with associations of physicians, which are paid periodic per capita amounts, according to each fund's membership. Then, the medical association reviews and pays the fees charged by physicians. If, in a quarter year, the fees charged exceed the money available, less than the full amount of each fee may be paid; alternatively, certain doctors (suspected of overservicing patients) may be underpaid. To safeguard the earnings of specialists in private practice, hospitals do not offer outpatient services, except for emergency cases.

The German pharmaceutical industry, largely an offshoot of the dye industry, is especially robust. Hundreds of new or slightly modified drugs are produced each year and dispensed by private pharmacies. The tragedy of thalidomide, which caused severe birth defects when taken by pregnant women, occurred in West Germany in the 1960s and led to more regulatory drug legislation in Germany and many other countries. On the other hand, the principle of chemotherapy originated in 1912 in Germany (Paul Ehrlich and "Salvarsan"), and the sulfonamides were first synthesized by German chemists.

In contrast to the United States, the entire health system in Germany required expenditure of 8.2% of the gross domestic product (GDP), as of 1987. Of this amount, 77% was derived from government programs, and only 23% came from the private sector. Most of the public sector funds came from the social insurance, administered by the sickness funds. In spite of Germany's period of brutal fascism and the experience of defeat in two world wars (1914–1918 and 1939–1945), the German health system has continued to serve well the great majority of the population to the present time.

Like the German system, the other welfare-oriented health systems of western Europe make use of many local insurance organizations to administer the health service financing. Each system, however, has certain unique characteristics. In France, for example, the patient must make payment for services directly to the physician and then seek reimbursement from his/her "caisse de maladie" according to a "nomenclature" (fees negotiated between the government and the medical association). Typically the reimbursement is for 80% of the charges, so that the patient copays 20%. Administrative mechanisms in Belgium, the Netherlands, and Austria differ in other ways.

The welfare-oriented health systems of Australia and Canada are more fully under the umbrella of government, without use of intermediary insurance agencies. Australia has no history of worker's insurance funds, so health insurance is managed by a single national government authority. In Canada, the key administrative bodies are the provincial governments, with partial funding by grants from the federal government. In both countries, funds come mainly from general revenues, rather than earmarked employer/employee contributions, to finance the programs. Most of the health services are still provided by private doctors who are paid by negotiated fees, and hospitals are paid by prospective global budgets. In Australia, most hospitals are sponsored by local governments; in Canada, the majority are controlled by churches or other voluntary bodies.

Among developing countries, there are many with welfare-oriented health systems. At the middle-income level, many are in Latin America, where social security programs have been organized for varying proportions of the population. Peru, with a national population of about 20,000,000 and a GNP per capita of $1153 in 1986, may be taken as illustrative.

Since 1960, Peru has become rapidly urbanized, to 67% of its residents in

1984; this has meant a reduced dependence on traditional healers, or "curanderos." It has also meant somewhat greater access of people to organized health programs, which are strongest in the cities. In 1968, the Peruvian government was seized by a military coup that, paradoxically, brought about agrarian land reforms and nationalized certain industries. In 1976, another, more conservative military group seized power; however, in 1980, a democratic civilian government was established, with national elections.

By 1985, the Peruvian Ministry of Health developed a national network of 612 health centers and 1700 health posts. Scores of charitable "beneficencia" hospitals were taken over by the MoH, which thus controls 55.2% of the hospital beds (1.56 per 1000 people). Along with the beds of other public agencies, government controls more than 80% of the total bed supply.

The country is divided into 17 health regions, and these into 57 health areas. The medical officers in charge of each jurisdiction are centrally appointed and are supposed to supervise all MoH services within their borders. The ambulatory care facilities give general primary care, including treatment of common ailments, although preventive maternal and child health services are emphasized.

Like nearly all Latin American countries, Peru has a social security program that provides medical care to 18.6% of the population. Unlike the Philippines or Germany, this social insurance program provides care in its own polyclinics and hospitals, staffed by salaried medical and allied personnel. In 1975, the two previously separate social insurance programs for manual and for white-collar workers were unified. Any covered person, however, willing and able to make substantial copayments, may consult private physicians and hospitals, and a small percentage does so.

Physicians in Peru numbered 17,500 in 1985, or 91.5 per 100,000 population. Some 70% of these physicians work in government agencies, but practice privately part-time, and 30% are wholly in private practice. There are seven medical schools, of which only one is private. Maldistribution of doctors is extreme, with 70% in 1985 located in Lima, where 16% of the population resides. Among dentists, public employment is less common, and 72% are entirely private. Out-of-hospital drug consumption is high, and more than half of household health expenditures in 1984 went for self-prescribed drugs.

The welfare-oriented policies in the Peruvian health system are probably best reflected by overall health expenditures. In 1984, 66.5% of expenditures came from government and 33.5% from private sources. The benefits of organized health services, in spite of general economic difficulties, are reflected in tuberculosis data. Ministry of Health reports indicated 225 cases per 100,000 population in 1962, and this rate was still 150 cases per 100,000 in 1983. However, the mortality rate declined from 37.8 tuberculosis deaths per 100,000 in 1970 to 17.6 deaths per 100,000 in 1984. Lives were saved by health service.

India is a very low income country with a welfare-oriented health system, having characteristics quite different from those in Peru. This huge country of more than 800,000,000 people had a GNP per capita of only $290 in 1986. Since winning independence from British rule in 1947, India has developed a national health system with thousands of publicly financed and publicly operated health facilities.

Continued from colonial times, India has 31 states and union territories, which carry major health service responsibilities. In each of these jurisdictions, there is a Ministry of Health and Family Welfare (MOHFW), responsible for personal and environmental health services. Within the states and territories, there are 408 districts, each containing an average of 2,000,000 people and headed by a Medical Officer of Health. Two thirds of MOHFW financing comes from the state level and one third from the national level—the latter mainly for family planning to control population growth.

Every district of India has a public hospital and several primary health centers—8000 of them in 1988. These are ideally staffed by one or two physicians plus allied health staff, but there are many medical vacancies. Around the primary health centers are more than 100,000 subcenters, staffed entirely by briefly trained auxiliary personnel. Because of the varying economic levels of the states, there are great differences in the amplitude of these several resources. Even peripheral to the subcenters, there are community health volunteers, who are trained for a few weeks to encourage sound health practices in the villages.

Although India is only slightly industrialized, it has a social security program covering employees of private firms and their dependents. In 1987, 28,000,000 people, or 3.5% of the population, were entitled to medical care through specially organized facilities or regular MOHFW resources under contract; in large cities, insured persons may be served by private general practitioners, paid by capitation. There is also a similar social insurance scheme, with organized medical services, for central government employees.

India's 125 medical schools, which are linked to universities, are almost entirely public and supervised by the Ministry of Education of each state. There are hundreds of voluntary health agencies, many of which are tied to foreign religious missions. The missions operate small hospitals with 26% of the national stock of hospital beds.

Of all modern physicians in India, 41% work for governmental health agencies, 12% for nongovernmental but organized health programs, and 47% are entirely in private practice. Altogether in 1987, there were about 325,000 modern physicians, or 41 per 100,000 population. A much greater number of traditional doctors, however, were almost entirely in private practice throughout India; this included some 400,000 Ayurvedic practitioners (many trained in government-run colleges) and 150,000 homeopathic doctors. Since the late 1970s, the government of India has stressed the training of multipurpose auxiliary health personnel.

Health centers and subcenters for ambulatory care are almost entirely governmental. Of the 550,000 hospital beds (0.71 per 1000 people), 70% were controlled by central or state governments and another 4.6% by local authorities. Regarding another resource, pharmaceutical products, India has successfully converted multinational into domestic production. In terms of the value of finished drug products, by 1972 government enterprises were producing 34%, private but domestically owned enterprises were producing 39%, and only 27% of finished products were produced by firms under foreign ownership.

In the early 1980s, total Indian health expenditures amounted to only 3% of the GNP. Of this, a 1970 study found that 84% came from private sources, and it is likely that the private sector still accounts for two thirds of the total (as in neighboring Pakistan). If so, one third of spending by the public sector constitutes an improvement in equity.

For the fight against certain diseases, the national and state MOHFWs in India conduct special campaigns—previously run vertically from the top, but now decentralized. These include the reduction of infant diarrhea (oral rehydration therapy), malaria control, tuberculosis control, the World Health Organization (WHO) "expanded program of immunization," leprosy control, and family planning. Improvements have resulted from all these campaigns. Life expectancy at birth in India has increased from 44 years in 1960 to 59 years in 1987. Even the crude birth rate, which contributes to India's huge population, has declined between these years from 42 to 32 per 1000 population.

COMPREHENSIVE HEALTH SYSTEMS

In several countries, national health systems that were welfare-oriented for some years underwent further political development after World War II and became comprehensive in type. This has meant that 100% of the national population has become entitled to complete health service, and the financial support has shifted almost entirely to general tax revenues. Larger proportions of doctors and other health personnel have come to work in organized frameworks on salary. Almost all health facilities have come under the direct control of government.

Great Britain adopted this comprehensive type of health system soon after World War II, pursuant to planning done during the war. The Scandinavian countries did likewise in the 1950s. Italy enacted national health service legislation in the 1970s, as did Greece and Spain, albeit somewhat less sweepingly. The British National Health Service (NHS), which has had worldwide impacts, well illustrates the comprehensive health system type.

Limited insurance for general practitioner services and drugs had covered low-wage manual workers in Great Britain since 1911. With the 1946 legislation, this program was expanded to provide all ambulatory treatment services and to become the first pillar of the NHS. Because of the war, British hospitals had been organized into regional groups, and these, headed by regional hospital boards, became the second organizational pillar. Local public health authorities, along with visiting nurse and ambulance services, became the third pillar. Finally, a special administrative channel was reserved for teaching hospitals, affiliated with medical schools. In this three- or four-part administrative structure, policies on professional remuneration varied pragmatically. General medical practitioners were paid by capitation, according to the persons enrolled with each one. Dentists were paid by fees for each unit of service. Hospital-based specialists (or consultants) were employed by the regional boards and paid salaries.

In 1974, the British NHS was reorganized to achieve greater administrative integration. After a preliminary period, all health services were placed under unified management in some 200 health districts. At this level, a well-trained management specialist was supported by a specialist in community medicine (including epidemiology). The regional hospital boards were converted into regional health boards and became the conduits for money from the central government. At all levels were community health councils, made up of leading consumers and providers, for advisory purposes.

Popular opinion in Great Britain has been highly favorable toward the NHS, although there are complaints about long waiting lists for elective (nonemergency) surgery in hospitals. The explanation for these delays is fundamentally that the resources provided by government for this large comprehensive health system are inadequate. In 1987, when the United States was spending 11.2% of gross domestic product on health and Sweden was spending 9.0%, Great Britain was spending only 6.1% of its smaller overall GDP. Of this expenditure, 87% came from government and 13% from the private sector. (In 1975, however, only 9% of British health expenditures had been private, and Conservative government policy has encouraged greater private spending.)

The development of comprehensive health systems in the Scandinavian countries was more gradual. The local workers health insurance funds were simply converted into branch offices of the national government, and services became available to everyone. The demand for health services in Norway and Sweden does not seem to be as high as in Great Britain, and yet both human and physical resources are relatively greater. In Sweden, for example, the health spending in 1987 amounted to 9.0% of GDP, of which 91% came from public sources and 9% from private. This was an increase from 8.0% of GDP in 1975, of which 10%, a slightly greater fraction, had previously come from private sources. The Swedish government, in other words, has responded to rising demand by strengthening the public sector.

Among developing countries, very few have achieved comprehensive health systems that have entitled 100% of their populations to complete health services. One of middle-income level is Costa Rica, which in 1948 abolished its military establishment and then gradually extended its social security coverage for medical care to everyone. Another such country, of very low-income level (GNP per capita of $400 in 1986), is Sri Lanka, a tropical island south of India.

In 1986, Sri Lanka had 16,100,000 people, with the same sort of vast disparities in family wealth as most developing countries: the richest 20% of households earned 50% of the total income, whereas the poorest 20% earned only 6%. Yet, the government health services made available to all these people are remarkably complete. For governance, the country is divided into 25 districts, each headed by a centrally appointed medical officer. Within each district, there are about ten divisions, averaging 60,000 people, with a medically staffed divisional health center. Even more peripherally, there are subdivisional health centers, staffed wholly by auxiliary personnel, including assistant medical practitioners with two years of training in primary health care. Voluntary health agencies are also strong in Sri Lanka, especially the Red Cross, the Cancer Society, and the Family Planning Association.

The supply of modern physicians in Sri Lanka is quite modest—13.4 per 100,000 in 1981—because many are Tamils, who faced ethnic discrimination and therefore emigrated. The stock of Ayurvedic practitioners is three times as great, and these are virtually all in private practice. Government health manpower needs in Sri Lanka are largely met by auxiliary personnel.

Nutrition policy in Sri Lanka has been a major factor contributing to health. Soon after independence in 1947, a weekly ration of rice was provided free to every family; even when this was altered in the 1970s, it was continued for very poor families, along with free lunches for all school children. General education has also had high priority in Sri Lanka. Nearly all girls, as well as boys, go to primary school; in 1985, adult literacy was 91 percent for men and 83% for women.

In the mid-1980s, the Sri Lankan Ministry of Health estimated that 93% of the population was readily accessible to health services. Because of the shortage of modern physicians, Ayurvedic practitioners are consulted extensively; many of these use penicillin and other scientific drugs in their practice.

Because Sri Lanka and India are geographically close and have cultural similarities, the health records of these countries have often been compared. In 1985, when India's infant mortality rate was 105 per 1000 live births, the rate in Sri Lanka was 36 per 1000. In 1987, life expectancy at birth was 59 years in India, and 71 years in Sri Lanka. Strong programs of nutrition and education have doubtless contributed importantly to these achievements, but the comprehensive health system has surely played a substantial part.

SOCIALIST HEALTH SYSTEMS

In countries that have had a revolution to install a socialist economic order, the health systems have become socialist in structure and function. This has meant that practically all physical and human resources have been taken over by government, and health services have theoretically become available to everyone. In 1989 and 1990, certain basic changes were brought about in these socialist economies, but conditions are described as they were shortly before this. (The patterns to be adopted after 1990 are far from clear.)

After the Russian Revolution of 1917, the Soviet Union became the first country with a socialist health system. These changes did not occur overnight, but were essentially completed by 1937. By then, virtually all doctors, nurses, and other health personnel had become public employees, and all hospitals and other health facilities were taken over by government. The private pharmaceutical industry was nationalized, and medical schools were removed from the universities and put under the Ministry of Health as academic institutes. Health science research was carried out in other special institutes, also under the Ministry of Health.

All services were free of charge to every Soviet resident, except drugs, which had to be purchased in government pharmacies. However, certain life-saving compounds and all drugs for military veterans, pensioners, and certain others were without charge. To provide accessible ambulatory care, hundreds of polyclinics, staffed by generalists, pediatricians, gynecologists, and others, were established in the cities, and hundreds of smaller health centers were constructed in rural areas. The Soviet "feldsher"—trained since the nineteenth century—was one of the world's earliest forms of medical assistant, serving mostly in rural areas where physicians were too few.

The Soviet health system has turned out enormous numbers of physicians; in 1986, there were 430 per 100,000 population. Nurses, midwives, and feldshers were also plentiful, but technicians were relatively less numerous than in other industrialized countries. Diagnostic and therapeutic equipment in hospitals was generally less developed than in western European countries—a deficiency that President Gorbachev's "perestroika" (restructuring) was expected to correct. Certain exceptionally well equipped and staffed hospitals and polyclinics, however, were established to serve high Communist Party officials. Although such preferred care is provided for "important persons" in most national health systems, it has caused much popular resentment in a theoretically egalitarian socialist society.

Since about 1960, private out-of-hospital health service has expanded slightly in the Soviet Union for people who can afford to pay private fees. These paying polyclinics are staffed by hospital-based specialists, who may work in them a limited number of hours per week. As a general back-up for all polyclinics and hospitals, all large Soviet cities have well-developed emergency services, staffed by physicians and feldshers and equipped with modern ambulances. Calls to a central telephone exchange lead to the dispatch of ambulances from various locations in large metropolitan areas.

The health of the population in the Soviet Union improved markedly after the 1917 Revolution for about 50 years. The infant mortality rate declined, and the life expectancy at birth increased significantly. Then, in the 1970s, these indices changed, and health conditions clearly deteriorated. Various explanations were offered, but most important seemed to be the Cold War and the vast military expenditures it entailed. The funds remaining for health services were seriously inadequate.

Soviet health system expenditures in the 1970s and 1980s were less than 4.0% of national wealth (as calculated by economists from international agencies). This was much lower than in any western industrialized country and far below the health needs. As part of perestroika, health expenditures were expected to increase, but the resultant effects would take time to see. In the other socialist countries of eastern Europe (Poland, Hungary, etc.), the health systems were largely modeled after the Soviet Union's, and the transformations toward a free-market pattern were occurring somewhat earlier in the 1980s, although the pace of change was slow.

Cuba, a middle-income developing country, had a social revolution in 1959 and then introduced a thoroughly socialist type of health system. Cuba's population is 10,100,000 and its GNP per capita in 1986 was just under $2000. The adult literacy attained by 1984 was 96%.

As in other socialist countries, practically all responsibility for health services are under the Ministry of Public Health. After several changes since 1959, the country has been divided into 14 health provinces, all headed by centrally appointed medical officers. Within the provinces are 169 urban or rural municipalities, which elect local assemblies, and these appoint municipal medical officers. Voluntary agencies are limited to mass organizations of women, farmers, workers, and youth who help out in health campaigns. There is virtually no market for private medical care, either modern or traditional.

Health manpower education was greatly expanded after the Cuban revolution to compensate for the 33–50% of physicians, dentists, and pharmacists who left the country. By 1968, the number of medical schools had increased from one to four, and by 1982 there were 17,000 active physicians (about half women, for a ratio of 170 per 100,000 population. Schools for nurses, dentists, and technicians were also expanded, but Cuba rejected the idea of the feldsher or general medical assistant. Leaders said that a revolutionary health system had no place for "second-class doctors" nor for other types of community health workers. Cuba has not even trained professional midwives; all childbirths are attended by physicians in hospitals.

Physical facilities were also greatly expanded in Cuba after the revolution. By 1982, there were 5.3 hospital beds per 1000 people, and their geographic distribution was largely equalized. Before 1959, metropolitan Havana had 62% of the beds, and the much larger rural population had 38%; in 1982, Havana had 39% of the beds and the rest of the country had 61%.

The most important physical structures in the Cuban health system are the 425 polyclinics, each serving about 25,000 people for general ambulatory care, preventive and curative. For every 5000 people, there is normally a team of four physicians (internist, pediatrician, obstetrician-gynecologist, and dentist), so that there would ideally be five such teams in each polyclinic. For preventive attention to cases with chronic disorders, patients are called back periodically for check-ups and counseling (a practice called dispensarization).

Since 1983, Cuba has been placing "family practitioners" at posts around the polyclinic to provide general primary health care to only 600–700 persons. These generalists are then backed up by the polyclinic medical teams. Cuba's attitude on family planning is not aggressive, because the country wants to increase its population; contraceptive advice and supplies, however, are freely available on request.

As a result of its overall socio-economic policies, as well as its health system, Cuba has attained the best health record of any country in Latin America, including several of much greater per capita wealth. The infant mortality rate was reduced to 15.0 per 1000 live births by 1986. Life expectancy at birth had been 61.8 years in 1960, and by 1982 it was extended to 73.5.

A last socialist country, which had a social revolution in 1949, is the People's Republic of China. With more than 1,100,000,000 people and a very complex social history, it is not easy to summarize China's health system, but we can examine the highlights. In spite of its socialist ideology, China's overall income level is so low (GNP of $300 in 1986) that government-financed health services for all have not yet been achieved.

Having passed through several major periods of political change since the earlier bourgeois revolution of 1911, by 1986 China had a ratio of 57 modern physicians per 100,000 population. There were also 32 traditional Chinese practitioners per 100,000 and, although official policy called for their integration into the government health services, the greater majority were in private practice. In addition, there are thousands of assistant doctors (45 per 100,000 people)—not to be confused with "barefoot doctors"—who are trained in secondary medical schools for three years. These secondary medical schools also train nurses, technicians, and pharmacy assistants. The barefoot doctor was a peasant trained for only a few months, principally during the period of the Cultural Revolution (1965–1975). At their peak, there were, 1,800,000 of these auxiliaries. After the death of Chairman Mao Tse-tung in 1976, they were upgraded to "village doctors," numbering 1,245,000 in 1989.

Hospitals were also vastly expanded in socialist China. By 1985, there were hospitals in all 2300 counties and a ratio of 2.1 beds per 1000 population. Formerly, the counties were organized into 27,000 communes, for local agricultural and other production, but these have been converted to townships. Each township, as well as the municipal districts, has health centers for general primary health care. In 1986, there were 48,100 such facilities, each serving an average of 22,000 people. In the cities, these were usually staffed by physicians, both Western and traditional; in small towns, they would have only assistant doctors of both types, plus allied health personnel. Finally, in the villages, there were small health stations, staffed with village doctors and aides, numbering in 1985 some 126,000 structures.

Through deliberate planning, China has developed 800 pharmaceutical plants that produce some 3000 modern drug compounds; in addition, it has 480 plants for manufacture of traditional drugs. These drugs are distributed through some 360 pharmaceutical warehouses in the provinces to hospitals, health centers, and some 20,000 local pharmacies; the latter were originally under the Ministry of Public Health, but many have become private since 1980.

The central Ministry of Public Health establishes general policies, but most responsibility is carried by corresponding agencies in each of the 21 mainland provinces (except Taiwan), 5 autonomous regions, and 3 centrally administered municipalities. Some 90% of financial support must come from within each province. Every county also has a Bureau of Public Health, headed by a modern physician, but below this level, the health service is managed by the health center staff.

To help meet the costs of medical care both in hospitals and health centers, several forms of health insurance have been developed: for central government employees (but not dependents), run by the Ministry of Finance; for workers in national or provincial enterprises, including dependents, handled by each enterprise and supervised by the Ministry of Labor; for workers in enterprises of the counties, municipalities, and townships, with some protection of dependents; and for farm families through local health cooperatives. The coverage of dependent costs in these insurance programs is usually for 50% of the official fees. According to a World Bank analysis, in 1987, all these forms of insurance accounted for 50% of health system expenditures; overall government revenues at all levels contributed 19%, and private individuals had to pay fees amounting to 32%. Health insurance covers about 40% of the national population with some protection.

Public health campaigns against malaria, schistosomiasis, tuberculosis, and other diseases are carried out by the Provincial Ministries of Public Health. Research, education of personnel, construction of facilities, and the management of all hospitals and health centers are all functions of government. It is the large recurrent expenditures for personal medical care in China that must be paid for privately or through health insurance. Also, since 1980, a growing proportion of modern physicians, and even village doctors, have undertaken private practice.

Family planning has been a major part of China's social policy since 1968. By 1987, the crude birth rate was reduced to 20 per 1000 people. Health achievements have likewise been impressive. Infant mortality was reduced from 150 deaths per 1000 live births in 1960 to 33 per 1000 in 1987. Life expectancy at birth over the same period was extended from 47 years to 70. Even though serious inequities persist in the operation of China's health system, its achievements have won world-wide admiration.

GENERAL TRENDS

In all four types of national health systems in industrialized and developing countries, certain general trends have been evident over the last 50 years. The resources, both human and physical, have been greatly expanded. As more people have survived to the older age groups and as educational levels have improved, the demands for personal health care everywhere have risen. Every country has responded by developing larger resources and new kinds of health personnel. Pharmaceutical products have also increased in quantity, variety, and effectiveness.

The organization of health systems, largely under government, has increased and grown more complex. Both public and private agencies have multiplied, and the strength and scope of Ministries of Health have generally been enhanced. Public health authorities have grown at various jurisdictional levels—local and provincial, as well as national. Nongovernmental voluntary agencies have also grown to promote health efforts regarding certain persons, disorders, or services.

As the interests of more groups of health-care providers and consumers become defined, the management of national health systems is becoming generally more sophisticated. Administrators are trained, record systems are formulated, consumers are given a stronger voice, and decision making has become a more democratic process. To limit abuses in the private market, regulatory powers have been extended. More and more aspects of health are being subjected to legislative intervention—from reducing the sale of harmful tobacco products to the mobilization of funds for supporting the costs of prevention and treatment.

As a share of national wealth, the money devoted to health systems has increased steadily, except perhaps in the European socialist countries. It has grown both in public and private sectors, although in all but a few countries more rapidly in the public sector. Of all health services, those in hospitals have absorbed the most rapidly expanding proportion, to provide the benefits of advanced technology to an aging population with chronic diseases. With the objective of meeting the health needs of more people, rural and urban, WHO has stressed everywhere a higher priority for primary health care.

In the patterns of delivery of health care, the key concept has become teamwork. The importance of this has long been recognized in hospitals, and it is now appreciated in ambulatory care, as well. The socialist countries first demonstrated the value of polyclinics and health centers to provide integrated preventive-curative services to general populations, and all countries with other types of health systems have, to some extent, acted likewise. There is a generally increased application of these organized frameworks, from the entrepreneurial to the welfare-oriented to the comprehensive and to the socialist types of health systems.

These developments in all components of national health systems add up to the attainment of greater health care equity in the world. In the words of the WHO's Constitution, it has long been agreed that "The enjoyment of the highest attainable standard of health is one of the fundamental rights of every human being, without distinction of race, religion, political belief, economic or social condition." Implementation of this ideal may lie in the future, but the developments in national health systems over the last 50 years give grounds for confidence about its ultimate achievement.

EPILOGUE

Since the above text was written in December 1990, the world has continued to undergo turbulent political changes. Reactions against social expenditures, designed to achieve equity, have occurred in many countries, including Great Britain and Sweden. These trends have been described as a "privatization" movement. Internal competitive markets have been introduced within the British NHS. The results of this strategy are not yet clear. Universal population coverage, nevertheless, has remained intact.

The most catastrophic changes have occurred in the countries of Eastern Europe and the Soviet Union, which had been their model. The socialist political structure has been vehemently rejected, and all these countries are attempting to convert to capitalism. The transformation from central planning to markets, and from public ownership to private, has been very difficult. The references to "socialist" health systems in the above accounts, therefore, have meaning only in a theoretical sense, which may regain viability at some future time.

The transformation of health systems, however, with the demise of socialism, is far from completed. Financial support in some countries is being changed from government revenues to social security. Public polyclinics still function, however, and only a few are changing to private group practices. Hospitals compete for patients, although their control remains governmental. Pharmacies in some Eastern European countries have been privatized.

China, although politically socialist, did not have a socialist health system. There was extensive use of social insurance for different population groups, and insured people were much better served than others. After the death of Mao Tse-tung in 1976, and the introduction of the "four modernizations," private medical practice was encouraged. In rural townships (formerly communes), the health centers and health stations had to be economically self-supporting.

In spite of these crucial changes in many health systems, the world trends toward organization continue. This means organization of all major components of health systems: resources, programs, economic support, management, and delivery of services. Whether the overall political structure is entrepreneurial, welfare-oriented, comprehensive, or socialist, increasing organization of the health system occurs. In most countries, the initial strategy for change is the organization of economic support, from which many others changes follow. The pace of health system organization, therefore, is heavily influenced by economic conditions throughout the world.

Bibliography

1. Bosch, P. F. 1990. *Textbook of International Health*. New York: Oxford Univ. Press
2. Elling, R. H. 1980. *Cross-National Study of Health Systems*. New Brunswick, NJ: Transaction Books
3. Org. for Econ. Coop. and Dev. 1990. *Health Care Systems in Transition*. Paris, OECD
4. Pannenborg, C. O., van der Werff, A. Hirsch, G. B., Bernard, K. 1984. *Reorienting Health Services: Application of a Systems Approach*. New York: Plenum
5. Raffel, M. W., ed. 1984. *Comparative Health Systems: Descriptive Analyses of Fourteen National Health Systems*. University Park, Penn: Penn. State Univ. Press
6. Roemer, M. I. 1991. *National Health Systems of the World*. New York: Oxford Univ. Press
7. Saltman, R. B., 1988. *The International Handbook of Health-Care Systems*. Westport, Conn: Greenwood Press

Annu. Rev. Publ. Health 1993. 14:355–77

POVERTY AND CULTURAL DIVERSITY: Challenges for Health Promotion Among the Medically Underserved

Jon F. Kerner
Division of Cancer Control, Department of Epidemiology and Biostatistics, Memorial Sloan-Kettering Cancer Center, New York, NY 10021

Linda Dusenbury
Institute for Prevention Research, Department of Public Health, Cornell University Medical College, New York, NY 10021

Jeanne S. Mandelblatt
Division of Cancer Control, Department of Epidemiology and Biostatistics, Memorial Sloan-Kettering Cancer Center, New York, NY 10021

KEY WORDS: health, race, ethnicity, SES

INTRODUCTION

As we approach the end of a decade, a century, and a millennium, two characteristics of the human condition will increasingly influence the health and well-being of the citizens of the United States and the world: poverty and cultural diversity. Both social class and ethnic/racial group membership are predictors of physical and mental health status. Both are associated with lifestyle, environmental, and occupational factors (e.g. tobacco and alcohol, air and water pollution, asbestos and lead exposure) and access to health-promoting and health-protecting resources (e.g. adequate and varied foodstuffs, sanitation) and preventive medical services (e.g. prenatal care, childhood immunization, chronic disease screening). Although poverty and cultural diversity have always been important determinants of health status, they are

0163-7525/93/0510-0355$02.00

now even more important in our efforts to promote health through the year 2000.

Poverty in the US increased during the 1980s. In 1979, 26.1 million Americans (11.7%) lived below the official poverty income cutoff ($7412), and 36.6 million (16.4%) lived below the 125% of poverty income cutoff ($9265). A decade later, 31.9 million Americans (13.1%) lived below the official poverty income cutoff ($12,092), and 42.6 million (17.5%) lived below the 125% poverty level (62). Although the number appeared to peak in 1984, a higher percentage of Americans are living below the poverty line today than in 1969. Moreover, as Brown & Gershoff (13) note, the total amount by which poverty incomes are below the poverty line increased by more than 50% from 1977 to 1986. In addition, the gap between rich and poor families grew larger through 1986. The richest fifth of the US population received 43.7% of the national pretax family income, and the poorest two fifths received 15.4%. From 1980 through 1986, only the richest fifth of the US population experienced an increase in their percentage of after-tax family income; all other income quintiles experienced a decline (13).

Compounding the income differential in the US, there have been rapid increases in ethnic and racial diversity from 1980 to 1990. Nationwide, the US experienced a 107.8% increase in population among Asian Americans, a 53% increase in population among Latin Americans, and a 13.2% increase in population among black Americans—all of which exceeds the overall US population growth of 9.8% since 1980 (62). In addition, regional cultural diversity and the diversity within local communities are even greater than reflected by national data.

In Europe and Asia, the breakdown of totalitarian socialist rule, increasing ethnic and racial group conflict, emigration from within, and immigration from the economically underdeveloped nations of Africa and South Asia, have created new socioeconomic and public health problems. Many of these problems have not been previously experienced by the relatively culturally homogeneous countries of Europe and the republics within what was the Soviet Union. Thus, like the US, they now face new public health challenges from increasing societal pluralism.

Ethnic and racial diversity are linked with both absolute and relative poverty. Although the largest number and percentage of poor Americans are white, Table 1 shows that a disproportionate percentage of US black and Latin American populations, particularly children, live below the poverty line (62). For example, in 1987, 51.5% of black children in the Midwest and 52.9% of Latin American children in the Northeast lived below the poverty line (62). The short- and long-term health consequences of such pervasive poverty among the multi-ethnic youth in our communities is one of the principal

Table 1 Percentage of all persons and children living below the poverty line in 1987 by race/ethnicity.

Population	White	Black	Latino
All persons	10.4%	32.6%	28.1%
Children (<18)	15.0%	45.1%	39.3%

challenges for those concerned with promoting health among high-risk populations.

Another reason that poverty and cultural diversity are so important is that the potential channels for promoting health far exceed, in number and complexity, the resources that society has been willing to invest in health promotion to low socioeconomic status (SES) and multi-ethnic populations. Such channels include television, radio, regional daily newspapers, small, local weeklies, and thousands of magazines with both broad and narrow readerships (3). Further, many institutional settings (e.g. schools, work places, religious institutions) can be used to channel health promotion messages.

Finally, various intermediary groups, such as the Shriners and the Urban League, serve as leaders of different segments of the target populations. These groups may have to be recruited to become "stakeholders" in national, regional, or local health promotion campaigns (38). Considering the diversity of these channels, both in terms of the complexity of targeting a health promotion campaign to diverse high-risk populations and in terms of the resources needed to take advantage of the multitude of channels for reaching the target populations, we will need to reformulate our health behavior change models and recalculate our health promotion budgets.

Limited availability and quality of primary care and diagnostic, treatment, and follow-up care within the "resource-limited" health-care settings that serve low SES and multi-ethnic populations also create significant barriers to health promotion. These barriers include reduced access to preventive medicine services and ambivalence or negative attitudes toward the use of health services in these settings. This, in turn, may reinforce delay and nonadherence behaviors among high-risk populations who have been recommended for surveillance and/or treatment of early-stage disease. As increasingly poor and culturally diverse populations demand more of resource-limited health-care facilities, the interaction between the health-care system and the people it serves may increase the barriers to promoting health among these high-risk populations.

In this paper, we review recent literature on each of the four issues outlined above. We examine the current approaches to health promotion and assess how well they apply to an increasingly multi-cultural, economically disadvantaged, and medically underserved US population. Health promotion is viewed as one of three dimensions to primary prevention; the remaining two are disease prevention and health protection (60). Although this review focuses on the implications of cultural diversity and poverty for health promotion, the interdependence of these different approaches to primary prevention is recognized.

POVERTY AND HEALTH PROMOTION

Because different ethnic and racial groups in the US experience different levels of social, economic, and educational status, the issue arises whether SES is the most important factor for predicting the health and well-being of multi-ethnic populations. In reviewing the disparities in health status among black Americans, Latin Americans, Asian Americans, and Native Americans, the executive summary of the US Department of Health and Human Services (DHHS) secretary's task force report on black and minority health (28) concluded:

> Only limited information exists to determine the possible association between health status and socioeconomic factors, such as income and education. Greater awareness of this relationship would make it possible to target existing resources more effectively toward the areas of greatest need in the various minority populations at risk (page 85).

In contrast, Tomatis (54) notes:

> When one reviews the literature, it is rather depressing to encounter the same observations, the same results, and the same conclusions and recommendations over the years. Although there is not much to be found that is new, poverty continues to be rediscovered. . . . Sanitary conditions are worse, mortality is higher, survival rates of cancer patients lower, and life expectancy shorter in developing countries than in industrialized countries. Similar if not identical differences can still be seen within industrialized countries between the socioeconomically less and more favored population groups.

These different views of our knowledge base about the relationship between poverty and health suggest that views on this issue may, in part, be determined by political perspective. There are broad and diverse sets of relationships between poverty and different health indices (1). Our review presents an example of the conceptual change, from a minority population focus to an SES focus, that has recently occurred in the prevention and control of one disease: cancer.

In 1979, the oldest and largest US disease-specific voluntary organization, the American Cancer Society (ACS), formed a National Advisory Committee on Cancer in Minorities. This action stemmed from a growing awareness that cancer incidence, mortality, and survival data pointed to the heavier cancer burden experienced by black Americans and other minorities as compared with white, non-Latino populations (18). A little more than six years later, this same committee was reconstituted as the National Advisory Committee on Cancer in the Socioeconomically Disadvantaged (SED).

This change in focus was based on two factors. First, a special report commissioned by the ACS (23) identified low SES as a common barrier to cancer prevention and control experienced by many minority groups. Second, a broader national consensus and response from the state and local divisions of the ACS was anticipated with a focus on the ubiquitous phenomenon of poverty, rather than a focus on the concerns of any specific ethnic or racial group (H. P. Freeman 1989, personal communication). Both the growing literature since 1985 on cancer in SED populations (20), and the positive response of the national office and state and local ACS divisions to the challenges of cancer prevention and control in low SES communities support the change from an exclusively minority focus to a poverty focus.

The literature on cancer and SES shows that incidence and mortality rates vary by SES level, regardless of the variable used to estimate SES (16). Recent analyses of Surveillance, Epidemiology, and End Results (SEER) cancer incidence data (39) indicate that, when SES was considered, black-white incidence rate differences were eliminated for several cancer sites (breast, cervix, esophagus, male lung, pancreas, and stomach). Racial differences persisted after adjusting for SES for cancers of the bladder, prostate, uterine corpus, and multiple myeloma. A possible mediator of the relationship between SES and cancer is working conditions (16). Although several studies have investigated work-site exposures to carcinogens, only limited research has been done on how different SES groups' occupational patterns may be linked to greater risk of developing cancer (40). Baquet et al (5), in a similar analysis of black-white and SES differences in SEER cancer incidence data, found that cancer at only one site (colon) was unrelated to race. Although overall cancer incidence differentials between blacks and whites were eliminated after controlling for SES, this study found that racial differences persisted for some cancers (e.g. prostate in blacks and rectum in whites).

One phenomenon that has linked low income and multi-ethnic populations has been the relative ineffectiveness of disseminating state-of-the-art health promotion and preventive medicine technologies to these high-risk populations. To understand this phenomenon, it is necessary to determine whether the interventions developed to date are largely insensitive to the needs and problems of these different target populations, whether these populations are not involved in the design or development of the interventions, or whether these populations are simply hard to reach with respect to changing their health behaviors. Another dilemma for institutions and organizations trying to promote health in multi-ethnic communities is the relative poverty experienced in many of these communities. Combined with the limited resources of the institutions and organizations that are trying to serve the needs of these communities, severe limits are placed on which programs and promotions can be tailored.

CULTURAL DIVERSITY AND HEALTH PROMOTION

Three components of cultural factors and diversity directly impact the success or failure of health promotion strategies. These components, described individually below, are ethnic/racial group variation in disease incidence and mortality, ethnic/racial group variation in risk factor exposures, and the role of cultural factors in influencing individual, family, organizational, and institutional/community health knowledge, attitudes, and behaviors. These components are described individually below.

Culture and Variation in Disease Incidence and Mortality

Despite a 31% reduction in all-cause, US, age-adjusted death rates from 1950 to 1980 (62), the US DHHS secretary's report (28) found that virtually every major illness index varied significantly by ethnic/racial group. For example, from 1950 through 1980, black males and females had 40–70% higher age-adjusted all-cause mortality rates compared with their white counterparts. Black infants had a 62% higher death rate within the first year of life compared with white infants in 1950; by 1980, the differential had risen to 92% (62). Blacks have the highest age-adjusted mortality rates from cardiovascular disease and cancer, the number one and two killers of all Americans.

Although national data suggest large disease variation among racial/ethnic groups, local data can magnify the size of these differences. Thus, McCord & Freeman (37) reported that the life expectancy of a black male growing up in Harlem, New York, is lower than that of a male growing up in Bangladesh. After age five, the same is true for black females in Harlem compared with females in Bangladesh. The authors suggested that the US consider communities like Harlem as health crisis zones. Substantial resources need to be invested to address these pervasive health and illness problems.

With respect to cancer incidence and mortality, large ethnic group and racial variations are observed within the US for all cancers combined. SEER data from the National Cancer Institute (4) point to significant ethnic group variation in site-specific cancer incidence, mortality, and survival rates. These differences are observed among and within Latin American, Native American, and Asian American populations. For example, although New Mexican and Puerto Rican Island Latinos have 26.5% and 36.9% lower overall age-adjusted cancer incidence rates, respectively, compared with US white populations, they have 96.2% and 131.2% higher stomach cancer incidence rates and

101.1% and 105.7% higher cervical cancer incidence rates, respectively, compared with non-Latino whites.

Moreover, studies of migrants to the US among Asian and Eastern European and Caribbean groups show changes in incidence and mortality rates from those in their place of birth. For example, Warshauer et al (61) examined 1975–1979 age-adjusted stomach and colorectal cancer incidence and mortality rates among Puerto Rican-born New York City residents, Puerto Rico residents, and nonwhite and other white New York City residents. The age-adjusted 1975–1979 mortality rates were compared with age-adjusted mortality rates within New York City from 1958–1962. The age-adjusted 1975–1979 incidence rates for New York City Puerto Ricans and other whites were compared with Spanish origin and other white age-adjusted incidence rates from New Mexico (1973–1977) and Los Angeles County (1972–1977).

For colorectal cancer, a dramatic 200% increase in male mortality and a 50% increase in female mortality over a 20-year period among Puerto Rican-born New York City residents was observed. Cross-sectional incidence patterns indicated that Puerto Rican New York City rates were twice as high as the incidence rates observed in Puerto Rico, but remained one half to two thirds of those of other whites in New York City. These intermediate incidence rates were similar to those observed in New Mexico and Los Angeles. These data, like previous migration studies, pointed to the important role that dietary change may play among first-generation immigrants to the US.

Culture and Variation in Risk Factor Exposures

Risk factor exposure among different racial and ethnic groups includes personal health practices and differential exposure to environmental toxins. Black Americans have higher self-reported prevalence rates of smoking, of being 30% or more above desirable weight, and of sleeping six hours or less per night (62). Conversely, blacks are less likely to report having had five or more drinks on any day in the past year and are more likely to report being physically active than whites or other nonwhites.

With respect to cigarette smoking, although both black and white smoking prevalence rates have dropped from 43% and 40%, respectively, in 1965, to 33.5% and 28.3% in 1987, the gap in smoking prevalence has widened. Marcus & Crane (32) reviewed the literature on smoking among US Latin Americans. They noted that various studies reveal consistent gender differences in smoking prevalence relative to non-Latino whites. Latin American males have higher smoking prevalence rates than other whites and blacks, and Latino females have lower rates than the other two groups.

The likelihood of alcohol use also differs significantly across racial/ethnic subgroups. Black Americans in national survey data are least likely to report drinking, with 34% reporting abstinence from all alcohol compared with 24%

abstinence reported by whites (43). When Latin Americans are divided into two crude acculturation groups, based on the in-home use of English (more acculturated) or Spanish (less acculturated), abstinence from alcohol varies greatly. Less acculturated Latin Americans are three times more likely to report abstaining from alcohol (27%) compared with those that are more acculturated (9%).

No differences in frequency of drinking were reported across racial/ethnic groups in this study. However, both more acculturated and less acculturated Latinos reported drinking larger quantities of alcohol compared with black and Anglo-American groups, which reported similar quantities of alcohol consumption. The differences were only statistically significant for the less acculturated Latinos and were tested after adjusting for the potentially confounding effects of age, income, education, gender, marital status, place of residence, and region (43).

Ethnic group differences in patterns of cardiovascular disease and cancer morbidity and mortality have been partly attributed to differences in dietary intake. In a series of papers reviewing nutrient intakes of whites, blacks, and Mexican Americans, Newell and colleagues (14, 15, 44) have reported on nutritional component variation among these ethnic/racial groups living in the same region of East Texas. With respect to fat and fiber intake, blacks of both genders had the highest cholesterol intakes, and black males had the highest saturated fat intakes of all groups. Mexican American total fat intake was significantly lower than Anglo-Americans. Black Americans also had significantly lower mean fiber values than whites or Mexican Americans (44).

In terms of sources of fat and fiber, Mexican Americans consumed a greater percentage of their saturated fat and cholesterol intake from meats, particularly beef, organ meats, and pork, as compared with whites and blacks (14, 15). Blacks obtained a higher percentage of their saturated fat from poultry, sausage, and cold cuts than did whites or Mexican Americans. Mexican Americans obtained the largest percentage of their dietary fiber (28.8%) from legumes, followed by grains and grain products (21.2%) and vegetables (20.1%). Blacks obtained the largest percentage of their dietary fiber from grains (25.3%), followed by vegetables (22.5%) and fruits (17.2%).

Finally, the number one source of dietary fiber for Anglo-Americans was vegetables (27.2%), followed by grains (25.8%), fruits (12.2%), and mixed dishes and sandwiches (12.2%). Significant ethnic group variation in quantities consumed and sources of fats and fiber suggests that nutritional health promotion campaigns must tailor their messages to reinforce good food purchase and eating habits in contrast, or in addition, to promoting uniform recommendations for dietary change.

Cigarette smoking, alcohol consumption, and dietary intake are all complex sets of individual behaviors. However, these behaviors are reinforced by a variety of family, institutional, and community informational and motivational forces. Of particular importance to health promotion planners who try to influence risk factor prevalence is that many of these behaviors are positively supported by tobacco, alcohol, and food industry advertising campaigns that spend billions of dollars every year to promote their products, support sporting and community events, and provide budgetary support for many of the key intermediary organizations that represent the ethnic and racial groups at greatest risk of dying from preventable diseases. As we turn to how cultural factors influence the knowledge, attitudes, and behaviors of high-risk populations, we must focus on how these elements may have been, and may continue to be, used to counter health promotion campaigns.

Culture and Knowledge, Attitude, and Behavior Variation

Cigarette smoking and dietary habits have already been described as risk factors that vary markedly by racial and ethnic group. Several studies have focused on acculturation among Latin American migrant populations to the US, by relating it to cigarette smoking behavior (35, 36, 50). Marin et al (35) present the strongest data supporting the link between acculturation, as measured by English and/or Spanish language usage in various social, family, and professional settings, and adult cigarette smoking behavior. In their survey, smoking prevalence was higher among less acculturated males and higher among more acculturated females. National Health Interview Survey 1987 Data (J. F. Kerner 1991, unpublished analysis) confirmed the link between English language use (higher acculturation) and higher smoking prevalence rates among a national sample of Latina females. However, no relationship was observed between acculturation and smoking prevalence among Latino males.

Studies from the Southwest (36, 50) have not observed any consistent relationship between smoking prevalence and acculturation among predominantly Mexican American populations. Recently, Samet et al (50) reported that, although acculturation was not a predictor of smoking, like non-Latino whites and blacks, Latin Americans in the Southwest who have less education and less income are more likely to smoke and should be targeted for smoking prevention and cessation programs.

These different and contradictory findings on the links between acculturation and cigarette smoking have several possible explanations. First, measurement of acculturation through language usage may be too crude to encompass the various psychosocial dimensions that may differentiate male and female Latin American populations with respect to cigarette smoking. Marin et al (34) have identified several attitudes and expectancies about cigarette smoking that differentiated 263 Latino smokers from 150 non-Latino white smokers. Latin Americans were less likely to report smoking as relaxing than non-Latino whites. Latin Americans were more concerned about the health consequences of their smoking for their children and the consequences of their quitting, with respect to improving the health of their children. Conceivably, these and other attitudes and beliefs may be related to different aspects of acculturation for different Latin American groups.

Community and social support for English and/or Spanish language use may also vary for different regional and/or urban and rural Latin American populations. This may partly explain the regional differences observed in the aforementioned studies. Finally, acculturation needs to be linked with cigarette smoking in other immigrant populations to understand completely the relationship between acculturation and smoking cessation in adult multi-ethnic populations.

Dusenbury et al (19) have reported that the same set of predictors of adolescent smoking apply to Latin American, black, and other white populations of sixth and seventh grade students in New York City public and parochial schools. Latin American students differ somewhat from other groups in the relative importance of family smoking as a predictor of adolescent smoking. The importance of familial influences among Latino populations is consistent with a finding from Markides et al (36), which indicated that Latina girls were more likely to be influenced by the smoking behavior of their parents than were Latino boys. The influence of peer group smoking may be greater for boys.

Bettes et al (8) examined differences among black, white, Puerto Rican, and Dominican adolescents in terms of the relationship between cigarette smoking and alcohol use and psychosocial functioning. Varying relationships between psychosocial antecedents of cigarette and alcohol use were observed among different ethnic groups. For example, high negative self-esteem increased the likelihood that a Dominican adolescent would experiment with alcohol to a greater degree than adolescents from other ethnic groups. In a similar vein, preferences for risk-taking increased alcohol use among Puerto Rican and Dominican adolescents relative to blacks and Anglos. For black students, psychological well-being was observed to be a protective factor for tobacco use.

Cultural factors also influence knowledge, attitudes, and behaviors related to AIDS risk. Marin (33) has identified the need for new ways of reaching high-risk Latin American populations. Survey data on Latinos show that they are less knowledgeable than non-Latino adults about AIDS and about the prevention of HIV infection. Marin (33) notes the significance of this knowledge gap because the interviews were conducted exclusively in English. Thus, English-speaking Latino respondents, who are more likely to have been exposed to AIDS and HIV information campaigns, which are usually conducted in English, were observed to be less knowledgeable than other English-speaking groups.

Latin Americans surveyed in San Francisco demonstrated a relatively high prevalence of misconceptions about the transmission of HIV, including toilet seats, blood donation, and drinking glasses. Cultural barriers to prevention efforts stem from several factors. Many Latin American males engaging in sexual relations with other males may not consider themselves homosexual and, thus, are not reached through aggressive gay organization efforts to promote HIV protective sexual practices. Many Latin Americans have strong anti-homosexual attitudes that may prevent some men from accepting or attending to AIDS prevention information (33). Culturally inappropriate services for Latino intravenous drug users and relatively low prevalence rates of condom use, combined with an unknown frequency of using prostitutes, have all been identified as potential barriers to preventing HIV transmission among Latino populations.

Exposure to health risks among different racial and ethnic groups includes both personal health practices and differential exposure to environmental toxins. One such environmental hazard, lead poisoning, has long been associated with environmental sources, such as lead paint in homes, nearby smelters, contamination from the fumes of leaded gasolines, and direct and indirect occupational exposures (29, 31). Efforts to reduce these exposures have tended to focus on health protection measures, such as legislative and regulatory requirements to reduce the exposure levels of lead in the environment. However, anthropological studies that focus on the culturally related knowledge, attitudes, and behaviors that may be sources of lead poisoning are also important (56).

For example, in a review of the literature from various cultures worldwide, and a report of his own ethnographic survey of Mexican American populations in the lower Rio Grande Valley of Texas, Trotter (56) identified three culturally shaped sources of lead exposure in human societies: food habits, culturally defined health beliefs, and beauty practices. With respect to food habits, previous research (57, 58) on folk remedies had identified a lead oxide glazing compound, called greta, as being commonly used in two types of traditional earthenware pots (jarro and casuela), which in turn are used for cooking and serving several staples of the Mexican American diet in the area. A survey of a convenience sample of patients from three local community clinics indicated that about 27% of the households used jarros purchased in Mexico, whereas 37% used casuelas. Lead levels from .33 μg Pb/mL to 3620 μg Pb/mL were found in an analysis of the inner surfaces of a sample of pots purchased from the same market areas.

Virtually everyone interviewed was aware that the pots were a potential source of lead poisoning. Various techniques were reported to test the safety of individual pots. Tapping the pot and listening for a dull sound, smelling the pot, and looking for bubbles in glaze were all reported as techniques for differentiating low-risk from high-risk pots. Some reported a final test that either neutralized the lead poisoning threat or identified the pot as unsafe for use. This involved filling the pot with vinegar and letting it stand for a day or two. Although none of these folk tests were shown to reduce the risk from lead, they clearly reduced the fear of the risk. Supporting the continued use of these pots was a strong shared belief that food cooked in them tasted much better than food cooked in modern pots and pans.

Beyond food preparation practices, lead-laced substances are used in a wide variety of cultures as folk medicines. Among Mexican Americans, both lead oxide (greta) and lead tetroxide (azarcon) have been linked to a commonly used treatment of an intestinal folk illness called empacho. A lead-based folk remedy has also been reported to be used for colds, flu, and other ailments by Hmong refugees in Minnesota (30). Finally, Middle Eastern, Asian, and Nigerian cosmetics are described as potential sources for elevated lead levels in children.

Trotter closes by describing knowledge deficiencies, communication resistance, cultural reinterpretations, and the cultural incongruity of mainstream explanatory models as sources of resistance to reducing cultural vectors of lead poisoning. A particularly interesting observation included the herb shop owner in Mexico, whose shop stocked many lead-based folk remedies. He explained that although Anglos were particularly susceptible to lead poisoning, his people were not. Thus, these remedies remained good medicine for them, given their resistance to its toxic effects.

Health promotion programs may have to address the varying needs of multi-ethnic audiences within the relatively uniform framework of a classroom, clinic, or work site. However, culture-specific approaches must be carefully considered in these settings before implementation to avoid a patchwork quilt of program components that address no individual groups' needs comprehensively. Health promotion programs in settings with multiethnic audiences will have to address a range of knowledge, attitudes, and behaviors that have varying levels of salience for any cultural, SES, or ethnic group. As an alternative, health promotion programs can also reach out to different, but relatively homogenous, ethnic and/or racial communities. Thus, programs can be tailored to fit the specific set of social and cultural reinforcers and communication channels for that group. Although this approach potentially increases the effectiveness of promoting health among diverse target populations, it also greatly increases the costs.

INTERVENTION CHANNELS FOR HEALTH PROMOTION

Green & Kreuter (25) have defined health promotion as:

> The combination of educational and environmental supports for actions and conditions of living conducive to health. The "actions" or behavior in question may be those of individuals, groups, or communities, of policy makers, employers, teachers, or others whose actions control or influence the determinants of health (page 321).

Although all may agree that health promotion focuses on lifestyle change, two philosophical camps exist about the definition of lifestyle. For some, a lifestyle is consciously chosen individual behavior. For others, it is "a composite expression of the social and cultural environment that condition and constrain behavior, in addition to the personal decisions the individual might make in choosing one behavior over another" (25). Green & Kreuter (25) reject both the "victim-blaming" school of total personal responsibility and the "system-blaming" school that would dictate uniform health-promoting policies. Rather, they embrace a health-promotion model that centers on the many and varied communities, with their diverse organs of communication and influence, that exist within pluralistic, democratic societies. In this approach, they focus our attention on the multiple channels through which individuals, families, groups, and communities can be heard, can participate in the process of setting health priorities, and thus, can be influenced to change (e.g. increase dietary fiber) or remain the same (e.g. prevent cigarette smoking).

The multiple community channels include the various organs of the mass media, work sites, schools, religious institutions, political and community organizations, voluntary agencies, and health-care settings. If we choose any public health problem, any disease prevention effort, or any lifestyle change campaign, we will find a plethora of programs, materials, and messages that target different segments of the health information consumer marketplace. Although a variety of theoretical models are described as the underpinnings for many of these efforts, in several ways health promotion reveals a parallel with product marketing and management approaches (24). Health is "marketed" to a culturally and economically diverse audience of potential "customers." But, there is ample evidence that public health is not competing for "shelf-space" with other concerns and priorities of low-income and multi-ethnic communities; is not being culturally and reading level appropriate; or being delivered through the channels that reach the target audiences without a substantial increase in health promotion resources.

With respect to competition, health in general and any disease in particular are not necessarily high priorities for low-income populations and all cultural groups. When unemployment, inferior or inadequate housing, violence, crime, and other major community problems are competing with health, it is difficult to predict which issue or set of issues will become the rallying point for community action at any moment in time. Moreover, the disease-specific institutes of the National Institutes of Health and the disease-specific voluntary agencies are competing to promote their particular message, be it early detection of breast cancer, AIDS prevention, or hypertension control.

Thus, the meaning of health being promoted to culturally diverse and low-income communities has to be at least as confusing to the target populations as the process is to any observer of these public health initiatives.

Yet, if a free market of ideas is the framework for health promotion in a pluralistic democracy, this illness-defined approach may be necessary, if only to ensure the opportunity for different individuals, families, organizations, and communities to buy into the health issue or issues of greatest concern to them.

Clearly, the process of consuming health information and making health behavior choices also competes with the efforts of some industries (e.g. tobacco and alcohol) that spend billions to promote their products without regard for the health of their consumers. Many of these advertising campaigns focus on black media outlets. The largest group of ads in black newspapers is for cigarettes, and such magazines as *Ebony* (9% of ad pages) and *Essence* (8% of ad pages) also get their share (51).

These corporations also discovered long ago that they could attract allies and silence potential foes through their financial support of political leaders and civil rights, educational, and community organizations that represent the concerns and aspirations of low-income and multi-ethnic communities (17, 45, 49). For example, R. J. Reynolds sponsors Salem Spirit Street Scenes at black neighborhood festivals and distributes More cigarettes, which are positioned to appeal to young women. Brown & Williamson Co., previously known for supporting the Kool Jazz Festival, also sponsored Kool achiever awards for people who have improved life in the inner city (51).

Of equal concern to health-promotion advocates is the hard-to-document phenomenon of tobacco companies being long-standing supporters of such black American organizations as the United Negro College Fund and the NAACP. In 1986, the NAACP was involved with Philip Morris to lobby against clean-air laws on the grounds that such legislation discriminates against black smokers (51). Public health advocacy and health-promotion campaigns, which try to use these same channels of influence, should not be surprised if they meet resistance or apathy, because some of these leaders, institutions, and organizations may be as addicted to tobacco dollars as tobacco product users are addicted to nicotine.

If the tobacco and alcohol companies are so successful in selling their products with culturally and educationally appropriate promotional campaigns, why has it been so difficult for health promotion campaigns to reach the same low-income and culturally diverse communities with their message? First, inadequate resources are spent on formative research in these communities. Whereas national health survey data provide a gross look at cultural and income variation on a diversity of health beliefs and behaviors, national probability samples, by necessity, homogenize and severely undersample local and regional populations of interest.

Recently, the National Cancer Institute funded a three-year needs assessment study that involved the completion of 16 focus groups to develop a telephone survey instrument for 400 US-born, 400 English-speaking Caribbean-born, and 200 Creole-speaking Haitian-born blacks as well as 400 Puerto Rican, 400 Dominican, 400 Colombian, and 400 Ecuadorian Latin American New York City residents (J. F. Kerner, R01 CA53083). When the survey is completed, it will provide a major opportunity to explore how cultural diversity, in addition to SES, predicts smoking and quitting, alcohol, and cancer screening behaviors; food knowledge; and barriers to health care in a multi-ethnic community.

Second, low SES, ethnic, and low literacy populations are three major groups that are often labeled "hard-to-reach." In describing certain audiences, this term may reflect more about the frustrations of current health promotion program planners than they do about the audiences themselves. Freimuth & Mettger (21) reflect on several preconceptions about the hard-to-reach. These groups are often characterized by a sense of fatalism, poor information processing skills, limited access to communication channels, and distrust of dominant institutions.

Upon careful assessment, some of these preconceptions may indeed prove true for specific populations in relation to specific health issues. For example, if every cancer patient known to a particular low SES individual had died of the disease, fatalism about cancer might be realistic given his/her experience. However, Freimuth & Mettger suggest (21) that through more and different formative research techniques, more sophisticated population segmentation techniques, and new roles for mass media, deficits can be reframed into differences and can be addressed more creatively in health-promotion campaigns.

Schools and work sites are channels where health-promotion efforts will increasingly be reaching new and expanding audiences (25). However, one is struck by the fact that virtually all the major health-promotion campaigns through either of these channels have been carried out in relatively resource-rich environments. Major corporations have recognized the cost-effectiveness of wellness promotion in terms of reduced absenteeism and health insurance claims. They have invested heavily in these programs, thus fostering a growing wellness promotion industry.

Although some of these programs may have begun to move from the white-collar office to the blue-collar shop floor, work-site health promotion among small businesses is rare (59). Yet, small businesses represent the largest number of work settings for low-income and multi-ethnic populations. The potential of such programs may appear promising. Unfortunately, many small businesses cannot even afford health insurance for their small number of employees and would be hard pressed to make time available at work or otherwise financially support health-promotion efforts in the work site. Thus, it will likely be left to the limited resources of the public health sector to devise cost-effective strategies for promoting health in the small business community.

Some promising examples of health promotion and health education programs are being initiated in schools that serve multi-ethnic student populations (10, 11, 12, 27). However, the majority of risk factor-prevention programs have been tested in relatively homogenous, white middle-class school districts, with necessary resources available to incorporate the multiple teaching components of the best-designed programs. From an evaluation research perspective, the internal validity of the research design and the likelihood of successful implementation are much higher in these settings and make them more desirable for testing the model.

Moreover, these school settings may be the only ones with the resources to incorporate health promotion programs into their ongoing curriculum permanently. For example, numerous well-tested smoking and substance abuse, school-based, prevention programs exist in the marketplace. Unfortunately, many schools are struggling to deliver core academic curricula and address accountability issues in terms of academic criteria. They have only limited resources to devote to these health-promotion priorities, which are often relegated to the status of secondary goals or future plans in these resource-limited educational systems.

THE HEALTH-CARE SYSTEM AND HEALTH PROMOTION

The health-care system represents another potential channel for promoting health in low-income and multi-ethnic communities. As health advocates, health-care providers and institutions can protect the health of the communities they serve (47). They can use their professional expertise and institutional resources to influence policy-makers, the media (3), and community leaders to promote the health and well-being of the populations they will eventually serve as patients.

Providers and institutions can choose to focus on providing more primary care and preventive medicine services to the patients they are already serving (inreach). They can also focus these services toward reaching out to the community from where their patient populations come (6). Finally, they can invest their reputations and institutional resources to develop health-promotion programs for their patients, their employees, and their community. In so doing, health-care providers and institutions could dramatically change the view that a health-care setting is the place to go only when one is threatened by illness or expected to die.

Three sets of barriers exist for health-care settings that are considering an investment in health promotion and preventive medicine services. The first is resources. For many US publicly funded health-care settings, the challenge of making it through the periodic evaluation and accreditation process by the Joint Commission Accrediting Health-Care Organizations is a major effort and achievement. Second, although grants may exist for such programs, many of these institutions find that the grants themselves represent a mixed blessing.

Grant funds usually require the preparation of a competitive application, which in turn requires an institutional investment that may have little chance of any return (i.e. funding). If funded, the projects require staff, space, and resources. These are usually in limited supply and are hotly contested by different factions within the institution. The funding, as often as not, may be time-limited. After raising hopes and expectations, the funding ends, even if the program was judged successful. Finally, grant funds may be counted as part of the total resource base when budget cuts are forced on these publicly funded institutions. Because the grant programs are usually immune from these "hard-money" cuts, the institution is forced to make even larger cuts from the nongrant-supported programs to achieve the percentage reduction targeted for the overall institutional resource base.

The second barrier is leadership from within the health-care setting. In a 1986 survey of 732 Canadian hospitals, the lack of a leader to implement health-promotion programs was named as the third most frequent barrier by the hospitals chief executive officers (6). Inadequate funding and staff support were the two most frequent barriers. Even clinical prevention programs may have some difficulty being successfully implemented in resource-limited health-care settings. These programs address persons identified to be at risk for particular health problems. Thus, specific clinical services (e.g. genetic counseling, prenatal care, screening for curable disease) can be delivered to the highest risk populations who need them most. Yet, even where low-income populations are regular users of the health-care system, opportunities to prevent illness or detect it in a potentially curable stage of development are missed repeatedly (22).

The third barrier is based on the interaction between two factors: the unwillingness of many low-income and multi-ethnic populations to make use of their health-care facilities until absolutely necessary, and the variable quality of the clinical services provided in these community-based health-care settings. Access to services and their use, of course, is partly defined by insurance status.

Uninsured Latin Americans are less likely than those insured to have a regular source of medical care (55). They are less likely to have seen a physician in the past year, and they are less likely to report their health status as good or excellent. Moreover, among those without health insurance, Mexican Americans were three times more likely than Puerto Ricans and almost four times more likely than Cuban Americans to report never having had a physical examination. Physician involvement with uninsured patients is estimated to be well below the proportion of the general population that is uninsured, and this varies considerably by specialty (9).

When low-income and ethnically diverse patients do receive care, what does the health-care system say to them? "When I went into the system [with a cancer symptom] I knew I was poor, but then the system made me feel poor." This quotation was typical of the experiences reported by cancer patients and their families in a series of national hearings held by the ACS in 1989 (2). Biopsy appointments canceled by the providers, clinical follow-up scheduled three or more weeks after a sign or symptom of cancer is detected, onerous financial and medical clearances for diagnostic and treatment procedures, and the inability to communicate with the provider are all significant barriers. These quality-of-care barriers are all too common in the health-care systems that serve low-income and culturally diverse populations.

From the provider's perspective, a survey of family practice residents regarding health care and poor patients indicated that a majority of residents (73%) believed that poor patients are more likely than others to miss appointments, are more likely to be late for appointments (51%), and are less knowledgeable about their illnesses (80%) (48). One in four residents believed that poor patients did not appreciate the work of their physicians and nurses, and 43% claimed that the poor are more difficult patients. Finally, 72% indicated that the poor are unlikely to practice preventive health behaviors or comply with their medical regimens (60%); 41% indicated that poor people care less than others about their health.

Low SES and ethnically diverse patients see the health-care system as cold, unfriendly, and insensitive to their particular cultural needs. Providers view these patients as noncompliant and unappreciative. Given these conditions, the prospects for promoting health to populations within or outside these institutions would appear dim. Yet, low-income patients, in particular, view physicians and health-care professionals as one of their most valued sources of health information (E. Calle 1989 unpublished presentation).

For example, women with a regular provider are more likely to have had a mammogram in the past year than women without a regular provider. The most frequently stated reason for never having had a mammogram is that the physician never recommended it (42). The solutions for promoting health through health-care settings center on providing better quality and more culturally sensitive health care and health information to those populations already being served (inreach). In addition, support for more primary care providers is required. Reformulating the community's image of its health-care settings can be achieved by directing new and expanded resources toward community-based health promotion programs, either centered in or associated with the community-based health-care settings.

SUMMARY AND SOLUTIONS

The issues that must be addressed, if we are to succeed in promoting health in low-income and culturally diverse multi-ethnic communities, can be summarized by three words: resources, strategy, and cooperation. In terms of resources, as poverty and cultural diversity increase, the need for additional resources to address growing gaps in the health status of different Americans will also grow. For example, with or without a more comprehensive federal approach to health-care financing, access to health-care services will continue to depend on the public health resources of state and local governments (52), which may choose to invest in primary care programs for the poor or other medically underserved ethnic groups. But even when they do, only a relatively small percentage of the needs in medically underserved areas, or counties designated as health manpower shortage areas, can be met (7).

New federal resources will be required. Three approaches can be taken to a renewed investment in the health and well-being of all Americans. First, we can simply increase the amounts spent through the existing networks of federal health programs. However, as we have noted above, many of the existing programs fail to address the numerous barriers to preventing disease and promoting health in low-income and culturally diverse communities. Second, we can invest heavily in understanding the diversity of needs and resources within these communities and make new efforts to tailor programs to meet these many and varied needs. This will require the support and involvement of existing community resources, in culturally sensitive and community-approved programs, which will vary from one community to another.

Third, it may be necessary, in our most economically depressed areas, to recognize that even more may be accomplished if health promotion and disease prevention are linked to educational opportunity, housing development, economic development, and community-based crime control programs. Human health is often highly dependent on community health, as measured by good housing, safe streets, and good jobs. We will continue to limit our abilities to make a difference and convince the communities that we are serious about change until we address this reality. Whatever path we take, equity of health status may not be a realistic goal for most health-promotion programs. Until sufficient resources are invested to achieve equal opportunity to achieve good health, health status equity will remain an enlightened fantasy.

Turning to strategies, two types of problems face health-promotion programs trying to be sensitive and appropriate to multi-ethnic and diverse SES communities. First, the information we have on the health priorities of different ethnic and SES groups is extremely limited. National data collection initiatives tend to homogenize groups. For example, national programs developed for Latin Americans may or may not be relevant to the many and varied Latino immigrant groups living in the US. For Asian Americans, this lack of data is an even more formidable barrier.

Second, if and when such data do lead to a better understanding of ethnic and SES group differences, we face a different problem. We can choose to deliver health promotion interventions in settings (e.g. schools, work sites, clinics) where culturally diverse groups share the same resources. Or, we may choose to reach out to different and culturally homogenous communities by tailoring the programs to meet the needs of that particular ethnic community.

Do we invest our limited health promotion resources in developing multicultural health education and promotion programs that create a menu of integrated opportunities for health behavior change? If so, different groups may focus on those components and messages that are of particular relevance to them. Or, do we begin to develop different health promotion modules targeted at specific ethnic, racial, or SES groups? Each group would then have its own set of programs, particularly relevant to its needs. With sufficient resources, components of both approaches would be ideal. The former strategy might best be conducted at the national level, whereas state and local resources could be better directed to developing programs tailored to the needs of their own particular high-risk populations.

Finally, in terms of cooperation, we have emphasized the importance of cultural sensitivity and community ownership of health promotion programs. Health promotion programs in multi-ethnic groups face numerous potential barriers (46), including inappropriate language, role models, and messages for a particular group. For written materials, reading level is frequently too difficult in medically underserved communities. Given overwhelming social and political needs, health promotion may seem irrelevant or secondary. The community may perceive themselves as powerless. Specific cultural practices or factors may complicate attempts at health promotion. Finally, there are potential philosophical barriers relating to the individual's right to control his/her own destiny, as well as the potential for distrust of the medical or government establishment. For example, many members of the black community cite the Tuskegee syphilis study of the 1930s as reason for continued distrust of the federal public health establishment (53).

Although the community must be involved in developing health promotion programs to overcome these potential barriers, the health professional also has an important role in determining health promotion priorities. Indeed, although the community must be involved in identifying needs and developing health promotion interventions, the health professional brings a theoretical orientation as well as a wealth of empirical experience to expedite program development. In the field of smoking and drug abuse prevention, for example, there is an abundance of evidence that scare tactics are not effective (26).

Nevertheless, scare tactics do have intuitive appeal. It has been common in our experience for community groups to propose scare tactics as an intervention. The health professional can help to shape and direct interventions from the standpoint of prevention theory and technology.

Ultimately, a cooperative partnership must be forged between the health professional and the community. Both bring essential expertise to the development of effective health promotion programs in multi-ethnic communities. What must be achieved is a respectful collaboration between the two, where the contribution of each is viewed as necessary, but not sufficient.

ACKNOWLEDGMENTS

The authors would like to express their deep appreciation to Ms. Kathleen Cagney, Community Program Analyst, Division of Cancer Control, Memorial Sloan-Kettering Cancer Center, for her assistance in identifying the literature for the review and for copy editing the manuscript.

Literature Cited

1. Black, D., Morris, J. N., Smith, C., Townsend, P. 1985. *Inequalities in Health: The Black Report*. Harmondsworth, England: Penguin
2. Am. Cancer Soc. 1989. Cancer and the poor: a report to the nation. Findings of regional hearings conducted by the Am. Cancer Soc.
3. Arkin, E. B. 1990. Opportunities for improving the nation's health through collaboration with the mass media. *Public Health Rep*. 105(3):219–23
4. Baquet, C. R., Ringen, K., Pollack, E. S., Young, J. L., Horm, J. W., et al. 1986. Cancer among Blacks and other minorities: statistical profiles. Bethesda, Md: Natl. Cancer Inst. NIH Publ. No. 86-2785
5. Baquet, C. R., Horm, J. W., Gibbs, T., Greenwald, P. 1991. Socioeconomic factors and cancer incidence among Blacks and Whites. *J. Natl. Cancer Inst*. 83(8):551–57
6. Baskerville, B., LeTouzé, D. 1990. Facilitating the involvement of Canadian health care facilities in health promotion. *Patient Educ. Couns*. 15(2): 113–25
7. Begley, C. E., Aday, L. U., McCandless, R. 1989. Evaluation of a primary health care program for the poor. *J. Community Health* 14(2):107–20
8. Bettes, B. A., Dusenbury, L., Kerner, J., James-Ortiz, S., Botvin, G. J. 1990. Ethnicity and psychosocial factors in alcohol and tobacco use in adolescence. *Child Dev*. 61:557–65
9. Blumenthal, D., Rizzo, J. A. 1991. Who cares for uninsured persons? A study of physicians and their patients who lack health insurance. *Med. Care* 29(6):502–20
10. Botvin, G. J., Batson, H., Witis-Vitale, S., Beri, V., Baker, E., Dusenbury, L. 1989. A psychosocial approach to smoking prevention for urban black youth. *Public Health Rep*. 104:573–82
11. Botvin, G. J., Dusenbury, L., Baker, E., James-Ortiz, S., Botvin, E. M., Kerner, J. F. 1992. Smoking prevention among urban minority youth: assessing effects on outcome and mediating variables. Health Psychol. 11(5):In press
12. Botvin, G. J., Dusenbury, L., Baker, E., James-Ortiz, S., Kerner, J. F. 1989. Skills training approach to smoking prevention among Hispanic youth. *J. Behav. Med*. 12:279–96
13. Brown, J. L., Gershoff, S. N. 1989. The paradox of hunger and economic prosperity in America. *J. Public Health Policy* 10(4):425–43
14. Borrud, L. G., McPherson, R. S., Nichaman, M. Z., Pillow, P. C., Newell, G. R. 1989. Development of a food frequency instrument: ethnic differences in food sources. Nut. & Ca. 12(3):201–11
15. Borrud, L. G., Pillow, P. C., Allen, P. K., McPherson, R. S., Nichaman,

M. Z., Newell, G. R. 1989. Food group contributions to nutrient intake in whites, blacks, and Mexican Americans in Texas. *J. Am. Diet. Assoc.* 89(8):1061–69
16. Can. Cancer Soc. 1991. Report from the panel on cancer and the disadvantaged.
17. Coughlin, D. 1992. Smoking guns. Black reps are high on funding from tobacco and alcohol PACs. *Village Voice*. Apr. 21: Metro 1
18. Devesa, S. S., Diamond, E. L. 1983. Socioeconomic and radial differences in lung cancer incidence. *Am. J. Epidemiol* 118(6):818–31
19. Dusenbury, L., Kerner, J. F., Baker, E., Botvin, G., James-Ortiz, S., Zauber, A. 1992. Predictors of smoking prevalance among New York latino youth. *Am. J. Public Health* 82(1):55–58
20. Freeman, H. P. 1991. Race, poverty and cancer (editorial). *J. Natl. Cancer Inst.* 83:526–27
21. Freimuth, V. S., Mettger, W. 1990. Is there a hard-to-reach audience? *Public Health Rep.* 105(3):232–39
22. Fruchter, R. G., Boyce, J., Hunt, M. 1980. Missed opportunities for early diagnosis of cancer of the cervix. *Am. J. Public Health* 70:418–20
23. Funch, D. P. 1985. *A report on cancer survival in the economically disadvantaged.* Prepared for Am. Cancer Soc. subcomm. of health care of econ. disadvantaged patients
24. Grace, V. L. 1991. The marketing of empowerment and the construction of the health consumer: a critique of health promotion. *Int. J. Health Serv.* 21(2): 329–43
25. Green, L. W., Kreuter, M. W. 1990. Health promotion as a public health strategy for the 1990s. *Annu. Rev. Public Health* 11:319–34
26. Goodstadt, M. S. 1974. Myths and methodology in drug education: a critical review of the research evidence. In *Research on Methods and Programs of Drug Education,* ed. M. S. Goodstadt. Toronto: Addic. Res. Found.
27. Harris, M. B., Davis, S. M., Ford, V. L., Tso, H. 1988. The checkerboard cardiovascular curriculum: a culturally oriented program. *J. School Health* 58(3):104–7
28. Heckler, M. M. 1985. *Report of the secretary's task force on black and minority health, executive summary.* Washington, DC: USDHHS
29. Landrigan, P. J. 1982. Occupational and community exposures to toxic metals: cadmium, mercury, and arsenic. *West J. Med.* 137:531–39
30. Levitt, C., Duvall, K., Godes, J., Dean, A. G., Roberts, J., Egenberger, J. 1983. Folk remedy-associated lead poisoning in Hmong children-Minnesota. *Morbid. Mortal. Wkly. Rep.* 32(42):555–56
31. Mahaffey, K. R. 1983. Sources of lead in the urban environment. *Am. J. Public Health* 73(12):1357–58
32. Marcus, A. C., Crane, L. A. 1985. Smoking behavior among US latinos: an emerging challenge for public health. (commentary) *Am. J. Public Health* 75:169–72
33. Marin, G. 1989. AIDS prevention among Hispanics: needs, risk behaviors, and cultural values. *Public Health Rep.* 104(5):411–15
34. Marin, G., Marin, B. V., Perez-Stable, E. J., Sabogal, F., Otero-Sabogal, R. 1990. Cultural differences in attitudes and expectancies between Hispanic and non-Hispanic white smokers. *Hisp. J. Behav. Sci.* 12(4):422–36
35. Marin, G., Perez-Stable, E. J., Marin, B. V. 1989. Cigarette smoking among San Francisco Hispanics: the role of acculturation and gender. *Am. J. Public Health* 79:196–98
36. Markides, K. S., Coreil, J., Ray, L. A. 1987. Smoking among Mexican Americans: a three-generation study. *Am. J. Public Health* 77(6): 708–11
37. McCord, C., Freeman, H. P. 1990. Excess mortality in Harlem. *N. Engl. J. Med.* 322(3):173–77
38. McGrath, J. C. 1991. Evaluating national health communication campaigns: formative and summative research issues. *Am. Behav. Sci.* 34 (6):652–65
39. McWhorter, W. P., Schatzkin, A. G., Horm, J. W., Brown, C. C. 1989. Contribution of socioeconomic status to Black/White difference in cancer incidence. *Cancer* 63(5):982–87
40. Michaels, D. 1983. Occupational cancer in the black population: the health effects of job discrimination. *J. Natl. Med. Assoc.* 75(10):1014–18
41. Deleted in proof
42. Natl. Health Interview Survey. 1988. Provisional estimates from the national health interview survey: supplement on cancer control—United States, 1987. *Morbid. Mortal. Wkly. Rep.* 37:418–19
43. Neff, J. A. 1986. Alcohol consumption and psychological distress among US

anglos, hispanics and blacks. *Alcohol Alcohol.* 21(1):111–19
44. Newell, G. R., Borrud, L. G., McPherson, R. S., Nichaman, M. Z., Pillow, P. C. 1988. Nutrient intakes of whites, blacks, and Mexican Americans in southeast Texas. *Prev. Med.* 17:622–33
45. Novak, V. 1989. Courting black power. *Common Cause Mag.* Mar/Apr:17–22
46. Orlandi, M. 1986. Community-based substance abuse prevention programs: a multi-cultural perspective. *J. School Health* 56(9):394–401
47. Pineault, R., Baskerville, B., LeTouzé, D. 1990. Health promotion activities in Quebec hospitals: a comparison of DSC and non-DSC hospitals. *Can. J. Public Health* 81(3):199–203
48. Price, J. H., Desmond, S. M., Snyder, F. F., Kimmel, S. R. 1988. Perceptions of family practice residents regarding health care and poor patients. *J. Fam. Pract.* 27(6):615–21
49. Raspberry, W. 1990. The black community and the tobacco problem. *Daily News.* Jan. 30:26
50. Samet. J. M., Howard, C. A., Coultas, D. B., Skipper, B. J. 1992. Acculturation, education, and income as determinants of cigarette smoking in New Mexico Hispanics. *Cancer Epidemiol. Biomark. Prev.* 1:235–40
51. Schultz, E. 1987. Where there's smoke . . . a campaign by cigarette makers to woo black smokers has sparked a heated debate. *Adweek* Apr. 6:32, 34
52. Sundwall, D. N., Tavani, C. 1991. The role of public health in providing primary care for the medically underserved. *Public Health Rep.* 106 (1):2–5
53. Thomas, S. B., Quinn, S. C. 1991. Public health then & now: the Tuskegee syphilis study, 1932 to 1972. *Am. J. Public Health* 81(11): 1498–1505
54. Tomatis, L. 1992. Poverty and cancer (editorial). *Cancer Epidemiol. Biomark. Prev.* 1:167–75
55. Treviño, F. M., Moyer, M. E., Valdez, R. B., Stroup-Benham, C. A. 1991. Health insurance coverage and utilization of health services by Mexican Americans, mainland Puerto Ricans, and Cuban Americans. *J. Am. Med. Assoc.* 265(2):233–37
56. Trotter, R. T. II. 1990. The cultural parameters of lead poisoning: a medical anthropologist's view of intervention in environmental lead exposure. *Environ. Health Persp.* 89:79–84
57. Trotter, R. T. II, Ackerman, A., Rodman, D., Martinez,, D. Sorvillo, F. 1983. Azarcon and greta: ethnomedical solution to an epidemiological mystery. *Med. Anthropol. Q.* 14(3):3–18
58. Trotter, R. T. II. 1985. Greta and azaracon: a survey of episodic lead poisoning from a folk remedy. *Hum. Org.* 44:64–72
59. Yenney, S. L. 1984. Small businesses and health promotion: the prospects look good. Off. of Dis. Prev. Health Promot., Public Health Serv., US Dep. Health Hum. Serv., pp. 35
60. Wallack, L., Winkleby, M. 1987. Primary prevention: a new look at basic concepts. *Soc. Sci. Med.* 25(8): 923–30
61. Warshauer, M. E., Silverman, D. T., Schottenfeld, D., Pollack, E. S. 1986. Stomach and colorectal cancers in Puerto Rican-born residents of New York City. *J. Natl. Cancer Inst.* 76(4):591–95
62. US Bur. of Census. 1990. *Statistical Abstract of the United States 1990.* Washington, DC. 991 pp. 110th ed.

Annu. Rev. Publ. Health. 1993. 14:379–411

A REVIEW OF SMOKING IN PREGNANCY: Effects on Pregnancy Outcomes and Cessation Efforts[1]

R. Louise Floyd
Prenatal Smoking Cessation Program, Program Services and Development Branch, Division of Reproductive Health, National Center for Chronic Disease Prevention and Health Promotion, Centers for Disease Control, Atlanta, Georgia 30333

Barbara K. Rimer
Cancer Control Research Program, Duke Comprehensive Cancer Center, Duke University Medical Center, Durham, North Carolina 27710

Gary A. Giovino
Epidemiology Branch, Office on Smoking and Health, National Center for Chronic Disease Prevention and Health Promotion, Centers for Disease Control, Atlanta, Georgia 30333

Patricia D. Mullen
School of Public Health, University of Texas, Houston, Texas 77225

Susan E. Sullivan
Cancer Control Research Program, Duke Comprehensive Cancer Center, Duke University Medical Center, Durham, North Carolina 27710

KEY WORDS: prenatal, substance use, interventions

INTRODUCTION

Prenatal smoking has become one of the most-studied risk factors in contemporary obstetrics. Kramer's (53) recent meta-analysis of determinants of low birthweight identified 121 studies published during the 1970s and early

1980s that dealt with smoking during pregnancy. Interest in this subject began in 1957, when Simpson (87) reported a significantly lower birthweight for infants born to mothers who smoked than for those born to mothers who did not. Since then, findings from case-control epidemiologic studies have consistently shown an association between smoking and a 150–250 g reduction in birthweight (88), with strong evidence of a dose response relationship (63). In the past 20 years, research has also brought to light additional smoking-related reproductive risks (32).

Table 1 Pregnancy-related cigarette smoking behaviors—United States, 1985 and 1990[a]

	Smoked during the 12 months before the birth		Quit after learning of pregnancy		Smoked after learning of pregnancy	
	1985 (%)	1990 (%)	1985 (%)	1990 (%)	1985 (%)	1990 (%)
All women[b]	31.8	23.7	21.2	22.6	25.1	18.3
18–24 years	40.1	29.3	21.1	23.4	31.6	22.4
25–29 years	34.4	25.7	23.6	26.3	26.3	18.9
30–34 years	24.3	21.1	18.9	19.4	19.7	17.0
35–44 years	23.4	17.7	16.7	17.4	19.5	14.6
Education						
Less than 12 years	46.0	35.5	14.8	13.5	39.2	30.7
12 years	35.8	28.1	20.2	24.2	28.6	21.3
13–15 years	24.0	19.7	29.4	28.3	16.9	14.1
16 years or more	13.4	7.8	37.5	32.2	8.4	5.3
Race						
White	33.2	25.3	21.7	22.3	26.0	19.7
Black	27.5	19.0	17.9	25.8	22.6	14.1
Hispanic origin						
Hispanic	16.8	12.1	38.9*	34.1*	10.3	8.0
Non-Hispanic	33.4	25.5	20.4	21.9	26.6	19.9
Marital status						
Currently married	29.8	21.2	22.5	24.0	23.1	16.1
Formerly married	40.1	36.9	14.3*	18.8	34.4	30.0
Never married	41.0	31.4	19.2	19.7	33.1	25.2

[a] Percent of US women 18–44 years of age who had given birth to a child within the past five years who reported having smoked cigarettes at any time in the 12 months preceding the birth. Of these, the percent who quit smoking after learning they had become pregnant and the percent who smoked at all after learning they had become pregnant are listed. Data were collected by the 1985 and 1990 National Health Interview Surveys. Source: CDC, unpublished data.

[b] Includes women with unknown sociodemographic characteristics.

*Figure does not meet standards of reliability or precision (more than 30% relative standard error in numerator of percent).

Note: Denominator for each cell excludes unknown.

Despite the volume of evidence amassed over the years that clearly shows the harmful effects of smoking during pregnancy (47), about one of five pregnant women continue to smoke (Table 1; 78). Prenatal smoking cessation could make significant contributions to the improvement of maternal and infant health (50) and could save the health-care system millions of dollars (58). Smoking abstinence during pregnancy appears in *Healthy People 2000* (91) as one of six key maternal and infant health risk reduction objectives, having a national goal of 90% abstinence by the year 2000.

This article provides an overview of the problems related to smoking during pregnancy and a discussion of the research trials conducted to promote prenatal smoking cessation. We pay particular attention to intervention approaches, emerging issues, and implications for policy and practice.

MAJOR HEALTH EFFECTS OF PRENATAL AND POSTNATAL SMOKING

The results of well-designed epidemiologic studies leave little doubt that smoking during pregnancy exerts an independent, adverse effect upon numerous reproductive outcomes. Reported relative risks of spontaneous abortion among pregnant smokers ranges from 1.1 to 1.8, depending upon the amount of smoking (45, 51, 81). Reported relative risks for other complications among women who smoke at least one pack of cigarettes a day include 2.0 for placenta previa, 1.8 for abruptio placenta, and 1.6 for bleeding during pregnancy. Although lower risks are reported for women who smoke less than one pack per day, these risks are still higher than those of the same complications among nonsmokers (59).

Low Birthweight and Intrauterine Growth Retardation

Of primary interest is a twofold increase in the risk among smokers of having an infant born weighing less than 2500 g (92). This lower birthweight primarily results from intrauterine growth retardation (IUGR), observable at all gestational ages. Estimates of the relative risk for IUGR among women who smoke range from 2.41 to 4.0 (53, 93). The IUGR associated with prenatal smoking is characterized by decreased biparietal diameter, decreased crown-to-heel length, and decreased chest and shoulder circumferences (64). Murphy et al (68) found that fetal biparietal diameter measurements are significantly lower from 21 weeks' gestation onward among women who are smokers than among women who are nonsmokers. Early onset of IUGR with normal proportioning and overall decreases in weight and length is consistent with symmetrical IUGR, which is characterized by consistent suboptimal growth (2). Studies of cessation patterns show that if a woman quits smoking early in pregnancy (before the sixteenth week), her chances of having a low birthweight baby are similar to that of a nonsmoker (10). Women who quit later in pregnancy continue to be at higher risk of having a low birthweight baby than women who have never smoked (93). Another study found the disparity in biparietal growth to be more pronounced in the last trimester (75). This effect is consistent with asymmetrical IUGR or rapid slowing of growth near term (2). Considered as a whole, research findings suggest that the IUGR associated with smoking is symmetrical, but aspects of asymmetrical IUGR have been documented among some infants born to smokers.

Low Birthweight and Preterm Delivery

Preterm delivery accounts for some of the low birthweight associated with smoking, but its significance is much less than that of IUGR. Kramer's (53) meta-analysis identified seven studies that addressed the effect of smoking on gestational age. Two studies found significant associations, but the effect was small (i.e. a reduction of 3.5 days). When data from four of the studies were combined, a calculated relative risk emerged of 1.41. Another study from the National Institute of Child Health and Human Development found a significant effect of smoking on preterm births. The study also found the most significant association among infants whose gestational age was less than 33 weeks (86).

Infant Respiratory Infections and Postnatal Smoking

With regard to the health effects of passive smoke exposure of the infant, numerous studies have documented the increased rates of respiratory infections, including pneumonia, bronchitis, tracheitis, laryngitis, and otitis media (20, 94). Rates of hospitalizations for these conditions are three times higher than for infants of nonsmokers (44). Several studies have documented the increased rates of Sudden Infant Death Syndrome (SIDS) among women who smoked during pregnancy (92); more recent studies have reported up to a twofold increase (43). The mechanism of this effect is not well understood, and the relative contribution of prenatal versus postnatal exposure is unclear.

SCOPE OF THE PROBLEM

Since 1965, cigarette smoking prevalence has declined substantially among women of reproductive age (WRA), or women 18–44 years old. In 1965, 38% of women 18–24 years old, 44% of those 25–34 years old, and 44% of those 35–44 years old smoked cigarettes. In 1990, prevalence was 23%, 28%, and 25% in each respective age category (69), and 26% of WRA overall (11).

The average number of cigarettes smoked each day by WRA increases as age increases (14 cigarettes per day for 18–24-year-olds, 16 cigarettes per day for 25–34-year-olds, and 19 cigarettes per day for 35–44-year-olds) (11).

Heavier smoking among older WRA smokers has also been reported elsewhere (12).

Smoking Prevalence and Race

In 1987 and 1988, cigarette smoking prevalence among WRA overall was 30% for whites, 31% for blacks, 9% for Asians, and 36% for Native Americans. Among Hispanics and non-Hispanics, prevalence was 20% and 30%, respectively (13). The rate of decline has been especially high in black women aged 18–24 years, for whom prevalence was 37% in 1965 and 10% in 1990 (69). In 1990, prevalence among black and white women was lower in the 18–24-year-old category (10% for blacks, 25% for whites), was about 29% for both races in the 25–34-year-old category, and was higher for blacks in the 35–44-year-old category (36% for blacks, 25% for whites) (69).

Smoking Prevalence and Women's Education

Prevalence of smoking decreases as women's education increases. The 1989 Behavioral Risk Factor Surveillance System generated standardized (by age and race) prevalence estimates for WRA: 44% of those with less than a high school education, 33% of those with a high school diploma, and 19% of those with at least some college were smokers (12).

Smoking Initiation Among Young Teenaged Women

Smoking initiation by young women is an important health concern in general, as well as a future reproductive risk factor for this population. Among female high school seniors, the percentage who smoked an average of at least one cigarette a day declined for all subgroups between 1976–1979 and 1980–1984 (4). For most subgroups, however, the decline has slowed in recent years. Among black females, a sharp decline continued throughout the 1980s. In general, the rate of decline has been less substantial among white females than among their nonwhite counterparts. Prevalence of daily smoking from 1985 to 1989 among female high school seniors was 34% among Native Americans, 23% among whites, 13% among Puerto Ricans and Latin Americans, 9% among Asians, 8% among Mexican Americans, and 7% among blacks. Data from the 1989 Teenage Attitudes and Practices Survey, a household survey of youths aged 12–18 years, indicate that, among young women, 17% of whites, 12% of Hispanics, and 5% of blacks smoked during the 30 days preceding the survey (14). In addition, a national survey of the nation's high school students showed a similar pattern: Among female students, smoking prevalence was highest in whites, intermediate in Hispanics, and lowest in blacks (15).

Smoking Prevalence Among Pregnant Women

The descriptive epidemiology of smoking is similar for WRA and pregnant women. The limited data available from pregnant women suggest that cigarette smoking among this group has decreased in recent years. Among married women aged 20 years and older who had a live-birth in 1967, 40% of whites and 33% of blacks reported smoking during their pregnancy. In 1980, 25% of white mothers and 23% of black mothers (20–44 years old) reported smoking during their pregnancy (49). The smoking rate did not decrease for white or black teenaged mothers during the same time frame. In 1985, 25% of women who had given birth during the previous five years reported that they had smoked after pregnancy was confirmed; in 1990, 18% of such women reported smoking (Table 1). Birth certificate data from 43 states and the District of Columbia indicated that 20% of mothers who gave birth in 1989 reported that they had smoked during their pregnancy (16). Other survey data show that 18% of pregnant women reported that they were smokers at the time of their 1989 interview (12).

Smoking prevalence during pregnancy decreases as maternal age and education increases (Table 1) (49, 89) and increases as birth order increases (89). Unmarried women are more likely to smoke while pregnant than are married women (Table 1) (89). Smoking prevalence is lower among young black mothers than among older black mothers and young white mothers (70). For all age groups, cigarette smoking prevalence during pregnancy is slightly higher among whites than among blacks (Table 1) (16). Prevalence is lower among Hispanic than non-Hispanic women (Table 1) (16). Women who drink during their pregnancy (78) and low-income women (28) are more likely to smoke during pregnancy.

Among WRA, regardless of marital status, about 25% of mothers who smoke before learning that they are pregnant quit smoking shortly after learning of the pregnancy (Table 1) (30). Among white women aged 20–44 years, another 12% stop smoking later during the pregnancy (30). The likelihood of quitting increases as education increases (Table 1) (30); the likelihood of quitting is lower for heavier smokers than for light smokers (30).

Among those who quit smoking upon learning that they are pregnant (spontaneous quitters), 21–35% may relapse before the end of their pregnancy. Maintenance of cessation in this group is associated with higher self-efficacy, stronger belief in the harmful effect of maternal smoking, primigravida status, and greater frequency of nausea (80). One encouraging study documented a cessation maintenance rate of 37% at six months' postpartum in a group of women receiving care through a health maintenance organization (HMO) (67). Overall, about 70% of women who quite smoking during pregnancy relapse within one year of delivery, and the relapse appears to be independent of the mother's education level (30). Risks to both mother and infant (as well as the continued prevalence of smoking during pregnancy) point to the need to identify effective behavioral interventions aimed at cessation. Maintaining cessation during pregnancy is as important among spontaneous quitters as is maintaining cessation after delivery among all who have quit. Insights into the reasons why women continue to smoke during and after pregnancy may be gained by understanding the reasons why women begin to smoke initially.

Beliefs About the Health Effects of Smoking During Pregnancy

Several studies have addressed the beliefs about the health effects of cigarette smoking during pregnancy. In 1985, 75% of US WRA responded that cigarette smoking during pregnancy increased the risk of a miscarriage, 68% replied that it increased the risk of a stillbirth, 76% responded that it increased the risk of premature birth, and 85% stated that it increased the risk of a low birthweight baby (33). The perception of risk increases with increasing education, both overall and for current smokers only (11, 17).

WHY WOMEN SMOKE

Women began to smoke more openly during World War II and increased their smoking through the 1960s (72). The increase in smoking prevalence paralleled the expansion of women's professional roles and their growing independence. When smoking was considered socially unacceptable for women, rates for men and women were more divergent (100). Thus, social disapproval may have inhibited women's smoking for at least the first third of the twentieth century. Fueled by, or perhaps fueling, the growing acceptance of smoking by women were media and marketing ads designed by the cigarette companies to appeal to women (27, 29, 41, 72).

Smoking to Relieve Stress

The increasing stress of women's multiple roles may have encouraged women to use smoking as a coping mechanism. Biener et al (8) found that, after controlling for age, women who reported that they had high-stress jobs were more likely to be smokers than those who reported that they had low-stress jobs. Pederson & Stavraky (74) suggested that both high and low levels of emancipation may be stressful for women and therefore related to smoking behavior. For women with children, smoking may be perceived as a way of coping with the demands of their children. One qualitative study found smoking was one of the most often identified strategies for coping with children (36). Biener (7) presents some evidence that female adolescents perceive smokers as more socially skilled, self-confident, and outgoing than those who do not smoke. This finding may partly explain the motivation for smoking initiation in this age group.

Smoking Because of Addiction

Both men and women smoke, in large part, because they are addicted to nicotine (95). However, evidence suggests that women derive important benefits from smoking that would be expected to continue during pregnancy. Some studies suggest that women use smoking to reduce anxiety and negative affect, to enhance pleasure, and to relax (7, 56, 85, 92, 100).

Smoking to Control Weight

Perhaps the most pervasive benefit that women perceive of smoking is its use in controlling weight (38, 41, 77). Tobacco use is inversely related to body weight, and many women smoke to control weight (7, 39, 41, 100). Concern over body weight and controlling it through cigarette smoking has long been an issue for women. The cigarette companies recognized this concern as early as 1928, when they urged female smokers to "reach for a Lucky instead" (of a sweet) (29, 38).

Smoking to Combat Depression

Two studies that investigated the relationship between smoking and depression are especially relevant. Frerichs et al (34) examined data from a large cross-sectional study in Los Angeles County. They conducted multivariate analyses and found that smoking and depression were not significantly related. However, in a more recent analysis using National Health and Nutrition Examination Survey (NHANES I) and Epidemiologic Follow-Up Study (NHEFS) data, Anda and associates (3) found that depressed smokers were 40% less likely than nondepressed smokers to have quit smoking. In neither study did gender differences hold up after completion of multivariate analyses. In view of the higher prevalence of depression among women, researchers must gain a better understanding of the role depression may play in smoking initiation, maintenance, and cessation.

Gender Differences in Quitting Behavior

Some studies have explored gender differences in quitting behavior. One study concluded that, compared with men, women are less interested in quitting and less persistent in their attempts to quit (9); another found women to be less successful in quitting than men (31). However, studies investigating gender differences in cessation have not always controlled for use of other forms of tobacco, such as smokeless tobacco, cigars, and pipe smoking. After controlling for all forms of tobacco use, differences in quit ratios between men and women are negligible (93).

Other Reasons for Smoking Behavior

Despite the above research, much remains unexplained as to why, in the face of clear evidence about the health risks, women continue to smoke during pregnancy. One study showed an association between smoking and the level of personalized beliefs regarding potential risks (6). Kruse et al (54) documented the importance of adverse health outcomes as a motivation for quitting. O'Campo et al (71) interviewed 847 women to assess their beliefs before, during, and after pregnancy. The most frequently mentioned reasons for quitting before or during pregnancy were fear of adverse pregnancy outcome and infant health problems (75%), advice from family or physician (8%), and illness or nausea from smoking (6%). Research from McBride & Pirie (60) provides additional support that physiological experiences during pregnancy affect smoking. In their study, women who had quit experienced morning sickness longer during pregnancy than those who had not quit. In one study, women who intended to breastfeed were more likely to quit smoking during pregnancy (71).

One of the few studies attempting to document reasons for continued smoking during pregnancy found that, among 599 low-income women, high levels of stress, social isolation, and distress were associated with continued smoking (61). Physical fatigue and other pregnancy-related stressors may also contribute to continued smoking (40). Women whose husbands or coworkers smoke are more likely to continue smoking through pregnancy (6, 18, 19). Lighter smokers, younger women (<25 years), and women who are having their first child are more likely to quit (60, 101). The same demographic factors that predispose women to smoke before pregnancy continue to exert an impact during pregnancy. Thus, women with lower levels of education and income and those married to smokers are more likely to continue smoking during pregnancy (19, 60). However, when O'Campo et al (71) used logistic regression to analyze responses from the women in their study, they found that the association between education and smoking cessation remained significant only for white women.

In summary, women continue to smoke during pregnancy for many of the same reasons they smoked before pregnancy: their addiction to nicotine and the pleasure and perceived benefits derived from smoking. Despite limited data, we can reasonably conclude that the affect regulation afforded by cigarettes may be especially important during pregnancy, with its new stresses and strains. Desire for a healthy pregnancy and infant appear to be the most salient motivation for cessation, but there is little research to explain what compels some women to believe that smoking may jeopardize a healthy pregnancy outcome whereas other women do not. Too little is known about the unique constellation of demographic, psychologic, sociocultural, and nicotine-related factors that result in continued smoking among pregnant smokers. The moderate success of many of the programs discussed below may reflect a need to understand better this constellation of factors as antecedents to intervention.

SMOKING CESSATION INTERVENTION TRIALS IN PREGNANCY

Many randomized controlled trials of prenatal smoking cessation interventions have been conducted in the United States, Canada, England, and Sweden. We review 13 of these studies and summarize their critical aspects in Tables 2 and 3. Although we used methodological standards to select these studies, we did not evaluate study quality. Such critiques are available elsewhere for several of them (65, 101). For this review, we selected studies of acceptable quality that added in a formative or cumulative way to the body of knowledge about prenatal smoking cessation. All studies represented in the tables, with the exception of Kendrick et al (48), were published in peer-reviewed journals and either experimental or quasi-experimental in design. Researchers have used increasingly sophisticated methodologies over time, and such issues as biochemical validation and nondisclosure, which were not considered in formative research studies, were of central importance in later studies (48). Earlier studies not employing biochemical validation methods were grouped in Table 2, and later studies that did use these methods were grouped in Table 3.

Definitions of smoking status varied among the studies reviewed. One study defined a smoker as anyone who had smoked in the past seven days (102), another defined it as anyone who smokes at least one cigarette a day (46), and yet another defined a smoker as anyone who was smoking at least ten cigarettes a day just before she learned that she was pregnant (83). To reconcile these variations, we have reported quit rates of current smokers at enrollment first, then of combinations of current smokers and spontaneous quitters (women who were smoking when they learned they were pregnant, but who had quit by the time they enrolled in care) (Tables 2 and 3).

Population characteristics of clients attending public health clinics in this country differ markedly from public prenatal clients in other countries. In this country, public clients are predominantly of lower income, whereas in England, for example, all socioeconomic levels are represented among those attending public clinics (23, 57). The studies are reviewed in chronological order, which generally follows the order in which they appear in Tables 2 and 3.

The first study reviewed, conducted by Baric et al (6) in England, addressed the basic issue of whether health education interventions could be effective

Table 2 Prenatal smoking cessation intervention studies without biochemical validation of self-reported endpoint measures

Primary author	Population characteristics	Design/Sample size	Selection criteria	Smoking measurement/Data points	Intervention characteristics	Quit rates/Other outcomes (measures of significance)
Baric et al (6)	Prenatal clinic patients.	RCT E = 63 C = 47	≤20 weeks gestation; Current smoker.	Self-reported smoking behavior at enrollment and 11 weeks later.	Cessation advice and counseling by M.D.	Quit rates *E = 14% (9) †C = 14% (2) Reduction, quits, quit attempts E = 60% C = 15% Significance levels not reported.
Donovan (23)	Prenatal clients from three hospital maternity units.	RCT E = 263 C = 289	≥5 cigarettes/day <30 weeks gestation.	Self-reported smoking behavior at enrollment and 48 hours' postpartum.	Cessation advice and counseling by M.D. at each prenatal visit.	Reduction E = −7.9 cigarettes/day C = +1.7 cigarettes/day No difference in birthweight of E's and C's. Significance levels not reported.

Table 2 *(Continued)*

Primary author	Population characteristics	Design/Sample size	Selection criteria	Smoking measurement/Data points	Intervention characteristics	Quit rates/Other outcomes (measures of significance)
Ershoff et al (24) Aaronson et al (1)	Prenatal clients attending an HMO.	Quasi-experimental E = 35 C = 44	<24 weeks gestation.	Self-reported smoking behavior at enrollment and two months' postpartum. Thiocyanate assays of urine samples for experimental group at the sixth month of pregnancy.	Self-help cessation materials introduced in clinic and mailed biweekly thereafter for seven weeks. Encouraged to access taped telephone messages about booklets.	Quit rates E = 28%* C = 14% *Rates exclude women who quit before intervention exposure. (Significance levels not reported.)
Bauman et al (5)	Public prenatal clients 56% black 36% in first trimester 46% in second trimester.	Quasi-experimental (randomization by clinic) E = 46 C = 36	Attendance at prenatal clinic.	Self-reported smoking status and carbon monoxide measure at initial visit and six weeks later.	Prepared script describing smoking, carbon monoxide, and harmful consequences of smoking. Both groups heard script. Experimental group got CO measurement.	CO levels ≥ 9 ppm at six weeks after initial visit. E = 76% C = 77% (NS)

Langford et al (55)	Participants in prenatal classes offered through six health departments.	RCT E1 = 40 C2 = 37 C = 39	Daily smoker during pregnancy or smoked three months before pregnancy 28 weeks' gestation.	Self-reported smoking behavior at enrollment, four months' postpartum and 12 months' postpartum.	C = Standard prenatal classes, no additional emphasis on smoking. E1 = Presentation on smoking and pregnancy plus brochure on smoking. E2 = Presentation, brochure and follow-up home visit.	<u>% Non-smokers</u> four months' postpartum E1/E2 combined = 22.1% C = 15.4% (NS) 12 months' postpartum E1/E2 = 23.4% C = 5.1% ($p = 0.02$).
MacArthur et al (57)	Prenatal clients in a large maternity hospital.	RCT E = 493 C = 489	Current smoker.	Self-reported status at enrollment and in the hospital after delivery.	Cessation advice by M.D. or midwife and written materials.	<u>Quit Rates</u> E = 9% C = 6% (Significance levels were not reported) Among primiparas E = 13% C = 7% <u>Infant Size</u> Among first borns, E's weighed 68 grams more ($p < .06$) and were .75 cm longer ($p < .01$) than controls.

Table 2 (*Continued*)

Primary author	Population characteristics	Design/Sample size	Selection criteria	Smoking measurement/Data points	Intervention characteristics	Quit rates/Other outcomes (measures of significance)
Mayer et al (59)	Public prenatal clients in one county 49% in second trimester 28% in third trimester.	RCT E/MC = 72 (Multi-component) E/RI = 70 (Risk information) C = 77	Attendance in WIC clinic. Current smokers.	Self-reported smoking behavior at enrollment, ninth month (recalled at postpartum) and postpartum.	E/MC: 20-minute counseling session including risk information and behavioral change component with self-help manual E/RI: 10-minute counseling session including risk information only. Interventions provided by a health educator.	Quit Rates ninth Month: E_{MC} = 11% E_{RI} = 7% C = 2.6% Postpartum: E_{MC} = 6.9% E_{RI} = 7.1% C = 0% (Partial biochemical validation of ⅓ of sample at postpartum visit (r = .25 for self-report + thiocyanate verification).

RCT = randomized controlled trial.
E = experimental group.
C = control group.

Table 3 Prenatal smoking cessation intervention studies without biochemical validation of self-reported endpoint measures

Primary author	Population characteristics	Design/Sample size	Selection criteria	Smoking measurement/Data points	Intervention characteristics	Quit rates/Other outcomes (measures of significance)
Sexton & Hebel (83) Sexton et al (84)	Prenatal clients from two private obstetrical practices, and one hospital obstetrical clinic.	RCT E = 463 C = 472	≥10 cigarettes per day at onset of pregnancy; <18 weeks' gestation.	Self-reported smoking behavior and salivary thiocyanate at enrollment and eighth month.	Special counselor provided education & support, ≥1 home visits, information and homework assignments mailed biweekly, telephone calls.	Quit rates Current smokers E = 32% C = 7% urrent smokers/Recent quitters E = 43% C = 20% ($p < .001$) Infant size Mean birthweight for E's was 92 grams heavier than C's $p < .05$) Length was 0.6 cm greater ($p < .05$)

Table 3 (*Continued*)

Primary author	Population characteristics	Design/Sample size	Selection criteria	Smoking measurement/Data points	Intervention characteristics	Quit rates/Other outcomes (measures of significance)
Windsor et al (102)	Prenatal clients in public clinics.	RCT E1 = 103 E2 = 102 C = 104	≤32 weeks' gestation.	Self-reported smoking behavior and salivary thicyanate at enrollment, 4–8 weeks after first visit, and ninth month or within 48 hours of delivery.	E1 = 10-minute counseling session, brochure on consequences of smoking during pregnancy and self-help manual geared specifically to pregnant smokers. E2 = same 10-minute counseling session and brochure with self-help manual for smokers in general.	Quit rates 95% CI E1 = 14% (0.07–0.21) E2 = 6% (0.01–0.11) C = 2% (0.00–0.05) Quit or reduced E1 = 31% (0.22–0.40) E2 = 20% (0.12–0.28) C = 9% (0.03–0.15)
Ershoff et al (25) Ershoff et al (26)	Prenatal clients in an HMO.	RCT E = 126 C = 116	≤18 weeks' gestation; ≥7 cigarettes/week.	Self-reported behavior at enrollment and the twenty-sixth week. Urine cotinine verification at multiple time points.	Serialized self-help program. Brochures mailed biweekly for seven weeks.	Quit rates 95% CI E = 22.2% (03.0–20.0) C = 8.6% Mean birthweight E = 3,366 NS C = 3,309 NS IUGR E = 1.7% ($p < .05$) C = 7.3%

Haddow et al (42)	Clients receiving care in private physicians offices and being screened for AFP.	RCT E = 1343 C = 1357	≥10 cigarettes per day 15–20 weeks' gestation.	Serum cotinine at 15–20 weeks. E = repeat serum cotinine one month later.	Experimental group received one interpreted measure of cotinine, a self-help smoking cessation booklet, and one follow-up measure after a month. Intervention provided by physician or physician office staff.	Among infants delivered by physicians in the experimental group who submitted repeat serum samples, birthweight was 66 g higher than in the control group ($p < 0.03$) and the low birthweight rate was 30% lower.
Hjalmarson et al (46)	Prenatal clients in public clinics.	RCT E = 417 C = 231	Current smoker <12 weeks Swedish speaking.	Self-reported smoking behavior at initial visit, 12–14 weeks, 30–34 weeks and 8 weeks after delivery. Blood thiocyanate at 30–34 weeks and 8 weeks after delivery.	Intervention consisted of a self-help manual given by the physician at the first visit.	Continuously abstinent* — OR (95% CI) E = 10.4% — 2.08(1.0–4.4) C = 5.2% 30–34 weeks' postpartum E = 12.6% — 1.53(0.8–2.8) C = 8.6% *OR and 95% CI were recalculated by authors.

Table 3 (*Continued*)

Primary author	Population characteristics	Design/Sample size	Selection criteria	Smoking measurement/Data points	Intervention characteristics	Quit rates/Other outcomes (measures of significance)
Kendrick et al (48)	Prenatal clients in public clinics in two states.	Quasi-experimental (Randomization by clinic) State 1: E = 236 C = 301 State 2: E = 378 C = 381	<32 weeks' gestation >0 cigarettes per week at enrollment.	Self-reported number of cigarettes at enrollment, eighth month, six weeks after delivery. Urine cotinine verification at these times.	Individualized counseling at each prenatal visit reinforced with brochure and audio-visual materials.	Quit rates State 1: E = 8% C = 10% ($p = 0.64$) State 2: E = 3.2% C = 3.4% ($p = 0.60$)
Windsor et al (103)	Public prenatal clients.	RCT E = 400 C = 414	<32 weeks' gestation ≥1 puff of cigarette in last seven days.	Self-reported smoking at intake, 4–8 weeks after intake, and approx. 32 weeks. Cotinine verification at these times.	15-minute individual session by trained counselor at first visit plus self-help manual; medical provider letter one week later; "buddy" materials and quarterly newsletter.	Quit rates E = 14.3% C = 8.5% ($p < .01$) >50% reduction E = 16.8% C = 12.3% ($p = 0.07$)

in promoting smoking cessation among pregnant women (Table 2). Physicians provided a brief one-on-one intervention by advising their clients to quit smoking. Sixty percent of the women in the intervention group made some type of change in their smoking behavior (they reduced consumption, attempted to quit, or quit), whereas only 15% of the control group had made such changes. Although significance levels were not reported in this study, the results were most encouraging for this new educational intervention that targeted pregnant smokers. A second study from England, conducted by Donovan (23), incorporated individualized counseling regarding the adverse consequences of prenatal smoking into the ongoing maternity care routine to demonstrate an increased birthweight among women who receive antismoking counseling. No difference in birthweight between the two groups was detected, and no quit rates were reported; however, those in the intervention group reduced average cigarette consumption by 7.9 cigarettes per day, and those in the control group increased consumption by 1.7 cigaretttes per day. The contribution of these two early studies was to establish the notion that prenatal smoking cessation counseling could be incorporated into routine prenatal care. Both studies relied on self-reported smoking status.

The next two US studies investigated the effects of innovative approaches to intervention content and format. In 1983, Ershoff et al reported the results of a prenatal smoking cessation intervention provided to clients concurrently receiving a nutritional counseling program in an HMO (1, 24). The methodological innovation of this study was the introduction of a laboratory method for confirming client reports of smoking behavior. Biochemical validation of self-reported smoking status was established for the treatment group at the initial visit, but no validation was provided for self-reported endpoint measures in either intervention or comparison groups. At two months postpartum, self-reported quit rates were 28% for the intervention group and 14% for the comparison group.

In another US study conducted about this same time, Bauman et al (5) attempted to assess the impact of the incorporation of a biological measure of smoking exposure [carbon monoxide (CO) monitoring] into the intervention, thus making it an intervention component as well as an impact measure. Subjects in the experimental group observed the measurement of their CO levels as well as the CO levels of others, including nonsmokers, in the orientation session. Subjects in the control group did not receive the CO measurement at enrollment. Carbon monoxide levels were measured in both groups six weeks after the orientation session. No differences were found in the CO levels of experimental and control subjects at the time of the second measurement. Self-reported quit rates were not reported.

In the Ershoff et al study (24), the serialized contact with the client, through mailed brochures, apparently contributed to some enhancement important to cessation. In the Bauman et al study (5), the client was given limited, one-time information followed by a voluntarily, self-administered, biological test aimed at reinforcing the verbal messages. Timing of initial exposure to the intervention was comparable for both studies. One could speculate that the ongoing program contact provided by the serialized mailing in Ershoff et al's study constituted a key ingredient in the program's success. The one-time-only contact, and the brevity of the intervention provided by Bauman and colleagues, may have accounted for its lack of impact. However, Gillies (35) also used CO measurement as a prenatal intervention component and found no significant difference in cessation rates during pregnancy among subjects who were current smokers at the time of enrollment (experimental group, 8%; control group, 5.6%). They did, however, find a significant difference in nonsmoking rates postpartum when they combined early quitters (those who stopped before they came for prenatal care) with those who were smoking at enrollment.

Another study by Langford et al (55) examined the issue of timing of intervention with a health education intervention provided late in pregnancy (seventh month) as a component of prenatal education classes. No significant differences were detected between the two groups until one year after delivery, at which time 23.4% of the experimental groups (groups 1 and 2 were combined for analysis) and only 5.1% of the control group were nonsmokers. Rates must be interpreted cautiously because of the small sample size; however, the notion of a delayed or postpartum impact of the prenatal intervention cannot be dismissed.

In 1984, Sexton & Hebel (83) conducted a study at the University of Maryland and reported highly encouraging quit rates (experimental group, 32%; control group, 7%) **and** an increase in birthweight (67 g) among women in the experimental group over that of women in the control group (Table 3). This study used a more intensive, multicomponent intervention that included one or more individual counseling sessions, home visits, periodic mailings of self-help materials, and follow-up telephone calls. Interventions were provided by trained counselors who actively engaged subjects in the cessation process during pregnancy. This landmark study provided some of the strongest evidence to date of the potential impact of systematic prenatal smoking cessation efforts.

In the mid-1980s, prenatal smoking cessation trials focused on efficacy and replicability. Efforts were also directed toward populations known to be at higher risk for smoking during pregnancy. Windsor and colleagues (102) conducted a well-designed study that sought to delineate the type of materials that were most effective in assisting pregnant women to stop smoking. The study targeted clients receiving care in public prenatal clinics. As described in Table 3, the intervention received by experimental groups 2 and 3 differed only in that the self-help manual given to group 2 was directed toward the general public, whereas the manual given to group 3 specifically addressed smoking cessation for pregnant women. Results showed higher quit rates for group 3 (14%) than for group 2 (6%); however, the quit rates for both surpassed that for the control group (2%).

A distinguishing methodological characteristic of these last two studies is that both used salivary thiocyanate (SCN) to verify self-reported smoking status among subjects. The Sexton et al (183) study compared mean thiocyanate levels for control and treatment groups. The researchers calculated differences in thiocyanate levels at baseline and eighth month for subjects in both control and treatment groups. Mean thiocyanate levels were significantly lower for the treatment group at the eighth month than for the control group. In addition, the decrease in thiocyanate levels from baseline to eighth month was significantly greater among subjects in the treatment group as compared with those in the control group.

In Windsor et al's (102) study, successful cessation was defined as a change in self-reported status from smoker at midpoint to nonsmoker at endpoint; this change in status was biochemically validated by a decrease in the level of SCN. All women lost to follow-up at either midpoint or endpoint were considered intervention failures and counted as smokers. These two studies demonstrated that the application of systematic, multicomponent, prenatal interventions by dedicated providers who used materials designed specifically for pregnant women resulted in much higher quit rates than those found in "usual care," or control clinics. In the Sexton et al (83) study, the intervention effect extended not only to smoking cessation, but also to a demonstrable improvement in pregnancy outcome. These two studies served as prototypes for many of the studies that followed and set a methodological standard requiring biochemical validation of self-reported quitting behaviors.

As research progressed in the field of prenatal smoking cessation, demonstration of an improvement in birthweight as a consequence of a systematic cessation program became an important study objective. Following the study by Sexton et al, MacArthur and colleagues (57) attempted to demonstrate such an impact in their study (Table 2). Women attending a large maternity hospital clinic were randomly assigned to experimental and control groups; women in the experimental group received individualized counseling by a physician and midwife, as well as written materials that reinforced the counseling. No significant differences in quit rates or birthweights were noted overall; however, an intervention effect was noted among women having their first baby. Women in the experimental group who were having their **first** baby were almost twice as likely as their control counterparts to stop smoking (13% versus 7%); their infants were 68 g heavier ($p = < .06$) than infants in the control group. The authors reported that the intervention varied within the study population in general, in that first-time pregnancies received the most complete exposure. Although these results were encouraging and supportive of Sexton et al's results, biochemical confirmation of self-reported behavior was lacking.

Ershoff and colleagues (25) replicated their earlier study by enlarging it. They focused solely on prenatal smoking cessation and looked at many prenatal outcomes (Table 3). For women who reported quitting before the twentieth week of gestation, all urine samples from the reported time of quitting to the twenty-sixth week were tested for cotinine (a metabolite of nicotine). Confirmation of a self-reported quit required at least one sample with a cotinine level less than 10ng/ml. For this group, an additional confirmation was obtained on a urine sample taken at 34 weeks. Quit rates therefore reflected continuous abstinence from some point before the twentieth week through delivery. As noted in Table 3, quit rates were almost three times higher for the experimental group than for the control group. It is difficult to determine the level of intervention exposure required to stimulate quitting (i.e. how many pamphlets). However, the majority of those who quit before the twentieth week received most of the mailings dealing with motivation for quitting, reasons for quitting, and strategies for quitting. The average number of booklets read was 5.8. A significantly lower rate of IUGR was noted in the experimental group (1.7%), and infants born of experimental mothers weighed more than those born of mothers in the control group. This study contributed significantly to the field, as it demonstrated a high rate of continuous abstinence in response to an intervention requiring a minimum level of provider time, as well as a significant decrease in the rate of IUGR among those receiving the intervention.

The majority of prenatal smoking cessation studies were implemented within the context of the prenatal care visit. In 1990, Mayer et al (59) reported a small, randomized controlled trial in a large Special Supplemental Food Program for Women, Infants, and Children (WIC) clinic in Michigan (Table 2). The highest self-reported quit rate was found in the group receiving risk information and a multicomponent intervention (11%.) Those receiving only risk information had a self-reported quit rate of 7%; the control group's quit rate was 2.6%. This study demonstrated that prenatal smoking cessation interventions were well accepted by WIC clients (81%) and that WIC clinics offered another setting for prenatal smoking cessation activities. Major limitations of the study included a small sample size, which limited its ability to detect small differences, and the lack of complete biochemical validation.

Two studies of note were published in 1991: one from the United States and one from Sweden (Table 3). Haddow et al (42) published the results of a randomized control trial in which a prenatal smoking cessation intervention was incorporated into an existing state program that screened pregnant women for alpha-fetoprotein (AFP). Overall, the intervention had no detectable effect on birthweight; however, in the group of women whose physicians submitted a second blood sample for testing one month after the initial intervention, a significant effect was observed. The mean birthweight for women in this group was 66 g higher than that for women in the control group ($p = 0.03$), and the proportion of low birthweight was 30% lower ($p = 0.08$). Self-reported quit rates were not reported, and the study did not control for maternal weight gain during pregnancy or for history of previous poor pregnancy outcomes. The contribution of this study was its creative use of an existing program as a vehicle for prenatal smoking cessation and its use of physicians as providers of the intervention.

Hjalmarson et al (46) also conducted a well-designed study by using physicians who instructed clients in the cessation process and provided them with a self-help manual. The authors defined continuous abstinence as self-reported cessation at 12–14 weeks' gestation, 30–34 weeks' gestation, and 8 weeks' postpartum. Self-reported quitting was verified by blood thiocyanate measures at 30–34 weeks. Results showed that women in the treatment group were twice as likely to maintain abstinence at all three measurement points than women in the control group. Although the rates of decreased consumption for treatment and control groups did not differ statistically, overall women decreased their smoking consumption by about 40% between the prepregnancy period and the first trimester.

In a more recent study, Kendrick and colleagues (48) presented preliminary results from two of three states involved in a randomized trial conducted in public prenatal and WIC clinics. The providers of the intervention were existing staff, including nurses, health educators, and in some cases WIC paraprofessionals. Early results based on self-reported data indicated that the intervention resulted in higher quit rates within the treatment groups. However, when self-reported data were matched with urinary cotinine values, the researchers determined that, at enrollment, 21% of self-reported nonsmokers in one state and 36% in another had cotinine values consistent with smoking. Nondisclosure continued to be a problem at the eighth month and appeared to be enhanced by treatment group status. These results were similar to those found by Windsor et al (103) (Table 3), who used the same biochemical confirmation test in a trial involving public prenatal clients. Windsor et al again demonstrated the efficacy of a multicomponent intervention that included a self-help manual, which was part of their earlier trial (102). An important contribution of these last two studies was to call attention to the high rates of nondisclosure among public prenatal clients. Recent studies have also documented nondisclosure, although at a lower level, among prenatal clients in multispeciality groups serving working and middle-class populations (25, 66).

CONCLUSIONS

The lack of biochemical validation of self-reported data in some reviewed studies mandates caution in summarizing the research in prenatal smoking cessation as a whole. Nevertheless, of the 13 studies reviewed, all but three reported some type of intervention effect. All provided, in varying degrees, one-on-one education with or without cessation counseling, delivered by a physician or other health-care provider in the context of the prenatal health care visit. The more successful programs reinforced the advice and counseling through printed materials, home visits, and/or telephone contacts (24, 25, 83, 102). Risk information alone may increase cessation activity above that resulting from usual care, but the addition of components to teach cessation skills produces higher reported quit rates (59), as do materials specifically targeting the pregnant smoker (102).

Studies that showed an intervention effect were distinguished by their use of "designated providers" whose specific job was providing intervention counseling (59, 83, 102). Minimal contact programs that relied on existing staff to deliver the intervention met with mixed success. Some studies reported no impact on cessation or outcome of pregnancy (23, 55, 102). However, Hjalmarson et al (46) found a significant cessation effect in a study in which physicians provided cessation advice and a self-help manual at the first prenatal visit. Given the scarce resources in many health-care environments, using existing providers may be the only option.

Haddow et al (42) found no overall effect on birthweight among experimental and control groups, but did find a significant increase in birthweight in infants born to women in the experimental group whose physicians adhered most closely to the study protocol. MacArthur et al (57) found no overall effect on quit rates, but did find a significant effect on birthweight and cessation among first time pregnancies. In their study, however, women expecting their first baby also received the most complete exposure to the intervention. Baric et al (6) found that, although all women in their study had heard about the dangers of smoking during pregnancy, women who had been pregnant before were more skeptical about accepting this information than women who were pregnant for the first time.

Cessation trials involving predominantly private populations or clients who attend HMOs apparently achieve greater cessation effects than those involving public health clients. Among the experimental groups of trials reviewed, the highest quit rate for current smokers at enrollment was 32% in a study population that consisted of clients from two private obstetrical practices and one hospital obstetrical clinic (66). Ershoff et al reported quit rates of 28% in their earlier study of HMO clients (24) and 22.2% in their later, more rigorous trial (25). Among public prenatal and WIC clients, studies reported quit rates of 3–14% percent (48, 59, 102). Studies from England conducted among client populations with representation from all socioeconomic levels reported quit rates ranging from 9% to 14% (6, 57). No data are available concerning the sociodemographics of public prenatal clients in the study by Hjalmarson and colleagues (46), which achieved a continuous abstinence rate of 10.4% through eight weeks' postpartum among experimental subjects.

Some studies showed a stronger intervention effect among women entering prenatal health care early (59, 102). This finding might suggest that either women are more open to cessation earlier in pregnancy or early entry to health care leads to an increase in the number of intervention exposures that results in increased cessation activity. Alternatively, women who enter health care earlier may be more prevention-oriented. Ershoff et al (25) found that among women in the experimental group who were smoking at enrollment, 22.2% stopped smoking before the twentieth week, but only 4% quit afterward. A stronger intervention effect among lighter smokers (< 10 cigarettes per day) has also been noted by some researchers (25, 102).

Some researchers found no significant effects of intervention on cessation during pregnancy, but later found significant differences in the proportion of nonsmokers in experimental groups versus those in control groups during the postpartum period (35, 55). This delayed effect on cessation rates is not well understood. One possible explanation is that some studies include both current smokers and recent quitters, and that the antismoking information and advice provided to the recent quitters during pregnancy contributed to a higher rate of long-term cessation maintenance among these women, thus contributing to an overall higher quit rate in the experimental group.

As a final point, questions about the degree and sources of error associated with various methods for ascertaining smoking status and issues to be considered in selecting ascertainment methods are of considerable importance to practitioners and researchers. Point prevalence measures of at least one week should be used to determine smoking status at entry into prenatal health care and to determine prepregnancy smoking status. Early quitting and continuous abstinence would be the measure of choice for end-of-pregnancy assessment; however, multiple measures throughout the course of pregnancy may not be practical.

Self-report is the most direct, practical, and widely used method. A wide range of strategies for obtaining self-report are available, from simple verbal inquiry on a single occasion about present smoking status to more complex inquires on several occasions about longer time sequences and multiple aspects of behavior within specific definitional boundaries. Velicer and associates (98) recommend that the decision to rely on self-report be based on the type of program, type of population, and demand characteristics of the situation. With respect to prenatal, care-based smoking cessation programs, all three of these factors could contribute to increasing nondisclosure. Because smoking presents a danger to the fetus and not just to the woman herself, she may be more reluctant to reveal her true smoking status to a caregiver. Both the intervention and the request for disclosure come from the clinic, and intervention group participants may feel a greater demand to claim a nonsmoking status. Thus, some form of biochemical validation is recommended. At a minimum, validation of self-reported quitters at endpoint (or a statistical sample thereof) would seem in order.

However, rates of disclosure among self-reported smokers can be improved by using multiple-choice questions that allow respondents to choose partially favorable answers, such as "I smoke now, but I have cut down since I found out I was pregnant." In a randomized trial, the multiple-choice format improved disclosure of smoking at the first prenatal care visit by 40% over that of a dichotomous question, "Do you smoke?" (66).

Biochemical measures generally have superior sensitivity and specificity over self-reported measures; however, they are not without problems. Administration can present difficulties, and where consent is required, pregnant women may be increasingly unwilling to allow urine samples, in particular, to be tested because of concern about drug and HIV testing. Biochemical ascertainment methods also involve additional expense.

Several biochemical measures, such as carbon monoxide, thiocyanate, and cotinine, which have been used to confirm self-report, have been the subject of previous reviews (37, 52, 73, 90, 98). One of these measures, thiocyanate, has lost acceptance as a suitable alternative (98), although it has been used in previous evaluations of prenatal smoking cessation (83, 102). Expired-air CO can be measured with easily operated, portable, and relatively inexpensive equipment. (Carbon monoxide can also be measured in hemoglobin, but this procedure is less practical with pregnant women from whom blood would have to be drawn specially in late pregnancy.) The sensitivity of exhaled CO for classifying active smoking ranges from 80% to 85%, but it can vary with time of day, e.g. in the morning, measures have a greater likelihood of missing smokers. Carbon monoxide has a short half-life, a factor that makes its sensitivity poor for light smokers (76, 99). Because many pregnant women reduce smoking and may smoke irregularly, this drawback could lead to underestimation of rates of smoking. Specificity is also affected by environmental pollution, including secondhand smoke and indoor combustion sources (37), and by lactose intolerance (62). The environmental factors may be more likely to affect women of lower socioeconomic status women, the same women who are more likely to smoke during pregnancy. Lactose intolerance has relatively high prevalence in black and Hispanic women.

Cotinine, a metabolic by-product of nicotine, has a longer half-life than that of CO. Cotinine, which is highly specific to tobacco users, is present in several bodily fluids. Urine is the most practical bodily fluid to measure cotinine during pregnancy, because urine specimens are given at every prenatal care visit. Although cotinine concentrations are influenced by nicotine gum, alternative nicotine delivery sources are viewed as contraindicated during pregnancy. At present, cotinine analyses must be conducted in a laboratory, and those analyses are relatively expensive.

Of the biochemical measures available, cotinine has superior specificity and sensitivity, but currently is more expensive than CO testing. Anonymous urine samples can be taken from self-reported nonsmokers without consent. However, when circumstances require informed consent for biochemical measures, selection bias can be a problem. Nevertheless, recent experience and scientific opinion suggest that some form of biochemical measure, at least on a sampling basis, should be used in conjunction with self-report measures to estimate the magnitude of the population of smokers who should be targeted for intervention and to estimate treatment effectiveness among smokers who receive interventions. The use of biochemical screening tests at the time of entry into care has been unexplored in prenatal populations; however, studies aimed at decreasing nondisclosure in this population have had encouraging results (66).

SUMMARY IMPLICATIONS FOR POLICY AND PRACTICE

Intervention trials in diverse populations that have measured the effect of prenatal smoking cessation counseling on birthweight confirm an improvement for infants whose mothers received systematic programs (25, 57, 83). The effect on birthweight was directly proportional to the effect on smoking. Cost-benefit analyses based on simulations (58, 103) and actual study data (26) indicate a savings of at least \$3 on the costs of neonatal care for every \$1 spent on prenatal smoking cessation intervention. Longer-term savings raise this ratio from over 5:1 (58) to as much as 17:1 (103).

The level of evidence to support prenatal smoking cessation as a recommended preventive service for all pregnant smokers meets the criteria established by the Expert Panel on the Content of Prenatal Care (65, 96) and by the US Preventive Services Task Force (97). Costs of intervention to the health-care provider in 1992 dollars would range from about \$6.50 (103) to \$13.00 (26) for a brief counseling session by a nonphysician health-care professional plus reinforcing materials. The structure of care determines whether the approximately \$3 in immediate savings are captured by the organization providing the service. In cases where prenatal and newborn hospital care are paid by the same entity, as with Medicaid, indemnity insurers, or HMOs, can recoup their intervention costs and save on neonatal care costs in the same year, thus making an unusually strong economic case for a preventive service (82).

The most successful prenatal smoking cessation study reviewed used a multicomponent intervention that employed designated providers who delivered one-on-one, individualized counseling to clients in the first or early second trimester and henceforth throughout the pregnancy (83). The most successful minimal contact (at least one contact) program in the literature was one conducted in an HMO that used serial mailings after an initial five-minute counseling session (25). Among exclusively low-income populations, only programs using designated providers and self-help manuals have produced cessation rates higher than those found in usual care clinics (59, 102).

A notable fact about prenatal smoking cessation trials as a whole is that even with the best results, the vast majority of women continue to smoke throughout pregnancy despite their knowledge of the increased risks of adverse consequences to themselves and to the developing fetus. Evidence suggests that continued smoking may be associated with high levels of stress, resulting from a job or the demands of child care. Some pregnant women may use cigarettes to limit weight gain; whereas others may use them to cope with depression. Some would argue that women who continue to smoke while pregnant are those who are most addicted to nicotine and who will require intensive intervention efforts to achieve cessation. Some of these arguments may explain the difficulty in achieving higher cessation rates among lower socioeconomic populations. Another contributing factor among low socioeconomic women is the high prevalence of smoking among others in the household. Minimal contact programs are less successful in this population; the more successful approaches use designated providers and multicomponent interventions. Successful programs that target lower socioeconomic women should include individualized counseling and follow-up, frequent cessation cues from multiple sources, and self-help materials. Among higher socioeconomic groups, minimal contact programs with serialized mailings of materials and telephone follow-up have been promising, low-cost strategies.

Few programs targeting pregnant women have been specifically designed for smokers who are in the precontemplative (not seriously thinking of quitting in the next six months) stage of behavior change (22). This lack may be due to the fact that the window of time for change is rather narrow for pregnant women; however, recent studies indicate that pregnant women who are precontemplators hold fewer positive attitudes about the benefits of cessation than do pregnant women who are contemplators (those who are seriously thinking of quitting in the next six months). Both groups lack self-efficacy with regard to their beliefs about achieving cessation (21). Recent research by Prochaska et al (79) demonstrates that moving smokers from precontemplation to contemplation requires a shift in the decisional balance of the pros and cons of smoking. These newer studies argue for more interventions that focus on the specific needs of the prenatal smoker, as defined by her current attitudes and beliefs, as well as her level of readiness to change her smoking behavior. Given the sustained prevalence of smoking among young, nonblack women, prenatal smoking apparently will continue to be a risk factor for many women for some time to come. Therefore, prenatal smoking cessation is an area in which continued inquiry is indicated for researchers, and application and persistence are indicated for clinicians.

ACKNOWLEDGMENTS

The authors acknowledge the following persons for their assistance in the development and preparation of this manuscript: Gary S. Stuart, Juliette S. Kendrick, Pattie Tucker, S. Christine Zahniser, Joyce Bryant-Adams, and Rhonda Gilley.

Literature Cited

1. Aaronson, N., Ershoff, D. H., Danaher, B. G. 1985 Smoking cessation in pregnancy: a self-help approach. *Addict. Behav.* 10:103–8
2. Altman, D. G., Hytten, F. E. 1989. Assessment of fetal size and fetal growth. In *Effective Care in Pregnancy and Childbirth,* ed. I. Chalmers, M. Enkin, M. J. N. C. Keirse, pp. 411–18. Oxford: Oxford Univ. Press. 1478 pp.
3. Anda, R. F., Williamson, D. F., Escobedo, L. G., Mast, E. E., Giovino, G. A., Remington, P. L. 1990. Depression and the dynamics of smoking. *J. Am. Med. Assoc.* 264 (12):1541–45
4. Bachman, J. G., Wallace, J. M., O'Malley, P. M., Johnston, L. D., Kurth, C. L., et al. 1991. Racial/ethnic differences in smoking, drinking, and illicit drug use among American high school seniors, 1976–89. *Am. J. Public Health* 81:372–77
5. Bauman, K. E., Bryan, E. S., Dent, C. W., Kock, G. G. 1983. The influence of observing carbon monoxide level on cigarette smoking by public prenatal patients. *Public Health Rep.* 98:536–47
6. Baric, L., MacArthur, C., Sherwood, M. 1976. A study of health education aspects of smoking in pregnancy. *Int. J. Health Educ.* 19(suppl) (2):1–16
7. Biener, L. 1987. Gender differences in the use of substances for coping. In *Gender and Stress,* ed. R. Barnett, L. Biener, G. Baruch, pp. 330–49. New York: Free Press
8. Biener, L., Abrams, D. B., Follick, M. J., Hitti, J. 1986. *Gender differences in smoking and quitting.* Presented at Soc. of Behav. Med., San Francisco
9. Blake, S. M., Klepp, K. I., Pechacek, T. F., Folsom, A. R., Luepker, R. V., et al. 1989. Differences in smoking cessation strategies between men and women. *Addict. Behav.* 14:409–18
10. Butler, N. R., Goldstein, H. 1973. Smoking in pregnancy and subsequent child development. *Br. Med. J.* 4:573–75
11. Cent. Dis. Control. 1990. Unpubl. data from the 1990 Nat. Health Interviews Surv. Atlanta: CDC
12. Cent. Dis. Control. 1991. Cigarette smoking among reproductive-aged women—Behavioral Risk Factor Surveillance System, 1989. *Morbid. Mortal. Wkly. Rep.* 40:719–23
13. Cent. Dis. Control. 1988. Unpubl. data from 1987 and 1988 Nat. Health Interview Surv. Atlanta: CDC
14. Cent. Dis. Control. 1991. Cigarette smoking among youth—United States, 1989. *Morbid. Mortal. Wkly. Rep.* 40: 712–15
15. Cent. Dis. Control. 1991. Tobacco use among high school students—United States, 1990. *Morbid. Mortal. Wkly. Rep.* 40:617–19
16. Cent. Dis. Control, Natl. Cent. Health Stat. 1992. Advance report of the new

data from the 1989 birth certificate. *Mon. Vital Stat. Rep.*, Vol. 40(12) Suppl.

17. Cent. Dis. Control. 1985. Unpubl. data from the 1985 Natl. Health Interview Surv. Atlanta: CDC
18. Cnattinguis, S. 1989. Brief report. Smoking habits in early pregnancy. *Addict. Behav.* 14:453–57
19. Cnattinguis, S., Thorslund, M. 1990. Smoking behavior among pregnant women prior to antenatal care registration. *Soc. Sci. Med.* 31(11):1271–75
20. Colley, J. R. T., Holland, W. W., Corkhill, R. T. 1974. Influence of passive smoking and parental phlegm on pneumonia and bronchitis in early childhood. *Lancet* 1:529–32
21. de Vries, H. 1992. *Smoking cessation for pregnant women: determinants and a pilot study*. Presented at 8th Int. Conf. on Smoking or Health. Buenos Aires
22. DiClemente, C. C., Prochaska, J. O., Fairhurst, S. K., Velicer, W. F., Velasquez, M. M., Rossi, J. S. 1991. The process of smoking cessation: an analysis of precontemplation, contemplation, and preparation stages of change. *J. Consul. Clin. Psychol.* 59 (2):295–304
23. Donovan, J. 1977. Randomized controlled trial of antismoking advice in pregnancy. *Br. J. Soc. Med.* 31:6–12
24. Ershoff, D., Aaronson, N., Danaher, B., Wasserman, F. 1983. Behavioral, health, and cost outcomes of an HMO-based perinatal health education program. *Public Health Rep.* 98:536–47
25. Ershoff, D. H., Mullen, P. D., Quinn, V. P. 1989. A randomized trial of serialized self-help smoking cessation program for pregnant women in an HMO. *Am. J. Pub. Health* 79(2):182–87
26. Ershoff, D. H., Quinn, V. P., Mullen, P. D., Lairson, D. R. 1990. Pregnancy and medical cost outcomes of a self-help prenatal smoking cessation program in an HMO. *Public Health Rep.* 105(4): 340–47
27. Ernster, V. L. 1987. A social history of cigarette smoking and advertising. *Not Far Enough: Women vs. Smoking,* A Workshop for Women's Group and Women's Health Leaders, USDHHS, pp. 4–10
28. Fichtner, R. R., Sullivan, K. M., Zyrkowski, C. L., Trowbridge, F. L. 1990. Racial/ethnic differences in smoking, other risk factors, and low birth weight among low-income pregnant women, 1989–1988. *Morbid. Mortal. Wkly. Rep. CDC Surveill. Summ.* 39(3):13–21
29. Fielding, J. E. 1987. Smoking and women. *N. Engl. J. Med.* 317(21): 1343–45
30. Fingerhut, L. A., Kleinman, J. C., Kendrick, J. S. 1990. Smoking before, during, and after pregnancy. *Am. J. Public Health* 80:541–44
31. Fiore, M. C., Novotny, T. E., Pierce, J. P., Giovino, G. A., Hatziandreu, E. J., et al. 1990. Methods used to quit smoking in the United States. *J. Am. Med. Assoc.* 263(20):2760–65
32. Floyd, R. L., Zahniser, C. S., Gunter, E. P., Kendrick, J. S. 1991. Smoking during pregnancy: prevalence, effects, and intervention strategies. *Birth* 18(1): 47–52
33. Fox, S. H., Brown, C., Koontz, A. M., Kessel, S. S. 1987. Perceptions of risks of smoking and drinking during pregnancy: 1985 NHIS findings. *Public Health Rep.* 102:73–79
34. Frerichs, R. R., Aneshensel, C. S., Clark, V. A., Yokopenic, P. 1981. Smoking and depression: a community survey. *Am. J. Public Health* 71(6): 637–40
35. Gillies, P. 1992. Anti-smoking interventions during pregnancy impact on smoking behavior and birthweight. In *Effects of Smoking on the Fetus, Neonate and Child,* eds. D. Poswillo, E. Alberman. London: Oxford Univ. Press. In press
36. Graham, H. 1987. Women's smoking and family health. *Soc. Sci. Med.* 25(1):47–56
37. Grabowski, J., Bell, C. S. 1983. *Measurement in the analysis and treatment of smoking behavior,* US DHHS Monogr. Washington, DC: GPO
38. Gritz, E. R. 1991. Smoking. *Women's Cancer Screening: Guidelines and Effect on Mortality*. Syntex Annu. Women's Healthcare Roundtable, pp. 59–76
39. Gritz, E. R., Klesges, R. C., Meyers, A. W. 1989. The smoking and body weight relationship: implications for intervention and postcessation weight control. *Ann. Behav. Med.* 11(4):144–53
40. Gritz, E. R., Kristeller, J. L., Burns, D. M. High-risk groups and patients with medical co-morbidity. *Nicotine Addict.* In press
41. Grunberg, J. E., Winders, S. E., Wewers, M. E. 1991. Gender differences in tobacco use. *Health Psychol.* 10(2):143–53
42. Haddow, J. E., Knight, G. J., Kloza,

E. M., Palomake, G. E., Nicholas, J. W. 1991. Cotinine-assisted intervention in pregnancy to reduce smoking and low birthweight delivery. *Br. J. Obstet. Gynecol.* 98:859–65
43. Haglund, B., Chattingius, S. 1990. Cigarette smoking as a risk factor for sudden infant death syndrome: population-based study. *Am. J. Public Health* 80:29–32
44. Harlap, S., Davies, A. M. 1974. Infant admissions to hospital and maternal smoking. *Lancet* 1:529–32
45. Himmelberger, D. U., Byron, W. B., Cohen, E. N. 1978. Cigarette smoking during pregnancy and the occurrence of spontaneous abortion and congenital abnormality. *Am. J. Epidemiol.* 108: 470–79
46. Hjalmarson, A. I., Hahn, L., Svanberg, B. 1991. Stopping smoking in pregnancy: effect of a self-help manual in controlled trial. *Br. J. Obstet. Gynecol.* 98(3):260–64
47. Inst. of Med. 1985. *Preventing Low Birthweight*. Washington, DC: Natl. Acad. Press
48. Kendrick, J. S., Zahniser, S. C., Floyd, R. L., Gargiullo, P. M., Salas, N. M., et al. 1991. *Nondisclosure of smoking status in intervention programs for public prenatal clients*. Abstr. presented at 1991 Annu. Meet. of Am. Public Health Assoc., Atlanta
49. Kleinman, J. C., Kopstein, A. 1987. Smoking during pregnancy, 1967–80. *Am. J. Public Health* 77:823–25
50. Kleinman, J. C., Pierre, M. B., Madans, J. H., Land, G. H., Schramm, W. F. 1988. The effects of maternal smoking on fetal and infant mortality. *Am. J. Epidemiol.* 127:274–82
51. Kline, J., Stein, Z. A., Susser, M., Warburton, D. 1977. Smoking: a risk factor for spontaneous abortion. *N. Engl. J. Med.* 297:793–96
52. Kozlowski, L. T., Herling, S. 1988. Objective measures. In *Assessment of Addictive Behaviors,* ed. D. M. Donovan, G. A. Marlatt, pp. 214–35. New York: Guilford
53. Kramer, M. S. 1987. Determinants of low birth weight: methodological assessment and meta-analysis. *Bull. WHO* 65(5):663–737
54. Kruse, J., Le Fevre, M., Zweig, S. 1986. Changes in smoking and alcohol consumption during pregnancy: a population-based study in a rural area. *Obstet. Gynecol.* 67(5):627–32
55. Langford, E. R., Thompson, E. G., Tripp, S. C. 1983. Smoking and health education during pregnancy. Evaluation of a program for women in prenatal classes. *Can. J. Public Health* 74:285–89
56. Livison, N., Leino, E. V. 1988. Cigarette smoking motives: factorial structure and gender differences in a longitudinal study. *Int. J. Addict.* 23(6): 535–44
57. MacArthur, C., Newton, J. R., Knox, E. G. 1987. Effect of anti-smoking health education on fetal size at birth: a randomized clinical trial. *Br. J. Obstet. Gynecol.* 94:295–300
58. Marks, J. S., Koplan, J. P., Hogue, C. J. R., Dalmat, M. E. 1990. A cost-benefit/cost-effectiveness analysis of smoking cessation for pregnant women. *Am. J. Prev. Med.* 6:282–89
59. Mayer, J. P., Hawkins, B. Todd, R. 1990. A randomized evaluation of smoking cessation interventions for pregnancy women at a WIC clinic. *Am. J. Public Health* 80:1:76–78
60. McBride, C. M., Pirie, P. L. 1990. A brief report. Postpartum smoking relapse. *Addict. Behav.* 15:165–68
61. McCormick, M. C., Brooks-Gunn, J., Shorter, T., Holmes, J. H. Wallace, C. Y., et al. 1990. Factors associated with smoking in low-income pregnant women: relationship to birth weight, stressful life events, social support, health behaviors and mental distress. *J. Clin. Epidemiol.* 43(5):441–48
62. McNeil, A. D., Owen, L. A., Belcher, M., Sutherland, G., Fleming, S. 1990. Abstinence from smoking and expired-air carbon monoxide levels: lactose intolerance as a possible source of error. *Am. J. Public Health* 80:1114–15
63. Meyer, M. B., Jonas, B. S., Tonascia, J. A. 1976. Perinatal events associated with maternal smoking during pregnancy. *Am. J. Epidemiol.* 103:464–76
64. Miller, H. C., Hassanein, K., Hensleigh, P. A. 1976. Fetal growth retardation in relation to maternal smoking and weight gain in pregnancy. *Am. J. Obstet. Gynecol.* 125:55–60
65. Mullen, P. D. 1990. Smoking cessation counseling in prenatal care. In *New Perspectives on Prenatal Care,* eds. I. R. Merkatz, J. E. Thompson, P. E. Mullen, R. L. Goldenberg, 11:161–76. New York: Elsevier. 656 pp.
66. Mullen, P. D., Carbonari, J. P., Tabak, E. R., Glenday, M. 1991. Improving disclosure of smoking by pregnant women. *Am. J. Obstet. Gynecol.* 165: 409–13
67. Mullen, P. D., Quinn, V. P., Ershoff, D. G. 1990. Maintenance of nonsmoking postpartum by women who stopped

smoking during pregnancy. *Am. J. Public Health* 80(8):992–94
68. Murphy, J. F., Drumm, J. E., Mulcahy, R. 1980. The effect of maternal cigarette smoking on fetal birthweight and on growth of the fetal biparietal diameter. *Br. J. Obstet. Gynaecol.* 87:462–66
69. Natl. Cent. Health Stat. 1992. *Health, United States, 1991*. Hyattsville, Md: Public Health Serv.
70. Natl. Cent. Health Stat., Schoenborn, C. A. 1988. Health promotion and disease prevention: United States, 1985. *Vital and Health Statistics,* Ser. 10., No. 163. DHHS Publ. No. (PHS) 88-1591. Public Health Serv. Washington, DC: GPO
71. O'Campo, P., Faden, R. R., Brown, H., Glien, A. C. 1992. The impact of pregnancy on women's prenatal and postpartum smoking behavior. *Am. J. Prev. Med.* 8(1):8–13
72. Orlandi, M. A. 1986. Gender differences in smoking cessation. *Women Health* 11(3/4):237–51
73. Pechacek, T. F., Fox, B. H., Murray, D. M., Lueper, R. V. 1984. Review of techniques for measurement of smoking behavior. In *Behavioral Health: A Handbook of Health Enhancement and Disease Prevention,* ed. J. D. Matarazzo, S. M., S. M. Weiss, J. A. Herd, N. E. Miller, pp. 729–54. New York: Wiley
74. Pederson, L. L., Stavraky, K. M. 1987. Relationship of smoking to lifestyle factors in women. *Women Health* 12(2):47–65
75. Persson, P. H., Grennert, L., Gennser, G., Kullanders, S. 1978. A study of smoking and pregnancy with special reference to fetal growth. *Acta Obstet. Gynecol. Scand. Suppl.* 78:33–39
76. Petitti, D. B., Friedman, G. D., Kahn, W. 1981. Accuracy of information of smoking habits provided on self-administered research questionnaires. *Am. J. Public Health* 71:308–11
77. Pomerleau, C. S., Pomerleau, O. F., Weinstein Garcia, A. 1991. Biobehavioral research on nicotine use in women. *Br. J. Addict.* 86:527–31
78. Prager, K., Malin, H., Spiegler, D., Van Natta, P., Placek, P. J. 1984. Smoking and drinking behavior before and during pregnancy of married mothers of live-born infants and stillborn infants. *Public Health Rep.* 99:117–27
79. Prochaska, J. O., Velicer, W. F., Guadagnoli, E. Rossi, J. S., DiClemente, C. C. 1991 Patterns of change: dynamic typology applied to smoking cessation. *Multivariate Behav. Res.* 26(1):83–107
80. Quinn, V. P., Mullen, P. D., Ershoff, D. H. 1991. Women who stop smoking spontaneously prior to prenatal care and predictors of relapse before delivery. *Addict. Behav.* 16:29–40
81. Risch, H. A., Weiss, N. S., Clarke, E. A., Miller, A. B. 1988. Risk factors for spontaneous abortion and its recurrence. *Am. J. Epidemiol.* 128:420–30
82. Russell, L. B. 1986. *Is Prevention Better than Cure?* Washington, DC: Brookings Inst.
83. Sexton, M., Hobel, J. R. 1984. A clinical trial of change in maternal smoking and its effect on birth weight. *J. Am. Med. Assoc.* 25:911–15
84. Sexton, M., Hebel, J. R., Fox, N. L. 1987. Postpartum smoking. In *Smoking and Reproduction,* ed. M. J. Rosenberg. Littleton, MA: PSG. 239pp
85. Shiffman, S. 1982. Relapse following smoking cessation. A situational analysis. *J. Consult. Clin. Psychol.* 50:71–86
86. Shiono, P. H., Klebanoff, M. A., Rhoads, C. G. 1986. Smoking and drinking during pregnancy. *J. Am. Med. Assoc.* 255:82–84
87. Simpson, W. J. 1957. A preliminary report on cigarette smoking and the incidence of prematurity. *Am. J. Obstet. Gynecol.* 73:808–15
88. Stein, Z., Kline, J. 1983. Smoking, alcohol and reproduction. *Am. J. Public Health* 73:1154–56
89. Stockbauer, J. W., Land, G. H. 1991. Changes in characteristics of women who smoke during pregnancy: Missouri, 1978–1988. *Public Health Rep.* 106: 52–58
90. Stookey, G. K., Katz, B. P., Olson, B. L., Drook, C. A., Cohen, S. J. 1987. Evaluation of biochemical validation measures in determination of smoking status. *J. Dent. Res.* 66(10): 1597–1601
91. US Dep. Health and Hum. Serv. 1990. *Healthy People 2000:* National Health Promotion and Disease Prevention Objectives. DHHS publ. no. (PHS) 91-50213. Washington, DC: US Dep. Health Hum. Serv.
92. US Dep. Health and Hum. Serv. 1980. *The Health Consequences of Smoking for Women: A Report of the Surgeon General*. Washington, DC: US Dep. Health Hum. Serv., Public Health Serv., Cent. Dis. Control., Cent. Chron. Dis. Prev. Health Promot., Off. Smoking Health
93. US Dep. Health and Hum. Serv. 1990.

The Health Benefits of Smoking Cessation: A Report of the Surgeon General. Washington, DC: US Dep. Health Hum. Serv., Public Health Serv., Cent. Dis. Control., Cent. Chron. Dis. Prev. Health Promot., Off. Smoking Health. DHHS publ. no. (CDC) 90-8416

94. US Dep. Health and Hum. Serv. 1986. *The Health Consequences of Involuntary Smoking. A Report of the Surgeon General*. DHHS publ. no. (CDC) 87-8398. Washington, DC: US Dep. Health Hum. Serv., Public Health Serv., Cent. Dis. Control., Cent. Chron. Dis. Prev. Health Promot., Off. Smoking Health
95. US Dep. Health and Hum. Serv. 1980. *Reducing the Health Consequences of Smoking, 25 years of Progress: A Report of the Surgeon General*. DHHS publ. no. (CDC) 89-8411. Washington, DC: US Dep. Health Hum. Serv., Public Health Serv., Cent. Dis. Control., Cent. Chron. Dis. Prev. Health Promot., Off. Smoking Health
96. US Dep. Health and Hum. Serv. 1989. *Caring for Our Future: The Content of Prenatal Care. A Report of the Public Health Service Expert Panel on the Content of Prenatal Care*. Washington, DC: US Dep. Health Hum. Serv., Public Health Serv.
97. US Prev. Serv. Task Force. 1989. *Guide to Clinical Preventive Services: Report of the US Preventive Services Task Force*. Baltimore: Williams & Wilkins
98. Velicer, W. F., Prochaska, J. O., Rossi, J. S., Snow, M. G. 1992. Assessing outcome in smoking cessation studies. *Psychol. Bull.* 111:23–41
99. Vogt, T. M. 1982. Questionnaires versus biochemical measures of smoking exposure. *Am. J. Public Health* 72:93
100. Waldron, I. 1991. Patterns and causes of gender differences in smoking. *Soc. Sci. Med.* 32(9):989–1005
101. Windsor, R. A., Orleans, C. T. 1986. Guidelines and methodological standards for smoking cessation intervention research among pregnant women: improving the science and art. *Health Educ. Q.* 13:131–61
102. Windsor, R. A., Cutter, G., Morris, J., Reese, Y., Manzella V., et al. 1985. The effectiveness of smoking cessation methods for smokers in public health maternity clinics: a randomized trial. *Am. J. Public Health* 75:1389–92
103. Windsor, R. A., Lowe J. B., Perkins, L. L., Smith D. Y., Artz, L., et al. 1993. Behavioral impact and cost benefit of health education methods for pregnant smokers in public health maternity clinics: the birmingham trial ii. *Am. J. Public Health*. In press

Annu. Rev. Publ. Health. 1993. 14:413–50

HARM REDUCTION: A Public Health Response to the AIDS Epidemic Among Injecting Drug Users

Don C. Des Jarlais
Beth Israel Medical Center, New York, NY 10013

Samuel R. Friedman and Thomas P. Ward
National Development and Research Institutes, Inc. (formerly Narcotic and Drug Research, Inc.), New York, NY 10013

KEY WORDS: HIV, prevention programs

INTRODUCTION

Human use of psychoactive drugs precedes recorded history, and human misuse of such drugs is probably almost as old. Within the last century, laboratory techniques for strengthening drug preparations and the invention of injection equipment as a method of administration have greatly increased the potential for harmful consequences of psychoactive drugs. The intense effects from intravenous administration of highly refined drugs creates a higher likelihood of developing both tolerance and dependence—and of overdosing, if the quantity of drug is greater than the amount usually taken. Nonsterile injections may also lead to abscesses and diseases, such as endocarditis. Furthermore, multiperson use of drug injection equipment has spread such infections as hepatitis B.

The HIV/AIDS epidemic, however, has created an adverse consequence that is qualitatively different from the previously experienced problems associated with the injection of psychoactive drugs. In many countries, this difference has led to a conceptual reevaluation of how to approach the problems associated with psychoactive drug use. There are several components of the difference between AIDS and other adverse consequences of drug

0163-7525/93/0510-0413$02.00

use. First (given the currently available medical treatments), HIV infection is almost uniformly fatal.[1] HIV infection thus has the potential to negate the very possibility of other life goals for the individual, such as abstinence from illicit drugs, raising children, or social and vocational rehabilitation. Second, AIDS/HIV infection is a particularly unpleasant way to die, typically involving a long period of pain, physical debilitation, and sometimes mental deterioration. It is also an expensive way to die, consuming considerable portions of the finite medical resources that an ethical society would provide to persons in ill health. Third, because HIV can be transmitted both sexually and perinatally, not only the drug injectors themselves are at risk, but also their sexual partners and potential children. Hence, HIV infection is an adverse consequence of drug use that is not limited to the drug users themselves, but can spread from drug users to become a threat to the health of the entire community. Fourth, the transmission of HIV among drug injectors occurs through multiperson use of the injection equipment, rather than through the drugs themselves. Thus, at both an individual and a societal level, prevention of HIV transmission without necessarily having to cease drug use or even drug injection is possible.

Because of this urgent need to prevent HIV infection among injecting drug users (IDUs), many different prevention programs have been developed. A conceptual perspective, most commonly called "harm reduction," which unifies and guides many (though certainly not all) of these different prevention programs, has also emerged. Elements of the harm-reduction perspective existed before the AIDS epidemic among IDUs (5), but the epidemic has served as the catalyst for a fuller intellectual elaboration of the perspective and has been the primary reason why previously unresponsive political leaders have implemented harm-reduction programs (3, 33).

Harm-reduction programs, unlike other current approaches to the problem of drug abuse, consider reducing adverse consequences of drug use without necessarily reducing the drug use itself to be not only possible, but desirable. The prevention of HIV infection among persons who continue to inject illicit drugs is thus an especially instructive instance of harm reduction as praxis. We will discuss in detail the harm-reduction perspective, which has led to implementation and elaboration of numerous harm-reduction-based programs, after a discussion of the HIV epidemic among IDUs.

[1]Intensive research is being conducted to develop treatments for both HIV infection and the opportunistic infections that occur in the presence of HIV-related immunosuppression. Given the nature of HIV infection, potentially successful treatments would probably require maintenance treatment, which in turn requires multiple expensive drugs with substantial toxicities. Thus, even though HIV infection would no longer be fatal, there still would be a great public health need to prevent HIV infections.

EARLY EPIDEMIOLOGY OF HIV INFECTION AMONG IDUs

AIDS was first noted among IDUs in New York City in late 1981 (15). This discovery was in itself strong evidence that an infectious agent was likely to be the etiologic agent for AIDS. However, the first cases of AIDS among IDUs did not generate a great deal of public health concern. The perception at that time was that these cases were confined to one geographic area, that the absolute number of cases was relatively small (only 1353 cases had been reported through 1984), and, of course, that they were occurring in a group that was both highly stigmatized and without political power.

Soon thereafter, however, the development of tests for detection of the antibody to HIV (then called either LAV or HTLV-III) dramatically changed our understanding of the scope of the AIDS problem among IDUs. Although there was still only a modest number of cases of fully developed AIDS among IDUs in the New York area, these tests revealed that approximately half of the IDUs in New York (21, 68) and northern New Jersey (107) had been infected with the virus. At about the same time, testing of sera collected from IDUs in western Europe found substantial HIV infection among IDUs in many different areas, with a moderate (approximately 30%) seroprevalence rate among IDUs in Amsterdam (100) and high rates (approximately 50%) in Edinburgh (83) and in parts of Italy (4). As a result, the scope of AIDS among IDUs was recognized as having rapidly changed from a "small" New York City problem to a large problem in several cities, and a moderate but growing problem in numerous other cities.

During 1984–1986, it was generally believed that AIDS would develop in only a fraction, perhaps 10–30%, of persons infected with HIV. As more follow-up studies were conducted, however, it became clear that almost everyone who was infected with HIV would develop AIDS (although the average time period from initial infection to development of AIDS appeared to be ten years) (105).

HETEROSEXUAL AND PERINATAL TRANSMISSION FROM IDUs

Studies of AIDS and HIV infection among the (noninjecting) sexual partners and children of IDUs showed that the virus was being transmitted both heterosexually and perinatally (26, 30). In most developed countries, including the United States, IDUs quickly became the most common source for HIV infection among heterosexual partners and children. AIDS was becoming a "family disease" among drug injectors—often with the father, mother, and younger (but not older) children all becoming infected, and then dying.

As we discuss below, after this evidence of heterosexual and perinatal transmission became clear, AIDS prevention programs targeted to IDUs increasingly emphasized condom use. Relatively great difficulties have been encountered, however, in attempting to change their sexual behavior.

RAPID TRANSMISSION OF HIV AMONG IDUs

Studies with historically collected sera of IDUs confirmed the possibility of very rapid transmission of HIV within a population of IDUs. Table 1 lists areas that have undergone rapid transmission (here defined as at least a 20% increase in seroprevalence within a two-year period). In some of these areas (e.g. Edinburgh, Bangkok, Manipur), the spread has been extremely rapid, with seroprevalence increasing by 40–50% within a two year-period.

Behavioral studies suggest at least two components that account for such rapid spread of HIV within a population of IDUs. First, all known instances of very rapid spread have occurred among populations that were previously unaware of a local threat of HIV/AIDS. In some cities, e.g. New York (35), this was because the virus began spreading rapidly in the 1970s, long before anyone was aware of AIDS and HIV infection. In other areas, however, spread occurred after AIDS among IDUs in other places had been well-described, but the local drug injectors either did not know of AIDS, or if they did, still did not believe that it would become a local problem. And, of course, without recognition of HIV/AIDS as a local threat, IDUs were not motivated to change their behavior. Moreover, the limited number of studies that have examined

Table 1 Areas that experienced rapid spread[a] of HIV among IDUs

Location	Reference
New York	Des Jarlais et al (35)
Sardinia	Farci et al (41a)
Rio de Janiero	Lima et al (65a)
Bangkok	Choopanya (19a)
Bologna	Titti et al (98a)
Milan	Titti et al (98a)
Padua	Bortolotti et al (6a)
Geneva	Robert et al (82a)
Vienna	Loimer et al (66a)
Edinburgh	Peutherer et al (79a)
Tours	Goudeau et al (51a)
Manipur (India)	Naik et al (72a)

[a] "Rapid Spread" was defined as an increase of 20% or greater in HIV seroprevalence within two years. Note that sampling comparability was not considered in constructing this listing.

multiperson use of injection equipment before AIDS suggest that sharing of injection equipment had been close to universal (36).

The second component of very rapid spread of HIV among a population of IDUs is a mechanism for "efficient mixing." Efficient mixing occurs when any individual drug injector can share injection equipment with a high percentage of the total population of drug injectors.[2] A "shooting gallery," where injection equipment is rented to a drug injector, used, and then returned to the gallery owner for rental to the next injector, is a prime example of a mechanism to provide efficient mixing. Shooting galleries have frequently been linked with HIV transmission (32, 68, 88). Another example is "dealer's works." Here, drug dealers lend injection equipment to customers; hence, the equipment is used by many different customers, which then may cause rapid transmission (83). In cities with centralized drug-distribution markets, IDUs may often gather in large numbers to pool resources to purchase drugs. (Street drug prices are often lower for larger purchases.) This large group may then use the same injection equipment, thus leading to yet another mode of efficient mixing. Indeed, such sharing with large numbers of other injectors has also been associated with rapid transmission of HIV (20).

NON-AIDS ILLNESSES ASSOCIATED WITH HIV AMONG IDUs

Cases of AIDS, as reported under the Centers for Disease Control (CDC) surveillance definition, are often used as a best measure of the scope of the AIDS problem. AIDS cases may, however, be a poor measure of overall HIV-related morbidity and mortality among IDUs. The original US studies of AIDS were conducted almost exclusively with homosexual/bisexual men. These studies identified both "persistent generalized lymphadenopathy" and "AIDS-related complex," as well as the opportunistic infections and neoplasms that made up the original CDC surveillance definition of AIDS. The opportunistic definitions that were included in the original surveillance definition, as well as those included in subsequent revised definitions, were all highly specific to cell-mediated immune function.

Studies of HIV infection among IDUs and their sexual partners, however, suggested a much wider spectrum of illnesses associated with HIV infection among those groups (89, 90, 94). HIV infection is now recognized to be associated with a wide spectrum of infectious diseases, not just the opportu-

[2]Under circumstances of perfectly efficient mixing, any individual injector would have an equal probability of sharing equipment with any other injector in the total population. The efficiency of mixing within the population is reduced when sharing occurs primarily within ethnic or friendship groups.

nistic infections that are part of the current surveillance definition of AIDS. Table 2 lists diseases likely to occur with increased incidence and/or increased severity in the presence of HIV infection. Incidence of these illnesses in the presence of HIV is increased by a factor of two to four, and thus not of the order of magnitude of the increased incidence of those opportunistic infections that are part of the AIDS surveillance definition (where the increase is by a factor in the thousands). So far, the increase in severity associated with some of these infections cannot be even roughly quantified.

The increased incidence and/or increased severity of these illnesses in the presence of HIV infection have important implications both for the clinical care of HIV-infected drug injectors and the epidemiology of HIV infection among IDUs. The studies from New York City (89, 94) showed not only that HIV-infected IDUs were developing these non-AIDS illnesses at a higher rate than HIV-negative IDUs, but that a substantial proportion of the IDUs died from these illnesses. The illnesses were thus of great clinical importance. They also tended to reduce the numbers of IDUs who, if they had survived these other illnesses, would later have developed AIDS. The Stoneburner study estimated that the additional number of HIV-positive drug injectors in New York who died from these non-AIDS illnesses was approximately equal to the number who died of AIDS.

More recently, a study of bacterial pneumonia among IDUs in Holland found the expected increase in incidence among HIV-infected subjects, yet did not find any increase in resultant fatalities (69). The authors attributed this finding to the superior overall health care that IDUs regularly receive in Amsterdam, as compared with New York. This interpretation, if correct, clearly indicates an urgent need for dramatically improved health care for HIV-infected drug injectors in the many parts of the world where IDUs currently do not even receive adequate health care.

The increased incidence of tuberculosis among HIV-infected drug users also deserves comment. Until recently, tuberculosis was generally considered to be well on its way to being conquered throughout the industrialized countries. Over the last two years, however, there has been an excess of

Table 2 HIV-related non-AIDS infections among injecting drug users

	Incidence	Severity	Reference
Bacterial pneumonia	yes	yes	Selwyn et al (89)
Tuberculosis	yes	yes	Stoneburner et al (94)
Endocarditis	yes	yes	Stoneburner et al (94)
Vaginal candidiasis	?	yes-?	??
Cervical cancer	?	yes-?	Vermund et al (102a)
Pelvic inflammatory disease	?	yes-?	Minkoff & DeHovitz (71)

28,000 (or 26,000) cases of tuberculosis over what would normally have been expected in the United States (92). There are probably several reasons for this unexpected increase—among other things, funding for tuberculosis control efforts had been reduced over the previous several years—but, HIV infection is now known to be "the strongest risk factor" among recent cases of tuberculosis (92).

HIV infection can lead to increases in tuberculosis in several ways. Many poor persons, including many IDUs, have been exposed to tuberculosis, but the disease was otherwise controlled by their immune systems. However, when HIV infection reduces the competence of the immune system, the tuberculosis emerges as an active disease. HIV-immunosuppressed persons are also more susceptible to contracting tuberculosis and developing active disease if they should be exposed. Living in crowded and confined places, such as prisons and homeless shelters, as many IDUs in the US now do, would also lead to high rates of transmission to others from HIV-positive persons with active tuberculosis.

One particularly disturbing aspect of the emerging tuberculosis/HIV connection has been the rapid increase in multidrug-resistant tuberculosis. In New York City, approximately 15–22% of the new tuberculosis cases involve multidrug-resistant strains (New York City Department of Health, June 1992, personal communication). Treatment of these strains is quite expensive, with an individual case costing $100,000–180,000; yet, treatment is not likely to be effective for many HIV-immunosuppressed persons, with fatal outcomes occurring in 70–90% of the cases (17, 40, 90, 91).

Multidrug-resistant strains of tuberculosis have arisen because persons with active tuberculosis failed to take complete courses of medication. The solution to this problem will require intensive research. Directly observed therapy, although not inexpensive, would appear to be highly cost-effective when compared with the consequences of failing to complete treatment. Providing directly observed therapy, however, is likely to be difficult for persons without a regular residence and with a drug-dependence problem. Involuntary confinement is probably possible under the public health laws in most states (although the laws in most states are seriously outdated with respect to current scientific knowledge of tuberculosis). However, the matter of whether involuntary confinement, even if used as a method of last resort, would be an effective method for public health control of tuberculosis is not clear. The potential need for involuntary confinement of HIV-positive tuberculosis patients also has the potential for reducing the small amount of mutual trust that now exists between many persons with or at risk for HIV infection and public health authorities.

Because tuberculosis can be transmitted through aerosols, it exacerbates the already very difficult problems of providing health care for HIV-positive persons. The risk of illness to persons who provide health care to persons infected with HIV has always been real, albeit small and relatively inexpensive to control. However, the increasing incidence of tuberculosis among HIV-positive persons may radically change that. An expert committee convened by the American Foundation for AIDS Research (AmFAR) estimated that more than $400 million in construction work would be needed to renovate existing health-care facilities to provide adequate infection control for tuberculosis in the US (D. Kirby, AmFAR 1992, personal communication).

One additional set of non-AIDS illnesses believed to be associated with HIV deserves special mention. Table 2 lists several gynecological conditions, including cervical cancer, pelvic inflammatory disease, and vaginal candidiasis. Women diagnosed with AIDS in the US have shorter survival times than men, even after statistically controlling on other relevant risk factors (86). One reason for this may be that women seek medical treatment later in their HIV illness because of other responsibilities, e.g. child care. Another possible reason is that there is relatively little information about the natural history of HIV infection in women (71). In the US, most women with AIDS are either IDUs themselves or the sexual partners of IDUs (18). Large-scale studies of the natural hsitory of HIV infection in women are just now beginning.

As more has been learned about HIV infection, the number of illnesses that appear to be associated with HIV infection has greatly increased. Many of the associations have been relatively modest in strength, although clearly important for the clinical care of HIV-positive persons. To avoid continuous revision of the surveillance definition of AIDS with new opportunistic infections (and particularly with weakly opportunistic infections), CDC has proposed that the surveillance definition for AIDS be revised to include all persons with CD4 cell counts of less than 200 per cubic millimeter of blood. Diagnosing AIDS would be greatly simplified, and most persons with severe manifestations of HIV immunosuppression would be included. The new definition would not, however, preclude the need for additional research on the outcomes of HIV infection in male and female IDUs and their sexual partners.

SPREAD OF HIV AMONG IDUs IN DEVELOPING COUNTRIES

During most of the 1980s, HIV infection among IDUs was considered to be a problem only for North America and western Europe, the traditional consumer countries for heroin and cocaine. Unfortunately, the well-documented rapid spread of HIV among drug injectors in Thailand during 1988 (20, 80, 102) demonstrated that the problem could also occur in industrializing countries. Since then, HIV infection among IDUs has been documented as a major public health problem in other parts of south Asia, South America, and eastern Europe. Table 3 lists countries where HIV infection among IDUs is considered a major public health concern. The problem is found at all levels of economic development and in countries with great differences in culture, the primary drug injected, and political systems.

Understanding the spread of HIV among IDUs in such a wide range of countries requires understanding of a group of interrelated problems: How does the nonmedical use of potentially injectable psychoactive drugs spread from country to country (or arise independently in different countries)? How does injection become a preferred method of administration? How does HIV spread across national borders to reach new populations of IDUs?

The World Health Organization (WHO) has coordinated a multisite international study that will provide data relevant for some of these questions (M. Carballo 1992, personal communication). At present, however, we have only working hypotheses rather than answers. Nonmedical psychoactive drug use has been noted in almost all cultures studied. The use of potentially

Table 3 Countries where HIV among IDUs is a public health problem

Europe[a]	*North America*	*Asia*
Austria	Canada	China
Belgium	United States	India
Denmark		Myanmar
Finland	*South America*	Thailand
France	Argentina	
Germany	Brazil	
Greece		*Australia*
Ireland		
Israel		
Italy		
Luxemburg		
Netherlands		
Poland		
Portugal		
Norway		
San Marino		
Spain		
Sweden		
Switzerland		
Turkey		
United Kingdom		
Yugoslavia		

[a]Source: European Centre for the Epidemiological Monitoring of AIDS. *AIDS Surveillance in Europe, Quarterly Report No. 28,* 31 December 1990 (Geneva, WHO-EC Collaborating Centre on AIDS).

injectable drugs, primarily heroin and cocaine, appears to follow drug distribution routes from producing regions to transshipment to consumer countries.[3] One geographic band of heroin use follows the land-transportation distribution route across southern Europe (Yugoslavia, Austria, Switzerland, northern Italy, southern France, Spain); another branches out from the "Golden Triangle" (Thailand/Laos/Myanmar) westward to northern India and eastward across China to Hong Kong. And, a cocaine land-distribution route runs south from northern Brazil to Rio de Janeiro, Sao Paulo, and Santos. With modern air transportation, distribution channels no longer have to follow land or sea routes. For instance, western Africa has become a major transshipment point for heroin from southeast Asia to Europe and the United States; thus, a local consumption problem has developed in western Africa.

Leakage from a distribution route into local consumption provides for a relatively inexpensive supply of drugs, because the marginal cost of adding additional drugs from further up the supply route is usually very low. A local consumption market can also serve as a buffer against economic losses for distributors if demand should become slack further down the supply route.

A potential inexpensive supply of injectable drugs is at best only a partial explanation for why a substantial degree of psychoactive drug injection might develop in a country. In several ways, illicit drug injection can be seen as an aspect of economic modernization. As suggested above, the improvements in transportation systems, such as highways, airports, and seaports, can also make drug-smuggling into the country much easier. Economic modernization often involves rapid urbanization and economic dislocations, which can create both large numbers of persons willing to use psychoactive drugs and sufficient numbers of persons willing to engage in the illicit distribution of the drugs.

Increased law-enforcement activities, based on international conventions and occasionally coordinated police work, have been the primary response to the spread of injectable drug use throughout the world. Law enforcement can also result in an increase in the use of injection as a route of administration. In several documented historical instances, law enforcement could suppress traditional, noninjecting methods of psychoactive drug use, such as opium smoking, rather easily, thereby creating at least a subset of previous users who then change to injecting (20, 31). Law-enforcement pressures also lead both drug distributors and drug users toward injection of psychoactive drugs. Both the illegal status of the drugs and intensified law enforcement (which

[3]The traditional distinction between producer and consumer countries is losing much of its meaning, as nonmedical psychoactive drug use has been dramatically increasing in the producer areas. The capability for local production of cannabis, amphetamines, hallucinogens, and "designer" narcotics in the traditional consumer countries has also blurred the distinction. The increasing psychoactive drug use in traditional transshipment countries further illustrates the need for a new conceptualization and a new terminology.

reduces supplies) tend to increase the price greatly. In this context, injection becomes the most cost-efficient method of administering psychoactive drugs, because a more intense drug effect is produced and because almost all of the drug is actually consumed. Drug distributors make their greatest profits from highly refined drugs, because they tend to be both injectable and the least bulky (which is important for concealing and transporting the drugs).

With modern air travel, distributors commonly respond to law-enforcement pressure simply by creating new distribution routes. The profits to be made from transporting illicit injectable drugs are sufficiently high that there is no longer any need to take direct routes from the production areas to the developed countries with their higher consumption rates. Moreover, with the increasing leakage at transshipment points into local consumption, international law enforcement may now have the additional side-effect of dispersing injectable drug use to many different countries.

Although there is relatively little scientific data on the causes of the spread of both drug use and drug injection into different countries, we have considerably more knowledge about how HIV spreads to IDUs in different countries. In some instances, HIV has spread to IDUs from other groups in the same area. In New York City, for example, HIV spread from noninjecting male homosexuals to IDUs with male homosexual drug injectors serving as a bridge group (35). A similar process apparently occurred in Rio de Janeiro (65). Moreover, despite the stereotype that drug injectors are too poor to travel, current data suggest that they engage in a substantial amount of travel. Preliminary data from the WHO study of HIV and drug injection in 13 different cities indicates that approximately one fifth of the IDUs in each of the cities not only had traveled outside of the home city, but had injected drugs outside of the home city.

SUMMARY OF EPIDEMIOLOGY

Much has been learned about the epidemiology of HIV infection among IDUs since the discovery of the first cases of AIDS among this population ten years ago. The problem of HIV infection among IDUs is already a world-wide problem. Moreover, there is every reason to expect further spread of injecting drug use to additional countries, with HIV infection among the IDUs likely to follow. Once HIV has entered a local population of IDUs, extremely rapid spread of the virus is possible, with up to half of the group becoming infected within several years. In addition, once drug injectors are infected with HIV, they are not only subject to developing the opportunistic infections and neoplasms that constitute the surveillance definition of AIDS, but are also more likely to develop a wide variety of other potentially fatal illnesses, such as bacterial pneumonia and tuberculosis.

All of the epidemiology in the field to date thus points to an urgent need for the prevention of HIV infection among IDUs wherever groups of IDUs are found.

THE HARM REDUCTION PERSPECTIVE ON PREVENTION OF HIV INFECTION AMONG IDUs

Programs to prevent HIV infection among IDUs have by now been implemented in most of the countries where illicit drug injecting is known to occur. These programs vary greatly in their content, intensity, and coverage of the drug-injecting population. The urgent need to prevent HIV infection and the great diversity in the programs themselves have created a need for a framework to organize the programs conceptually. The most common framework is called the "harm reduction" or "harm minimization" approach to the problems of drug use.

Harm reduction is in an ongoing process of development as a perspective on the problems of psychoactive drug use. The concept has received the most consideration and development in Holland, the United Kingdom, and Australia (8–11, 38, 93, 109). However, specialists in the field are still trying to formulate a brief but inclusive definition of what constitutes harm reduction (9, 95), and it may be premature even to attempt a formal definition at this time. Yet, despite the difficulties in trying to provide a concise and permanent definition of a field that is still undergoing rapid growth, some fundamental tenets of the approach, particularly with respect to preventing HIV infection, can be listed.

The basic premise of the harm-reduction perspective concerns the sense in which psychoactive drug use should be considered a problem. In some perspectives, the basic problem is simply the use of the illicit psychoactive drugs as such; thus, all efforts need to be concentrated upon reducing current use of the drugs and preventing new persons from ever starting to use them. The harm-reduction perspective, in contrast, sees the problem not so much as the drug use itself, but rather as the harmful consequences of some types of drug use. Harm reduction simply calls for reducing the harmful effects of drug use. If reducing the drug use is the only way in which harmful consequences can be reduced, then reduction is necessary. For many types of drug-related harm, however, it is possible to reduce at least a substantial part of the harm without necessarily eliminating (or even reducing) the drug use itself. HIV infection among IDUs is a readily comprehensible example of this type of harm. Because the multiperson use of injection equipment is the actual mode of HIV transmission, it is certainly possible to have many types of illicit drug use that do not involve HIV transmission. Within the harm-reduction perspective, therefore, reduction of the drug use itself becomes not the fundamental public goal, but merely one possible means to a multitude of public goals.

In addition to the shift from defining reduction of drug use as the fundamental goal to perceiving it as merely one possible means to other goals, harm reduction is, above all, a pragmatic approach to psychoactive drug use. Emphasis is on attainable short-term results over utopian long-term goals. The ideal method for reducing the harm associated with illicit psychoactive drug use would simply be to prevent any further use. Obviously, no one would be sharing injection equipment if heroin, cocaine, amphetamines, and other injectable drugs were not being illicitly used. However, because complete elimination of illicit drug use is extremely unlikely to occur in the foreseeable future, a harm-reduction approach focuses instead upon what can be done to reduce HIV transmission through the sharing of injection equipment.

The answer to this pragmatic question leads us to another characteristic of the harm-reduction perspective; namely, that it is based on multiple, complementary solutions operating simultaneously, rather than some single best solution. That is, there are usually many things that can be done simultaneously to reduce the specific harm, even if some of these activities might appear at first to be in conflict with each other. With respect to the prevention of HIV transmission among IDUs, for example, drug abuse treatment programs can be established to reduce the use of psychoactive drugs, while IDUs are being encouraged to use drugs either without injection or by practicing safer injection. At the same time, sterile injection equipment can be provided at no cost (or sold cheaply), so that sharing of equipment is not necessary. And, disinfectants, such as bleach, can be provided so that, whenever sharing does occur, the equipment can be disinfected before multiperson use.

Although harm-reduction offers several approaches simultaneously, no individual drug user will be involved in all of these programs at the same time. This apparent inconsistency can create troublesome complications for some political leaders, who have tended to see illicit drug users as one homogenous group that should be encouraged (or coerced) to change its behavior in a single way. Harm-reduction practitioners, on the other hand, have no difficulty in recommending a relative hierarchy of choices to individual drug users, usually in the same order of preference in which the different activities are presented above. Individual drug users are thus enabled to make informed choices as to which type of harm reduction they will follow, with the understanding that their specific choices may change over time.

Indeed, the very idea that an illicit drug user is capable of a rational, informed choice—and will exercise that choice to reduce harm both to the individual and to society as a whole—distinguishes the harm-reduction perspective from other perspectives in the drug abuse field. Other perspectives tend to emphasize the limitations on rational choice that occur when a person is physically or psychologically dependent upon psychoactive drugs. (Another common assumption is that, because illicit drug users by definition have chosen to break the laws regarding drug use, they cannot be trusted to make any decisions that will benefit society as a whole.)

The final characteristic of the harm-reduction perspective that needs to be discussed here is its concern with overcoming the marginalization of illicit drug users by the dominant society. A substantial amount of the harm incurred by illicit drug users results not so much from the use of illicit drugs themselves, but from the associated social marginalization and stigmatization. With respect to HIV prevention, harm-reduction programs need to address the compounded stigmatization associated with both illicit drug injection and AIDS itself. This double stigmatization has created multiple new problems, as well as exacerbating numerous older problems. For instance, especially earlier in the AIDS epidemic, it has impeded community action against AIDS among some ethnic minority communities in the United States (48, 81). It has also increased the distrust between IDUs and public health authorities, thus making implementation of prevention programs that much more difficult (14). Finally, the fear of stigmatization has led some IDUs to deny their risk of transmitting AIDS to their sexual partners (A. Abdul-Quader 1991, personal communication). The harm-reduction framework responds to such stigmatization by insisting that IDUs are recognized as full members of the community, that safeguarding the public health of the entire community requires providing adequate health services to all of its members, and that IDUs should be encouraged to participate actively in AIDS prevention projects. Moreover, because HIV is transmitted from IDUs to their sexual partners and their children, the framework further emphasizes the linkage between the health of drug users and the health of the community as a whole.

HIV PREVENTION PROGRAMS FOR IDUs

The harm-reduction perspective has emerged as a unifying theoretical expression of a multitude of different HIV prevention programs that have been practiced in many different countries. In keeping with the perspective, different prevention programs have usually been implemented simultaneously to provide for the specific needs of different subsets of IDUs.

However, in those instances in which many different prevention programs have become operational at approximately the same time in the same place, evaluation of the distinct effects of each individual prevention program has been extremely difficult. Moreover, this has been only one of the methodological problems in drawing conclusions about the effectiveness of AIDS prevention programs for IDUs. Program evaluations have also tended to use different units of measurement for the relevant AIDS risk behaviors, thus making it all the more difficult to compare different programs. Similarly, the demographic and behavioral characteristics of the IDUs who participate in the different programs have usually been only briefly described in the evaluation reports, so that it has not been possible to control statistically for the differences among the participants in different programs. Finally, most evaluations have relied upon simple pre-post experimental designs, even though a large percentage of IDUs, once aware of AIDS, will already have changed their behavior in the absence of formal prevention programs (34). (Attempting to use a control group that was "protected" from learning about AIDS would, of course, be a highly unethical research procedure.)

Nonetheless, despite these numerous methodological difficulties, the present state of evaluation research on AIDS prevention programs for IDUs does permit some generalizations about the actual and potential effectiveness of the different programs. Table 4 presents results from several studies for each of the major types of AIDS prevention programs for IDUs. This table is not meant to be comprehensive; rather, studies were selected to illustrate the variety of programs in different geographical locations and in different time periods.

The syringe exchange is perhaps the prototypical harm-reduction method for preventing HIV infection among IDUs. In a syringe-exchange program, IDUs can, at no cost, exchange their used needles and syringes for new, sterile injection equipment (10, 33, 55, 56, 66, 76). In addition, by collecting the used injection equipment, syringe exchanges also provide for safe disposal of potentially HIV-contaminated equipment. Because the exchange is conducted on a face-to-face basis, syringe exchanges also provide an opportunity for delivery of other services to IDUs. Syringe exchanges typically provide AIDS education and counseling, distribute condoms (to prevent sexual transmission of HIV), and make referrals to drug abuse treatment or other medical and social services that may be desired by the participants. Many also distribute alcohol swabs (to reduce the likelihood of developing abscesses and other infections) and bleach for disinfecting injection equipment in the event it is used by more than one person. Some even do on-site testing for tuberculosis and sexually transmitted diseases.

In addition to differences in the number and kind of extra services that are offered on-site or by referral, exchanges also vary in their locations (fixed versus "roving" sites), hours of operation, the variety of needles and syringes distributed, and most notably the allowed number of syringes to be exchanged. That is, some organizations exchange only a limited number of syringes at one time, whereas others exchange without any limit. Persons exchanging large numbers at a single time—up to several hundred syringes, in some cases—are clearly exchanging for others. Some exchange workers believe

Table 4 Results from studies of various types of AIDS prevention programs for IDUs

Author	Sample	Mechanism of change	Results
Klee et al (63)	North-West of England: 169 IDUs (46 female, 123 male) recontacted for structured questionnaire 6–9 months after previous interview as part of larger (n = 303) sample.	Unspecified, although overall AIDS awareness was high, and many subjects had already sought HIV testing on their own initiative.	Changes from intake to follow-up: 32/169 (19%) had stopped all drug use; 29/137 (21%) had switched from injecting to other modes of drug-taking; 46 were borrowing used equipment less frequently, or not at all; 50 were passing on used equipment less frequently, or not at all.
Neaigus et al (75)	New York City: 121 street-recruited IDUs (65% male, 35% female) reinterviewed at a mean of 4.5 months after intake. 58% black, 31% Latino, 11% white.	Outreach intervention including AIDS information, condom distribution, and referral to HIV testing.	Changes from intake to follow-up: 44% (vs. 22% at intake) had not injected within the previous 30 days; Of 68 still injecting at follow-up, percent of injections at shooting galleries declined from 13% to 7%.
Martin et al (68a)	Verona, Italy: Of 189 subjects at intake, 73 IDUs (21 HIV+, 52 HIV−) interviewed 6 months after HIV testing and counseling, and AIDS education session.	25-minute audiovisual presentation in which subjects were "not exhorted to change behaviour but rather encouraged to carefully evaluate risks."	Changes from intake to follow-up: Needle sharing declined from 66/189 (35%) to 9/73 (12.3%). At-risk sex during previous six months declined from 38.6% to 32.9%; Average number of at-risk encounters declined from 23.7 to 18.9—for HIV+, from 25.2 to 16.3; Average % of times using condoms during at-risk encounters increased from 48.7% to 70.2%.

Hart et al (55)	London, UK: 133 clients of the syringe-exchange scheme of Middlesex Hospital interviewed 1 month after entry, with 76 contacted for 3-month follow-up.	Syringe exchange with AIDS education.	Changes from intake to follow-up: Frequency of injections per month declined from a median of 56 to a median of 48.5; Percent sharing equipment declined from 32/133 (15%) to 17/76 (11%).
Kall & Olin (62a)	Stockholm: 2 groups of IDUs detained at the Remand Prison were interviewed and given HIV serum tests: 156 subjects from May–Sept. 1987; 268 subjects from July–Dec. 1988. A majority used amphetamine as their main drug.	No specific intervention, but overall AIDS awareness was high, as indicated by the fact that 80% of subjects during 1987 interview period had already been tested for HIV.	Differences between 1987 and 1988 samples: 1987: 15% never shared needles; 1988: 27% never shared needles. 1987: 16% of HIV- subset never shared; 1988: 26% of HIV- subset never shared. In a subset of 39 subjects who participated in both years, 21 (54%) shared less often.
Watters et al (106)	San Francisco: 2114 IDUs were interviewed and HIV tested in 6 cross-sections from 1986 to 1989. Convenience samples drawn from 3 detox clinics and 3 street locales.	An aggressive prevention campaign directed at IDUs from mid-1986 and thereafter, including street outreach and bleach distribution.	Changes from 1986 to 1989: 1986: 8.8% reported no needle sharing; 1989: 34.5% reported no needle sharing. 1986: 13% reported safe needle-hygiene; 1989: 73.3% reported safe needle-hygiene. Among subset of needle-sharers, 3% reported bleach use in 1986, 85.8% in 1989.

Table 4 *(Continued)*

Author	Sample	Mechanism of change	Results
Stephens et al (92a)	Cleveland: 322 IDUs were interviewed about risk behaviors before, and again 3–5 months after, an educational intervention.	Educational intervention presented in one-on-one format by professional health educator, typically lasting 45 minutes to an hour, including bleach demonstration and other risk reduction.	Changes from intake to follow-up: % sharing works declined from 67.4 to 24.3; % injecting drugs declined from 92.2 to 70.5; Among the subset still injecting, % using bleach increased from 33.5 to 62.2.
Nicolosi et al (75a)	Northern Italy: Of 933 IDUs—64% enrolled from detox clinics, 36% from other clinics—460 participated in at least 2 follow-up interviews, at a mean of 10.4 months after enrollment.	In addition to a national mass-media campaign since 1988, an intervention involving HIV counseling and testing was administered to the detox patients.	At intake, all 933 subjects were injecting; At follow-up, 128/460 (28%) had stopped injecting. At intake, 71.7% of subjects shared needles; At follow-up, only 214/460 (46.5%) shared.
Pomeroy et al (80a)	Dublin: 60 IDUs (47 male, 13 female) in a methadone program interviewed regarding previous and present behavior.	Methadone program and overall AIDS awareness.	Although 58 (97%) admitted to previously having shared needles, only 13 (22%) reported sharing within the previous 6 months.
Haemmig et al (52a)	Bern, Switzerland: 113 IDUs were given an anonymous, self-administered questionnaire at a street site.	Sterile injection equipment freely available. Moreover, modes of HIV transmission were correctly identified by >90%.	Within the past 3 years, 30% shared needles, but only 14% in the past 6 months. 55% said they would never borrow, and 67% said they would never lend equipment.
Tross et al (98b)	New York: 420 IDUs at a Lower East Side outreach program storefront were interviewed and then reinterviewed 4 months later.	Outreach intervention based on self-efficacy and social peer support models, using ex-IDU outreach workers.	% sharing needles decreased from 74% at intake to 33% at follow-up.

Donoghoe et al (39a)	UK multisite: Questionnaire survey, with reinterview after 2–4 months, of 142 clients (120 male, 20 female) of syringe exchanges.	Syringe exchange AIDS education.	Changes from intake to follow-up: Number of sexual partners: No partner—23% to 31%; Multiple partners—26% to 21%; Regular partner—49% to 52%. Any condom use: 38% to 30%. Non-IDU partner: 36% to 39%; 46% to 55% for sexually active subset.
Wyld et al (110)	Edinburgh: 115 HIV+ IDUs and their heterosexual partners—30 of the couples both HIV+, 85 couples serologically discordant—were interviewed every 6 months over a 3-year period about their sexual histories since 1983.	HIV testing and repeated counseling.	Report any condom use: 2% in 1983, 48% in 1989; Couples reporting a pregnancy: 23/89 (26%) in 1987, 9/78 (11.5%) in 1989.

Table 4 (*Continued*)

Author	Sample	Mechanism of change	Results
Friedman et al (46a)	Brooklyn: 243 IDUs (158 males, 85 females) who were sexually active during 6 months before intake and mean 7.8 months before follow-up. 43% black, 41% Latino, 16% white—also, 26% prostitutes.	Peer pressure for risk reduction mobilized through group meetings, one-on-one counseling, and while distributing condoms, bleach, etc.	Changes from intake to follow-up: Percent always using condoms—24–33%; Mean proportion of sex acts in which condom was used—39–48%; Of 185 not always using condoms at intake, 39 (21%) were always using condoms at follow-up. Group attendance in re: always using condoms: 51% of attenders vs. 25% of nonattenders always used condoms; Among prostitutes, 61% of attenders vs. 32% of nonattenders always used condoms; Among nonprostitutes, 42% of attenders vs. 26% of nonattenders always used condoms.
Liebman & Sepulveda-Irene (64)	Philadelphia: Community health outreach workers made contact with 6629 high-risk individuals (54% IDUs, 9% prostitutes, sexual partners of IDUs—percent unspecified): 29% female, 71% male; 57% black, 28% Hispanic, 14% white.	Face-to-face conversation about AIDS risk and referral to treatment and services in the course of distributing condoms and bleach kits.	82% of all contacts accepted condoms; 90% of prostitutes accepted condoms; 84% of males accepted condoms; 74% of females accepted condoms.

Poole et al (80b)	San Francisco: Project AWARE followed up 40 HIV+ females at 6- and 12-month intervals. 16 were IDUs, 16 had an HIV+ sex partner, 4 had a high-risk partner, 3 had no identified risk.	Social influence through peer group organization.	Changes from intake to follow-up: Average number of sex partners—from 5.2 to 2.1 (6 mo.) to 4.0 (12 mo.); Percent with fewer partners—40% (6 mo.), 50% (12 mo.); Percent abstinent—35% (6 mo.), 8% (12 mo.) Percent having vaginal sex without condom—from 75% to 37% (6 mo.) to 37% (12 mo.).
Vanichseni et al (101)	Bangkok: 601 in-treatment IDUs: 336 with no previous HIV test (NPT), 73 who had tested positive (PT+), 148 who had tested negative (PT−).	HIV testing and counseling.	Frequency of condom use w/primary partner: Always—PT+ 29%; PT− 11%; NPT 9%; Sometimes—PT+ 43%; PT− 17%; NPT 20%; Never—PT+ 29%; PT− 71%; NPT 72%. Any contraception in past 6 months: PT+ 89%; PT− 73%; NPT 60%. Frequency of condom use w/casual partner: Always—PT+ 57%; PT− 30%; NPT 33%; Sometimes—PT+ 14%; PT− 22%; NPT 22%; Never—PT+ 29%; PT− 48%; NPT 46%.
Jain et al (61)	Sacramento: 671 IDUs recruited from treatment programs, hospital and jail. 150 of these returned for follow-up.	Intensive education/prevention program targeted to IDUs and their sexual partners, including HIV testing.	Changes from intake to follow-up: % never using condoms—from 68% to 62%; % often or always using condoms—from 22% to 26%; Average number of sex partners, last 6 mos: from 11 to 5.6.

that such large-volume exchangers defeat some of the secondary purposes, because there is no personal contact possible between the staff and the anonymous persons who are indirectly served through the large-volume exchangers. Limiting the number of syringes exchanged at one time, however, reduces the availability of sterile injection equipment among the local IDU population and the number of AIDS workers among the IDU population. In one study of an exchange (with a limit of five on the number of syringes that could be exchanged), IDUs persisted in passing on used equipment to others (63). At other programs, however, the large-volume exchangers are considered to be "satellite" workers, who increase the overall coverage of the exchange among the local population of IDUs. A few exchanges have even begun training these satellite workers to provide AIDS education and referrals (52).

Syringe exchanges have not led to an increase in illicit drug use, as many opponents had feared (70). Indeed, all evaluations to date have shown that illicit drug use does not increase among participants in the exchanges and there is no detectable increase in the number of new drug injectors in any given locality where syringe exchanges have been implemented. In some American cities, such as Portland (78), Tacoma (53), and New Haven (76), the syringe exchanges have also proven to be major referral sources for helping persons into drug abuse treatment programs.

However, the precise extent to which syringe exchanges have reduced HIV transmission among IDUs is difficult to determine. The methodological concerns noted above also apply to almost all syringe-exchange studies. All evaluations have shown some reduction in AIDS risk behavior, particularly in multiperson use of injection equipment, but these have often been of a modest magnitude, and no study to date has shown complete elimination of multiperson use. On a more positive note, however, implementation or large-scale expansion of syringe exchanges has been followed by stabilization of HIV seroprevalence among IDUs in several cities (see discussion below)—and by actual reductions in hepatitis B transmission among IDUs in Amsterdam (11), San Francisco (98), and Tacoma (54)—which suggests a substantial impact on reducing the transmission of blood-borne viruses among IDUs.

Although syringe-exchange programs have so far received the most public attention as a harm-reduction strategy for preventing HIV infection, over-the-counter sale of sterile injection equipment probably can reach a very high percentage of IDUs. Before the AIDS epidemic, there was great variation in the laws regulating the sale and possession of injection equipment. In the United States, almost all states criminalized the possession of equipment for injecting illicit drugs, and the states with large numbers of IDUs also tended to require prescriptions for the sale of injection equipment. In Europe, most countries did not have laws criminalizing possession or requiring prescriptions, but many pharmacists unofficially chose not to sell injection equipment to suspected IDUs. In fact, in Amsterdam, the decision of one central-city pharmacist to stop selling injection equipment to suspected IDUs that led to organized demands from IDUs for the establishment of the world's first syringe-exchange program in 1984—even before concern about AIDS among IDUs in that city. In Edinburgh, police persuaded pharmacists not to sell injection equipment in 1982, at about the time that HIV was being introduced into the local community of IDUs (83). HIV then spread rapidly among the group—reaching 50% seroprevalence within approximately two years—an experience that served as a powerful example of the dangers of restricting legal access to sterile injection equipment.

In Innsbruck, Austria, before concern about AIDS, pharmacists would sell needles and syringes only in lots of at least 100 (50). This requirement for a large-volume minimum purchase was meant to, and indeed did, discourage IDUs from purchasing injection equipment in the pharmacies. As the AIDS threat became evident, however, public health officials convinced the pharmacists to sell needles and syringes to IDUs and educated the IDUs about the need to use sterile equipment. HIV seroprevalence among drug injectors in that city has subsequently stabilized. Similarly, in Glasgow, Scotland, pharmacists were persuaded to sell injection equipment to IDUs, and an evaluation study has since shown a decrease in multiperson use of injection equipment among the IDUs (51). Before the AIDS epidemic, France required prescriptions for the sale of injection equipment. Because of concern about AIDS, the law was changed, and a national program was established to train pharmacists in how to sell injection equipment to IDUs while providing information on how to use the equipment safely. Several evaluation studies showed that, after the change in the law and the training of the pharmacists, multiperson use of injection equipment by IDUs in France declined substantially (41, 60). In yet another scenario, preexisting pharmacy availability of syringes made it possible for AIDS education and counseling for IDUs to lead to rapid behavior change. This happened in Bangkok after HIV had already spread rapidly within the group. The education program was followed by rapid behavior change; indeed, studies indicate that the majority of IDUs stopped sharing injection equipment, with 80% of them now obtaining sterile injection equipment from pharmacies. This large-scale behavior change was then followed by reduced seroconversion and stabilization of HIV seroprevalence among IDUs in Bangkok (20).

Rather than thinking of these two approaches as competitive, we should emphasize that most places that have implemented syringe-exchange programs have simultaneously implemented over-the-counter sales of injection equipment to IDUs (if they did not already have legal sales). As noted above, this is consistent with the harm-reduction approach of providing multiple means toward the same specific goal. It does, however, present formidable problems for evaluation research (as also noted above). Many IDUs who are not using syringe exchanges, and who thus might have served as a comparison group for IDUs, are obtaining their injection equipment from pharmacies. Because both the exchanges and the pharmacies are providing sterile injection equipment, there is obviously no strong rationale for expecting differences in AIDS risk behavior between participants in one program or the other.

In the United States, laws enacted before AIDS—and continuing political opposition to providing legal access to injection equipment for IDUs—have combined to limit greatly both syringe exchange and over-the-counter sales as AIDS prevention activities. Despite these impediments, there are a number of legal and underground exchanges currently operating (3, 33, 53, 76, 78), and there has been a marked increase in both legal and underground exchanges over the last several years. Still, in the absence of a national system of legal syringe-exchange programs, AIDS prevention for IDUs in the US has instead emphasized drug abuse treatment (discussed below) and outreach/bleach-distribution programs. The outreach programs typically (although not exclusively) use trained ex-addicts who go into high-drug-use areas and conduct face-to-face AIDS education, as well as provide referrals to other services, such as drug abuse treatment and HIV counseling and testing. The outreach workers also typically distribute small bottles of bleach for disinfecting used injection equipment, along with condoms to reduce sexual transmission of HIV. Evaluations of the outreach/bleach-distribution programs to date have shown large pre-post reductions in drug-injection risk behavior (16, 64, 75, 106), although not complete risk elimination. Moreover, stabilization of HIV seroprevalence has been noted in several cities after the implementation of outreach/bleach-distribution programs (106). Nonetheless, although proper use of bleach clearly can kill HIV, it is still not clear whether using bleach has a protective effect under field conditions. Indeed, the self-reported use of bleach was not associated with reduced HIV seroconversions in a Baltimore study (104).

Providing increased drug abuse treatment has been advocated not only in countries that have adopted a harm-reduction perspective (e.g. Australia and the Netherlands), but also in countries that have not adopted the perspective (e.g. the United States). Studies of methadone maintenance treatment have shown that if IDUs enter high-dosage treatment before an epidemic of HIV in the local community—and remain in treatment during the epidemic—they are substantially less likely to be infected with HIV (1, 6, 88). These results are hardly surprising, given the previously well-documented ability of drug abuse treatment to reduce (though not eliminate) illicit drug use as such for many persons (23, 59). Nevertheless, there are still important areas of disagreement regarding drug abuse treatment as a method of preventing HIV infection among IDUs.

One concern is whether drug abuse treatment can be provided on a sufficient scale, and made attractive enough, to enroll enough IDUs to prevent an HIV epidemic among IDUs in a given local community. Treatment clearly can protect individuals from HIV infection, but it is not yet clear whether treatment systems can be rapidly developed on a scale large enough to prevent community-wide HIV epidemics. Methadone maintenance is probably the most attractive treatment for persons with heroin dependence, but, because methadone itself is a narcotic, is often very unpopular with political leaders. Even in areas where concern about AIDS has led to increased methadone treatment, there have been some instances when not enough treatment capacity has been available, when persons have been prematurely terminated from treatment, and when insufficient treatment dosages have been used. In fact, a recent study of the "low threshold" methadone maintenance program in Amsterdam, which uses low methadone dosages, did not show a protective effect against HIV seroconversion from being in the program (99).

Using treatment to prevent HIV infection for persons injecting cocaine is even more problematic, because there is not yet any maintenance chemotherapy (equivalent to methadone for heroin users) for persons dependent upon cocaine. Despite these important limitations of drug abuse treatment as a method of preventing HIV infection, such treatment will probably be a critical part of both harm-reduction and non-harm-reduction approaches to HIV prevention among IDUs. Providing treatment has considerable political appeal (as against syringe exchange or over-the-counter sales), because it promises to reduce other harms associated with illicit drug injection, not just HIV infection. Even workers in "safer injection" programs, such as syringe exchange, feel a strong need to be able to refer IDUs to drug abuse treatment when asked (27). The ability to provide such services also helps to legitimate outreach and syringe-exchange work both to the IDUs and community leaders.

With a few exceptions, HIV counseling and testing has not been adopted as a major AIDS prevention measure, whether or not the country in question has adopted an overall harm-reduction perspective. Several studies have shown that HIV testing and counseling lead to reduced AIDS risk behavior (13, 84, 87, 101), but the amount of research on this topic has been relatively small, considering the number of IDUs who have by now been counseled and tested in research projects alone. Part of the difficulty with using this approach as an AIDS prevention measure has been the need to keep the counseling and testing truly confidential and voluntary. Loss of confidentiality or anonymity can lead to severe discrimination against HIV-positive persons, and coercive testing would violate the principle of "public health officials working with IDUs to prevent AIDS," which has always been a major component of harm reduction.

Sweden has utilized HIV counseling and testing among IDUs as a prevention strategy to the greatest extent. The results from Sweden would suggest that counseling and testing generally have had a positive effect—or at least not a discernible negative one (7, 77). Particularly now that it is possible to provide some effective treatment for HIV infection, as well as prophylaxis for opportunistic infections, the possibility of using HIV counseling and testing as one part of larger integrated systems for HIV prevention among IDUs increases.

Another approach to HIV prevention is the encouragement of drug users' organizations that promote risk-reducing changes in drug-injector subcultures. This approach is congruent with harm-reduction perspectives in that it is based on respect for users' ability and willingness to take responsibility for issues of public health. It is also based on the finding that peer influence and peer norms are related to risk reduction (2, 29, 45, 58, 67, 73).

The first users' organizations formed in the Netherlands in the early 1980s, where the drug users' unions *(junkiebonden)* developed mechanisms to protect users from "bad dope" being sold on the streets and where their pressure led to reforms in the way some drug treatment programs treated clients, as well as bringing about the establishment of the first syringe exchange (to prevent hepatitis B). Later, when drug users became convinced that AIDS was a threat to them, the *junkiebonden* became involved in a wide range of educational and peer-influence projects that served to delegitimate the sharing of potentially infected syringes (25, 43, 44). Drug users' organizations have been a major component in Australian AIDS policy where, in addition to contributing ideas and influence in program development, they are actively involved in risk-reduction efforts. Many European countries, including Germany, the United Kingdom, Italy, and Spain, also have users' organizations. These organizations have sent representatives and held meetings of their own at both the Second (Barcelona, 1991) and Third (Melbourne, 1992) International Conferences on the Reduction of Drug-Related Harm.

In the United States, the high level of hostility toward drug users, the Federal requirements for drug-free workplaces, and the extreme levels of impoverishment in which many users live have prevented any widespread establishment of drug users' organizations. *Street Voice,* a newsletter published by IDUs in Baltimore, is a major exception, although it also has faced many problems because of the destitution of many of its members. In two of the National AIDS Demonstration Research projects, efforts have been made to organize drug injectors against AIDS in Minneapolis-St. Paul (12) and in

Brooklyn. The Brooklyn project has reported widespread risk reduction among its participants, including greater use of bleach and condoms than in a comparison outreach project (47, 49, 62, 97).

HOW MUCH PREVENTION IS NEEDED FOR SUCCESS?

An almost universal finding in the studies of AIDS prevention programs for IDUs has been an outcome of substantial risk reduction, but never of complete risk elimination. Regardless of the type of program, or even the combination of programs in a given area, there still appears to be a substantial residual level of persistent risk behavior among the IDUs as a group. This residual risk behavior raises the question of whether prevention programs for IDUs will ever completely succeed. However, there are at least two localities where prevention programs for IDUs appear to be succeeding in preventing community-level HIV epidemics. The Skane province in southern Sweden has an estimated 3000 IDUs, of whom at least 90% have been tested for HIV (66). In addition to the widespread HIV counseling and testing, drug abuse treatment is also widely available (although methadone maintenance is limited). Moreover, there is a syringe-exchange program, and sterile injection equipment can be obtained from pharmacies in nearby Copenhagen. The HIV seroprevalence rate is approximately 2% and has remained stable over the last five years. Only 20% of the known HIV seropositives were infected locally (the others were infected outside of the province, and/or moved into the area after being infected).

Similarly, Australia has a wide variety of AIDS prevention programs for IDUs. There are numerous syringe exchanges, which also distribute bleach, and injection equipment is also sold over-the-counter. Treatment is sufficiently available to constitute a true treatment-on-demand situation. User groups have been supported by the government to implement prevention programs and provide policy advice. There are specialized prevention programs targeted at subgroups of IDUs, e.g. youth, gays, prisoners. As a result of all this, the HIV seroprevalence rate varies somewhat from city to city, but overall is less than 2%. And, the rate has been stable for the last several years in all of Australia's major cities (24).

These two examples suggest that it may be possible to prevent an epidemic of HIV among IDUs with currently available prevention programs. One critical factor appears to be starting prevention programs early enough. In both Skane and Australia, the prevention programs were begun before there was any rapid spread of HIV among IDUs. A second critical factor appears to be providing a variety of means for behavior change simultaneously, as soon as the IDUs themselves have recognized the threat of HIV and AIDS. Consistent with the harm-reduction perspective, different IDUs will avail themselves of different programs, and the same IDUs may utilize different programs at different times.

Much more research is clearly needed to determine precisely how much prevention and how much risk reduction is needed to prevent epidemics of HIV among IDUs. The current evidence indicates, however, that prevention of HIV epidemics should be considered a realistic, attainable goal.

HARM REDUCTION AND HIV PREVENTION: PRAGMATIC CONCERNS

Although the evidence strongly suggests that harm-reduction programs can reduce HIV transmission among IDUs, perhaps even preventing epidemics of HIV, there remain several difficult issues facing AIDS prevention efforts. Although almost all programs have achieved immediate reductions in AIDS risk behaviors, the problem of maintaining such behavior change has received little attention. It has long been well known that "relapse" back to drug use is the norm after drug abuse treatment. One New York study found that almost one third of street-recruited IDUs reported that they could not maintain their AIDS risk reduction (28). Fundamental questions about maintenance of behavior change, including the conditions that threaten maintenance—and whether failures to maintain will consist primarily of transient lapses or full relapses—have not been addressed.

Whether political leaders will fail to maintain support for AIDS prevention programming will also be important. If prevention programs are initially successful, this may, ironically, create the complacent perception that they are no longer needed. Termination or curtailment of prevention programs may then be followed by increased transmission of HIV. At present, not enough is known about the long-term dynamics of HIV epidemics among IDUs to make knowledgeable decisions about the consequences of reducing prevention efforts. The safest course would be to maintain full prevention efforts, but fiscal problems may lead political leaders to do otherwise.

One aspect of long-term dynamics that suggests an indefinite need for prevention programs is the continuing initiation of new persons into illicit drug injection. The fear that new persons might start injecting illicit drugs has often been raised as an objection to harm-reduction programs, such as syringe exchanges. All data from syringe-exchange studies indicate that they do not lead to such increases, but the larger question of why people would start to inject even after knowing about AIDS remains important. The National AIDS Demonstration Research studies, which have been conducted in the US since the late 1980s, found that approximately 20% of the subjects had begun injecting drugs since information about AIDS was widespread in American society (46). Studies of new injectors also suggest that their level of AIDS risk behavior has been declining as the AIDS epidemic continues (74, 103), but new injectors are still showing substantial levels of risk behavior, and clearly knowledge of AIDS is not in itself a sufficient deterrent. Initiation into drug injection is probably best conceptualized as a transition process, with multiple determinants, from previous noninjection drug use (29). The social and psychological conditions under which the process is most likely to occur, and the extent to which the process can be reversed, remain to be determined (96).

Although AIDS prevention programs have led to substantial changes in the drug-injection risk behaviors of IDUs, changes in sexual risk behaviors have generally been much more modest (22, 42, 61). Changes in sexual behavior with casual sexual partners and within prostitute-client relationships have been achieved through several prevention programs, but it has been particularly difficult to get IDUs to practice safer sex within primary sexual relationships. These difficulties in encouraging safer sex should not be seen as specific to IDUs. Encouraging homosexual men and heterosexual nondrug injectors to practice safer sex within primary relationships has proven to be as difficult (70). There are probably multiple reasons why committed couples are not likely to practice safer sex, including emotional denial of AIDS risk, fatalism with respect to HIV transmission, the implication of infidelity associated with condom use, lack of skills in discussing/negotiating safer sex, perceived loss of erotic pleasure associated with condom use, and, for heterosexual couples, the desire to have children despite risks of sexual and perinatal transmission. Given the difficulties in changing sexual behavior within primary partnerships, the most effective method for preventing sexual transmission of HIV among IDUs and their sexual partners is probably to prevent the initial transmission through multiperson use of injection equipment.

Crack cocaine use has been associated with "sex-for-drugs exchanges" and large-scale increases in sexually transmitted disease in the US (85), but has been associated with increased sexual transmission of HIV only in the northeastern US (19, 82). Presumably, the large concentration of HIV-infected drug injectors in the northeast, many of whom also use crack (39), are a reservoir for heterosexual transmission of HIV.

There are two types of geographical areas where AIDS prevention efforts face difficult challenges. In high-seroprevalence areas in the developed countries, even relatively low levels of risk behavior may lead to moderate-to-high rates of new HIV infections. City-background HIV seroprevalence was the strongest predictor of the rate of new HIV infections in the National AIDS Demonstration Research study (46). A second generation of prevention programs, which go beyond what is currently being done, may be required to reduce the number of new HIV infections in high-seroprevalence areas.

The second type of geographical area where AIDS prevention is likely to be quite difficult is in developing countries. Many leaders of developing countries are likely to see both AIDS and illicit drug injection as peculiarly western vices, and thus not likely to become problems in their countries. Even if the leaders see AIDS and illicit drug injection as likely problems, it may be culturally difficult to adopt anything other than punitive approaches to these potential problems in some countries. A harm-reduction response to these potential problems might be to favor traditional, noninjected forms of psychoactive drug use over injected drug use (108). It is difficult to envision how this might be done, however, other than simply not attempting to suppress traditional noninjecting methods of psychoactive drug use.

In addition to the policy problems in implementing AIDS prevention in some developing countries, simple lack of monetary resources may be a very important obstacle. Providing sterile injection equipment to persons illicitly using drugs would not be a viable option in countries with inadequate supplies of injection for medical uses. In such situations, the most likely course of effective action may be widespread use of materials, like bleach, to disinfect injection equipment between users (Jo Kittelson, WHO, 1991, personal communication).

HARM REDUCTION AND HIV PREVENTION: PHILOSOPHIC CONCERNS

As discussed above, the harm-reduction approach to preventing AIDS among IDUs, their sexual partners, and their children faces some formidable practical challenges. The challenges at the philosophical level are probably equally important. Many harm-reduction-based prevention programs, such as syringe exchanges, are opposed not on the basis of their potential effectiveness, but because they appear to condone illicit drug use within the community. It is argued that such programs are a "surrender in the fight against drugs," and that "they send the wrong message about drugs to our children" (3, 37, 70, 79).

Even proponents of the harm-reduction approach to AIDS prevention have noted that the perspective is limited in its ability to project ideals for society with respect to psychoactive drug use (57), and that it is very difficult to state just what the perspective is, as opposed to stating what the perspective is not (95). It may be particularly helpful to have US contributions to the practice and conceptualization of harm reduction. The United States clearly has the largest set of psychoactive drug problems of any country in the world. It may thus have the most to gain from a harm-reduction approach, and if harm reduction were successful on a large scale in the US, it would be a powerful example for other countries.

An adaptation of the harm-reduction perspective to the United States setting is beyond the scope of this article, but we would like to suggest an outline of how harm reduction might be incorporated into thinking about the US drug problem. Musto (72) has analyzed the US approach to psychoactive drug use in terms of an historical alternation between two fundamentally opposed conceptualizations of the role of psychoactive drug use in human society that have shaped opinion and policy. The first perspective celebrates the positive effects of psychoactive drugs. Nonmedical psychoactive drug use is seen as aiding in the fulfillment of positive human potential. Drug use, in this view, not only provides pleasure, but leads to social solidarity, self-knowledge, enhanced work productivity (including intellectual and artistic accomplishment), and spiritual development.

According to Musto, the uncritical celebratory approach to nonmedical use of psychoactive drugs leads to excessive use and clear evidence of harmful effects. A social backlash then develops, leading to a prohibitionist (or zero tolerance) perspective, which then becomes dominant. Within the prohibitionist approach, nonmedical psychoactive drug use is seen not only as leading to numerous harms to the individual user and to society, but the drug use itself is viewed as immoral. Information that drugs may have some positive effects for the individual is systematically suppressed, and efforts are made to stigmatize drug users socially. Even those drug users whose own use is evidently not causing harm to themselves are held to be responsible for the larger harm caused to others.

The one-sidedness of the prohibitionist approach leads to a societal amnesia regarding both the positive and negative consequences of nonmedical psychoactive drug use. When a new generation discovers the positive aspects of drug use, the official dogma on drugs is easily discredited, and the social stage is set for the next cycle of a celebratory period.

The harm-reduction perspective, properly articulated, may offer a more satisfactory and stable alternative to this cycling back and forth between the one-sidedly celebratory or the prohibitionistic periods that Musto described. Indeed, harm reduction could become a kind of Hegelian synthesis of the celebratory perspective (thesis) and the prohibition perspective (antithesis). Harm reduction acknowledges the positive experiences that can result from psychoactive drug use, without attempting to either deny or exaggerate the harmful consequences that can also occur. For harm reduction to become a true synthesis, however, it must do more than simply incorporate some elements of the celebratory and some elements of the prohibition perspective. Harm reduction, both in theory and in practice, will need to become a sum greater than the parts taken from the other two perspectives, particularly because of the many obvious conflicts between the other two perspectives. Harm reduction, in its attempt to integrate multiple aspects of psychoactive drug use, may be the most appropriate perspective on psychoactive drug use in present-day complex societies. In a complex society, achieving universal compliance with a single, socially approved way of using (or not using) drugs is highly unlikely.

Before harm reduction is accepted as a basis for drug policy in many countries, however, it will be necessary to show that harm-reduction approaches can succeed in controlling the spread of HIV among drug users. Over the course of the first decade of the AIDS epidemic among IDUs throughout the world, it has become increasingly clear that the attendant problem was much worse than anyone would have expected in 1981. The AIDS epidemic has thus created a sense of public health emergency that has led many otherwise reluctant political leaders to experiment with harm-reduction approaches. Such approaches have shown considerable success in leading to risk reduction among IDUs, but whether the international HIV epidemic among IDUs can effectively be brought under public health control is still an open question. If these efforts should fail, the entire harm-reduction perspective would probably lose political credibility.

ACKNOWLEDGMENTS

The research was supported by grant DA03574 from the National Institute on Drug Abuse. The views expressed in this paper do not necessarily reflect the positions of the granting agency or of the institutions by which the authors are employed.

Literature Cited

1. Abdul-Quader, A. S., Friedman, S. R., Des Jarlais, D. C., Marmor, M., Maslansky, R., Bartelme, S. 1987. Methadone maintenance and behavior by intravenous drug users that can transmit HIV. *Contemp. Drug Prob.* 14:425–34
2. Abdul-Quader, A. S., Tross, S., Friedman, S. R., Kouzi, A. C., Des Jarlais, D. S. 1990. Street-recruited intravenous drug users and sexual risk reduction in New York City. *AIDS* 4:1075–79
3. Anderson, W. 1991. The New York needle trial: the politics of public health in the age of AIDS. *Am. J. Public Health* 81:1506–17
4. Angarano, G., Pastore, G., Monno, L., Santantonio, F., Luchera, N., Schiraldi, O. 1985. Rapid spread of HTLV-III infection among drug addicts in Italy. *Lancet* 8467:1302
5. Berridge, V. 1992. *Harm reduction: An historical perspective.* Presented at 3rd Int. Conf. on Reduct. of Drug-Relat. Harm, Melbourne
6. Blix, O., Gronbladh, L. 1988. *AIDS and IV heroin addicts: the preventive effect of methadone maintenance in Sweden. Presented at 4th Int. AIDS Conf.,* Stockholm (abstr. #8548)

6a. Bortolotti, F., Cadrobbi, P., Crivellaro, C., Menenghetti, F., Carretta, M., et al. 1989. The changing epidemiology of acute type B hepatitis: results of an 11-year prospective study in Padua (Northern Italy). *Infection* 17:364–68

7. Bottiger, M., Forsgren, M., Grillner, L., Biberfeld, G., Eriksson, G., Janzon, R. 1988. *Monitoring of HIV infection among IV drug users in Stockholm.* Presented at 4th Int. AIDS Conf., Stockholm (abstr. #4709)
8. Bowtell, B. 1992. *Development of policy relating to the prevention of HIV among injecting drug users.* Presented at 3rd Int. Conf. on Reduct. of Drug-Relat. Harm, Melbourne

9. Brettle, R. P. 1991. HIV and harm reduction in injection drug users. *AIDS* 5:125–36
10. Buning, E. C. 1989. *The role of the needle exchange project in preventing HIV infection among drug users in Amsterdam*. Presented at What Works Conf: An Int. Perspect. on Drug Abuse Treat. and Prev. Res. New York
11. Buning, E. C., van Brussel, G. H. A., van Santen, G. 1988. Amsterdam's drug policy and its implications for controlling needle sharing. In *Needle Sharing Among Intravenous Drug Abusers: National and International Drug Perspectives*, ed. R. J. Battjes, R. W. Pickens, pp. 59–74, Res. Monogr. 80. Rockville, Md: Natl. Inst. on Drug Abuse
12. Carlson, G., Needle, R. 1989. *Sponsoring addict self-organization (Addicts Against AIDS): A case study*. Presented at 1st Annu. Natl. AIDS Demonstr. Res. Conf., Rockville, Md.
13. Casadonte, P. P., Des Jarlais, D. C., Friedman, S. R., Rotrosen, J. P. 1990. Psychological and behavioral impact among intravenous drug users of learning HIV test results. *Int. J. Addict* 25:409–26
14. Casriel, C., Des Jarlais, D. C., Rodriguez, R., Friedman, S. R., Stepherson, B., Khuri, E. 1990. Working with heroin sniffers: clinical issues in preventing drug injection. *J. Subst. Abuse Treat.* 7:1–10
15. Cent. Dis. Control. 1982. Update on the acquired immune deficiency syndrome (AIDS)—United States. *Morbid. Mortal. Wkly. Rep.* 31:507–14
16. Cent. Dis. Control. 1990. Update: reducing HIV transmission in intravenous drug users not in drug treatment—United States. *Morbid. Mortal. Wkly. Rep.* 39:529, 535–38
17. Cent. Dis. Control. 1991. Nosocomial transmission of multidrug-resistant tuberculosis among HIV-infected persons—Florida and New York. *Morbid. Mortal. Wkly. Rep.* 40:585–91
18. Cent. Dis. Control. 1992. *HIV/AIDS Surveillance, Year-End Edition. US AIDS Cases Reported Through December 1991*. Atlanta: CDC
19. Chiasson, M. A., Stoneburner, R. L., Hildebrandt, D. S, Ewing, W. E., Telzak, E. E., et al. 1991. Heterosexual transmission of HIV-1 associated with the use of smokable freebase cocaine (crack). *AIDS* 5:1121–26
19a. Choopanya, K. 1989. Report prepared for WHO multi-center study. Geneva: WHO
20. Choopanya, K., Vanichseni, S., Plangsringarm, K., Sonchai, W., Carballo, M., et al. 1991. Risk factors and HIV seropositivity among injecting drug users in Bangkok. *AIDS* 5:1509–13
21. Cohen, H. W., Marmor, M., Des Jarlais, D. C., Spira, T., Friedman, S. R., et al 1985. *Behavioral risk factors for HTLV-III/LAV seropositivity among intravenous drug abusers*. Presented at 1st Int. AIDS Conf., Atlanta
22. Cohen, J. 1991. Why woman partners of drug users will continue to be at high risk for HIV infection. *J. Addict Dis.* 10:99–110
23. Cooper, J. R. 1989. Methadone treatment and acquired immunodeficiency syndrome. *J. Am. Med. Assoc.* 262: 1664–68
24. Crofts, N., Stevenson, E. 1992. *The epidemiology of HIV infection among injecting drug users in Australia*. Presented at 3rd Int. Conf. on Reduct. of Drug-Related Harm, Melbourne
25. de Jong, W. M. 1986. *De sociale beweging van opiatengebruikers in Nederland*. Doctoraal-scriiptie sociol., Erasmus Univ., Rotterdam
26. Deren, S. 1985. *A Description of Methadone Maintenance Patients and Their Children*. New York: NY State Div. of Subst. Abuse Serv.
27. Des Jarlais, D. C. 1989. AIDS prevention programs for intravenous drug users: diversity and evolution. *Int. Rev. Psychol.* 1:101–8
28. Des Jarlais, D. C., Abdul-Quader, A., Tross, S. 1991. The next problem: maintenance of AIDS risk reduction among intravenous drug users. *Int. J. Addict.* 26:1279–92
29. Des Jarlais, D. C., Casriel, C., Friedman, S. R., Rosenblum, A. 1992. AIDS and the transition to illicit drug injection: results of a randomized trial prevention program. *Br. J. Addict.* 87: 493–98
30. Des Jarlais, D. C., Chamberland, M. E., Yancovitz, S. R., Weinberg, P., Friedman, S. R. 1984. Heterosexual partners: a large risk group for AIDS. *Lancet* 2:1346–47
31. Des Jarlais, D. C., Courtwright, D. T., Joseph, H. 1991. The transition from opium smoking to heroin injection in the United States. *AIDS Public Policy J.* 6:88–90
32. Des Jarlais, D. C., Friedman, S. R. 1990. Shooting galleries and AIDS: infection probabilities and "tough" policies. *Am. J. Public Health* 80:142–44
33. Des Jarlais, D. C., Friedman, S. R. 1992. The AIDS epidemic and legal

access to sterile equipment for injecting illicit drugs. *Ann. Am. Acad. Polit. Soc. Sci.* 521:42–65

34. Des Jarlais, D. C., Friedman, S. R., Hopkins, W. 1985. Risk reduction for the acquired immunodeficiency syndrome among intravenous drug users. *Ann. Intern. Med.* 103:755–59
35. Des Jarlais, D. C., Friedman, S. R., Novick, D., Sotheran, J. L., Thomas, P., et al. 1989. HIV-1 infection among intravenous drug users in Manhattan, from 1977 through 1987. *J. Am. Med. Assoc.* 261:1008–12
36. Des Jarlais, D. C., Friedman, S. R., Strug, D. 1986. AIDS and needle sharing within the intravenous drug use subculture. In *The Social Dimensions of AIDS: Methods and Theory,* ed. D. Feldman, T. Johnson, pp. 111–25. New York: Praeger
37. Des Jarlais, D. C., Milliken, J., Lambert, B. Media coverage of the AIDS epidemic among intravenous drug users. In *Mass Media and Society: The Effects of Media on Human Behavior,* ed. S. Fischoff, W. J. Laczek. APA
38. Des Jarlais, D. C., Sotheran, J. L. 1990. The public health paradigm for AIDS and drug use: shifting the time frame. *Br. J. Addict.* 85:348–49
39. Des Jarlais, D. C., Wenston, J., Friedman, S. R., Sotheran, J. L., Maslansky, R., Marmor, M. Crack cocaine use in a cohort of methadone maintenance patients. *J. Subst. Abuse Treat.* In press

39a. Donoghoe, M. C., Stimson, G. V., Dolan, K., Alldritt, L. 1989. Sexual behaviour of injecting drug users and associated risks of HIV infection for non-injecting partners. *AIDS Care* 1: 103–9

40. Edlin, B. R., Tokars, J. I., Grieco, M. H., Crawford, J. T., Williams, J., et al. 1992. An outbreak of multidrug-resistant tuberculosis among hospitalized patients with the acquired immunodeficiency syndrome. *N. Engl. J. Med.* 326:1514–21
41. Espinoza, P., Bouchard, I., Ballian, P., Polo DeVoto, J. 1988. *Has the open sale of syringes modified the syringe exchanging habits of drug addicts*. Presented at 4th Int. AIDS Conf., Stockholm (abstr. #8522)

41a. Farci, P., Novick, D. M., Lai, M. E., Orgiana, G., Strazzera, A., et al. 1988. Introduction of human immunodeficiency virus among parenteral drug abusers in Sardinia: a seroepidemiologic study. *Am. J. Epidemiol.* 127:1312–14

42. Fazey, C. S. J. 1990. *Preventing the Spread of HIV Infection: A Study of Drug Patients' Syringe and Condom Use*. Mersey Regional Health Authority, Studies of Drug Issues: Rep. No. 4, Liverpool
43. Friedman, S. R., de Jong, W. M., Des Jarlais, D. C. 1988. Problems and dynamics of organizing intravenous drug users for AIDS prevention. *Health Educ. Res.* 3:49–57
44. Friedman, S. R., de Jong, W. M., Des Jarlais, D. C., Kaplan, C., Goldsmith, D. S. 1987. *Drug users' organizations and AIDS prevention: Differences in structure and strategy*. Presented at 3rd Int. AIDS Conf., Washington, DC
45. Friedman, S. R., Des Jarlais, D. C., Sotheran, J. L., Garber, J., Cohen, H., Smith, D. 1987. AIDS and self-organization among intravenous drug users. *Int. J. Addict.* 22:201–19
46. Friedman, S. R., Jose, B., Deren, S., Des Jarlais, D. C., Myers, M., et al. 1991. *Preliminary analysis of HIV seroconversions among drug injectors in 13 cities*. Presented at 3rd Annu. Natl. AIDS Demonstr. Res. Conf., Rockville, Md.

46a. Friedman, S. R., Jose, B., Neaigus, A., et al. 1991. *Peer mobilization and widespread condom use by drug injectors*. 7th Int. Conf. on AIDS, Florence (abstr. #W.D.54)

47. Friedman, S. R., Neaigus, A., Jose, B., Sufian, M., Stepherson, B., et al. 1990. *Behavioral outcomes of organizing drug injectors against AIDS*. Presented at 2nd Annu. Natl. AIDS Demonstr. Res. Conf., Rockville, Md.
48. Friedman, S. R., Sotheran, J. L., Abdul-Quader, A., Primm, B. J., Des Jarlais, D. C., et al. 1987. The AIDS epidemic among Blacks and Hispanics. *Milbank Q.* 65(Suppl. 2):455–99
49. Friedman, S. R., Sufian, M., Curtis, R., Neaigus, A., Des Jarlais, D. C. 1992. Organizing drug users against AIDS. In *The Social Context of AIDS,* ed. J. Huber, B. E. Schneider, pp. 115–30. Newbury Park, Calif: Sage
50. Fuchs, D., Unterweger, B., Hausen, A., Reibnegger, G., Werner, E. R., et al. 1988. Anti-HIV-1 antibodies, anti-HTLV-1 antibodies and neopterin levels in parenteral drug addicts in the Austrian Tyrol. *J. AIDS* 1:65–66
51. Goldberg, D., Watson, H., Stuart, F., Miller, M., Gruer, L., Follett, E. 1988. *Pharmacy supply of needles and syringes—the effect on spread of HIV*

among intravenous drug misusers. Presented at 4th Int. AIDS Conf., Stockholm (abstr. #8521)

51a. Goudeau, A., Dubois, F., Barin, F., Choutet, P., Jusseaume, P., et al. 1986. *Emergence of HTLV-III/LAV and delta agent in a French intravenous drug abuser population: prospective study (1982–1985)*. 2nd Int. Conf. on AIDS, Paris (abstr. #169)

52. Guilfoile, A. 1991. *Boulder, Colorado needle exchange program*. Presented at 119th Annu. Meet. of Am. Public Health Assoc., Atlanta, Nov. 10–14 (session #2170)

52a. Haemmig, R. B., Minder Nejedly, M., Malinverni, R. 1991. Needle sharing and condom use among heavy intravenous drug users (IVDU) in Bern, Switzerland, 7th Int. Conf. on AIDS, Florence (abstr. #W.C. 3366)

53. Hagan, H., Des Jarlais, D. C., Purchase, D., Reid, T., Friedman, S. R. 1991. The Tacoma syringe exchange. *J. Addict. Dis*. 10:81–88

54. Hagan, H., Des Jarlais, D. C., Purchase, D., Reid, T., Friedman, S. R., Bell, T. A. 1991. The incidence of HBV infection and syringe exchange programs (letter). *J. Am. Med. Assoc*. 266:1646–47

55. Hart, G. J., Carvell, A. L. M., Woodward, N., Johnson, A. M., Williams, P., Parry, J. 1989. Evaluation of needle exchange in central London: behaviour change and anti-HIV status over one year. *AIDS* 3:261–65

56. Hartgers, C., Buning, E. C., Coutinho, R. A. 1989. *Evaluation of the needle exchange program in Amsterdam*. Presented at 5th Int. AIDS Conf., Montreal

57. Hawks, D. 1992. *Impediments to the adoption of harm reduction policies*. Presented at 3rd Int. Conf. on Reduct. of Drug-Relat. Harm, Melbourne

58. Huang, K. H. C., Watters, J., Case, P. 1989. *Compliance with AIDS prevention measures among intravenous drug users: health beliefs or social/environmental factors?* Presented at 5th Int. AIDS Conf., Montreal (abstr. #M.D.O.5)

59. Hubbard, R. L., Marsden, M. E., Rachal, J. V., Harwood, H. J., Cavanaugh, E. R., Ginzburg, H. M. 1989. *Drug Abuse Treatment: A National Study of Effectiveness*. Chapel Hill/London: Univ. North Carolina Press

60. Ingold, F. R., Ingold, S. 1989. The effects of the liberalization of syringe sales on the behaviour of intravenous drug users in France. *Bull. Narc*. 41:67–81

61. Jain, S., Flynn, N., Bailey, V., Sweha, A., Ding, D., Sloan, W. 1989. *IVDU and AIDS: more resistance to changing their sexual than their needle-sharing practices*. Presented at 5th Int. AIDS Conf., Montreal (abstr. #W.D.P.79)

62. Jose, B., Friedman, S. R., Neaigus, A., Sufian, M. 1990. *Condom use among drug injectors in an organizing project neighborhood*. Presented at 2nd Annu. Natl. AIDS Demonstr. Res. Conf., Rockville, Md.

62a. Kall, K., Olin, R. 1990. HIV status and changes in risk behavior among intravenous drug users in Stockholm 1987–88. *AIDS* 4:153–57

63. Klee, H., Faugier, J., Hayes, C., Morris, J. 1991. Risk reduction among injecting drug users: changes in the sharing of injection equipment and in condom use. *AIDS Care* 3:63–73

64. Liebman, J., Sepulveda-Irene, B. 1989. *Effectiveness of street outreach as an AIDS-prevention strategy for IV drug users, their sexual partners, and prostitutes in Philadelphia*. Presented at 1st Annu. Natl. AIDS Demonstr. Res. Conf., Bethesda, Md.

65. Lima, E. D. S., Bastos, F. I. P. M., Friedman, S. R. 1991. *HIV-1 epidemiology among IVDUs in Rio de Janeiro, Brazil*. Presented at 7th Int. AIDS Conf., Florence (abstr. W.C. 3287)

65a. Lima, E. S., Bastos, F. I., Friedman, S. R. 1992. Prospects for HIV infection among drug injectors in Rio de Janeiro: perspectives and unanswered questions. *Bull. Narc*. In press

66. Ljungberg, B., Christensson, B., Tunving, K., Andersson, B., Landvall, B., et al. 1991. HIV prevention among injecting drug users: three years of experience from a syringe exchange program in Sweden. *J. AIDS* 4:890–95

66a. Loimer, N., Presslich, O., Hollerer, E., Pakesch, G., Pfersman, V., et al. 1990. Monitoring HIV-1 infection prevalence among intrevenous drug users in Vienna 1986–1990. *AIDS Care* 2: 281–86

67. Magura, S., Grossman, J. I., Lipton, D. S., Siddiqi, Q., Shapiro, J., 1989. Determinants of needle sharing among intravenous drug users. *Am. J. Public Health* 79:459–62

68. Marmor, M., Des Jarlais, D. C., Cohen, H., Friedman, S. R., Beatrice, S. T., et al. 1987. Risk factors for infection with human immunodeficiency virus among intravenous drug

abusers in New York City. *AIDS* 1:39–44

68a. Martin, G. S., Serpelloni, G., Galvan, U., Rizzetto, A., Gomma, M., et al. 1990. Behavioural change in injecting drug users: evaluation of an HIV/AIDS education programme. *AIDS Care* 2: 275–79

69. Mientjes, G. H., van Ameijden, E. J., van den Hoek, A., Coutinho, R. A. 1991. Increasing morbidity without rise in non-AIDS mortality among HIV-infected intravenous drug users in Amsterdam. *AIDS* 6:207–12

70. Miller, H. G., Turner, C. F., Moses, L. E., eds. 1990. *AIDS: The Second Decade*. Washington, DC: Natl. Acad. Press

71. Minkoff, H. L., DeHovitz, J. A. 1991. Care of women infected with the human immunodeficiency virus. *J. Am. Med. Assoc.* 266:2253–58

72. Musto, D. F. 1991. Opium, cocaine, and marijuana in American history. *Sci. Am.* 265:40–47

72a. Naik, T. N., Sarkar, S., Singh, H. L., Bhunia, S. C., Singh, V. I., et al. 1991. Intravenous drug users—a new high-risk group for HIV infection in India. *AIDS* 5:117–18

73. Neaigus, A., Friedman, S. R., Curtis, R., Des Jarlais, D. C., Furst, R. T., et al. 1993. *HIV Risk Networks and Social Networks Among Drug Injectors,* NIDA Rev. Monogr. Rockville, Md: Natl. Inst. of Drug Abuse. In press

74. Neaigus, A., Friedman, S. R., Stepherson, B., Jose, B., Sufian, M., et al. 1991. *Declines in syringe sharing during the first drug injection*. Presented at 7th Int. AIDS Conf., Florence (abstr. #M.D.4057)

75. Neaigus, A., Sufian, M., Friedman, S. R., Goldsmith, D., Stepherson, B., et al. 1990. Effects of outreach intervention on risk reduction among intravenous drug users. *AIDS Educ. Prev.* 2:253–71

75a. Nicolosi, A., Molinari, S., Musicco, M., et al. 1991. Positive modification of injecting behavior among intravenous heroin users from Milan and Northern Italy 1987–89. *Br. J. Addict.* 86:91–102

76. O'Keefe, E., Kaplan, E., Khoshnood, K. 1991. *Preliminary Report: City of New Haven Needle Exchange Program*. New Haven, Conn: Off. of Mayor Daniels

77. Olin, R., Käll, K. 1989. *HIV status and changes in risk behavior among arrested and detained intravenous drug abusers in Stockholm 1987–1988*. Presented at 5th Int. AIDS Conf., Montreal (abstr. #W.D.P. 76)

78. Oliver, K. J., Maynard, H., Des Jarlais, D. C. 1991. *Portland, Oregon needle exchange program*. Presented at 119th Annu. Meet. of Am. Public Health Assoc., Atlanta, Nov. 10–14 (session #2170)

79. Pear, R. 1992. US drug official urges mayors to forgo needle-swap programs. *NY Times* June 3:B3.

79a. Peutherer, J. F., Edmond, E., Simmonds, P., Dickson, J. D. 1986. *HTLV-III infection in intravenous drug abusers in Edinburgh*. 2nd Int. Conf. on AIDS, Paris (abstr. #167)

80. Phanuphak, P., Poshyachinda, V., Uneklabh, T., Rojanapithayakorn, W. 1989. *HIV transmission among intravenous drug abusers*. Presented at 5th Int. AIDS Conf., Montreal (abstr. T.G.O.25)

80a. Pomeroy, L., O'Connor, J., Barry, J. 1991. *Needle sharing and sexual behavior amongst attenders at a methadone program in Dublin*. 7th Int. Conf. on AIDS, Florence (abstr. #W.C.3314)

80b. Poole, L.E., Cohen, J. B., Lyons, C. A., et al. 1989. *Behavior changes to reduce HIV transmission risk in a prospective study of seropositive women*. 5th Int. Conf. on AIDS, Montreal (abstr. #W.D.P.53)

81. Quimby, E., Friedman, S. R. 1989. Dynamics of Black mobilization against AIDS in New York City. *Soc. Prob.* 36:403–15

82. Ratner, M., Inciardi, J., Bourgois, P., Dunlap, E., Boyle, K., et al. 1991. *Crack Pipe as Pimp: An Eight-City Ethnographic Study of the Sex-for-Crack Phenomenon. Draft final report*. Rockville, Md: Natl. Inst. on Drug Abuse

82a. Robert, C.-F., Deglon, J.-J., Wintsch, J., Martin, J.-L., Perrin, L., et al. 1990. Behavioural changes in intravenous drug users in Geneva: rise and fall of HIV infection, 1980–1989. *AIDS* 4:657–60

83. Robertson, J. R., Bucknall, A. B. V., Welsby, P. D., Roberts, J. J. K., Inglis, J. M., et al. 1986. Epidemic of AIDS related virus (HTLV-III/LAV) infection among intravenous drug users. *Br. Med. J.* 292:527–29

84. Roggenburg, L., Sibthorpe, B., Tesselaar, H. 1990. *IDUs' perception of the effect of HIV counseling and testing*

on behavior. Presented at 2nd Annu. NADR Natl. Meet., Bethesda, Md., Nov. 28–30

85. Rolfs, R. T., Goldberg, M., Sharrar, R. G. 1990. Risk factors for syphilis: cocaine use and prostitution. *Am. J. Public Health* 80:852–57
86. Rothenberg, R., Woelfel, M., Stoneburner, R., Milberg, J., Parker, R., Truman, B. 1987. Survival with the acquired immunodeficiency syndrome. *N. Engl. J. Med.* 317:1297–1302
87. Rugg, D. L., MacGowan, R. J. 1990. *Assessing the effectiveness of HIV counseling and testing: A practical guide*. Backgr. paper for WHO Global Programme on AIDS (GPA), Geneva, Nov. 13–16
88. Schoenbaum, E. E., Hartel, D., Selwyn, P. A., Klein, R. S., Davenny, K., et al. 1989. Risk factors for human immunodeficiency virus infection in intravenous drug users. *N. Engl. J. Med.* 321:874–79
89. Selwyn, P. A., Feingold, A. R., Hartel, D., Schoenbaum, E. E., Alderman, M. H., et al. 1988. Increased risk of bacterial pneumonia in HIV-infected intravenous drug users without AIDS. *AIDS* 2:267–72
90. Selwyn, P. A., Hartel, D., Lewis, V. A., Schoenbaum, E. E., Vermund, S. H., et al. 1989. A prospective study of the risk of tuberculosis among intravenous HIV-infected patients. *N. Engl. J. Med.* 319:545–50
91. Shafer, R. W., Chirgwin, K. D., Glatt, A. E., Dahdouh, M. A., Landesman, S. H., Suster, B. 1991. HIV prevalence, immunosuppression, and drug resistance in patients with tuberculosis in an area endemic for AIDS. *AIDS* 5:399–405
92. Snider, D. E. 1992. *Testimony before the National Commission on AIDS regarding The future of the HIV epidemic: Potential for change*. Washington, DC, Jan. 14

92a. Stephens, R. C., Feucht, T. E., Roman, S. W. 1991. Effects of an intervention program on AIDS-related drug and needle behavior among intravenous drug users. *Am. J. Public Health* 81: 568–71

93. Stimson, G. V. 1990. *The prevention of HIV infection in injecting drug users: recent advances and remaining obstacles*. Presented at 6th Int. AIDS Conf., San Francisco
94. Stoneburner, R. L., Des Jarlais, D. C., Benezra, D., Singh, T., Sotheran, J. L., et al. 1988. A larger spectrum of severe HIV-1-related disease in intravenous drug users in New York City. *Science* 242:916–19
95. Strang, J. 1992. *Harm reduction: responding to the challenge*. Presented at 3rd Int. Conf. on Reduct. of Drug Relat. Harm, Melbourne
96. Strang, J., Des Jarlais, D. C., Griffiths, P., Gossop, M. 1992. The study of transitions in the route of drug use: the route from one route to another. *Br. J. Addict.* 87:473–83
97. Sufian, M., Friedman, S. R., Neaigus, A., Stepherson, B., Rivera-Beckman, J., Des Jarlais, D. C. 1990. The impact of AIDS on Puerto Rican intravenous drug users. *Hisp. J. Behav. Sci.* 12: 122–34
98. Taylor, F. 1991. Decline in hepatitis B cases. *Am. J. Public Health* 81:221–22

98a. Titti, F., Lazzarin, A., Costigliola, P., Oliva, C., Nicoletti, L., et al. 1987. Human immunodeficiency virus (HIV) seropositivity in intravenous (IV) drug abusers in three cities of Italy: possible natural history of HIV infection in IV drug addicts in Italy. *J. Med. Virol.* 23:241–48

98b. Tross, S., Abdul-Quader, A., Silvert, H. M., et al. *Determinants of needle-sharing change in street-recruited New York city IV drug users*. 7th Int. Conf. on AIDS, Florence (abstr. #W.D.4115)

99. van Ameijden, E. J. C., van den Hoek, A., Coutinho, R. A. 1991. *Risk factors for HIV seroconversion in injecting drug users in Amsterdam, the Netherlands*. Presented at 7th Int. AIDS Conf., Florence (abstr. #Th.C.104)
100. van den Hoek, J. A. R., Coutinho, A., van Haastrecht, H. J. A., van Zadelhoff, A. W., J. Goudsmit. 1988. Prevalence and risk factors of HIV infections among drug users and drug-using prostitutes in Amsterdam. *AIDS* 2:55–60
101. Vanichseni, S., Choopanya, K., Des Jarlais, D. C., Plangsringarm, K., Sonchai, W., et al. 1992. HIV testing and sexual behavior among drug injectors in Bangkok, Thailand. *J. AIDS* 5:1119–23
102. Vanichseni, S., Sakuntanaga, P. 1990. *Results of three seroprevalence studies for HIV in IVDU in Bangkok*. Presented at 5th Int. AIDS Conf., San Francisco (abstr. F.C.105)

102a. Vermund, S. H., Kelley, K. F., Klein, R. S., Feingold, A. R., Schreiber, K., et al. 1991. High risk of human papillomavirus infection and cervical squamous intrapithelial lesions among women with symptomatic human immunodeficiency virus infection. *Am. J. Obstet. Gynecol.* 165:392–400

103. Vlahov, D., Anthony, J. C., Celentano, D., Solomon, L., Chowdhury, N. 1991. Trends of HIV-1 risk reduction among initiates into intravenous drug use, 1982–1987. *Am. J. Drug Alcohol Abuse* 17:39–48

104. Vlahov, D., Celentano, D. D., Munoz, A., Cohn, S., Anthony, J. C., Nelson, K. E. 1991. *Bleach disinfection of needles by intravenous drug users: association with HIV seroconversion*. Presented at 7th Int. AIDS Conf., Florence (abstr. #M.C.49)

105. Ward, J. W., Hardy, A. M., Drotman, D. P. AIDS in the United States, 1987. In *AIDS and Other Manifestations of Human Immunodeficiency Virus Infection* ed. G. P. Wormser, R. Stahl, E. Bottone, pp. 18–35. Park Ridge, NJ: Noyes. 1103 pp.

106. Watters, J. K., Cheng, Y., Segal, M., Lorvick, J. Case, P., Carlson, J. 1990. *Epidemiology and prevention of HIV in intravenous drug users in San Francisco, 1986–1989*. Presented at 6th Int. AIDS Conf., San Francisco (abstr. #F.C.106)

107. Weiss, S. H., Ginzburg, H. M., Goedert, J. J., Biggar, R. J., Mohica, B. A., et al. 1985. *Risk for HTLV-III exposure and AIDS among parenteral drug abusers in New Jersey*. Presented at 1st Int. AIDS Conf., Atlanta

108. Wodak, A. *The prevention of further spread of HIV infection among and from injecting drug users: An outline for national approaches*. Rep. to Global Programme on AIDS. Geneva: WHO

109. Wodak, A. 1992. *Implementation of policy into programs*. Presented at 3rd Int. Conf. on Reduct. of Drug Relat. Harm, Melbourne

110. Wyld, R., Davidson, S., Brettle, R., et al. 1991. *Changes in sexual behavior amongst drug users: Edinburgh 1983–1989*. 7th Int. Conf. on AIDS, Florence (abstr. #W.C.3106)

Annu. Rev. Publ. Health 1993. 14:451–67

HETEROSEXUAL TRANSMISSION OF HIV: The Role of Other Sexually Transmitted Infections and Behavior in Its Epidemiology Prevention and Control[1]

Sevgi Okten Aral
Division of STD/HIV Prevention, Centers for Disease Control, Atlanta, Georgia 30333

KEY WORDS: STD/HIV interaction, gender difference in HIV acquisition, gender-specific HIV/AIDS prevention, socio-economic factors and HIV

INTRODUCTION

The human immunodeficiency virus (HIV) is a sexually transmitted pathogen that is inefficiently transmitted by sexual exposure (35). Despite this relative inefficiency, the numbers of new cases of HIV infection continue to increase. The growth rates of acquired immunodeficiency syndrome (AIDS) cases escalated as rapidly, or more rapidly, in societies where the virus was introduced more recently than in those where the epidemic had started earlier. And, the spread rate of HIV was highly variable across societies and transmission groups (71).

HIV transmission patterns were also heterogeneous and changing (72, 78). The majority of adult cases of AIDS in North America and Europe occurred among male homosexuals and injecting drug users. However, as early as 1984, descriptions of AIDS epidemiology in Africa have indicated that, globally, heterosexual transmission of HIV is more common than transmission by homosexual contact or injecting drug use (70, 73, 74, 78). During 1986, in the United States, only 4% of all cases reported in adults were classified as having acquired AIDS by heterosexual contact (13). However, heterosexual patients without any other risk factors comprised the fastest growing group of AIDS cases in the US, thus increasing the proportion of cases in this transmission group over time. Of the first 100,000 persons infected with AIDS, 5% were attributed to heterosexual transmission, compared with 7% among the second 100,000 persons. This represents a 44% increase (16). Of all AIDS cases reported among women, 34% were attributed to heterosexual transmission. Similar shifts in transmission groups among AIDS cases have occurred in other areas. For example, in the early years of the epidemic in Brazil (1982–1985), an overwhelming majority of AIDS cases were highly educated homosexual men; since 1988, more cases of AIDS have been reported among women, persons with less education, and injecting drug users (18).

At the individual level, as well, HIV epidemiology is marked by heterogeneity and change. The estimated risk of acquiring HIV infection in the United States ranges from 1 in 500 to 1 in 5 billion, depending on the risk group of the sex partners (4). From April 1991 to March 1992, the reported number of AIDS cases per 100,000 persons varied between 0.2 in North Dakota and 42.4 in Florida, and was as high as 122.4 in the District of Columbia (17). In 1981, only 189 cases of AIDS were reported; in 1990, this number climbed to 43,339 (17.2 per 100,000 population) (15). This variability and increase are reflected in individual probabilities of exposure to a sex partner who was infected with HIV. The marked heterogeneity and change in the rate of transmission, pattern of transmission, and risk of acquisition of

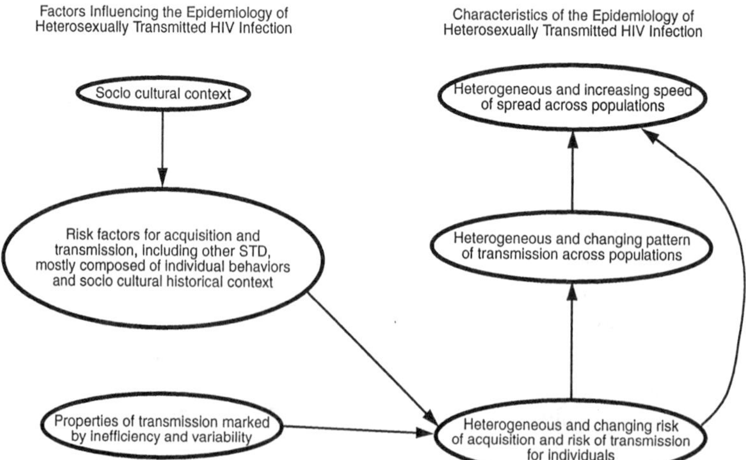

Figure 1 Characteristics of the epidemiology of heterosexually transmitted HIV infection and factors influencing the epidemiology.

HIV all result largely from the inherent properties of HIV transmission, the distribution and change of risk factors for such transmission, and the behavioral and societal variables influencing these (Figure 1).

This paper focuses on heterosexual transmission—the largest and fastest growing component of HIV spread. Its properties, associated risk factors, and the effects of societal context on these factors are reviewed. The methodological difficulties involved in establishing causal links between potential risk factors and HIV transmission, and in evaluating the efficacy and population impact of alternative prevention and control strategies, are summarized, and a consideration of available strategies for the prevention and control of heterosexually transmitted HIV is outlined.

PROPERTIES OF HETEROSEXUAL TRANSMISSION

Compared with other sexually transmitted diseases (STD), the efficiency of sexual transmission of HIV is relatively low (35). The risk of transmission of *N. gonorrhea* from an infected female prostitute to a serviceman in a single sexual exposure has been estimated to be 22–25% (38, 39). Approximately 20–27% of steady sex partners of persons infected with hepatitis B were also infected with the same virus (41, 61). Of persons who had sexual contact with individuals infected with syphilis, 30% become infected (12). With HIV, only 15% of the regular sexual contacts of 1600 HIV-1 infected persons in North America and Europe were infected with HIV (35).

Heterosexual transmission in both directions, i.e. male-to-female and female-to-male, has been well documented. The efficacy of male-to-female transmission appears to be up to fourfold higher than female-to-male transmission (20, 80).

The probability of HIV transmission during a single sexual encounter is highly variable. Maximum and minimum rates of HIV transmission per single sexual encounter have been estimated to be very low compared with other STDs (35). Based on earlier studies (34, 66, 69), per contact infectivity for male-to-female transmission appears to be 0.2% or less. Nevertheless, some individuals become infected after a single or a few sexual encounters, whereas others remain uninfected even after hundreds of unprotected sexual exposures (69, 71). Although some individuals appear to be highly infectious and perform as effective transmitters of HIV (23, 64), others do not infect their partners despite sexual contract (21).

The probability of HIV transmission during a single sexual encounter is influenced by the intrinsic properties of the transmitter, the virus, and the susceptible. And, it may depend on many factors, including T-helper lymphocyte counts, T-suppressor cell counts, the presence or absence of HIV antigen, and the presence or absence of HIV antibody (30, 31, 47, 62, 84, 89).

The duration of infection influences the probability of an infected individual transmitting HIV to sex partners (35, 71). Persons with a more advanced clinical stage of disease or a more profound immunodeficiency are more infectious to their sex partners (30, 45, 48). In addition, immediately following acquisition of infection, people are apparently highly infectious. Viral strains of HIV may also vary considerably in their ability to infect a new host. Some viral isolates appear to replicate more efficiently in vitro, whereas others may be more infective in vivo (35, 71).

Other factors, such as infection with other sexually transmitted pathogens, specific sexual practices, lack of male circumcision, dry sex or the use of desiccants in the vagina, and sexual intercourse during menstruation, affect the probability of HIV transmission. These factors are discussed below.

RISK FACTORS FOR HETEROSEXUAL TRANSMISSION

An individual's risk of becoming infected with HIV involves the likelihood of having sexual intercourse with an infected partner and the likelihood of transmission during sexual intercourse with an infected partner. Personal protection against HIV infection necessitates lowering one or the other of these risks.

Likelihood of Exposure to an Infected Partner

For men, the likelihood of exposure to an infected partner is increased if the partner uses injectable drugs, has had sexual intercourse with bisexual men, has had sexual intercourse with injecting drug users, has received blood from transfusions between 1978 and 1985, or has had more than ten lifetime sex partners (14, 52, 67, 68).

A woman's sex partner is more likely to be infected if he is bisexual, uses injectable drugs, has hemophilia, has had sexual intercourse with women who used injectable drugs, has received blood transfusions between 1978 and 1985, or has had more than 20 lifetime sex partners (67).

The probability of exposure to an infected partner is also higher if the partner has used crack cocaine (58, 81). This particular risk behavior is strongly associated with other risk behaviors, including exchange of sex for cocaine or money, sex with multiple partners, sex with anonymous partners, and a history of STDs.

Geographic differences in rates of HIV infection are also reflected in the probability of exposure to infected partners. The likelihood of exposure to such a partner increases if the partner is from an area marked by a high prevalence of HIV. Some states have manifold higher prevalence rates than others. Moreover, HIV is concentrated in certain cities within states and in certain neighborhoods within cities (67). In 1989, 1 in 200 women giving birth in New York state was HIV infected, whereas none of 17,273 women giving birth in New Hampshire were (67, 83). Although the overall rate of seroprevalence in 26 hospitals, in 21 cities in 1988–1989 was 1.3%, it ranged from 0.1% in some hospitals, to 7.8% in others, and was as high as 18% and 22% for 25–44-year-old men in two hospitals in the communities with the highest prevalence of AIDS (83).

The facts surrounding differential probabilities of exposure to infected partners appear straightforward. However, as Peterman et al (67) point out, gathering the relevant information on potential sex partners under real-world conditions is difficult. For example, among 422 sexually active college students, 32% of the men and 23% of the women were sexually involved with multiple partners; in 60% or more of the cases, their sex partners did not know about their sexual involvement with others (21). Similarly, 38% of 52 female partners of infected bisexual men did not know that their partner was bisexual, despite being in long-term relationships with them (63). Thus, use of the above information for personal protection is problematic.

Perhaps because information regarding heterosexual transmission of HIV in Europe and North America lagged behind information on homosexual transmission, compared with gay men, heterosexuals in the US appear to be relatively less concerned about their chances of exposure to an infected partner. Only 12% of 63 heterosexuals who had been previously tested in a Miami STD clinic had ever asked a partner about his/her HIV status (42). In contrast, 23% of one cohort of gay men had asked sex partners about their HIV status (93).

Likelihood of Acquiring HIV Infection When Exposed to an Infected Partner

For men, the risk of acquiring HIV infection during heterosexual intercourse is increased if sexual contact occurs during menses (24, 56). The presence of HIV-infected blood cells in the vagina could explain the increased risk associated with sexual contact during menses. The presence of clinical and biological symptoms of HIV infection in the infected female partner also increases men's risk of acquiring HIV infection (24). The number of sexual exposures is also positively associated with men's risk of acquiring HIV infection (56). Insertive anal intercourse does not appear to be a high risk practice for heterosexual men.

Uncircumcised men are more likely to be seropositive (8). Circumcision appears to be protective against other STDs, as well (2). However, without controlled studies, it is difficult to rule out completely the potential confounding effects of sexual behavior in the association between circumcision and risk of HIV acquisition.

Condom use is protective against acquisition of infection (91). The magnitude of protection reported varies across studies. However, the specific magnitude of protection provided by condom use, as measured by most current studies, may not be meaningful, because condom use is a multidimensional behavior that is often inadequately measured.

For women, the risk of acquiring HIV through heterosexual contact with an infected partner increases with the length of the relationship and the frequency of intercourse (56). In studies that measure the number of sexual exposures (rather than the length of relationship and the frequency of intercourse), this variable is associated with risk of HIV acquisition (65).

Receptive anal intercourse emerges as an important risk factor for women as it does for men who have sex with men (51, 56). Studies of female partners of infected men suggest that women who reported having anal intercourse with their partners were two to four times more likely to be infected than women who only had vaginal intercourse (28, 86, 90). Oral sex appears to be a route of transmission in male-to-male (59) and female-to-female transmission (57) and, therefore, would be expected to be a risk factor for heterosexual transmission.

Inadequate lubrication of the vagina during sexual intercourse with an infected partner apparently increases the risk of acquiring HIV infection. The use of desiccants in the vagina has been suggested as a factor that may contribute to the high rates of heterosexual transmission of HIV in Africa (55, 67). The observation that older women may have a higher risk of acquiring HIV infection when exposed to an infected partner is also consistent with the dry sex hypothesis (35, 69). The suggestion that couples spend more time engaging in foreplay to ensure adequate lubrication of the vagina (1) may have a protective role to play in this context.

The awareness of partners' HIV status and condom use apparently protect women against acquiring HIV infection when exposed to an infected partner (51). Furthermore, an association between use of oral contraceptive pills and women's risk of acquiring HIV infection has been reported in the literature (51). However, whether the use of oral contraceptives increases or protects against the risk of acquiring infection is not clear.

Currently, our understanding of the risk factors for acquisition of HIV infection is limited. The realization that host infectiousness may vary over the course of the infection is recent, and the knowledge of patterns of infectiousness over time may be incomplete. Thus, most investigations of risk factors for acquiring HIV infection do not take the variability in infectiousness into consideration in their design. Often, information on the duration of infection in the host, the clinical stage of HIV disease, and/or biological markers is unavailable. Consequently, it is impossible to adjust for the potential confounding effects of host infectiousness in data analysis. As future studies control for indicators of infectiousness, findings on risk factors for acquiring HIV infection can be better understood and interpreted.

A second limitation to our understanding of risk factors for HIV infection results from an inadequate differentiation among risk factors for exposure to an infected partner, risk factors for acquiring infection when exposed to an infected partner, and the combined effect of these two, i.e. risk factors for being infected. Although most investigations of risk factors focus on infection status as the outcome, prevalent infection is easier to identify than incident infection.

Perhaps as a result of overlooking the differentiation between risk of exposure to an infected partner and risk of acquiring infection, some studies investigate risk behaviors in inappropriate populations. For example, studies of STD clinic populations often fail to identify risk factors for exposure to an infected partner, because STD clinic attendance selects for exposure to sexually transmitted pathogens (3). Such selection bias may be relatively more serious in studies of behavioral risk factors. Increasing awareness of the effects of study population on study findings will help facilitate the accumulation of more meaningful information.

The Role of Other STDs in the Acquisition of HIV Infection Through Heterosexual Transmission

The association between HIV infection and other STDs has been observed in many populations and has been particularly remarkable in urban populations in Africa and in inner city populations in the US. The potential causal links represented in the observed associations has been difficult to interpret, partly because of the complex nature of the relationship between HIV and other STDs. Behavioral risk factors are similar for all sexually transmitted infections, including HIV. As a result, coinfection with more than one sexually transmitted pathogen is frequent. Thus, attempts to understand the relationship between a given STD and HIV infection need to control for the potential confounding effects of sexual behavior and other STDs; they also need to specify the direction, magnitude, and nature of the STD-HIV effect. It is important to determine the role of other STDs in the transmission of HIV, the role of other STDs in the progression of HIV disease, and the role of HIV infection in alterations of natural history, diagnosis, or response to therapy of other STDs (92). The relationships between specific STDs and HIV apparently are not uniform. The relative importance of STDs in HIV transmission may depend on competing risk factors, such as circumcision or receptive anal intercourse, the prevalence of which varies with gender and sexual preference (92). In addition, the importance of STDs in HIV transmission may be magnified when they occur conjointly with some other risk factors, such as dry sex. The prevalence of these risk factors varies across societies and cultural groups, as well as by gender and sexual orientation.

Available data indicate that genital ulcer disease, including chancroid, syphilis, and genital herpes, is a risk factor for heterosexual transmission of HIV (6, 32, 44, 75, 82, 85). The results of prospective studies that control for the potential confounding effects of sexual behavior also support this hypothesis.

Studies of the relationship between syphilis and HIV infection show a two- to ninefold increase in HIV infection risk associated with syphilis (9, 10, 19, 23, 26, 33, 95). Even after controlling for the potential confounding effects of sexual behavior in prospective studies, this relationship is statistically significant. Although a statistically significant association between chancroid (Ig G antibody to *Hemophilus ducreyi*) and HIV seropositivity has been reported, effects of sexual behavior and other STDs were not controlled (74). Herpes simplex virus type 2 (HSV-2) infection may be associated with increased risk for HIV infection among homosexual men (36, 88), but some studies found no association (33, 43, 95).

Available data on the association between nonulcerative STDs and HIV infection are more limited. However, if nonulcerative STDs facilitate HIV transmission, they will account for greater proportions of HIV infection than genital ulcer disease in most societies. In many societies, chlamydial infection, gonorrhea, and trichomoniasis are more common than genital ulcers (92). Chlamydial cervicitis has been associated with a fourfold increase in the risk for HIV seroconversion in prospective studies (46, 75). Gonorrhea is apparently associated with a three- to ninefold increase in HIV risk in prospective studies of heterosexual populations (43, 95). Female prostitutes with trichomoniasis were at three times greater risk of HIV seroconversion compared with those without infection (46). Women with anogenital warts are three to four times more likely to have HIV infection (19, 77).

Other STDs may also be risk factors for the progression of HIV disease. The role of other STDs in the progression of HIV disease is not well studied. Most studies do not control for duration of HIV infection, baseline immunologic status, and age—all important confounders. At this time, results regarding the effect of other STDs on the progression of HIV disease are inconclusive (92).

Indirect relationships between HIV infection and other STDs may further reinforce the role of STDs as risk factors for HIV transmission, especially at the community level. Theoretically, HIV infection might change STD incidence and frequency of recurrences; lead to atypical presentations including larger, more numerous or more persistent lesions; or modify the natural history of STDs resulting in more frequent complications (92). Such changes in the presentation and epidemiology of STDs would further facilitate the heterosexual transmission of HIV.

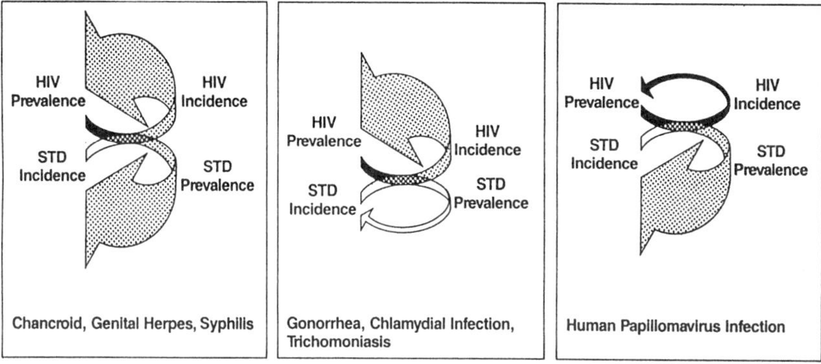

Figure 2 HIV infection and other STDs—the Wasserheit loops.

Apparently, HIV infection results in decreased responsiveness to standard therapy among persons with chancroid (7, 54) and early infection with syphilis (5, 25, 40). Atypical presentation with both chancroid and syphilis in the presence of HIV infection, including larger and extragenital lesions, have also been reported (4, 11, 50, 76). Severity of herpes simplex type 2 lesions and their frequency of recurrence increase in the presence of HIV infection (22, 79, 87); resistance to therapy may also increase in such cases (27, 96).

In summary, the relationships between HIV infection and other STDs may be different for different STDs. According to Wasserheit (92), genital ulcer disease and HIV infection reinforce each other. These STDs facilitate HIV transmission, and HIV infection may simultaneously prolong or augment the infectiousness of individuals with genital ulcer disease. Discharge syndromes, including gonorrhea, chlamydial infection, and trichomoniasis, seem to promote HIV transmission without a synergistic increase in their own prevalence or incidence. Human papillomavirus infection may be an opportunistic infection, the expresssion and progression of which are augmented by HIV (Figure 2).

SOCIETAL CONTEXT: Effects of Society and Culture on Risk Factors for Heterosexual Transmission of HIV and Effects of HIV Disease on Society

Globally, incidence of heterosexually transmitted HIV is strongly associated with patterns of heterosexual networking; prevalance and incidence of STDs, such as chancroid, syphilis, gonorrhea, and chlamydial infection; and prevalence of specific sexual practices and other behavioral risk factors discussed earlier, such as male circumcision and the use of desiccants in the vagina. As a result, societal factors that influence patterns of heterosexual networking,

STD prevalence, and the other related behaviors affect the incidence of heterosexually transmitted HIV in indirect but important ways.

Two prototypes of heterosexual networking have been described (49). In pattern I, marital stability is strong, women are dependent on their husbands, social structure is often patrilineal, and men have premarital and extramarital sex with a small number of women who themselves have many partners. In pattern II, marital stability is weaker, women are more independent and may return easily to their original families with their children, both men and women have fluid networks of sexual partnerships, and the role of prostitution is less apparent. Pattern I is exemplified by Kigali, Rwanda, where the prevalence of HIV infection in young adults has risen to 20% or higher. Pattern II is exemplified by Kinshasa, Zaire, where prevalence of HIV infection has leveled off at 7–8% in young adults (37).

Several societal factors apparently affect patterns of heterosexual networking. A youthful population composition; urbanization with dominant rural-to-urban migration streams of young, single adults; economic underdevelopment accompanied by high rates of unemployment; low levels of literacy and education; a subordinate status for women, as reflected in the social, political, economic, and legal systems; and a double standard for sexual conduct all seem to reinforce heterosexual network patterns conducive to HIV transmission (37).

Prevalence and incidence of STDs in a society are affected by patterns of heterosexual networking. In addition, they are affected by factors that help or hinder the early and appropriate diagnosis and treatment of curable bacterial STDs. These factors include the availability and accessibility of health care services and their utilizaition, which is affected by STD symptom recognition and health care seeking. Delayed diagnosis and treatment of curable bacterial STDs increase the probability of HIV transmission for the individual and the incidence of HIV in the community.

Effects of heterosexually transmitted HIV on the society are major. The economic system is negatively impacted through the very high health care costs for HIV disease and the large numbers of productive years of life lost. HIV infected babies and children add significantly to this burden. Early death of parents result in large numbers of orphans who need care. Some of these children may themselves have HIV disease. In societies where incidence of heterosexually transmitted HIV is high, the composition of the population may be altered significantly, and whole communities may disappear.

METHODOLOGICAL ISSUES

Studies of heterosexually transmitted HIV infection involve difficult issues of measurement and design. Moreover, inaccuracies of measurement may hinder the internal validity of results (60).

Measurement of incident HIV requires repeated screening of uninfected persons at relatively short intervals. Often, the exact timing of seroconversion and infection is difficult to determine. Identification of prevalent infection, although relatively easier, is less helpful in determining risk factors. Determination of other biologic and immunologic charcteristics at the time of infection may not be possible.

Measurement of incident infection with other sexually transmitted pathogens may also be difficult, particularly in women who often are asymptomatic with many sexually transmitted infections. Diagnosis of STDs is problematic, especially in resource-poor settings that lack appropriate diagnostic technologies; however, STD diagnosis may involve considerable misclassification error, even in the most developed clinical settings. Moreover, among HIV infected persons, STD diagnosis appears to be particularly subject to misclassification errors.

Sexual behaviors constitute the major risk factors for exposure to infected partners and acquisition of infection when exposed to an infected partner. Measurement of sexual behaviors presents an important challenge because they are difficult to validate. Use of infection with other STDs as biological markers for sexual behavior is desirable, but provides only a partial solution to the problem, as the relationship between sexual behavior and infection with even the most frequent STD is neither perfect nor well understood.

Sexual behaviors and other STDs that comprise the risk factors for heterosexually transmitted HIV are strongly correlated among themselves. Thus, the potential for serious confounding in observed associations is great. Furthermore, often the collinearity among these variables is such that controlling for confounding through analytic techniques may not be possible.

In the light of the measurement and design issues mentioned above, the need for conducting prospective studies and, where possible, intervention studies is clear.

IMPLICATIONS FOR PREVENTION AND CONTROL

Several program and policy implications emerge based on the above considerations. First, targeted behavioral interventions to reduce risk of exposure to infected partners and risk of acquiring infection when exposed to infected partners should be implemented urgently. Due to effectiveness and cost considerations, these interventions must be targeted to persons at high risk. In many societies, risk of exposure to and acquisition of HIV in the general population are low, and universal behavioral interventions are not warranted.

Second, STDs are among the most readily modifiable risk factors for the spread of HIV. Therefore, STD services must be strengthened and then coordinated with HIV services for reinforcement in all societies. This is particularly important in areas of high STD prevalence, such as many parts of Africa and Asia.

Third, persons infected with other STDs constitute a most readily identifiable high-risk group for HIV infection. They should be targeted in behavioral intervention and health promotion efforts.

Fourth, a multipronged approach to the means of prevention should be adopted in all societies. Condom use, discriminating selection of sex partners, and decreased number of sex partners should be viewed as complementary methods and not as mutually exclusive alternatives. In light of the remarkable variability of HIV prevalence and patterns of sexual networking across population groups, different means of prevention will clearly be more suitable to different groups. Decreasing number of sex partners threatens the economic survival of prostitutes, but may bc a viable means of prevention for married men who have many extramarital partners. A discriminating selection of sex partners may be a realistic approach for many members of societies in which HIV infections are confined to particular geographic, demographic, or occupational groups.

Fifth, behavioral interventions should be located in the community so that individuals do not have to go outside their daily routine to receive the interventions. In many societies, the workplace may be the best site for the implementation of behavioral interventions.

Sixth, epidemiologic and prevention research should focus on questions with widespread prevention implications. For example, the role of oral contraceptives in HIV transmission needs to be defined more clearly and considered in the formulation of prevention strategies. Similarly, evaluation research should explore the extent to which control of STDs will prevent HIV transmission.

Finally, in many societies, prostitutes and other subgroups have very high HIV infection rates, and efforts to change their sexual behaviors apparently fail to control HIV transmission. These situations clearly call for a societal self-examination that focuses on such factors as poverty, inequality, and women's subordination, all of which affect risk factors for heterosexual transmission, such as prostitution. Ultimately, the epidemiology, prevention, and control of all STD, including HIV, depend on the basic structure of society.

Acknowledgments

The author thanks Jeffrey Harris and Thomas Peterman for their invaluable input and Joye Blalock for her superb secretarial assistance in the preparation of this manuscript.

Literature Cited

1. Albert, A. E., Hatcher, R. A., Graves, W. 1991. Condom use and breakage among women in a municipal hospital family planning clinic. *Contraception* 43:167
2. Aral, S. O., Holmes, K. K. 1990. Epidemiology of sexual behavior and sexually transmitted diseases. In *Sexually Transmitted Diseases,* ed. K. K. Holmes, P.-A. Mardh, P. F. Sparling, P. J. Wiesner, W. Cates, et al, 2:31. New York: McGraw-Hill
3. Aral, S. O., Soskolne, V., Joesoef, R. M., O'Reilly, K. 1991. Sex partner selection as risk factor for STD: clustering of risky modes. *Sex Transm. Dis.* 18:10–17
4. Berger, J. R., Hensley, G., Moskowitz, L. 1989. *Syphilitic myelopathy with human immunodeficiency virus: a treatable cause of spinal cord disease.* 5th Int. AIDS Conf., Montreal (Abstr. W.B.P. 51)
5. Berry, C. D., Hooton, T. M., Collier, A. C., 1987. Neurologic relapse after benzathine penicillin therapy for secondary syphilis in a patient with HIV infection. *N. Engl. J. Med.* 316:1587–89
6. Cameron, D. W., Lourdes, J. D., Gregory, M. M., Simonsen, J. N., D'Costa, L. J., et al. 1989. Female to male transmission of human immunodeficiency virus type 1: risk factors for seroconversion in men. *Lancet* 2:403–7
7. Cameron, D. W., Plummer, F. A., D'Costa, L. J., Ndinya-Achola, J. O., Ronald, A. R. 1988. *Prediction of HIV infection by treatment failure for chancroid, a genital ulcer disease.* 4th Int. AIDS Conf., Stockholm (Abstr. 7637)
8. Cameron, D. W., Simonsen, J. N., D'Costa, L. J., Ronald, A. R., Maitha, G. M., et al. 1991. Female to male transmission of human immunodeficiency virus type 1: risk factors for seroconversion in men. *Lancet* 2:403
9. Cannon, R. O., Hook, E. W., Nahmnias, A. J., Lee, F. K., Glasser, D., Quinn, T. C. 1988. *Association of herpes simplex virus type 2 with HIV infection in heterosexual patients attending sexually transmitted disease clinics.* 4th Int. AIDS Conf., Stockholm (Abstr. 4558)
10. Cannon, R. O., Quinn, T., Rompalo, A., Glasser, D., Groseclos, S., Hook, E. 1989. *Syphilis is strongly associated with HIV infection in Baltimore STD Clinic patients independent of risk group.* 5th Int. AIDS Conf., Montreal (Abstr. Th.A.O. 18)
11. Caumes, E., Janier, M., Janssen, F., Rybojad, M., Dallot, A., Morel, P. 1989. *Atypical secondary syphilis in HIV seropositive patients.* 5th Int. AIDS Conf., Montreal (Abstr. W.B.P. 49)
12. Cent. for Dis. Control. 1979. *STD Fact Sheet,* pp. 79–8195. Atlanta; US Dep. of Health, Educ. Welf. Publ. CDC
13. Cent. for Dis. Control. 1986. Update: Acquired immunodeficiency syndrome—United States. *Morbid. Mortal. Wkly. Rep.* 35:756–66
14. Cent. for Dis. Control. 1989. *National HIV Seroprevalence Serosurveys: Summary of Results. Data from Serosurveillance Activities through 1989.* Atlanta: US Dep. of Health and Hum. Serv., Public Health Serv.
15. Cent. for Dis. Control. 1991. Update: Acquired Immunodeficiency Syndrome, United States 1981–1990. *Morbid. Mortal. Wkly. Rep.* 40(22):358–63
16. Cent. for Dis. Control. 1992. The second 100,000 cases of Acquired Immunodeficiency Syndrome, United States, June 1981–December 1991. *Morbid. Mortal. Wkly. Rep.* 41(2):28–29
17. Cent. for Dis. Control. 1992. Quarterly AIDS map. *Morbid. Mortal. Wkly. Rep.* 41(16):281
18. Chequer, P., Rodrigues, L., Castilho, E., Bergamashi, D. 1989. *Trend analysis of AIDS cases reported in Brazil, 1982–1988.* 5th Int. AIDS Conf., Montreal (Abst. M.G.O. 26)
19. Chiphangwi, J., Dallabetta, G., Saah, A., Liomba, G., Miott, D. 1990. *Risk factors for HIV-1 infection in pregnant women in Malawi.* 6th Int. AIDS Conf., San Francisco (Abst. Th.C 98)
20. Clemetson, D., Moss, G., D'Costa, L., Kreiss, J., Ndinya-Achola, J. 1990. *Incidence of HIV transmission within HIV discordant heterosexual partnerships in Nairboi, Kenya.* 6th Int. AIDS Conf., San Francisco 2:448 (Abstr. 3187)
21. Cochran, S. D., Mays, V. M. 1990. Sex, lies, and HIV. *N. Engl. J. Med.* 322:774
22. Corey, L. 1990. Genital herpes. In *Sexually Transmitted Diseases,* ed. K.

K. Holmes. New York: McGraw-Hill. 399 pp.

23. Darrow, W. W., Echenberg, D. F., Jaffe, H. W., Echenberg, D. F., Jaffe, H. W., et al. 1987. Risk factors for human immunodeficiency virus (HIV) infections in homosexual men. *Am. J. Public Health* 77:479–83
24. DeVincenzi, I., Ancelle-Park, R. 1989. *Heterosexual transmission of HIV: a European study. II. Female-to-male transmission*. 5th Int. AIDS Conf., Montreal, pp. 74 (Abstr. Th.A. 0.20)
25. Duncan, W. C. 1989. Failure of erythromycin to cure secondary syphilis in a patient infected with the human immunodeficiency virus. *Arch. Dermatol.* 125:82–84
26. Elifson, K., Soles, J., Sweet, H., Darrow, W. 1989. *Risk factors for HIV infection among male prostitutes in Atlanta*. 5th Int. AIDS Conf., Montreal (Abstr. W.A.P. 38)
27. Erlich, K., Mills, J., Chatis, P., Mertz, G. J., Busch, D. F., et al. 1989. Acyclovir-resistant herpes simplex virus infections in patients with the acquired immunodeficiency syndrome. *N. Engl. J. Med.* 320:293–96
28. European Study Group. 1989. Risk factors for male to female transmission of HIV. *Br. Med. J.* 298:411
29. Franzen, C., Albert, J., Biberfeld, G., Lidin-Janson, G., Lowhagen, G-B. 1988. *Natural history of heterosexual HIV infection in a Swedish cohort*. 4th Int. AIDS Conf., Stockholm (Abstr. 4021)
30. Goedert, J. J., Eyster, M. E., Biggar, R. J., Blattner, W. A. 1988. Heterosexual transmission of human immunodeficiency virus: association with severe depletion of T-helper lymphocytes in men with hemophilia. *AIDS Res. Hum. Retroviruses* 3:355–61
31. Goudsmit, J., Lange, J. M. A., Paul, D. A., Dawson, G. J. 1987. Antigenemia and antibody titers to core and envelope antigens in AIDS, AIDS-related complex, and subclinical human immunodeficiency virus infection. *J. Infect. Dis.* 155:558–60
32. Greenblatt, R. M., Lukehart, S. A., Plummer, F. A., Quinn, T. C., Critchlow, C. W., et al. 1988. Genital ulceration as a risk factor for human immunodeficiency virus infection. *AIDS* 2:47–50
33. Hayes, C. G., Manaloto, C. R., Basaca-Sevilla, V., Padre, L. P., Laughlin, L. W., et al. 1990. Epidemiology of HIV infection among prostitutes in the Philippines. *J. Acquired Immunodefic. Syndr.* 3:913–20
34. Hearst, N., Hulley, S. B. 1988. Preventing the heterosexual spread of AIDS. Are we giving our patients the best advice? *J. Am. Med. Assoc.* 259: 2428–32
35. Holmberg, S. D., Horsburgh, C. R. Jr., Ward, J. W., Jaffe, H. W. 1989. Biologic factors in the sexual transmission of human immunodeficiency virus. *J. Infect. Dis.* 160:116–25
36. Holmberg, S. D., Stewart, J. A., Gerber, A. R., Byers, R. H., Lee, F. K., et al. 1988. Prior herpes simplex virus type 2 infection as a risk factor for HIV infection. *J. Am. Med. Assoc.* 259:1048–50
37. Holmes, K. K., Aral, S. O. 1991. Behavioral interventions in developing countries. In *Research Issues in Human Behavior and Sexually Transmitted Diseases in the AIDS Era,* ed. J. N. Wasserheit, S. O. Aral, K. K. Holmes, pp. 318–66. Washington, DC: Am. Soc. for Microbiol.
38. Holmes, K. K., Johnson, D. W., Trostle, H. J. 1970. An estimate of the risk of men acquiring gonorrhea by sexual contact with infected females. *Am. J. Epidemiol.* 91:170–74
39. Hopper, R. R., Reynolds, G. H., Jones, O. G., Zaidi, A., Wiesner, P. J., et al. 1978. Cohort study of veneral disease. I. The risk of gonorrhea transmission from infected women to men. *Am. J. Epidemiol.* 108:136–44
40. Johns, D. R., Tierney, M., Felsenstein, D. 1987. Alteration in the natural history of neurosyphilis by concurrent infection with the human immunodeficiency virus. *N. Engl. J. Med.* 316:1569–72
41. Judson, F. N. 1981. Epidemiology of sexually transmitted hepatitis B infections in heterosexuals: a review. *Sex. Transm. Dis.* 8(Suppl.):336–43
42. Kamb, M. L., Otten, M. W., Guerena, F., Onorado, J., Wroten, J., et al. 1991. *Extensive HIV seropositivity among heterosexuals in an STD clinic*. 7th Int. AIDS Conf., Florence (Abstr. C.C. 99)
43. Kingsley, L. A., Armstrong, J., Rahman, A., Ho, M., Rinaldo, C. R. 1990. No association between herpes simplex virus type-2 seropositivity or anogenital lesions and HIV seroconversion among homosexual men. *J. Acquired Immunodefic. Syndr.* 3:773–79
44. Kreiss, J. K., Koech, D., Plummer, F. A., Holmes, K. K., Lightfoote,

M., et al. 1986. AIDS virus infection in Nairobi prostitutes. *N. Engl. J. Med.* 314:414–18

45. Laga, M., Nzila, N., Manoka, A. T. Kivuvu, M., Behets, F., et al. 1989. *High prevalence and incidence of HIV and other sexually transmitted diseases among 801 Kinshasa prostitutes.* 5th Int. AIDS Conf., Montreal (Abstr. Th.A.O.21)
46. Laga M., Nzila, N., Manoka, A. T., Malele, M., Bush, T. J., et al. 1990. *Non ulcerative sexually transmitted diseases (STD) as risk factors for HIV infection.* 6th Int. AIDS Conf., San Francisco (Abstr. Th.C. 97)
47. Laga, M., Taelman, H., Bonneux, L., Cornet, P. Vercauteren, G., Piot, P. 1988. *Risk factors for HIV infection in heterosexual partners of HIV infected Africans and Europeans.* 4th Int. AIDS Conf., Stockholm (Abstr. 4004)
48. Laga, M., Taelman, H., Van der Stuyft, P., Bonneaux, L., Vercauteren, G., Piot, P. 1989. Advanced immunodeficiency as a risk factor for heterosexual transmission of HIV. *AIDS* 3:361–69
49. Larson, A. 1989. Social context of human immunodeficiency virus transmission in Africa: historical and cultural bases of East and Central African sexual relations. *Rev. Infect. Dis.* 11:716–31
50. Latif, A. S. 1989. *Epidemiology and control of chancroid.* 8th Int. Soc. for Sex. Transm. Dis. Res., Copenhagen (Abstr. 66)
51. Lazzarin, A., Saracco, A., Musicco, M., Nicolosi, A. 1991. Man-to-woman sexual transmission, of the human immunodeficiency virus, risk factors related to sexual behavior, man's infectiousness, and woman's susceptibility. Arch. Intern. Med. 151(12): 2411–16
52. Lederman, M. M., Ratnoff, O. D., Evatt, B. L., McDougal, J. S. 1985. Acquisition of antibody to lymphadenopathy-associated virus in patients with classic hemophilia (factor VIII deficiency). *Ann. Intern. Med.* 102:753
53. Lifson, A. R., O'Malley, P. M., Hessol, N. A., Buchbinder, S. P., Cannon, L., Rutherford, G. W. 1991. HIV seroconversion in two hemosexual men after receptive oral intercourse with ejaculation: Implications for counseling concerning safe sexual practices. Am. J. Public Health 81:1509
54. MacDonald, K. S., Cameron, W., D'Costa, L. J., Ndinya-Achola, J. O., Plummer, F. A., Ronald. A. R. 1989. Evaluation of fleroxacin (RO 23-6240) as single-oral dose therapy of culture-proven chancroid in Nairobi, Kenya. *Antimicrob. Agents Chemother.* 33: 612–14
55. Mann, J. M., Nzilambi, N., Piot, P., Bosenge, N., Kalala, M., et al. 1988. HIV infection and associated risk factors in female prostitutes in Kinshasa, Zaire. *AIDS* 2:249
56. Marinacci, G., Costigliola, P., Ricchi, E., Chiodo, F. 1991. *Risk factors in heterosexual transmission of HIV.* 7th Int. AIDS Conf., Florence (Abstr. W.C. 3111)
57. Marmor, M., Weiss, L. R., Lyden, M., Weiss, S. H., Saxinger, W. C., et al. 1986. Possible female-to-female transmission of human immunodeficiency virus. *Ann. Intern. Med.* 105:969
58. Marx, R., Aral, S. O., Rolfs, R. T., Sterk, C. E., Kahn, J. G. 1991. Crack, sex, and STD. *Sex. Transm. Dis.* 18:92
59. Mayer, K. H., DeGruttola, V. 1987. Human immunodeficiency virus and oral intercourse. *Ann. Intern. Med.* 107–428
60. Mertens, T. E., Hayes, R. J., Smith, P. G. 1990. Epidemiological methods to study the interaction between HIV infection and other sexually transmitted diseases. *AIDS* 4:57–65
61. Mosley, J. W. 1975. The epidemiology of viral hepatitis: an overview. *Am. J. Med. Sci.* 270:253–70
62. Osmond, D., Bacchetti, P., Chaisson, R. E., Kelley, T., Stempel, R., et al. 1988. *Am. J. Public Health* 78:944–48
63. Padian, N. S. 1989. *Female partners of bisexual men.* Presented at the CDC Workshop in Bisexuality and AIDS, Atlanta, Oct. 1989
64. Padian, N. S., Marquis, L., Francis, D. P., Wiley, J., Anderson, J. E., et al. 1987. Male-to-female transmission of human immunodeficiency virus. *J. Am. Med. Assoc.* 258:788–90
65. Padian, N. S., Shiboski, S. C., Jewell, N. P. 1990. The effect of number of exposures on the risk of heterosexual transmission. *J. Infect. Dis.* 161(5): 883–87
66. Padian, N. S., Wiley, J., Winkelstein, W. 1987. *Male-to-female transmission of human immunodeficiency virus (HIV): current result, infectivity rates, and San Francisco population seroprevalence estimates.* 3rd Int. AIDS Conf., Washington, DC (Abstr. THP. 48)
67. Peterman, T. A., Cates, W. Jr., Wasserheit, J. N. 1993. Prevention of the sexual transmission of HIV. In

AIDS, ed. V. I. DeVita, Jr., S. Hellman, S. A. Rosenberg. Philadelphia: Lippincott. In press

68. Peterman, T. A., Lui, K. J., Lawrence, D. N., Allen, J. R. 1987. Estimating the risks of transfusion-associated acquired immunodeficiency syndrome and human immunodeficiency virus infection. *Transfusion* 27:371
69. Peterman, T. A., Stoneburner, R. L., Allen, J. R., Jaffe, H. W., Curran, J. W. 1988. Risk of human immunodeficiency virus transmission from heterosexual adults with transfusion-associated infections. *J. Am. Med. Assoc.* 259:55–58
70. Piot, P., Kreiss, J. K., Ndinya-Achola, J. O., Ngugi, E. N., Simonsen, J. N., et al. 1987. Editorial review: heterosexual transmission of HIV. *AIDS* 1:199–206
71. Piot, P., Laga, M., Ryder, R., Perriens, J., Temmerman, M., et al. 1990. The global epidemiology of HIV infection: continuity, heterogeneity, and change. *J. Acquired Immunodefic. Syndr.* 3: 403–12
72. Piot, P., Plummer, F. A., Mhalu, F. S., Lamboray, J. L., Chin, J., Mann, J. W. 1988. AIDS: an international perspective. *Science* 239:573–79
73. Piot, P., Quinn, T. C., Taelman, H. Feinsod, F. M., Minlangua, K. B., et al. 1984. Acquired immunodeficiency syndrome in a heterosexual population in Zaire. *Lancet* 2:65–69
74. Piot, P., Van Dyck, E., Ryder, R. W., Nzila, N., Laga, M. 1989. *Serum antibody to Haemophilus ducreyi as a risk factor for HIV in Africa, but not in Europe*. 5th Int. AIDS Conf., Montreal (Abstr. M.A.O.32)
75. Plummer, F. A., Simonsen, J. N., Cameron, D. W., Ndinya-Achola, J. O., Kreiss, J. K., et al. 1991. Cofactors in male-to-female transmission of HIV. *J. Infect. Dis.* 163:233–39
76. Quale, J., Tellitz, E., Augenbraun, M. 1990. Atypical presentation of chancroid in a patient infected with the human immunodeficiency virus. *Am. J. Med.* 88(5):43N-44N
77. Quinn, T. C., Glasser, D., Cannon, R. O., Matuszak, D. L., Dunning, R. W., et al., 1988. Human immunodeficiency virus infection among patients attending clinics for sexually transmitted diseases. *N. Engl. J. Med.* 318:197–204
78. Quinn, T. C., Mann, J. N., Curran, J. W., Piot, P. 1986. AIDS in Africa: an epidemiologic paradigm. *Science* 234:955–63
79. Quinnan, G. V., Masur, H., Rook, A. H., Armstrong, G., Frederick, W. R., et al. Herpes virus infections in the acquired immune deficiency syndrome. *J. Am. Med. Assoc.* 252:72–77
80. Rehmet, S., Staszewski, S., Helm, E. B., Doerr, H. W., Stille, W. 1991. *Cofactors of HIV transmission in heterosexual couples*. 7th Int. AIDS Conf., Florence (Abstr. W.C.3132)
81. Rolfs, R. T., Goldberg, M., Sharrar, R. G. 1990. Risk factors for syphilis: cocaine use and prostitution. *Am. J. Public Health* 80:853
82. Ryder, R., Hassig, S., Ndilu, M., Behets, F., Nanlele, K., et al. 1989. *Extramarital/prostitute sex and genital ulcer disease (GUD) are important HIV risk factor in 7068 male Kinshasa factory workers and their 4548 wives*. 5th Int. AIDS Conf, Montreal (Abstr. M.A.O.35)
83. St. Louis, M. E., Rauch, K. J., Petersen, L. R., Anderson, J. E., Schable, C. A., Dondero, T. J. 1990. Seroprevalence rates of human immunodeficiency virus infection at sentinel hospitals in the United States. *N. Engl. J. Med.* 323:213
84. Seage, G. R., Horsburgh, C., Hardy, A., 1988. *Increased suppressor T cells in probable transmitters of human immunodeficiency virus*. 4th Int. AIDS Conf., Stockholm (Abstr. 4561)
85. Simonsen, J. N., Cameron, D. W., Gakinya, M. N., Ndinya-Achola, J. O., D'Costa, L. J., et al. 1988. Human immunodeficiency virus infection among men with sexually transmitted diseases. *N. Engl. J. Med.* 319:274–78
86. Sion, F. S., Morais de Sa, C. A., Rachid de Lacerda, M. C., Quinones, E. P., Perei, R. A., et al. *The importance of anal intercourse in transmission of HIV to women*. 4th Int. AIDS Conf., Stockholm (Abstr. 4007)
87. Sooy, C. D., Mills, J. 1988. *Herpes virus infection presenting as giant herpetic nasal ulcers in AIDS*. 4th Int. AIDS Conf., Stockholm (Abstr. 7096)
88. Stamm, W. E., Handsfield, H. H., Rompalo, A. M., Ashley, R. L., Roberts, P. L., Corey, L. 1988. The association between genital ulcer disease and acquisition of HIV infection in homosexual men. *J. Am. Med. Assoc.* 260:1429–33
89. Staszewski, S., Rehmet, S., Hofmeister, W. D. 1988. *Analysis of transmission rates in heterosexual transmitted HIV infection*. 4th Int. AIDS Conf., Stockholm (Abstr. 4068)
90. Steigbigel, N. H., Maude, D. W.,

Feiner, C. J., Harris, C. A., Saltzman, B. R., Klein, R. S. 1988. *Heterosexual transmission of HIV infection*. 4th Int. AIDS Conf., Stockholm (Abstr. 4057)
91. Stone, K. M., Grimes, D. A., Magder, L. S. 1986. Personal protection against sexually transmitted diseases. *Am. J. Gynecol*. 155:180
92. Wasserheit, J. N. 1992. Epidemiological synergy: interrelationships between human immunodeficiency virus infection and other sexually transmitted diseases. *Sex. Transm. Dis*. 19(2):61–77
93. Wiktor, S. Z., Biggar, R. J., Melbye, M., Ebbesen, P., Colclough, G., et al. 1990. Effect of knowledge of human immunodeficiency virus infection status on sexual activity among homosexual men. *AIDS* 3:62
94. Van de Perre, P., Rouvroy, D., Lepage, P. Bogaerts, J., Kestelyn, P., et al. 1984. Acquired immunodeficiency syndrome in Rwanda. *Lancet* 2:62–65
95. VanRaden, M., Kaslow, R., Kingsley, L., Detels, R., Narer, J., et al. 1989. *The Multicenter AIDS Cohort Study. The role of ulcerative genital diseases in promoting acquisition of HIV-1 by homosexual men*. 5th Int. AIDS Conf. Montreal (Abstr. Th.A.O.17)
96. Youle, M. M., Hawkins, D. A., Collins, P. Shanson, D. C., Evans, R., et al. 1988. Acyclovir-resistant herpes in AIDS patients treated with Foscarnet. *Lancet* 2:341–42

Annu. Rev. Publ. Health 1993. 14:469–90

THE NEW PUBLIC HEALTH

Julio Frenk
National Institute of Public Health, Mexico; Center for Population and Development Studies, Harvard University, Cambridge, Massachusetts 02138

KEY WORDS: definition of public health, conceptual models, health research, human resource development, utilization of knowledge

---

INTRODUCTION

Health is a crossroad. It is where biological and social factors, the individual and the community, and social and economic policy all converge. In addition to its intrinsic value, health is a means for personal and collective advancement. It is, therefore, an indicator of the success achieved by a society and its institutions of government in promoting well-being, which is the ultimate meaning of development.

As a field of knowledge and as a social practice, public health has historically been one of the vital forces that have led to reflection on and collective action for health and well-being. However, there is a widespread impression that this leading role has been weakening and that public health is today experiencing a severe identity crisis, as well as a crisis of organization and accomplishment. A recent report prepared by a special committee of the Institute of Medicine opens with the following statement: "In recent years, there has been a growing sense that public health, as a profession, as a governmental activity, and as a commitment of society is neither clearly defined, adequately supported, nor fully understood" (8).

Like the societies of which they are a part, public health institutions all over the world are experiencing new tensions that have exacerbated problems, but have also created challenges for innovation. For nearly 80 years, we have had schools devoted to the teaching of public health. Over time, our schools have developed a valuable tradition that has made it possible to build a broad institutional basis. At the same time, departments and programs with other names have arisen. These departments share a great deal of the vision and mission of public health. However, problems have been mounting. In many

0163-7525/93/0510-0469$02.00

countries, schools and institutes of public health have become isolated from scientific progress and from efforts to organize better health systems. This has relegated them to a secondary role both in academia and in applied areas, thus generating a vicious circle between isolation and irrelevance.

Today more than ever, public health institutions need to redefine their mission in light of the increasingly complex environment in which they operate. Today more than ever, they must ask themselves about their social role, about the scope of their actions, and about the bases of their knowledge. In light of the magnitude of the problems, which have even led many to abandon the term "public health," we urgently need to propose for ourselves a renaissance that, by assimilating the most valuable aspects of our intellectual tradition, legitimately enables us to speak of a new public health. What are the conceptual principles that underlie this renaissance? What are its organizational challenges? What are the characteristics of the epidemiological and social context that establish the need for change and specify the limits of its feasibility? This article attempts to offer some preliminary answers to these questions. The purpose is to contribute to a process that will once again place public health at the center of the scientific and political debate on the future course of individual and social well-being.

ELEMENTS OF AN INTELLECTUAL TRADITION

To a large extent, the challenge to public health is to build and consolidate a vigorous intellectual tradition that both supports its efforts to create knowledge and guides its practical applications. Many generations of public health researchers, professors, and workers have made essential contributions along these lines. Like all living traditions, this one should involve a continuous process of building and renewal. From this point of view, we can organize our discussion by considering that the development of an intellectual field (4) is based on the following four elements (15, 23):

1. Conceptual base. This element establishes the limits of the specific area of research, teaching, and action. Hence, it involves rigorously defining what constitutes public health, and more specifically—in an effort to differentiate the previous uses of this term—the new public health.
2. Production base. This element refers to the set of institutions where a critical mass and a critical density of researchers come together to generate the body of knowledge that gives substantive content to the intellectual field.
3. Reproduction base. This element ensures the consolidation and continuity of the intellectual field—and thus the construction of an authentic tradition—through three principal vehicles: educational programs to train

new professionals and researchers, publications to disseminate results, and associations for the exchange of ideas and the aggregation of interests.

4. Utilization base. This element ensures the translation of knowledge into two types of products: technological developments (including new organizational schemes) and decision making based on research results. As we discuss later, the utilization base is of great importance for providing feedback to the individuals and institutions involved in the production and reproduction of knowledge.

In the rest of this article, we examine the challenges to the new public health by analyzing each of the above elements.

CONCEPTUAL BASE

Any project to renew public health would be useless if it did not take as its point of departure a systematic effort to specify its current meaning and to separate it from obsolete conceptions. In this section, therefore, we attempt first to define the two faces of public health: as a field of research and as a form of professional practice. In the case of research, we propose a typology and reflect on the role of the different scientific disciplines in public health. We also discuss the reasons why we believe that the term "public health" should continue to be used. Indeed, when defined rigorously, this term is better than the alternatives that have been proposed by other reform projects. The updating that public health requires today should be truly conceptual, not just a matter of terminology.

However, a complete conceptual development cannot be limited to definitions, but must also deal with the models that have guided public health. The second part of this section briefly reviews such models in order to introduce a subject that should receive much more attention in the effort to get the new public health off the ground.

Definition of Public Health

The term public health is charged with ambiguous meanings. Throughout its history, five connotations have been particularly prominent. The first equates the adjective "public" to governmental action, that is, the public sector. The second meaning is somewhat broader, as it includes not only government programs, but also participation of the organized community, i.e. the public. The third use identifies public health with "nonpersonal health services," that is, services that cannot be appropiated by a specific individual, because they are targeted at the environment (e.g. sanitation) or the community (e.g. massive health education). The next usage is slightly broader, because it adds a series of personal preventive services for vulnerable groups (e.g. maternal and child care programs). Finally, the expression "public health problem" is often used, especially in nontechnical language, to refer to diseases that are particularly frequent or dangerous.

There are also associations among these different meanings. In some industrialized countries, for example, the private sector has tended to provide most personal therapeutic services, whereas the public sector has assumed responsibility for preventive and nonpersonal services, which tend to deal with high-frequency problems. This has reinforced the notion of public health as a separate subsystem of services, provided by the state and parallel to the mainstream of high-technology curative medicine. This perspective largely permeates the aforementioned report by the special committee of the Institute of Medicine. Thus, its definition of the "substance" of public health limits it to "organized community efforts aimed at the prevention of disease and promotion of health" (10).

Recently, a more comprehensive conception of public health has emerged. According to this view, the adjective public does not designate a particular set of services, a form of property, or a type of problem, but rather a specific level of analysis: the population level. In contrast to clinical medicine, which operates at an individual level, and biomedical research, which analyzes the subindividual level, the essence of public health is that it adopts a perspective based on groups of people or populations. This population perspective inspires the two facets of public health: as a field of inquiry and as an arena for action (17).

PUBLIC HEALTH RESEARCH As a multidisciplinary field of research, the new public health can be defined as the application of the biological, social, and behavioral sciences to the study of health phenomena in human populations. This is why it encompasses two main objects of analysis: first, the epidemiological study of the health conditions of populations; second, the study of the organized social response to those conditions, in particular, the way in which such response is structured through the health care system.

To visualize the role of public health within the more general field of health research, we can relate the levels with the objects of analysis. This produces the typology shown in Figure 1 (21). For the first dimension of the typology—the objects of analysis—we define conditions as the biological, psychological, and social processes that constitute the levels of health in a given individual or population. By response we are not referring to the internal physiopathological reaction to a given disease process, but to the external response that society organizes for improving health conditions. For the second dimension, we recognize two levels of analysis: the first level ad-

LEVEL OF ANALYSIS	OBJECT OF ANALYSIS	
	Conditions	Responses
Individual and Subindividual	*Biomedical Research* (Basic biological processes; structure and function of the human body; pathological mechanisms)	*Clinical Research* (Efficacy of preventive, diagnostic, and therapeutic procedures; natural history of diseases)
Population	*Epidemiological Research* (Frequency, distribution, and determinants of health needs)	*Health Systems Research* (Effectiveness, quality, and costs of services; development and distribution of resources for care)

Figure 1 Typology of health research, with examples of phenomena to be studied. (Adapted from Ref. 21.)

dresses individuals or parts of individuals (i.e. organs, cells, or subcellular elements); the other is the aggregate level of groups or populations.

Crossing these two dimensions yields the three principal types of research that characterize the field of health: biomedical, clinical, and public health research. Thus, most biomedical research is concerned with the conditions, processes, and mechanisms of health and illness, especially at the subindividual level. Clinical research focuses primarily on studying the efficacy of the preventive, diagnostic, and therapeutic responses applied to the individual. The objects indicated above can also be analyzed at the population level. As shown in Figure 1, this is precisely what constitutes public health research, which is subdivided into two principal types: epidemiological research, which studies the frequency, distribution, and determinants of health needs, defined as those conditions that require care (11), and health systems research (HSR), which can be defined as "the scientific study of the organized social response to health and disease conditions in populations" (23).

To extend the typology, Figure 2 shows that epidemiological research may, in turn, be classified according to the point of departure for analysis. On the one hand, it is possible to start with a set of determinants to study their various consequences; this is the case of environmental, occupational, genetic, and social epidemiology. On the other hand, research may begin by examining some specific health condition (for example, positive health, infectious diseases, chronic and degenerative ailments, injury) to investigate its multiple determinants.

Health systems research also includes two major categories. The first can be called "research on health systems organization," which is focused on the

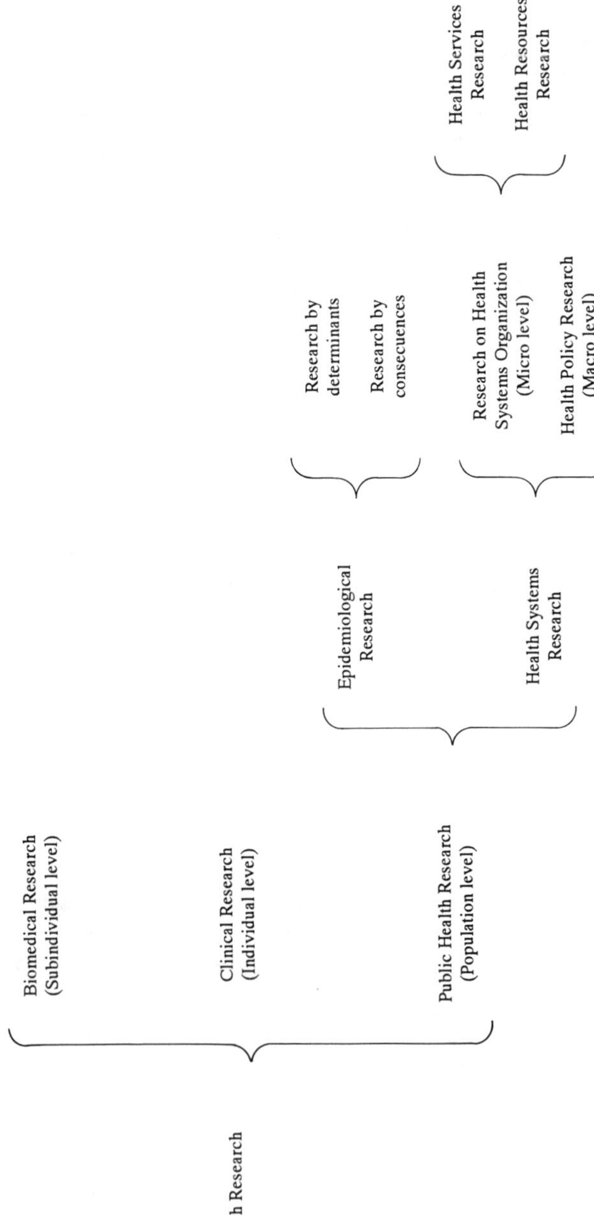

Figure 2 Classification of health research. (Adapted from Ref. 23.)

micro- and intra-organizational level of the health system. It studies the combination of various resources for producing health services of a given quality and technological content. Thus, it includes research on health resources and health services. As can be seen, health services research is part of HSR, as it seeks to analyze the primary products of the system, which are precisely the services. However, the literature still commonly uses the terms "health systems research" and "health services research" interchangeably.

The second category of HSR is called "health policy research." It focuses on the macro- and interorganizational level of the health system. Its purpose is to investigate the social, political, and economic processes that determine the specific forms adopted by the organized social response. Therefore, it studies the determinants, design, implementation, and consequences of health policies.

Naturally, the typologies proposed here represent mere abstractions for synthesizing distinctions that are never so clear-cut in real life. In particular, the four boxes in Figure 1 should not be seen as mutually exclusive compartments. On the contrary, there are numerous connections among the major types of health research. Thus, for example, various emerging fields, such as bioepidemiology, clinical epidemiology, decision analysis, and technology assessment, deal with interfaces among the four types. Indeed, the principal message of Figure 1 is integration: The essential difference between public health research, on the one hand, and biomedical and clinical research, on the other, is not in the objects but in the levels of analysis. A great part of the isolation of traditional public health might have resulted from a conception that postulated that it should study objects other than those examined by the biomedical and clinical sciences, thus erecting an insurmountable barrier. As we attempt to demonstrate further on, the future of public health will depend on its ability to build bridges with the other types of health research and to make its specific and irreplaceable contribution to this undertaking, namely, analysis at the population level. Thus, the challenge is to integrate levels and objects of analysis so as to achieve a full understanding of the broad health field. In the case of public health, this also requires integration among scientific disciplines.

THE ROLE OF THE DISCIPLINES The very definition of public health research involves an effort to achieve interdisciplinary integration. An important obstacle to such integration has been the tendency to identify each level of analysis with a given discipline. In particular, the resultant confusion suggests that the biological sciences are applicable only to the individual and subindividual levels, whereas the population level is the exclusive jurisdiction of the social sciences.

All human populations are organized in societies, which is why the social sciences are indispensable for fully understanding health in populations, i.e. public health. However, there is also a biological dimension of human populations, which is expressed, among other phenomena, in the distribution of genetic characteristics, herd immunity, and the interaction of humans with other populations, such as microorganisms. In particular, there is a broad field that could be called "bioepidemiology," which encompasses the study of the biological determinants, risk factors, and consequences of health processes in populations, as well as the use of methods and techniques derived from the biological sciences to characterize such phenomena. The examples of such applications include seroepidemiology and health surveys that require laboratory tests to measure the prevalence or incidence of a given condition; bromatological and somatometric studies, which are a key part of nutritional epidemiology; and the toxicological analysis of environmental risks. Thus, far from pertaining solely to the study of individual phenomena, the biological sciences also contribute to understanding human populations. The other side of the coin is that the biological sciences are just as essential to public health as are the social sciences.

In addition, there is a second reason why the biological scieces should be an integral part of public health. To achieve a proper understanding of any health condition in a population (a particular disease, for example), we must understand the biological processes that underlie the condition. The rich research tradition on the so-called tropical diseases offers innumerable examples of this type of linkage between biological and population phenomena.

We therefore postulate that an essential element of the public health renaissance is to reincorporate fully the teaching and research of the biological sciences, which many schools of public health have neglected in recent decades. Together with this reencounter, a broad, rigorous, and pluralist development of the social sciences is necessary; this has also been absent from many academic institutions devoted to health. This urgent need for interdisciplinary integration is one of the reasons why, in defining public health, we prefer to use the concept of population more than that of collectivity, which is found in such proposals as that of "collective health" in Brazil. The terms collectivity and community allude to a form of social organization. The term "population" is broader, because it includes both the social and biological dimensions of human groups.

This reasoning also underlies the need to preserve the term public health over those that have arisen in recent decades to designate certain innovative projects, such as "social medicine" or "sociomedicine." These terms are acceptable when studying only the social dimension of health (27), but are not valid as substitutes for the concept of public health, which, as we have just argued, is broader. Indeed, what defines the essence of the new public health is not the exclusive use of certain sciences over others. The biological reductionism of the past should not be replaced by a sociological reductionism. Rather, we need an effort of integration among scientific disciplines. This is precisely the conceptual opening that stems from defining public health by reference to its population level of analysis.

THE PRACTICE OF PUBLIC HEALTH As indicated above, public health is not only a field of inquiry, but also a space for professional practice. This dimension also requires conceptual clarification.

As an arena for action, the modern conception of public health goes beyond fragmentary dichotomies, such as personal versus environmental services, preventive versus curative activities, and public versus private responsibilities. Instead of lending itself to these dichotomies, the new public health addresses the systematic efforts to identify health needs and organize comprehensive services with a well-defined population base. It thus encompasses the information required for characterizing the conditions of the population and the mobilization of resources necessary for responding to such conditions. In this sense, the essence of public health is the health of the public. Therefore, it includes "the organization of personnel and facilities to provide all health services required for the promotion of health, prevention of disease, diagnosis and treatment of illnesses, and physical, social, and vocational rehabilitation" (32). Public health encompasses the more narrow concept of medical care, but not in its technical and interpersonal aspects as applied to individuals in clinical situations, but rather in its organizational dimension as related to well-defined groups of providers and users. In addition, public health includes coordination of those actions that have an impact on the health of the population, although they go beyond health services strictly speaking. This is the meaning of the definition offered by the special committee of the Institute of Medicine about the mission of public health: "The fulfillment of society's interest in assuring the conditions in which people can be healthy" (9).

An important factor in the emergence of this broad perspective on the practice of public health has been the growing involvement of the state in financing and providing all types of health services. Indeed, any original limitation placed on the public sector to organize only environmental or preventive services has been invalidated practically worldwide, as the state has assumed a dominant role in the health system, including personal medical care. Indeed, the largest share of resources currently spent by the public sector in almost all countries is earmarked for personal curative services, whether provided by private contractors or salaried government personnel (22).

THE UNIVERSE OF PUBLIC HEALTH Although we have defined research and practice separately, both refer to the same universe, which delimits the space for integrating the two faces of public health. This universe can be represented graphically as a three-dimensional matrix, as shown in Figure 3. Thus, the efforts to generate knowledge about health and then to act upon it can be expressed in various areas of application, which may be specific populations, such as children, pregnant women, the elderly, and migrants; particular problems, such as mental or dental health; or specific programs, such as environmental, occupational, and international health. Referring to the previous discussion on the objects of analysis, in each one of these areas of application, it is possible to do research and to act on health conditions or on the responses to them. In turn, the knowledge of such objects is based on applying the biological, social, and behavioral sciences.

Conceptions about the limits and contents of the universe of public health have varied throughout history. Likewise, the definitions that we have proposed for the two dimensions of public health result from a historical development in which different conceptual models of knowledge and action in this field have been taking shape. As the history of thought is not a mere progression of ideas, many of these models persist today. It is thus advisable to become familiar with them.

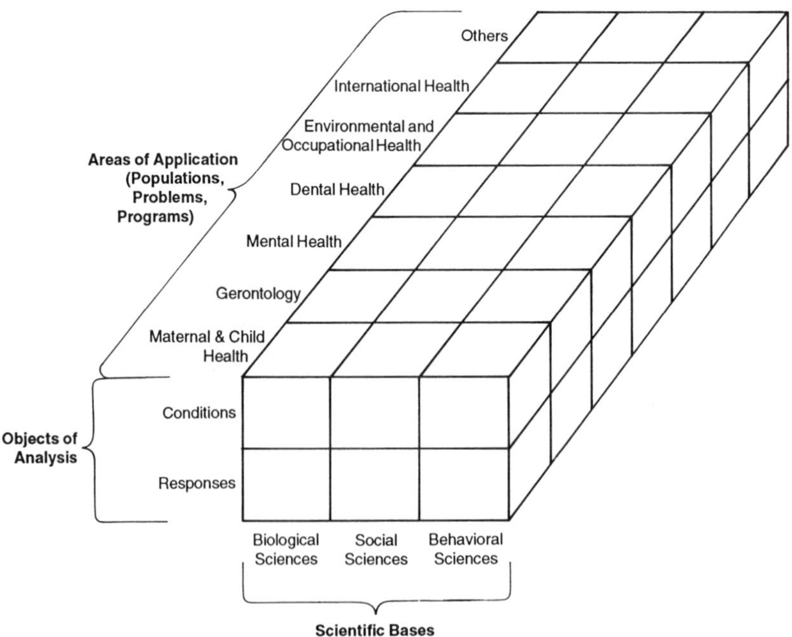

Figure 3 The universe of public health.

Conceptual Models in Public Health

Because the boundaries among fields of knowledge do not come from an intrinsic or predetermined division of reality, the first step in the development of a discipline or profession is, to quote Bourdieu et al (5), "to construct the object." As noted above, the health field includes two major objects of analysis: conditions and responses. This distinction is useful for identifying the principal conceptual models that have guided public health, as depicted schematically in Figure 4.

In simplified form, we suggest that conditions have historically been analyzed from two main perspectives: health and disease. The limits between the two are not always obvious; in fact, the most comprehensive conceptions go beyond this dichotomy. However, public health thinking has included two main currents that, as Dubos reminds us, go back to the worship of Hygeia versus Aesculapius (12). One focuses on the study of disease; the other, while not excluding disease, seeks to understand the determinants of health in a broad conception that includes human development and well-being.

The social response to health and disease conditions may be directed to different objects of intervention. Historically, the main objects have been the individual, including his or her immediate family surroundings, and the environment, which can be subdivided into the biological and physical components and the social components.

Crossing these two dimensions produces the typology of models shown in Figure 4. The names given to the models correspond to the main historical currents of thinking about health. For example, the "hygienist/preventive" model was developed considerably in the nineteenth century, when there was a movement to instruct the family on a series of rules for behavior that defined a "healthy life," and came to constitute what Foucault has called "a morality

SOCIAL RESPONSE: OBJECTS OF INTERVENTION	CONDITIONS: ANALYTICAL PERSPECTIVES	
	Health	Disease
Individual/Family	Hygienist/Preventive Model	Biomedical Model
Biophysical Environment	Sanitarist Model	Classical Epidemiologic Model
	Ecologist Model	
Social Environment	Sociomedical Model	Social Epidemiologic Model

Figure 4 Main conceptual models on public health. (Adapted from Ref. 17.)

of the body" (13). This model was displaced by the "biomedical model," which brought the control of specific diseases to the center of public health concerns (29), but eventually reappeared in programs aimed at changing individual behaviors and lifestyles as a basic strategy of health promotion (14).

Not all the conceptual models fit perfectly into the proposed categories. For example, the "ecologist model," whose principal exponent is Dubos (12), seeks to transform both the physical and social environments. The "socio-medical model" actually encompasses very diverse conceptions whose single common denominator is that they all attempt to explain health phenomena in society (6, 27, 30, 31).

It is beyond the scope of this paper to undertake an exhaustive analysis of each of the models proposed in Figure 4. Our purpose has simply been to show the wealth of intellectual traditions that have characterized public health. Each of them has implied a particular program of development for acquisition of knowledge and for action in public health (2). Therefore, they are an essential element for placing the bases of production, reproduction, and utilization of knowledge in their conceptual context.

PRODUCTION BASE

In this section, we analyze the generation of knowledge through public health research. The problem of translating research results into actions is discussed when we examine the utilization base.

A large part of the current crisis in public health is due to the weak basis of its scientific production. Indeed, public health research has taken a back seat to biomedical and clinical research (7). In addition to economic factors and the ways in which public health has been institutionalized, this lag may be due to the dominant mode of scientific production, which clashes with the spirit of integration that should characterize public health.

There is a conventional image that scientific progress necessarily implies a growing fragmentation of the objects of study and the consolidation of independent disciplines. No doubt the construction of specialized paradigms has made possible major progress in scientific knowledge by facilitating the identification of clear frontiers where the efforts of leading researchers are focused. Thus, the subspecialization of knowledge produces economies of scale by avoiding the dispersion of the limited human, material, and financial resources devoted to research. Moreover, working on narrow questions, while sacrificing breadth, attains greater depth. This process also facilitates the development of academic institutions, because it makes the consolidation of cohesive scientific communities possible in very specific fields.

Its advantages notwithstanding, the fragmentation of knowledge as a basis for organizing research has several limitations. The most important is that integrating knowledge becomes a no-man's land. Obviously, nature is not divided into the same categories as those through which researchers frame their questions. To the contrary, real phenomena have a comprehensive character that poses an essential challenge to scientific knowledge. Most of the development of science in the West has been based on a movement to fragment that comprehensive character analytically. But, we have lacked a parallel movement of synthesis. Therein lies perhaps the principal reason why science is often attacked as reductionist.

Fragmentation of knowledge poses severe obstacles to the potential users of research, who often have to provide a response to problems that do not recognize the arbitrary borders imposed by scientific subspecialization. This is manifested with particular clarity in a field like public health, which is closely associated with the problems of the population and with the institutions created to solve them. In applied fields, decision-makers face complex problems on which they demand comprehensive information, but scientific knowledge is provided to them in small parcels that are very difficult to aggregate. Thus, the gap between decision-making and research widens to the detriment of both.

One way to counteract the trend toward knowledge fragmentation in the health field is through "mission-oriented research" (3, 18). This concept refers to a research effort that attempts to modify some aspect of reality through the production of knowledge and technology. That modification of reality is precisely what defines the mission of research. Mission-oriented research is based on integration along three dimensions: levels of analysis, objects of analysis, and disciplines.

Integration among levels is possible because, as we saw when explaining the typology of health research (Figure 1), there is an essential unity of the objects. Indeed, the only difference between public health research and biomedical and clinical research is the level of analysis. This makes it possible to design comprehensive research programs that deal with specific problems from the subindividual level to the population level. In addition, it is necessary to integrate objects, so that both conditions and responses are studied. The challenge, then, is to select some areas of application among those that form the universe of public health (Figure 3) in order to develop research that combines biomedical aspects, technological developments, clinical trials, epidemiological field studies, and social and economic analyses of services. Naturally, neither of these two types of integration is possible without the third, integration of disciplines. Indeed, the richness of public health is that it lends itself to the conjunction of the biological, social, and behavioral sciences around a common problem.

Mission-oriented research has many advantages over the fragmentary model. Complete information on the problem is generated more rapidly and efficiently, because knowledge is integrated from the moment that research is planned, rather than at the end. The practical implications of research can be identified and translated into action more easily. Thus, the relationship between decision-makers and researchers is more a matter of agreement on a shared mission than confrontation based on differences in training and expectations. Setting priorities and forming groups are also easier when there is a well-defined focus of attention. Financing research is also facilitated when it is associated with a clear mission. Interinstitutional and multicentric collaboration becomes essential. Finally, knowledge advances more rapidly when approaches and disciplines are integrated around comprehensive problems.

All these advantages also pose an enormous challenge to the new public health: to break with isolation so as to open the way to creative interaction with biomedical research, clinical medicine, and the social sciences. In addition to this opening, the development of a solid basis for the production of knowledge requires an effort to create and consolidate institutions that include research among their essential missions. In this regard, the world consensus that appears to be emerging on the need to promote health research in underdeveloped countries is encouraging. This consensus is reflected in the report of the Commission on Health Research for Development (7). One of the Commission's main recommendations is to promote "essential national health research," i.e. research that every country, regardless of its level of development, must carry out if it aspires to advance independently in acquiring new knowledge of its own health problems and in closing the gap between current knowledge and action. Although the precise mix of projects will vary from country to country, mission-oriented research is especially relevant for carrying out this recommendation. The public health community must take advantage of the emerging consensus that the kind of research it promotes is precisely what the world requires today.

REPRODUCTION BASE

As noted above, intellectual traditions are reproduced through education, publications, and scientific and professional associations. The strengthening of the new public health requires a sustained effort to build better publications and more pluralistic and representative associations than we currently have. Of special concern are the problems affecting the development of human resources. In many countries of the world, public health education is experiencing a crisis that is manifested in a variety of ways: low quality, obsolescence of its organizational structures, separation from research and practice, limited relevance to the definition of health policies and decision-making, lack of standards that could provide guidance in defining new programs, limited sense of identity reflected in the disparate nomenclatures of programs and degrees, and lack of integrated systems for manpower development.

One of the roots of this crisis is that many schools of public health have not proved capable of changing at the same speed at which the reality of health has evolved in almost all countries. Indeed, both health conditions and the forms of social response have become much more complex in recent years (20). The challenge facing the schools is to learn to respond to this new complexity. To do so, schools should develop the capacity to assess their reality continuously through a dual effort: on the one hand, the ability to look outside, at the changing character of their environment; on the other hand, the introspection required to renew organizational schemes (16). To be successful, such an effort should harmonize two values: the academic excellence of programs and their relevance to decision-making. The balance between these two values is the key to a successful utilization of knowledge.

UTILIZATION BASE

Public health requires a new style of leadership. One of the key aspects is that it must be permanently open to its environment in two directions. First, public health must establish sensors to detect unmet needs and emerging opportunities in order to guide the selection of priorities. Second, it must develop effectors that facilitate the utilization of knowledge in new technological developments and in more rational decision-making processes. In this section, we focus on the second aspect, which is essential to the renewal of public health.

The creation of a solid utilization base requires differentiated structures in public health organizations, especially those responsible for generating new knowledge. Indeed, most of the barriers between decision-makers and researchers correspond to structural circumstances, not to mere differences in training or personality. Those barriers are rooted in the different kinds of logic and demands that researchers and decision-makers face in their respective areas of activity (19). The main barriers are summarized in Figure 5, together with some possible solutions for overcoming them. Before analyzing these barriers, certain concepts should be clarified. By "decision-maker" we mean any person who makes a decision to determine a course of action in response to a given health problem. Although a high proportion of decision-makers are public officials, these two terms should not be used interchangeably, as decision-makers include a broader range of people, such as leaders of community organizations and service providers. In all cases, they face problems whose solutions require decisions to be made on the basis of a diversity of factors. To ensure that research is relevant to decision-making,

POTENTIAL BARRIERS BETWEEN RESEARCHERS AND DECISION MAKERS	MEANS OF OVERCOMING THE BARRIERS
1. Priorities	- Education of "informed consumers" of research - Presence of decision makers in the governing or advisory bodies of research institutions
2. Time management	- Collaboration between researchers and decision makers since the planning stage of projects - Identification of intermediate products of research
3. Language and accessibility of results	- Executive summaries - "Translators" of research to policy - Joint seminars for discussing results
4. Perceptions about the final product of research: discovery vs. decision	- Explicit utilization objectives together with production-of-knowledge objectives
5. Integration of different findings on the same problem	- Meta-analysis - Mission-oriented research

Figure 5 Sources and solutions of possible barriers between researchers and decision makers. (Adapted from Ref. 19.)

there should be more than one solution, each with different effectiveness (1). In addition, there should be uncertainty as to the nature and effectiveness of the solutions. Research can then produce knowledge that reduces the uncertainty. Unfortunately, there are several circumstances that prevent this application of knowledge and result in decision-making that responds more to immediate pressures or to ideological preferences than to scientific evidence.

As shown in Figure 5, the first potential conflict revolves around the definition of priorities. The perception that decision-makers have of the most pressing problems may not coincide with the topics that researchers consider to be of greatest scientific interest. A possible solution to this barrier involves ensuring the presence of decision-makers in the governing or consultative bodies of research institutions, so that they can express their needs and identify opportunities in current projects.

Sometimes, the discrepancy reflects a distorted perception by decision-makers of the value of research. This distortion may take two forms: undervaluing the potential of research to help in decision-making or overestimating its potential, thereby generating unrealistic expectations. To overcome this barrier, decision-makers must be "informed consumers" of research products, which requires an educational effort that, to date, has been neglected. This effort involves introducing research topics in the educational programs for those who are not going to be researchers, but users of research. Such topics would have two essential purposes: to learn to value the contribution of research to decision-making and to gain a mastery of the minimum criteria for judging the quality of results. A strategy is needed to induce a greater and more informed demand for research products.

A second barrier reflects the real differences between political time and scientific time. In general, decision-makers are chronophobic, because time is one of the principal enemies to overcome; researchers, on the other hand, tend to be chronophilic, because time is one of the main ingredients of their research, allowing for the full expression of the processes under study. One way of overcoming this barrier is to ensure the collaboration between researchers and decision-makers from the earliest planning stages of the proposed research. This would open a space for negotiation and agreement on the time frames required for producing useful results. Differences in time management may also be addressed if researchers offer intermediate products, such as bibliographic reviews and progress reports, which are useful for decision-making even before the project has been completed.

Another set of important differences has to do with the language and accessibility of results. For the researcher, results must be communicated in precise terms, so that they enrich the paradigms of his or her own discipline. This means that language is often esoteric and that communication occurs in specialized publications, which often can only be retrieved through a bibliographic search. For the decision-maker, results must be expressed in an understandable language and be readily available.

Communication barriers can be reduced if, in addition to specialized articles, research projects also produce "executive summaries," which communicate in a nontechnical language the results most pertinent to decision-making. This would imply developing a dual system for presenting results: academic articles for peer scientists and executive summaries for decision-makers. The summaries could be complemented with joint seminars where decision-makers and researchers analyze results. To facilitate such an exchange between the two groups, "translators" could be trained who would consider the needs, values, and priorities of each (26). Such translators already exist for the general public, in the form of writers who are professionally devoted to the dissemination of scientific information. Equal importance should be accorded to professionals who facilitate communication between researchers and decision-makers, by translating the findings into recommendations for policy and action.

A fourth potential barrier is represented by the different perceptions about the nature of the final product of research. For the scientific community, the product is the published article and its potential impact on the ideas of others (as measured, for example, by the number of bibliographic citations). For the decision-maker, research has not come to a proper conclusion until it influences a decision. One means for overcoming this barrier is to specify, from the initial formulation of research proposals, a series of precise objectives for applying the results, alongside the strictly scientific objectives (D. Yach and J. Dick, Implementation of Research: The Key to Closing the Gap Between Public Health Knowledge and Action, unpublished document). The purpose is to ensure that utilization of knowledge stops being a random event and becomes instead a programmed phase of the research process. This would require that the scientific community give a specific weight to application efforts in its schemes for evaluating researchers' performance. Academic excellence should be defined not only as strict adherence to the highest standards of research and education, but also as the undertaking of all possible efforts to translate knowledge into action.

Finally, there is the problem of integrating different results on the same research question. The decision-maker requires integrated information that enables him or her to assess all the dimensions of a question so as to make a decision. In contrast, the way in which scientific work is usually organized leads to disaggregation of the objects of study. This problem has two aspects. The first has to do with those situations in which various research projects on a single topic do not yield conclusive results, or the results may even be mutually contradictory. In this case, one solution could be a detailed review of evidence and meta-analysis, which uses quantitative techniques for synthesizing data from several projects (24, 25, 33). The second aspect of the problem of integration has to do with those situations in which the decision-maker has results from several projects that have dealt with a single topic but at different levels of analysis. In this case, the solution is to carry out mission-oriented research, which has the advantages discussed earlier.

Much of the discussion on the utilization of knowledge leaves the implementation of solutions in the hands of individual actors. However, the current complexity in the production of knowledge requires organized solutions. Research institutions must have differentiated structures that make it possible to establish dynamic and creative linkages with their environment, especially the capacity for projecting scientific knowledge toward decision-making.

Otherwise, the barriers indicated in Figure 5 will continue to impoverish not only the utilization of knowledge, but also its production and reproduction. The failure to use results leads to inadequate public support for research. This, in turn, generates a decline of scientific production, which ends up reinforcing the vicious downward spiral in the use of research (34). Impoverished research, in turn, undermines the intellectual vitality of educational endeavors to reproduce knowledge.

This problem evidently affects all research. However, given its proximity to the decision-making process, the field of public health manifests in a particularly clear way the contradictions analyzed above and the need to come up with creative solutions.

CONCLUSIONS

As we approach the twenty-first century, our capacity to face the challenges of public health will depend on our ability to derive, from the rich intellectual traditions that nourish it, the definitions and comprehensive projects that will guide its future. The success of the new public health will require actions on the organizational front. In this respect, there is a need to pay attention to the three cardinal points of organization: design, development, and performance. Our discussion on the bases of production, reproduction, and utilization of knowledge has suggested new paths in this direction. After all, social development is based on the patient and thorough effort to establish solid institutions. Organizations are the vehicles for bringing together individual wills in order to attain a level that is higher than the simple sum of these wills. Following the metaphor taken from physics, what is most important is not only to form a critical mass of talent, but also to reach a critical density through which such talent can be mutually enriched within a shared institutional space. No doubt the future of public health will depend to a great extent on our ability to design and develop institutions and to assure their sound performance.

But, the internal organization of public health itself is not enough. A broad effort of linkage is needed, a commitment to the population's health and the services for improving it. The basic challenge in this regard is to modernize public health. Beyond the several meanings that changing political circumstances can attribute to this term, modernization should be understood above all as a process of opening. It is not a question of an irreflexive permeability that overlooks the advances of the past, but rather an effort to integrate tradition and progress. This is the meaning of the words spoken by the Mexican poet Octavio Paz (28) in his address to the Royal Swedish Academy the day before receiving the 1990 Nobel Prize for Literature:

> ... between tradition and modernity lies a bridge. Isolated, traditions are petrified and modernities are rendered volatile; together, each inspires the other, each responds to the other by giving it weight and gravity.

In the case of public health, modernization must be understood as a process of opening in at least seven directions. First, as we have emphasized, is decision-making. Research should provide scientifically validated information that is relevant to the problems of decision-makers at all levels. The second opening is toward the university. Together with relevance, research and higher education in public health should promote excellence. For this purpose, close links should be established with the broader university milieu. Third, public health should open up to the other fields of health, so that its population approach may find support in individual and subindividual phenomena. This effort to integrate levels of analysis should be accompanied by a parallel effort to link disciplines. Hence, the fourth opening is to the social, biological, and behavioral sciences. The specificity in time and space of many health phenomena requires a comparative approach that can only be attained through the following two openings: to the international sphere and to the future in order to adopt a strategic vision that enables us to anticipate problems and not just react when they have already occurred. Finally, all of the above should be guided by the essential opening process that gives meaning to public health: the permanent concern to understand the health needs of the population and to learn from them.

It is too soon to determine whether public health will prove capable of responding to the challenges of our time. What is certain is that the possibility of bringing about a renewal of health systems will depend, to a great extent, on the modernization of public health. Although their ultimate fate is associated with the broader social and economic development, health actions also have their own dynamics, whereby they can contribute to the general progress of nations. Because it is a crossroad, health makes it possible for the population to give a specific and daily meaning to the goals of reducing inequality and promoting social well-being. Therein lies the commitment that, if fulfilled, will make the new public health flourish.

Acknowledgments

This paper attempts to integrate various elements from my previous work. Therefore, the first debt of gratitude is to my coauthors of the articles cited in this text, especially José-Luis Bobadilla, Jaime Sepúlveda, Enrique Ruelas, and Lilia Durán. In addition, many ideas expressed in this document have benefited from exchanges with many people, most importantly Guillermo Soberón, José Laguna, Jaime Martuscelli, Avedis Donabedian, Harvey Fineberg, Carlos Santos-Burgoa, and Miguel Angel González-Block, as well as many researchers and students from the National Institute of Public Health of Mexico. Such gratitude notwithstanding, the responsibility for the content of this paper lies with the author alone.

An initial version was prepared at the request of the Pan American Health Organization (PAHO) and presented at the meeting on Development of the Theory and Practice of Public Health in the Americas, organized by PAHO together with the US and Latin American Associations of Schools of Public Health, New Orleans, October 21–24, 1991.

Literature Cited

1. Ackoff, R. L. 1978. *The Art of Problem Solving*, p. 12. New York: Wiley
2. Alvarado, C. A. 1976. Concepto de salud pública. In *Medicina Sanitaria y Administración de Salud*, ed. A. Sonis, pp. 1–5. Buenos Aires: El Ateneo
3. Bobadilla, J. L., Frenk, J., Sepúlveda, J., Martínez-Palomo, A. 1988. *Health research in Mexico: strengths, weaknesses and gaps*. Presented at 4th Meet. of Comm. on Health Res. for Dev., Mexico City
4. Bourdieu, P. 1976. *Some properties of fields*. Lecture at Ecole Normale Supérior, Paris. Cited in Ref. 27
5. Bourdieu, P., Chamboredon, J. C., Passeron, J. C. 1975. *El Oficio del Sociólogo: Presupuestos Epistemológicos*, pp. 51–81. Buenos Aires: Siglo XXI
6. Chave, S. P. W. 1984. The origins and development of public health. In *Oxford Textbook of Public Health*, Vol. 1: History, Determinants, Scope, and Strategies, ed. W. W. Holland, R. Detels, G. Knox, pp. 3–19. Oxford: Oxford Univ. Press
7. Comm. on Health Res. for Dev. 1990. *Health Research: Essential Link to Equity in Development*. New York: Oxford Univ. Press
8. Comm. for the Study of the Future of Public Health, Inst. of Med. 1988. *The Future of Public Health*, p. v. Washington, DC: Natl. Acad. Press
9. Comm. for the Study of the Future of Public Health, Inst. of Med. 1988. See Ref. 8, p. 40
10. Comm. for the Study of the Future of Public Health, Inst. of Med. 1988. See Ref. 8, p. 41
11. Donabedian, A. 1976. *Aspects of Medical Care Administration: Specifying Requirements for Health Care*. Cambridge, Mass: Harvard Univ. Press
12. Dubos, R. 1959. *Mirage of Health: Utopias, Progress, and Biological Change*. New York: Harper & Row
13. Foucault, M. 1976. La crisis de la medicina o la crisis de la antimedicina. *Educ. Med. Salud* 10:152–70
14. Frenk, J. 1979. Salud, educación y medicina: expectativas y limitaciones. *Cienc. Desarrollo* 26:133–38
15. Frenk, J. 1988. La investigación en salud pública: una nueva realidad. *Gac. Med. Mex.* 124:155–56
16. Frenk, J. 1988. La modernización de la salud pública. *Nexos* 122:57–58
17. Frenk, J. 1988. La salud puacblica: campo del conocimiento y ámbito para la acción. *Salud Publica Mex.* 30:246–54
18. Frenk, J. 1990. La salud perinatal como modelo para la investigación con misión. In *Memorias del Primer Congreso Nacional sobre Defectos al Nacimiento*, pp. 25–27. Mexico City: Grupo de Estudios al Nacimiento
19. Frenk, J. 1992. Balancing relevance and excellence: organizational responses to link research with decision making. *Soc. Sci. Med.* 35:1397–1404
20. Frenk, J., Bobadilla, J. L., Sepúlveda, J., López-Cervantes, M. 1989. Health transition in middle-income countries: new challenges for health care. *Health Policy Plan.* 4:29–39
21. Frenk, J., Bobadilla, J. L., Sepúlveda, J., Rosenthal, J., Ruelas, E. 1988. A conceptual model for public health research. *Bull. Pan. Am. Health Org.* 22:60–71
22. Frenk, J., Donabedian, A. 1987. State intervention in medical care: types, trends and variables. *Health Pol. Plan.* 2:17–31
23. Frenk, J., Durán, L. 1990. Investigación en sistemas de salud: estado del arte en México y perspectivas de desarrollo. *Cienc. (Mex.)* 41:15–25 (special issue)
24. Glass, G. V. 1976. Primary, secondary, and meta-analysis of research. *Educ. Res.* 5:3–8
25. Louis, T. A., Fineberg, H. V., Mosteller, F. 1985. Findings for public health from meta-analysis. *Annu. Rev. Public Health* 6:1–20
26. May, J. J. 1975. Symposium: the policy uses of research. Introduction. *Inquiry* 12:228–30
27. Mercer, H. 1987. La medicina social en debate. *Cuad. Médico-Soc.* 42:5–13
28. Paz, O. 1990. La búsqueda del presente. *La Jornada*, Dec. 9, pp. 29–31
29. Rosen, G. 1972. The evolution of social medicine. In *Handbook of Medical Sociology*, ed. H. E. Freeman, S. Levine, L. G. Reeder, pp. 30–60. Englewood Cliffs, NJ: Prentice-Hall. 2nd ed.
30. Terris, M. 1957. Concepts of social medicine. *Soc. Sci. Rev.* 31:164–78
31. Terris, M. 1964. On the distinction

between individual and social medicine. *Lancet* 26:653–55

32. Terris, M. 1985. Editorial: the distinction between public health and community/social preventive medicine. *J. Public Health Policy* 6:435–39
33. Thacker, S. B. 1988. Meta-analysis: a quantitative approach to research integration. *J. Am. Med. Assoc.* 259: 1685–89
34. World Health Org. 1986. *Improving Health Care Through Decision-linked Research: Application in Health Systems and Manpower Development*. Part II: options for implementation. Doc. No. HMD/86.4.2. Geneva: WHO

Annu. Rev. Publ. Health 1993. 14:491–513

BREATHING BETTER OR WHEEZING WORSE? THE CHANGING EPIDEMIOLGY OF ASTHMA MORBIDITY AND MORTALITY[1]

K. B. Weiss

Departments of Health Care Sciences and Medicine and the Center for Health Policy Research, George Washington University, Washington, DC 20037

P. J. Gergen

Office of Epidemiology and Clinical Trials, Division of Allergy, Immunology, and Transplantation, National Institute of Allergy and Infectious Diseases, National Institutes of Health, Rockville, Maryland 20892

D. K. Wagener

Environmental Studies Branch, Office of Analysis and Epidemiology, National Center for Health Statistics, Centers for Disease Control, Hyattsville, Maryland 20782

KEY WORDS: surveillance, prevalence, hospitalization

INTRODUCTION

During the past few decades, there has been great interest in the epidemiologic changes in asthma morbidity and mortality (8, 16, 27, 60, 62, 92). An active literature has attempted to synthesize an explanation for these changes (13, 37, 98, 105, 117). However, a critical comparison of trends in asthma morbidity and mortality with trends in known and possible risk factors, which is necessary to build sensible ecological hypotheses, has not emerged.

In this article, we provide an in-depth examination of US asthma morbidity and mortality trends, compare US and international trends, explore the concurrent trends in possible risk factors, and construct several plausible ecologic hypotheses. Finally, we propose an action plan for public health interventions that are needed to address this problem.

OVERVIEW OF ASTHMA SURVEILLANCE

It is essential to highlight a few of the technical aspects and limitations to data used to monitor asthma trends.

The Data Sets Used for Asthma Surveillance

In the United States, information on trends of asthma morbidity and mortality is found in the national health information systems maintained at the National Center for Health Statistics (109). Prevalence data are obtained from two population-based surveys, the National Health Interview Survey (NHIS) and the National Health and Nutrition Examination Survey (NHANES). The NHIS is a household interview survey that has provided information of asthma prevalence since 1970. The NHANES is a periodic interview and examination survey. Health-care utilization is tracked by two national surveys: the periodic (recently turned annual) National Ambulatory Medical Care Survey of nonfederal, office-based physicians, with data on asthma visits since 1974; and the annual National Hospital Discharge Survey of selected nonmilitary hospitals with six or more beds and average length of stays of less than 30 days, with data on asthma hospitalizations since 1967. US mortality records provide the longest perspective on asthma mortality trends. A complete national vital records system has been maintained since the early 1930s.

Cautions About International Comparisons

To obtain a broad epidemiologic perspective on trends, it is useful to compare US asthma morbidity and mortality with that of other countries. International comparisons of asthma, however, are limited by a lack of data or data collected with dissimilar instruments. Whenever possible, international data on related asthma morbidity trends are explored to provide a broad perspective for our study of US trends.

Changes in Diagnostic Coding and Accuracy of Death Certificates

It is customary to present epidemiologic data on asthma ambulatory care, hospitalization, and mortality by using recorded diagnostic information. These data are abstracted by using an international diagnostic classification scheme, the International Classification of Diseases (ICD) codes. Unlike most previous revisions, the coding change of asthma between the eighth and ninth revisions of the ICD in 1979 had an important effect on the diagnosis of asthma. Under the eighth revision, "bronchitis with mention of asthma" was coded as "bronchitis." Under the ninth revision, asthma coexistent with bronchitis was recorded as "asthma." Overall, there is an estimated 30% increase in deaths attributed to asthma between ICD-8 and ICD-9. However, for persons aged less than 45 years, the effect is estimated to be less than 5% (98). The potential implications of this coding change is highlighted later in the text.

The accuracy of the coding of asthma on death certificates has been of great concern. Studies from New Zealand (88), Britain (3), and the United States (10) have reported that the accuracy of the coding is dependent on the age of the decedent. For persons under age 35, the coding is virtually 100% accurate; by age 70, the accuracy approaches 50%. As a result, most of the reported literature on asthma mortality focuses on the younger age range.

TRENDS IN ASTHMA EPIDEMIOLOGY

Recent Trends in Asthma Prevalence

As seen in Figure 1, data on self-reported[1] asthma from the NHIS show that the prevalence of this condition has increased during the past decade. Close examination of the most recent prevalence data demonstrates that the increases are largest in younger age groups. Figure 1 illustrates that the greatest increase in prevalence is seen in persons under 18 years of age.

Previous reports of NHIS data indicated that the prevalence of asthma during the last 12 months before interview among children and adolescents, under 17 years of age, increased 23%, from 3.1 to 3.8 per 100 population, between 1970 and 1978–1980 (27). During the same time period, self-reported lifetime history of asthma among 6–11-year-old children interviewed in NHANES increased 58%, from 4.8 per 100 population in NHANES I (1971–1974) to 7.6 per 100 population in NHANES II (1976–1980) (32). Results from the special child health supplements to the NHIS, conducted in 1981 and 1988, show that the asthma prevalence for children under 18 years of age has increased 39%, from 3.2 to 4.3 per 100 population between 1981 and 1988 (36, 104).

There is evidence that asthma prevalence is increasing in other countries, as well. In Sweden, the prevalence of asthma increased 47% (1.9 to 2.8 per 100 population) among 18-year-old military conscripts between 1971 and 1981 (1). In Finland, the recorded asthma prevalence between 1966 and 1989 increased fivefold (0.29 to 1.79 per 100 population) among 19-year-old military conscripts (38). Two surveys, 26 years apart (1964 and 1990), of

[1]For children, data are parental-reported.

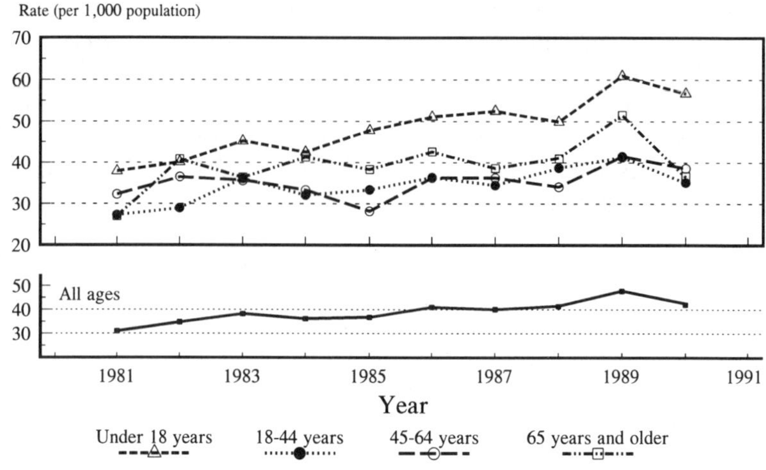

Figure 1 Trends in US asthma prevalence, 1981–1990.

7-year-old school children in Melbourne, Australia, found reported ever-asthma increased 141% (19.1 to 46 per 100 population) (81). Shaw et al (90) reported an increase in asthma prevalence for a rural adolescent population in New Zealand. Not all data on trends demonstrate an increase. For example, another study of Finnish children and adolescents reported no change in prevalence during the 1970s (77).

Conflicting data also exist in the trends in asthma prevalence in England. Burney et al (16) examined the reported prevalence of asthma or bronchitis in the last 12 months, and ever-wheeze over a 13-year period (1973–1986) among children 4–12 years of age. The asthma prevalence increased 138% among boys and 378% among girls. Persistent wheeze increased 74% among boys and 117% among girls. Anderson (5) reached a different conclusion after comparing results of prevalence studies of asthma conducted in the United Kingdom between 1964 to 1986: "...prevalence of wheezing over the last year or which was described as 'current' or 'recent' show little evidence of a trend..." However, in spite of these differences, there appears to be an increase in prevalence of "diagnosed" asthma over the recent decade.

Trends in Medical Care Utilization

TRENDS IN AMBULATORY CARE Asthma is commonly believed to cause mild morbidity, contributing to nearly 6.5 million office visits in 1985 (108).

Between 1975 and 1990, rates of ambulatory care visits for asthma increased from 2.71 to 2.85 visits per 100 population (Figure 2). This increase in rates appears to be limited to two age-specific groups, persons 15–44 years of age and those 65 years and older. From England, data on trends in general practice visits for asthma between 1971 and 1981 identified general increases across all age groups and gender (4).

Acute asthma exacerbations have been estimated to account for 1.8 million emergency room visits annually (108). However, there are no readily available estimates of US trends in use of emergency rooms for asthma.

TRENDS IN HOSPITALIZATIONS US asthma hospitalization rates have increased during the 1970s and leveled off during the 1980s for all but a few age groups (Figure 3). Although the most notable change occurred the year of the revision between ICD-8 and ICD-9, asthma hospitalization rates for the total population stayed relatively constant during a decade when hospitalization rates, in general, demonstrated dramatic declines (65). There were only two notable age-specific trends: a modest decline during the 1980s for persons aged 45–64 and a notable increase in hospitalization for children under age 15, a persistent 25-year trend.

During the 1980s, the increase among children appeared to be limited to those under age 5 (Figure 4). Trends during the same time period for children aged 5–17 and for adults were either stable or slightly decreasing. During the ten-year period, the younger cohort of children would have advanced into the next age group. Interestingly, the passage of these children into the older age group did not lead to a subsequent increase in hospitalization rates in the older age group.

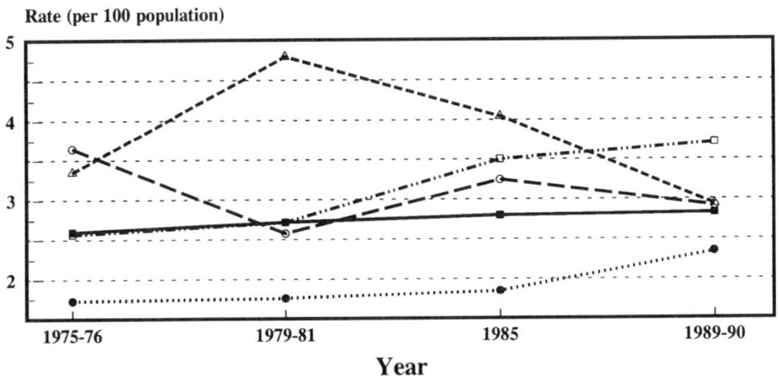

Notes: ICD-8 and ICD-9 = 493
Source: National Ambulatory Medical Care Survey, NCHS.

Figure 2 Trends in US ambulatory care visits to physicians' offices, 1975–1990.

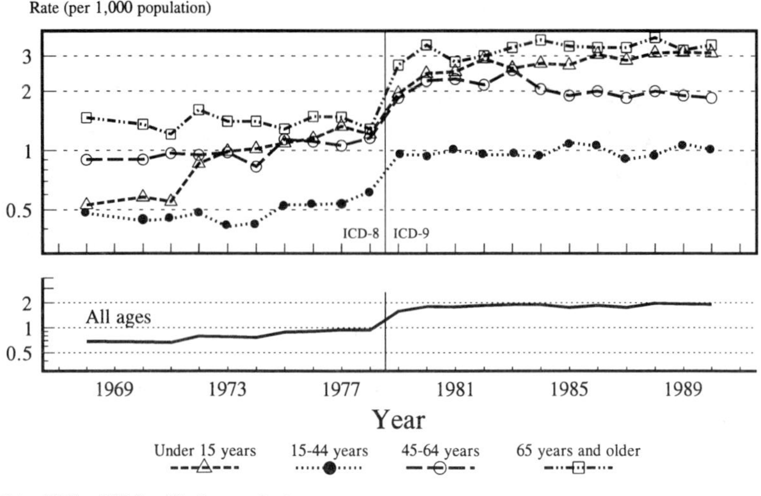

Notes: ICD-8 and ICD-9 = 493, all ages crude rate.
SOURCE: National Hospital Discharge Survey

Figure 3 Trends in US asthma hospitalizations, 1968–1990.

Limited data suggest that the severity of children who were hospitalized for asthma may have increased during the 1980s (33, 113). The percentage of hospitalizations for children under 18 years of age with severe respiratory failure leading to intubation or cardiopulmonary arrest increased from 0.11 to 0.50% between 1979 and 1987. In contrast, during the same time period,

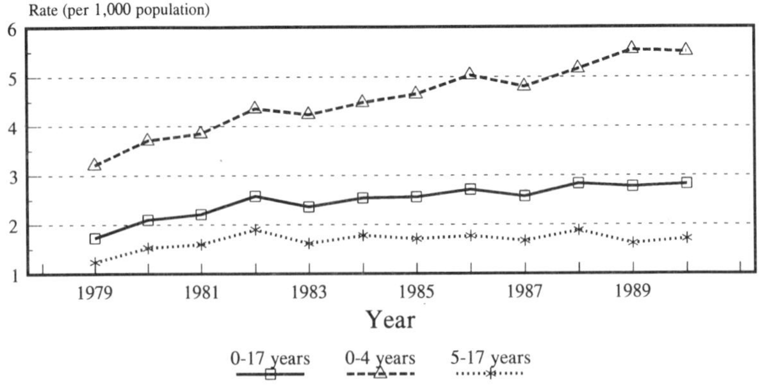

Notes: ICD-9 = 493, newborns excluded.
SOURCE: National Hospital Discharge Survey

Figure 4 Trends in US asthma hospitalization among children under 18 years of age, 1979–1990.

the length of stay for asthma decreased 0.5 days (which is less than for hospitalizations in general) (33).

Asthma hospitalization rates among children have also increased in several other countries. Between 1957 and 1984, the increase in hospitalization rates in England and Wales was primarily limited to younger persons, aged 0–4 years and 5–14 years (4). At the Royal Alexandra Hospital in Brighton, England, asthma hospitalizations among children increased eightfold between 1971 and 1985, with the greatest increase among children aged 0–4 (99). In New Zealand, asthma hospitalizations increased approximately 4.5-fold among the 0–13-year-old children between 1974 and 1989 (45). Since the 1960s, asthma hospitalizations among children aged 0–14 years increased tenfold in New Zealand, eightfold in Queensland, Australia, sixfold in England and Wales, fourfold in Canada, threefold in the United States, and threefold in Tasmania, Australia (61).

Trends in Asthma Mortality

The trends for US asthma mortality during the early portion of this century appear stable (Figure 5). There was, however, a dramatic increase during the late 1940s and early 1950s, followed by a steady decrease until the late 1970s. Since 1978, the rates appear to be increasing. Curiously, trends for the 5–34-year age group did not demonstrate the dramatic increase in the 1950s. During the 1980s, US asthma mortality within the 5–34 age range was similar between genders and across each ten-year age group.

Asthma mortality rates for persons aged 5–34 have increased since 1980 in the United States, Canada, England and Wales, and Japan (Figure 6).

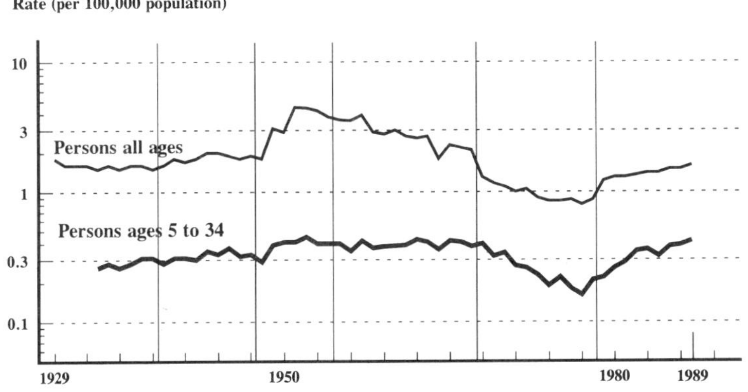

Note: crude rates.
Source: NCHS VSS

Figure 5 Trends in US asthma mortality, 1929–1989.

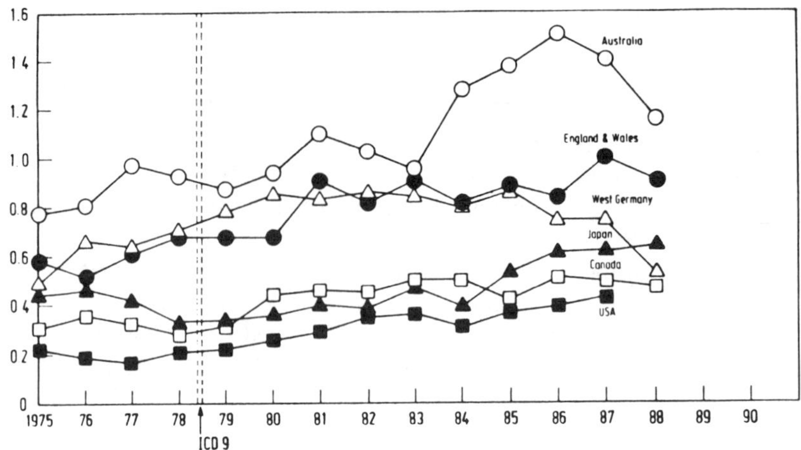

Figure 6 Mortality from asthma (rate per 100,00) in 5–34-year-old subjects in Australia, England and Wales, West Germany, Japan, Canada, and the United States. (Adapted from Ref. 85.)

During this same time period, asthma mortality in Australia demonstrated an increase followed by a decrease, and rates in West Germany declined (85, 86).

Comparing the Trends in Prevalence, Medical Care Utilization, and Mortality During the 1980s

The trends in asthma prevalence, medical care utilization, and mortality, when presented individually, suggest general increases. When viewed together, however, these trends depict a rather perplexing story. As shown in Table 1, data on recent trends in the United States (1979–1989) demonstrate that the ratio of asthma mortality to hospitalization appears to have been stable for children and steady or slightly increasing for adults, whereas hospitalizations as a percentage of prevalence decreased during this same period. Hence, the mortality as a percentage of prevalence may have actually decreased.

The trends in prevalence, hospitalization, and mortality appear different, thus making any single explanation of causes of these changes highly implausible. The most apparent increase in prevalence rates are for children and adolescents under age 18, notably among children aged 5–17 years. The increases in US hospitalization rates appear to be restricted to persons under age 5. US mortality seems to be increasing for persons of all ages.

The Effect of Race upon Asthma Morbidity and Mortality

Asthma prevalence and hospitalization and mortality rates vary by race, being consistently higher in blacks than whites. Throughout the 1980s, the trends

Table 1 Trends in asthma severity in the United States

	Mortality as a percent of hospitalization	Hospitalization as a percent of prevalence
Children	(aged 0–14 years)	(aged 0–17 years)
1979	0.09	—
1982	0.09	6.43
1985	0.10	5.46
1989	0.10	4.55
Adults	(aged 15–44 years)	(aged 18–44 years)
1979	0.21	—
1982	0.31	3.38
1985	0.27	3.29
1989	0.32	2.41

Source: Based on National Health Interview Survey (prevalence), National Hospitalization Discharge Survey (hospitalizations), National Vital Records Program (mortality), NCHS.

in asthma hospitalization rates also remained significantly higher for blacks than whites.

PLAUSIBLE EXPLANATIONS FOR THESE RECENT TRENDS

The most intriguing of the trends is the increase in hospitalization rates among younger children. It appears clear that the 0–4-year age group, which is exhibiting increased hospitalization rates, is not expressing increased morbidity as it becomes older.

Several explanations are plausible. A high case-fatality rate would explain this trend; however, this is extremely unlikely, as the number of deaths in the under 5 age group would have had to increase several hundredfold to accommodate the lack of increase in hospitalization trends for the older children and young adults. The death rate in children under age 5 has remained low during this period. A second explanation is that the disease-state is still present, but is being better controlled without the need for hospitalization. This would suggest that older children and young adults had been receiving increasingly better outpatient medical care. National data on outpatient care for asthma does not support this possibility. Alternatively, older persons with asthma are being removed from the agent or environment that is causing the more severe morbidity. Or, during the past decade, a large group of younger children was developing asthma or an asthma-like syndrome that remitted early in life, before age 5. Finally, this age-specific trend could represent an increasing tendency of physicians to admit young children who present to the hospital emergency room.

The two-phase mortality trend, from 1970 to 1990, could represent a trend in one single factor that first was associated with improvement and then a loss of improvement. It could also represent distinct factors: one associated with declining mortality in the 1970s, and another associated with increasing mortality during the 1980s.

Perhaps the most important question concerning these trends is, Are they real changes in population morbidity or are they an artifact of the way we diagnose, record, or analyze the health of the nation? Some of these recent trends may be artifacts introduced by changes in the process of monitoring asthma morbidity, including changes in diagnostic recognition and accuracy, diagnostic transfer, and the ICD revisions.

Changes in Diagnostic Recognition and Accuracy

Some or most of the changes in prevalence could be related to a change in the diagnostic recognition of asthma by either the general population or the health-care providers. Prevalence is generally self-reported. During the past 10–15 years, both physician and public awareness of the signs and symptoms of asthma may have increased. Therefore, an increasing asthma awareness could have led to an elevated number of reports without a true increase in the disease burden in the population, as much asthma is undiagnosed (93). It is less likely that diagnostic recognition would have been an important factor in either hospitalization or mortality trends. No new diagnostic technology has appeared that would have improved the recognition of asthma. For asthma mortality, the autopsy rate for children and young adults in the United States is relatively high (55.9% between 1979 through 1987) and has changed very little (110), which suggests that there has been little change in the diagnostic accuracy of in this outcome, as well.

Changes in Diagnostic Transfer

An increase could occur if there were a change in the way another disease was classified so that the disease was now being classified as asthma. This issue of diagnostic transfer—also called diagnostic fashion—has, in fact, been a central concern in recent asthma trends. It has been proposed that the diagnosis of asthma is being substituted for bronchitis, and that this substitution is artificially inflating the estimates of asthma (16, 33, 47).

Figure 7 shows the hospitalization rates for both asthma and bronchitis for children aged 0–14 during the 1970s and 1980s. As previously seen, rates for asthma in this age group steadily increased during this time period. From

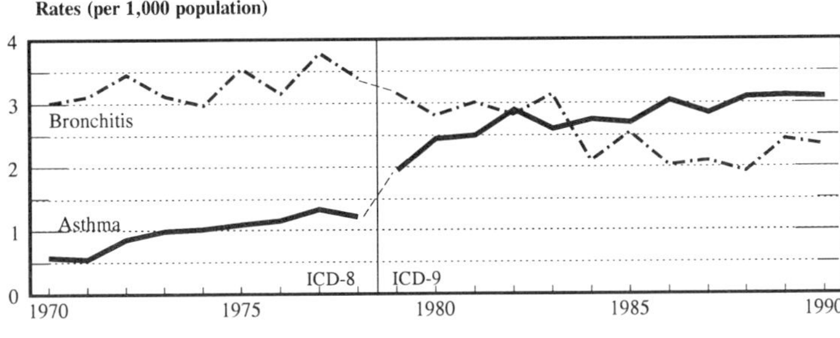

Note: ICD-8 and ICD-9 =493.
Source: NCHS, NHDS

Figure 7 Trends in US hospitalization rates for asthma and bronchitis, children aged 0–14 years, 1970–1990.

1970 to 1983, the rates for bronchitis remained essentially constant; in 1984, the rates dropped, as did hospitalization rates in general for children (51). After the one-year decrease in 1984, bronchitis hospitalization rates once again remained steady through 1990. Furthermore, during this time period—despite the decline in bronchitis—there had been an overall steady increase in the rates for these two conditions combined. These data strongly suggest that the recent increase in asthma hospitalizations in young children is largely unrelated to diagnostic transfer from bronchitis.

Effects of the ICD Revision

Change in ICD coding can create a dramatic one-year increase in both hospitalization (40) and mortality data (15, 27, 110). Although, coding reclassification probably did have some impact on rates, there is strong evidence that this coding change is not primarily responsible for the recent increases. The effects of the change in ICD coding would be seen primarily in the first year or after the change. This is reflected in the noted increase in asthma hospitalization rates between 1978 and 1979 (see Figure 3). Therefore, although some of these recent increases in asthma prevalence, morbidity, and mortality may have been artifacts of changes in diagnostic practices or changes in the health surveillance systems, it seems as though some true increase in the burden of this illness is occurring.

Changes in Risk Factors as Possible Links to Recent Asthma Trends

Several possible risk factors have been associated with asthma morbidity or mortality.

CHANGES IN RATES OF PREMATURITY The relationship between asthma and lung disease in the premature infant has been the focus of much study. Survivors of neonatal lung disease, especially its sequelae of bronchopulmonary dysplasia, have been reported to have increased levels of airway obstruction, hyperinflation, and bronchial reactivity in childhood (9). Low birthweight has been associated with decreased flow rates in childhood (19) and for persons with asthma (54). In another study, 7-year-old children, whose birthweights were under 2000 g, had more problems with cough but not wheezing, as compared with age-matched schoolmates (18).

More low birthweight infants are surviving. From 1971 through 1982, US perinatal mortality rates decreased for all birthweights for both blacks and whites (42). Are the increased numbers of surviving premature babies driving up the asthma rates? This is an intriguing possibility that deserves much more study.

CHANGES IN RATES OF BREASTFEEDING Prospective studies following infants for the first four (28) and five (103) years of life have found no effect of breastfeeding on development of asthma in children. This remained true whether or not there was a family history of atopy (28). The frequency of breastfeeding has followed somewhat of a cyclic course in the United States during the last several decades. Between 1971 and 1982 the initiation of breastfeeding increased from 24.7 to 61.9%. However, from 1982 through 1989, there has been a decline from 61.9 to 52.2% in the initiation of breastfeeding (83). The largest decreases from 1984 through 1989 occurred among black, young, and poor women. However, changes in breastfeeding probably have not played any role in the changing picture of asthma epidemiology.

CHANGES IN THE OUTDOOR ENVIRONMENT In Israel, asthma has been reported to be increased in polluted areas as compared with nonpolluted areas (35). A look at individual pollutants gives a similar picture. An increase in fine particulate pollution has been shown to be associated with increased hospitalizations for asthma and bronchitis in a localized area (76). Sulfur dioxide causes bronchoconstriction and asthma-like symptoms, even at low levels with chronic exposure (73, 91). Nitrogen dioxide, associated with gas stoves, has been implicated as a cause of respiratory disease and an inconsistent effect on pulmonary function (66). Ozone has been shown to increase bronchial reactivity (73). Airborne acidity has been associated with daily symptoms among moderate to severe asthmatics (70). Exposure to multiple pollutants may have important synergistic effects, e.g. ozone has been shown to potentiate the asthmatic response to sulfur dioxide (49).

During the 1980s, the trends in US air pollution have been uniformly down

(26). From 1981 to 1990, air concentrations of the following pollutants decreased: sulfur dioxide, carbon monoxide, nitrogen dioxide, ozone, and total suspended particles. Smaller size particles, less than 10 microns (PM-10), are more important for respiratory disease, but have been monitored only since 1989. Thus, nationwide, no evidence exists that supports the role of outdoor pollution levels as the primary factor driving the changes in the epidemiologic patterns of asthma morbidity.

CHANGES IN THE INDOOR ENVIRONMENT For the purposes of this discussion, we limit our analysis of indoor environmental factors to smoking, aeroallergens, viral agents, molds, and irritant gases.

Smoking is a well-recognized respiratory irritant and often has major impact on the quality of indoor air. Children whose parents smoke have been reported to have many more problems with wheezing, lower respiratory infections, and asthma than children of parents who do not smoke, especially in the first year of life (14, 67). This effect remains even after controlling for other predictors of childhood wheezing, such as daycare, season of birth, sharing a bedroom, and parental history of childhood respiratory trouble (118). Maternal smoking has consistently been reported to be most important, because of the greater exposure of the child to maternal than paternal smoke. The effect of maternal smoking can be seen even if the mother only smoked during pregnancy and quit before delivery, which suggests a congenital effect (102). Tobacco smoke has been implicated with an earlier onset of asthma (112), the development of asthma before age 12 (53), and increased severity of asthma (64, 112).

Between 1965 and 1985, the age-adjusted prevalence of current smoking decreased from 52 to 33% for men and from 34 to 28% for women (29). In the past, black women had a higher prevalence of smoking than white women (28); in the late 1980s, however, black women were smoking less than white women (20). Among women aged 20–24 years with a high school education or less, the prevalence of smoking increased from 40% in 1974 to 44% in 1985. By 1987, the rate had dropped to 37.6% in this group (72).

Do changes in smoking play a role in the changing morbidity and mortality of asthma? Smoking probably plays a role, but from the data now available it is not possible to indict smoking as the driving force for the observed increases in asthma. Morbidity and mortality data are not collected by education status of the mother; therefore, the effect of increased smoking among less-well-educated women cannot be assessed. However, the black-white difference in level of asthma morbidity and mortality may be partially explainable by racial differences in smoking.

Individual allergens, mostly indoor, are important epidemiologically in eliciting asthma. Dust mite (63, 74), alternaria (44, 69), cockroach (48, 75), cat (75, 87, 106), and pollens (ragweed and rye grass) (75, 87) have all been reported to elicit asthmatic symptoms. Dust mite antigen has been identified as being important etiologically in asthma onset (96), with higher levels of exposure in infancy associated with earlier onset of asthma. Alternaria has been implicated in fatal and near fatal asthmatic attacks (69). No information is available on trends in exposure to any of these allergens.

Viral infections are well recognized to be precipitating factors asthma attacks (57–59, 101). Bacterial infections do not seem to be important triggers of asthma (55, 59). However, sinusitis, regardless of etiology, is felt to make asthma difficult to control until it is adequately treated (79). Respiratory infections (e.g. croup, bronchiolitis, pneumonia), especially before the age of 2, have been reported to be associated with the later development of asthma (6, 12, 50, 78). No trends data exist that would provide the necessary information on the changing impact of respiratory viral infections.

US housing conditions have changed over the past few decades, becoming increasingly "energy efficient." This has meant that there is much less change for air exchange in the indoor air and a greater chance for the build up of allergens and irritant gases. The percentage of new homes with central heating and air-conditioning increased dramatically during the past two decades (43). During this time period, however, the percentage of gas-fueled forced-air heating remained essentially constant, while the percentage of homes with gas ranges used for cooking decreased (97). During the past decade, there have been many other changes in both residential and work indoor environments, such as increased insulation and wall-to-wall carpeting, that would appear to have an impact on indoor air quality.

Home dampness and the presence of molds in the home have been reported to be associated with an increased prevalence of respiratory symptoms, including asthma and wheeze, with odds ratios ranging for 1.2 to 1.8 (12, 24, 100). It has been suggested, based on the results of exercise provocation, that this association may partly be explained by a tendency of parents from homes with visible molds to over-report symptoms (100).

Thus, there are apparently several possible indoor air pollutants that may affect asthma prevalence and morbidity. However, there are few data that explicitly examine trends in indoor quality.

CHANGES IN SOCIOECONOMIC STATUS Socioeconomic status (SES) appears to have a modest effect on asthma prevalence (27, 84, 111) and a large effect upon the small area geographic variations in both hospitalization and mortality rates (17, 23, 52, 114). Figure 8 presents county-level asthma mortality rates by quintile of county median income. A clear inverse relationship between low SES and high asthma mortality rates emerged between the periods of 1969–1972 and 1979–1982; the relationship has

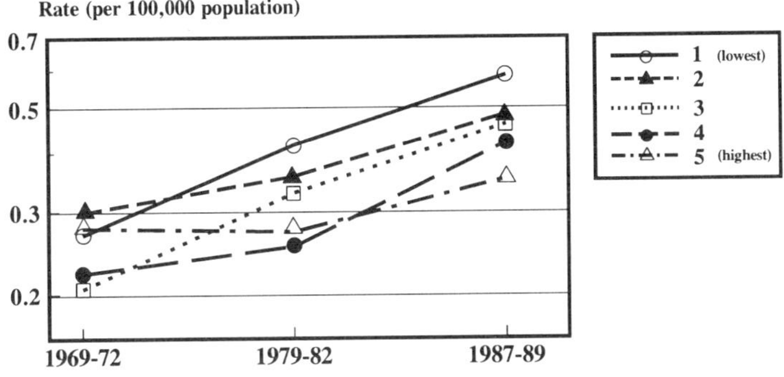

Note: ICD-8 and ICD-9 = 493.
Source: NCHS, VSS

Figure 8 Trends in US asthma mortality among persons aged 5–34; country rates by quintile of median income, multiyear averages.

persisted to the period 1987–1989. This relationship was not seen when examined by education.

Recent efforts to understand the relationship between asthma and SES have been focused on the inner city (107). During the past decade, the chances of a child being raised in families with only one parent and limited financial resources have increased (41). In 1987, nearly 50% of black children and 42% of Hispanic children under age 6 were poor, verses 10% of white children (25). Forty-six percent of all poor children in the United States lived in the central cities (30); from 1975 to 1987, the proportion of poor children living in areas of the central cities where 20% of the population or more is poor rose from 54 to 61% (30).

An increasingly disproportionate number of families in the inner city is headed by young, single, poorly educated women (116). In 1987, 20% of all children under age 6 lived with single mothers (25); the poverty rate among these children was 61%. Single mothers on welfare often have inadequate social supports to help them through the stresses of caring for a chronically ill child (39, 56). Social support moderates stress and encourages improved coping with illness (21, 31).

CHANGES IN THE MEDICAL CARE ENVIRONMENT In 1985, among children under age 6, 30% of the poor and 32% of the near-poor were without health insurance (30). Thirteen percent of those families who were more than 150% above the poverty line were uninsured. These poor, uninsured children made 38% fewer visits to a physician than those with insurance (71). Poor children are also twice as likely to report no regular source of pediatric care and are far more likely to receive their care from overburdened hospital outpatient and emergency departments rather than individual physicians (2).

During the past decade, there have been dramatic changes in the US health-care system. It is difficult, if not impossible, to examine most of these changes as they relate to the trends in asthma morbidity. Access and pharmacotherapy, however, do appear to frequent the asthma literature as possible links to morbidity. Therefore, we limit the following discussion of possible changes in the health-care system to these two factors.

Changes in access to medical care With the advent of Medicaid, access to medical care for poor children improved considerably (68). However, a growing number of uninsured families do not qualify for Medicaid because their income is above the Medicaid eligibility cutoff (133–185% above the poverty line) (25). Between 1979 and 1987, the percentage of asthma hospitalizations for children reporting either Medicaid or self-pay increased (33). Moreover, although Medicaid overcame an important barrier to care for previously uninsured children, it has established its own, less easily measured barriers, such as completing and processing forms, waiting in lines, and lack of access to office based physicians (115). In the state of Maryland, asthma hospitalization rates for children with Medicaid were both higher and slightly more likely to be emergent admissions (114). These reports suggest that Medicaid may not be providing an adequate access to good quality health care for such conditions as asthma.

Changing pharmacotherapy The past two decades have exhibited dramatic changes in the use of medications to control asthma symptoms (11, 34). These pharmaco-epidemiologic trends reflect increases in both the total use and the distribution of use among different classes of drugs. Data from the National Prescription Audit reported an increase of prescriptions of anti-asthma drugs (oral and inhaled bronchodilator and inhaled anti-inflammatory drugs) by approximately 9.5% per annum between 1981 and 1985. Sustained release theophylline formulations increased 138% during this time period, while other formulations of this drug decreased (11). From 1980 to 1986, prescriptions for inhaled sympathomimetics [metered dose inhalers (MDIs)] for the Michigan Medicaid population increased at a rate of 22% per annum (34).

During the past decade, there has been a dramatic increase in the use of MDIs as a principal pharmacotherapeutic agent for asthma symptom control (11). Also, methylxanthine use has shifted from immediate to sustained release preparations. This change may be an important trend in relation to recent trends in asthma morbidity. MDIs have been at the center of controversy twice during the two decades. It has been proposed that a high-dose inhaler (isoproterenol 0.2 mgs/puff) was responsible for a increase in deaths in England during the late 1960s (46, 94). More recently, there has been a controversy that Fenoterol, another MDI that is currently not used in the United States, is causing excess morbidity (22, 80). One study has proposed that regular versus occasional use of these MDIs may be correlated with risk of morbidity (89). Furthermore, results from a large pharmaco-epidemiologic study in Canada suggest that frequent use of MDIs along with theophylline and oral steroids can serve as an important epidemiology marker of death and near-death for asthma (95). The recent and dramatic changes in asthma drug therapy, when viewed in the context of the recent increases in asthma mortality, suggest that further studies are needed to examine whether these two trends represent a causal or coincident occurrence.

PUBLIC HEALTH IMPLICATIONS OF THE CHANGING PATTERNS OF ASTHMA EPIDEMIOLOGY

As with most issues in public health, a close examination reveals substantial complexity in what, at first blush, appears simple. There are at least three separate components to the recent trends in US asthma morbidity. Asthma prevalence has steadily increased during the past decade. However, this increase appears to be limited to persons under age 45, if not entirely limited to children and young adults. Asthma morbidity, as measured by physicians visits and hospitalizations, appears to have increased, as well. The increase in hospitalizations has been limited almost exclusively to children under 5 years of age, whereas physician visits have increased for the older age groups, 15–44 years and 65 years and older. Asthma mortality during the past decade has also demonstrated an increase, but only with certainty for persons under age 35, for whom the death certificates reflect accurate diagnosis. Furthermore, asthma mortality, unlike prevalence or hospitalization rates, has demonstrated an increase that was preceded by an entire decade of decline. It would be extremely difficult, and probably grossly incorrect, to ascribe these very different trends to a single underlying change.

It is possible, however, to highlight some of the more plausible explanations for each trend. The changing prevalence of asthma, even a few percent over a decade for such a large segment of the population (i.e. all persons under age 45), would require an increase in a broad-reaching exposure. There is no reported change in the outdoor environment, such as pollution, that would explain the change in prevalence. Changes in the indoor environment, caused by changes in indoor living, are a much more plausible pathway.

Enhanced diagnostic recognition is the most likely explanation for recent increases in asthma prevalence. The nature of the data on asthma prevalence, self-reported, is very susceptible to enhanced diagnostic recognition. During the past decade, the public and the US medical community have been exposed to the important message that an unexplained wheeze or chronic cough may be asthma, particularly for children. However, it is not apparent that diagnostic recognition can account for all of the recent changes.

Increases in asthma hospitalization rates have been limited to very young children, under age 5. It is unlikely that diagnostic transfer, at least in the United States, can explain all of the increase. Therefore, other explanations are needed. We emphasize that the increase in hospitalization rates in the children under age 5 has not resulted in a subsequent increase in hospitalization rates for older age groups, e.g. ages 5–14 years. The underlying explanation of recent hospitalization trends must reflect a disease expression that either is absolutely well controlled by age 5 or is an asthma-like syndrome that remits by this age.

One explanation for the recent increases in asthma hospitalization rates may be changes in exposures to respiratory viral infections. A decade's growth in the percentage of children under age 5 in daycare settings might provide the necessary exposure to produce an increase in wheezy illness that is being diagnosed as asthma in this population. A very different, and perhaps equally plausible, explanation for at least a portion of the recent trends in hospitalization rates relates to increasing numbers survivors of premature births with attendant transient bronchial hyperreactivity during early life.

The reasons for the decrease and then increase in asthma mortality during the past two decades is, perhaps, the most troubling trend to attempt to understand. It is not possible to ascribe the decrease in asthma mortality to any factor other than changes in pharmacotherapy during the early 1970s. This is a time in which methylxanthines were heavily used as the primary drug intervention. During the 1980s, pharmacotherapy changed once again. The use of inhaled beta-agonists became widely accepted, and the monitoring of theophylline levels to avoid toxicity became widely available. The use of steroids also began to increase. Aside from these dramatic changes in pharmacotherapy, there are, in the United States, no other known therapeutic trends would serve as a bases as a plausible explanation of recent trends.

STRATEGIES FOR PUBLIC HEALTH INTERVENTIONS

Because of the complex, multidimensional nature of the recent secular trends, there can be no single proposed public health intervention (7). Broad sweeping public education programs now in progress will increase awareness among physicians and the general public, thus leading to earlier diagnosis and hopefully better treatment. However, these programs will not move us closer to an understanding of the factors that are driving these important health trends.

A series of studies will need to be funded if we are to dissect this problem. As research dollars are increasingly competitive, it will be important to focus public health resources on very specific targetable goals. We will need to conduct more studies to identify the important risk factors and ways to intervene in the causal pathways toward morbidity and mortality. Studies of the long-term effect of low birthweight on the development of asthma or asthma-like morbidity and the impact of indoor air quality as it relates to asthma need to be further explored. Asthma morbidity in children under age 5 deserves special consideration. Longitudinal studies must be directed at this younger age group to increase our understanding of the pathogenesis of the disease, natural history, and disease control.

Both asthma hospitalization and mortality can serve as an important sentinel events (82) in understanding the failure of the medical care system to deliver optimal care. Given our state of knowledge, the public health sector should focus its limited resources on those at highest risk—persons living in poverty, especially those in the inner city. The complex public health problem that the recent unfavorable trends in asthma morbidity present are likely to be solved if broad public education programs are supplemented with appropriate targeted research and intervention strategies that are so badly needed.

Literature Cited

1. Aberg, N. 1989. Asthma and allergic rhinitis in Swedish conscripts. *Clin. Exp. Allergy* 19:59–63
2. Access to Health Care in the United States. 1987. Special Rep. No.2., pp.4–10. Princeton, NJ: Robert Wood Johnson Found.
3. *Accuracy of Death Certificates in Bronchial Asthma*. 1984. Accuracy of certification procedures during the confidential inquiry by the British Thoracic Association. *Thorax* 39:505–9
4. Alderson, M. 1987. Trends in morbidity and mortality from asthma. *Popul. Trends* 49:18–23
5. Anderson, H. R. 1989. Is the prevalence of asthma changing? *Arch. Dis. Child.* 1989;64:172–5
6. Anderson, H. R., Bland, J. M., Patel, S., Peckham, C. 1986. The natural history of asthma in childhood. *J. Epidemiol. Commun. Health* 40:121–29
7. Anthony, J. C. 1990. Prevention research in the context of epidemiology with a discussion of public health models. In *Conceptual Research Models for Preventing Mental Disorders*, ed. P. Muehrer, pp. 1–32. Rockville, Md: Natl. Inst. of Mental Health
8. Asthma—United States, 1980–1987. 1990. *Morbid. Mortal. Wkly. Rep.* 39: 493–96
9. Bader, D., Ramos, A. D., Lew, C.D., Platzker, A. C. G., Stabile, M. W., Keens, T. G. 1987. Childhood sequelae of infant lung disease: exercise and pulmonary function abnormalities after bronchopulmonary dysplasia. *J. Pediatr.* 110:693–99
10. Barger, L. W., Vollmer, W. M., Felt, R. W., Buist, A. S. 1988. Further investigation into the recent increase in asthma death rates: a review of 41 asthma deaths in Oregon in 1982. *Ann. Allergy* 60:31–39
11. Bosco, L. A., Knapp, D. E., Gerstman, B. B., Graham, C. F. 1987. Asthma drug therapy trends in the United States, 1972 to 1985. *J. Allergy Clin. Immunol.* 80:398–402
12. Brunekreef, B., Dockery, D. W., Speizer, F. E., Ware, J. H., Spengler, J. D., Ferris, B. G. 1989. Home dampness and respiratory morbidity in children. *Am. Rev. Respir. Dis.* 140: 1363–67
13. Buist, A. S., Vollmer, W. M. 1990. Reflections on the rise in asthma mor-

bidity and mortality. *J. Am. Med. Assoc.* 264:1719–20

14. Burchfiel, C. M., Higgins, M. W., Keller, J. B., Howatt, W. F., Butler, W. J., Higgins, I. T. T. 1986. Passive smoking childhood. Respiratory conditions and pulmonary function in Tecumseh, Michigan. *Am. Rev. Respir. Dis.* 133:966–73
15. Burney, P. G. 1986. Asthma mortality in England and Wales: evidence for a further increase, 1974–84. *Lancet* 2: 323–26
16. Burney, P. G., Chinn, S., Rona, R. J. 1990. Has the prevalence of asthma increased in children? Evidence from the national study of health and growth 1973–86. *Br. Med. J.* 300:1306–10
17. Carr, W., Zeitel, L., Weiss, K. 1992. Variations in asthma hospitalizations and deaths in New York City. *Am. J. Public Health* 82:59–65
18. Chan, K. N., Elliman, A., Bryan, E., Silverman, M. 1989. Respiratory symptoms in children of low birth weight. *Arch. Dis. Child.* 64:1294–1304
19. Chan, K. N., Noble-Jamieson, C. M., Elliman, A., Bryan, E. M., Silverman, M. 1989. Lung function in children of low birth weight. *Arch. Dis. Child.* 64:1284–93
20. Cigarette smoking among adults—United States, 1990. 1992. *Morbid. Mortal. Wkly. Rep.* 41:354–62
21. Cobb, S. 1976. Social support as a moderator of life stress. *Psychosom. Med.* 38:300–14
22. Crane, J., Flatt, A., Jackson, R., et al. 1989. Prescribed fenoterol and death from asthma in New Zealand, 1981–1983: case-control study. *Lancet* 1:917–22
23. Davis, P., Jackson, R., Pearce, N. 1985. Asthma mortality. *NZ Med. J.* 98:604
24. Dales, R. E., Zwanenburg, H., Burne, K. R., Franklin, C. A. 1991. Respiratory health effects of home dampness and molds among Canadian children. *Am. J. Epidemiol.* 134:196–203
25. *Data Sourcebook: Five Million Children,* p. 9. 1990. New York: Columbia Univ. Natl. Cent. for Child. in Poverty
26. Environ. Protect. Agency. 1991. National air quality and emissions trends report, 1990. Research Triangle Park, NC: Office of Air Quality Planning and Standards, EPA-450/4–91–023
27. Evans, R., Mullally, D. I., Wilson, R. W., Gergen, P. J., et al. 1987. National trends in the morbidity and mortality of asthma in the US. Prevalence, hospitalization and death from asthma over two decades: 1965–1984. *Chest* 91:65S–74S
28. Fergusson, D. M., Horwood, L. J., Shannon, F. T. 1983. Asthma and infant diet. *Arch. Dis. Child.* 58:48–51
29. Natl. Cent. for Health Stat. 1989. Health, United States, 1988. DHHS Publ. No.(PHS)89–1232. Public Health Serv. Washington, DC: GPO
30. *Five Million Children: A statistical profile of our poorest young citizens,* p. 22. 1990. New York: Columbia Univ. Natl. Cent. for Child. in Poverty
31. Ganster, D. C., Victor, B. 1988. The impact of social support on mental and physical health. *Br. J. Med. Psychol.* 61:17–36
32. Gergen, P. J., Mullally, D. I., Evans, R. III. 1988. National Survey of Prevalence of asthma among children in the United States, 1976 to 1980. *Pediatrics* 81:1–7
33. Gergen, P. J., Weiss, K. B. 1990. Changing patterns of asthma hospitalization among children: 1979 to 1987. *J. Am. Med. Assoc.* 264:1688–92
34. Gerstman, B. B., Bosco, L. A., Tomita, D. K., Gross, T. P., Shaw, M. M. 1989. Prevalence and treatment of asthma in the Michigan Medicaid patient population younger than 45 years, 1980–1986. *J. Allergy Clin. Immunol.* 83:1032–39
35. Goren, A. I., Hellmann, S. 1988. Prevalence of respiratory symptoms and diseases in school children living in a polluted and in a low polluted area in Israel. *Environ. Res.* 45:28–37
36. Weitzman, M., Gortmaker, S. L., Sobol, M. A., Perrin, J. M. 1992. Recent trends in the prevalence and impact of childhood asthma. *J. Am. Med. Assoc.* 268:2673–77
37. Gregg, I. 1983. Epidemiologic aspects. In *Asthma,* ed. T. J. H. Clark, S. Godfrey, pp. 242–84. London: Chapman & Hall
38. Haahtela, T., Lindholm, H., Bjorksten, F., Koskenvuo, K., Laitinen, L. A. 1990. Prevalence of asthma in Finnish young men. *Br. Med. J.* 301:266–68
39. Haggerty, R. J. 1980. Life stress, illness and social supports. *Dev. Med. Child Neurol.* 22:391–400
40. Halfon, N., Newacheck, P. W. 1986. Trends in the hospitalization for acute childhood asthma, 1970–84. *Am. J. Public Health* 76:1308–11
41. Helmick, S. A., Zimmerman, J. D. 1984. Trends in the distribution of children among households and families. *Child Welf.* 63:401–9
42. Hoffman, H. J., Bergsjo, P., Denman,

D. W. 1988. Trends in birth weight-specific perinatal mortality rates: 1970–83. In *Proc. of the Int. Collab. Effort on Perinatal and Infant Mortal.*, Vol. 2., pp.III-51–III-71. Hyattsville, MD: DHHS

43. *Homebuilders Assoc. Data Rep.* 1990. Washington, DC: Natl. Homebuilders Assoc.
44. Horst, M., Heiiaoui, A., Horst, V., Michel. F.-B., Bousquet, J. 1990. Double-blind, placebo-controlled rush immunotherapy with a standardized alternaria extract. *J. Allergy Clin. Immunol.* 85:460–72
45. Horwood, L. J., Dawson, K. P., Mogridge, N. 1991. Admission patterns for childhood acute asthma: Christchurch 1974–89. *NZ Med. J.* 104:277–79
46. Inman, W. H. W., Adelstein, A. M. 1969. Rise and fall of asthma mortality in England and Wales in Relation to use of pressurized aerosis. *Lancet* 2: 279–85
47. Jackson, R., Sears, M., Beaglehole, R., Rea, H. 1988. International trends in asthma mortality: 1970 to 1985. *Chest* 94:914–18
48. Kang, B., Chang, J. L. 1985. Allergenic impact of inhaled arthropod material. *Clin. Rev. Allergy* 3:363–75
49. Koenig, J. Q., Covert, D. S., Hanley, Q. S., van Belle, G., Pierson, W. E. 1990. Prior exposure to ozone potentiates subsequent response to sulfur dioxide in adolescent asthmatic subjects. *Am. Rev. Respir. Dis.* 141(2): 377–80
50. Konig, P. 1978. The relationship between croup and asthma. *Ann. Allergy* 41:227–31
51. Kozak, L. J., Norton, C., McManus, M., McCarthy, E. 1987. Hospital use pattern for children in the United States, 1983 and 1984. *Pediatrics* 80:481–90
52. Marder, D., Targonski, P., Orris, P., Persky, V., Addington, W. 1992. Effect of racial and socioeconomic factors on asthma mortality in Chicago. *Chest* 101:4265–95
53. Martinez, F. D., Cline, M., Burrows, B. 1992. Increased incidence of asthma in children of smoking mothers. *Pediatrics* 89:21–26
54. McCormick, M. C., Brooks, G. U., Workman, D. 1992. The health and development status of very low-birth-weight children at school age. *J. Am. Med. Assoc.* 267:2204–8
55. McIntosh, K., Ellis, E. F., Hoffman, L. S., Lybass, T. G., Eller, J. J., Fulginiti, V. A. 1973. The association of viral and bacterial respiratory infections with exacerbations of wheezing in young asthmatic children. *J. Pediatr.* 82:578–90
56. McLanahan, S., Garfinkel, I. 1989. Single mothers, the underclass, and social policy. In The ghetto underclass: social science perspectives, ed. J. W. Wilson. *Ann. Am. Acad. Polit. Soc. Sci.* 501:92–104
57. Minor, T. E., Baker, J. W., Dick, E.C., et al. 1974. Greater frequency of viral respiratory infections in asthmatic children as compared with their nonasthmatic siblings. *J. Pediatr.* 85: 472–77
58. Minor, T. E., Dick, E. C., Baker, J. W., Ouellette, J. J., Cohen, M., Reed, C. E. 1976. Rhinovirus and influenza type a infections as precipitants of asthma. *Am. Rev. Respir. Dis.* 113: 149–53
59. Minor, T. E., Dick, E. C., DeMeo, A. N., Ouellette, J. J., Cohen, M., Reed, C. E. 1974. Viruses as precipitants of asthmatic attacks in children. *J. Am. Med. Assoc.* 227:292–98
60. Mitchell, E. A. 1983. Increasing prevalence of asthma in children. *NZ Med. J.* 96:463–64
61. Mitchell, E. A. 1985. International trends in hospital admission rates for asthma. *Arch. Dis. Child.* 60:376–78
62. Mitchell, E. A., Jackson, R. T. 1989. Recent trends in asthma mortality, morbidity, and management in New Zealand. *J. Asthma* 26:349–54
63. Murray, A. B., Ferguson, A. C., Morrison, B. J. 1983. Diagnosis of house dust mite allergy in asthmatic children: what constitutes a positive history? *J. Allergy Clin. Immunol.* 71:21–28
64. Murray, A. B., Morrison, B. J. 1988. Passive smoking and the seasonal difference of severity of asthma in children. *Chest* 94:701–8
65. Natl. Cent. for Health Stat. 1991. *Health, United States, 1990,* p. 143. Hyattsville, Md: Public Health Serv.
66. Neas, L. M., Dockery, D. W., Ware, J. H., Spengler, J. D., Speizer, F. E., Ferris, B. J. J. 1991. Association of indoor nitrogen dioxide with respiratory symptoms and pulmonary function in children. *Am. J. Epidemiol.* 134:204–19
67. Neuspiel, D. R., Rush, D., Butler, N. R., Golding, J., Bijur, P. E., Kurzon, M. 1989. Parental smoking and post-infancy wheezing in children: a prospective study. *Am. J. Public Health* 79:168–71
68. Newacheck, P. W., Halfon, N. 1986.

Access to ambulatory care services for economically disadvantaged children. *Pediatrics* 78:813–19
69. O'Hollaren, M. T., Yunginger, J. W., Offord, K. P., Sombr, M. J., O'Connell, E. J., et al. 1991. Exposure to an aeroallergen as a possible precipitating factor in respiratory arrest in young patients with asthma. *N. Engl. J. Med.* 324:359–63
70. Ostro, B. D., Lipsett, M. J., Wiener, M. B., Selner, J. C. 1991. Asthmatic responses to airborne acid aerosols. *Am. J. Public Health* 81: 694–702
71. Parker, S., Greer, S., Zuckerman, B. 1988. Double jeopardy: the impact of poverty on early childhood development. *Pediatr. Clin. North Am.* 35: 1227–40
72. Pierce, J. P., Fiore, M. C., Novotny, T. E., Hatziandreu, E. J., Davis, R. M. 1989. Trends in cigarette smoking in the United States. Educational differences are increasing. *J. Am. Med. Assoc.* 261:56–60
73. Pierson, W. E., Covert, D. S., Koenig, J. Q. 1984. Air pollutants, bronchial hyperreactivity, and exercise. *J. Allergy Clin. Immunol.* 73:717–21
74. Platts-Mills, T. A. E., Mitchell, E. B., Nock, P., Tovery, E. R., Moszoro, H., Wilkins, S. R. 1982. Reduction of bronchial hyperreactivity during prolonged allergen avoidance. *Lancet* 2: 675–78
75. Pollart, S. M., Chapman, M. D., Fiocco, G. P., Rose, G., Platts-Mills, T. A. E. 1989. Epidemiology of acute asthma. IgE antibodies to common inhalant allergens as a risk factor for emergency room visits. *J. Allergy Clin. Immunol.* 83:875–82
76. Pope, C. A. III 1989. Respiratory disease associated with community air pollution and a steel mill, Utah valley. *Am. J. Public Health* 79:623–28
77. Poysa, L., Korppi, M., Pietikainen, M., Remes, K., Juntunen-Backman, K. 1991. Asthma, allergic rhinitis and atopic eczema in Finnish children and adolescents. *Allergy* 46:161–65
78. Pullan, C. R., Hey, E. N. 1982. Wheezing, asthma, pulmonary dysfunction 10 years after infection with respiratory syncytial virus in infancy. *Br. Med. J.* 284:1665–69
79. Rachelefsky, G. S., Spector, S. L. 1990. Sinusitis and Asthma. *J. Asthma* 27:1–3
80. Rea, H. H., Scragg, R., Jackson, R., Beaglehole, R., Fenwick, J., Sutherland, D. C. 1986. A case-control study of deaths from asthma. *Thorax* 41:833–39
81. Robertson, C. F., Heycock, E., Bishop, J., Nolan, T., Olinsky, A., Phelan, P. D. 1991. Prevalence of asthma in Melbourne schoolchildren: changes over 26 years. *Br. Med. J.* 302:1116–18
82. Rutstein, D., Berenberg, W., Chalmers, T. C., Child, C. G., Fishman, A. P., Perrin, E. B. 1976. Measuring the quality of medical care: a clinical method. *N. Engl. J. Med.* 294:582–88
83. Ryan, A. S., Rush, D., Krieger, F. W., Lewandowski, G. E. 1991. Recent declines in breast-feeding in the United States, 1984 through 1989. *Pediatrics* 88:719–27
84. Schwartz, J., Gold, D., Dockery, D. W., Weiss, S. T., Speizer, F. E. 1990. Predictors of asthma and persistent wheeze in a national sample of children in the United States. Association with social class, perinatal events, and race. *Am. Rev. Respir. Dis.* 142:555–62
85. Sears, M .R. 1991. International trends in asthma mortality. *Allergy Proc.* 12: 155–58
86. Sears, M. R. 1991. Worldwide trends in asthma mortality. *Bull. Int. Union Tuberc. Lung Dis.* 66:79–83
87. Sears, M. R., Herbison, G. P., Holdaway, M. D., Hewin, C. J., Flannery, E. M., Silva, P. A. 1989. The relative risks of sensitivity to grass pollen, house dust mite and cat dander in the development of childhood asthma. *Clin. Exp. Allergy* 19:419–24
88. Sears, M. R., Rea, H. H., DeBoer, G., Beaglehole, R., Gillies, A. J. D., et al. 1986. Accuracy of certification of deaths due to asthma. A national study. *Am. J. Epidemiol.* 124:1004–11
89. Sears, M. R., Taylor, D. R., Print, C. G., Lake, D. C., Li, Q., et al. 1990. Regular inhaled beta-agonist treatment in bronchial asthma. *Lancet* 336:1391–96
90. Shaw, R. A., Crane, J., O'Donnell, T. V., Porteous, L. E., Coleman, E. D. 1990. Increasing asthma prevalence in a rural New Zealand adolescent population: 1975–89. *Arch. Dis. Child.* 65:1319–23
91. Sheppard, D. 1988. Sulfur dioxide and asthma—a double-edged sword? *J. Allergy Clin. Immunol.* 82:961–64
92. Sly, R. M. 1989. Mortality from asthma. *J. Allergy Clin. Immunol.* 84: 421–34
93. Speight, A. N., Lee, D. A., Hey, E. N. 1983. Underdiagnosis and undertreatment of asthma in childhood. *Br. Med. J.* 286:1253–56

94. Speizer, F. E., Doll, R., Heaf, P., Strang, L. B. 1968. Investigation into use of drugs preceding death from asthma. *Br. Med. J.* 1:339–43
95. Spitzer, W. O., Suissa, S., Ernst, P., Horowitz, R. I., Habbick, B., et al. 1992. The use of beta agonists and the risk of death and near death from asthma. *N. Engl. J. Med.* In press
96. Sporik, R., Holgate, S. T., Platts-Mills, T. A. E, Cogswell, J. J. 1990. Exposure to house-dust mite allergen (Der p I) and the development of asthma in childhood. *N. Engl. J. Med.* 323:502–7
97. Statistical Highlights. Ten Year Summary. Washington, DC: Gas Appliance Manuf. Assoc.
98. Stewart, C. J., Nunn, A. J. 1985. Are asthma mortality rates changing? *Br. J. Dis. Chest* 79:229–34
99. Storr, J., Barrell, E., Lenney, W. 1988. Rising asthma admissions and self referral. *Arch. Dis. Child.* 63:774–79
100. Strachan, D. P. 1988. Damp housing and childhood asthma: validation of reporting of symptoms. *Br. Med. J.* 297:1223–26
101. Tarlo, S., Broder, I., Spence, L. 1979. A prospective study of respiratory infection in adult asthmatics and their normal spouses. *Clin. Allergy* 9:293–301
102. Taylor, B., Wadsworth, J. 1987. Maternal smoking during pregnancy and lower respiratory tract illness in early life. *Arch. Dis. Child.* 62:786–91
103. Taylor, B., Wadsworth, J., Golding, J., Butler, N. 1983. Breast feeding, eczema, asthma, and hayfever. *J. Epidemiol. Commun. Health* 37:95–99
104. Taylor, W. R., Newaheck, P. W. 1992. The impact of childhood asthma on health. *Pediatrics.* 90:657–62
105. Van Asperen, P. P. 1987. Annotation: is asthma really changing? *Aust. Paediatr. J.* 23:271–72
106. Van Metre, T. E., Marsh, D. G., Adkinson, N. F. J., et al. 1986. Dose of cat (Felis domesticus) allergen 1 (Fel d 1) that induces asthma. *J. Allergy Clin. Immunol.* 78:62–75
107. Weiss, K. B., Gergen, P. J., Crain, E. F. 1992. Inner-city asthma. The epidemiology of an emerging US public health concern. *Chest* 101:362s–67s
108. Weiss, K. B., Gergen, P. J., Hodgson, T. A. 1992. An economic evaluation of asthma in the United States. *N. Engl. J. Med.* 326:862–66
109. Weiss, K. B., Wagener, D. K. 1990. Asthma surveillance in the United States. A review of current trends and knowledge gaps. *Chest* 98:179S-84S
110. Weiss, K. B., Wagener, D. K. 1990. Changing patterns of asthma mortality. Identifying target populations at high risk. *J. Am. Med. Assoc.* 264:1683–87
111. Weitzman, M., Gortmaker, S., Sobol, A. 1990. Racial, social, and environmental risk factors for childhood asthma. *Am. J. Dis. Child.* 144:1189–94
112. Weitzman, M., Gortmaker, S., Walker, D. K., Sobol. A. 1990. Maternal smoking and childhood asthma. *Pediatrics* 85:505–11
113. Williams, M. H. 1989. Increasing severity of asthma from 1960 to 1987. *N. Engl. J. Med.* 320:1015–16
114. Wissow, L., Gittelshon, A. M., Szklo, M., Starfild, B., Mussman, M. 1988. Poverty, race, and hospitalization for childhood asthma. *Am. J. Public Health* 78:777–82
115. Wolfe, B. L. 1980. Childen's utilization of medical care. *Med. Care* 18:1196–1207
116. Wood, D. L., Valdez, R. B., Hayashi, T., Shen, A. 1990. Health of homeless children and housed, poor children. *Pediatrics* 86:858–66
117. Woolcock, A. J. 1986. Worldwide differences in asthma prevalence and mortality: why is asthma mortality so low in the USA? *Chest* 90:40S-45S
118. Wright, A. L., Holberg, C., Martinez, F. D., Taussig, L. M. 1991. Group Health Medical Associates. Relationship of parental smoking to wheezing and nonwheezing lower respiratory tract illness in infancy. *J. Pediatr.* 118:207–14

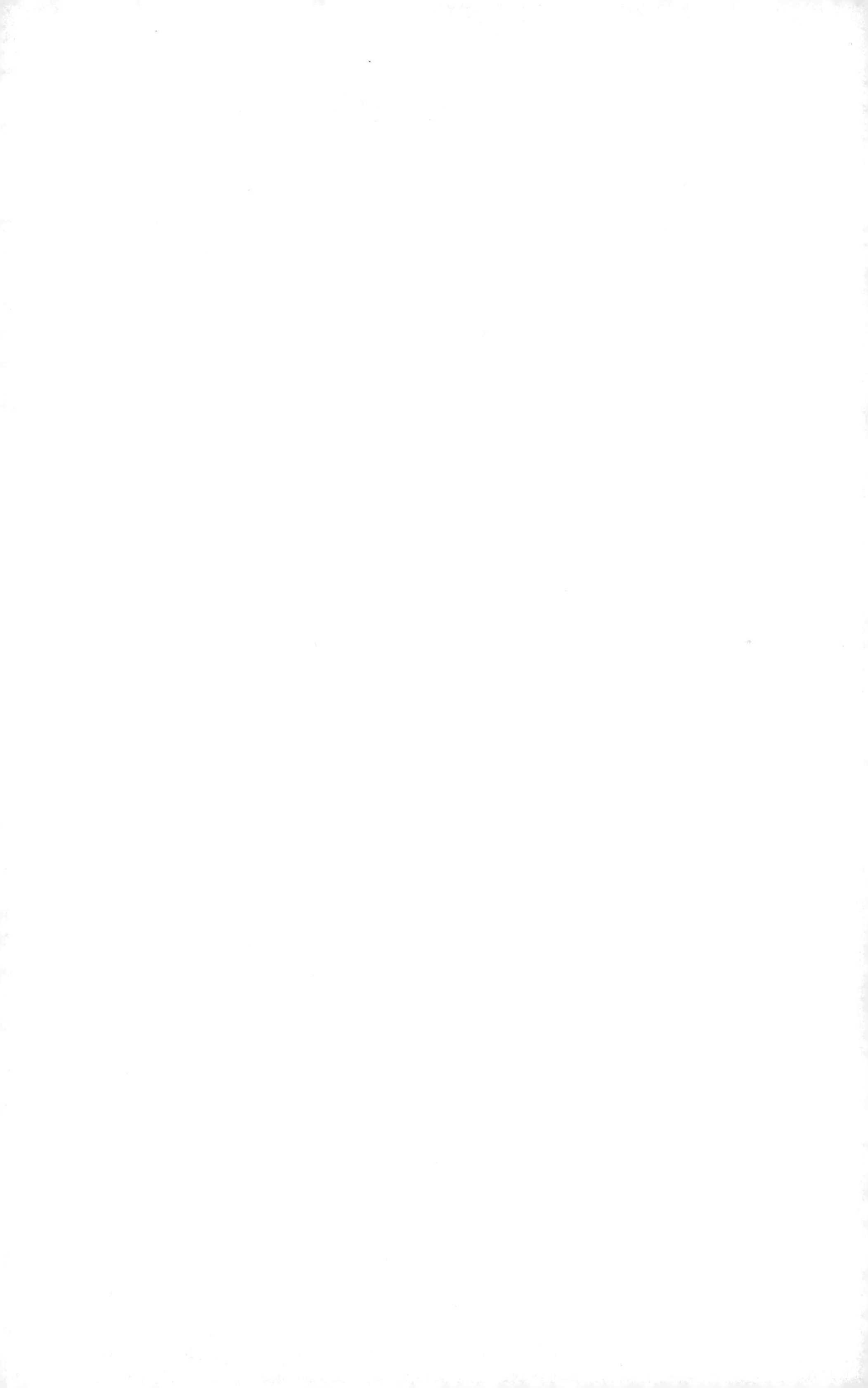

Annu. Rev. Publ. Health. 1993. 14:515–43

INJURIES FROM TRAFFIC CRASHES: Meeting the Challenge

John D. Graham

Injury Control Center, Harvard School of Public Health, Boston, Massachusetts 02115

KEY WORDS: automobile safety, transportation, injury control, highway safety, regulation

---

INTRODUCTION

In 1990, about 6.5 million traffic crashes were reported to police in the United States. Although 66% of the crashes resulted in no reportable injury to occupants, 28% resulted in minor or moderate injury and 6% in severe or fatal injury (67). Injury from motor vehicle crashes is the single largest cause of premature death among young people aged 1–30 (5, 66, 84). At current mortality rates, a baby born today has roughly 1 chance in 70 of ultimately dying in a traffic crash. Traffic crashes are also the largest cause of crippling injuries to the brain and spinal cord (84, 88). Recent estimates place the lifetime economic burden of motor vehicle injury at about $50 billion per year (84), not including the personal burden of the pain and suffering caused by traffic crashes.

Since World War II, the annual number of traffic fatalities in the United States has increased by 33%, from 34,800 in 1950 to 46,300 in 1990 (73). Although this rising burden of trauma is disconcerting, it resulted from the rapid motorization of American society. During this same period, the number of licensed drivers increased almost threefold; the number of registered vehicles, fourfold; and the number of vehicle miles driven, almost fivefold (107). Progress in reducing the traffic fatality rate, measured as the number of traffic fatalities per 100 million vehicle miles driven, has been steady and substantial. In total, the United States has cut this measure of the traffic fatality rate by almost 72% from 7.59 in 1950 to 2.15 in 1990 (73) (see Table 1).

The progress in traffic safety is remarkable when one considers the unfavorable factors that were operating to exacerbate the traffic fatality rate during this 40-year period. As the baby-boom generation moved through the

0163-7525/93/0510-0515$02.00

Table 1 The US traffic fatality rate, 1950–1990[a]

Years	Fatality rate[b]	Percentage change
1950	7.59	—
1950–1954	7.16	—
1955–1959	5.91	−17.46
1960–1964	5.37	− 9.31
1965–1969	5.47	+ 1.02
1970–1974	4.34	−20.62
1975–1979	3.40	−21.57
1980–1984	3.01	−11.47
1985–1989	2.47	−11.87
1990	2.15	—

[a] From Ref. 73.
[b] Fatalities per 100 million vehicle miles of travel.

risky teenage driving years in the 1960s, licensure rates among teenagers were rapidly increasing (78). The average size and weight of the passenger car fleet declined in response to fuel economy pressures, particularly from 1975 to 1990 (37, 72). Light and heavy trucks, which cause significant damage in two-vehicle crashes, have accounted for an increasing fraction of the total vehicle fleet and miles driven (72, 107). Average vehicle horsepower and travel speeds increased persistently, although the OPEC oil embargo of 1973–1974 led to temporary imposition of the national maximum 55-mile per hour speed limit. Average speeds on many highways dropped sharply in 1974 because of the slower legal maximum, but highway speeds have increased steadily from 1975 to 1990 (107). In addition, until about 1980, the per capita rate of alcohol consumption (and presumably the rate of drinking and driving) increased substantially, partly because of rising incomes and the declining real price of alcohol (24, 56, 93, 104, 117). Although all of these trends acted to increase the traffic fatality rate, the observed traffic fatality rate actually declined.

These facts suggest that some steps taken to improve the safety of motor vehicle travel since World War II were effective. This chapter examines the sources of safety progress, how opportunities were missed to make even more dramatic progress, and what pro-safety measures should be considered in the future. A cost-effectiveness framework is used to provide perspective about which traffic safety policies can produce the largest public health gains per dollar of investment.

Looking toward the year 2000, important changes in the characteristics of vehicles, highways, drivers, and pedestrians will present new safety challenges and require innovative solutions. The chapter describes these changes. The chapter also notes that the traffic safety community is not well prepared to meet these challenges because of persistent neglect of basic investments in traffic safety research. The chapter concludes on two notes of optimism: the consumer's increasing interest in vehicle safety, which is triggering competitive market forces on behalf of safety, and the public health community's increasing commitment to injury control, which promises to return traffic injuries to the governmental agenda, where it was briefly in the 1960s when Ralph Nader emerged as a political figure.

EXPLAINING THE PROGRESS, 1950–1980

Time-series models of long-term trends in fatality rates have provided useful insights into the causes of traffic safety progress. At the most abstract level, the declining fatality rate is associated with long-term increases in levels of household education and income, which would be expected to increase both the public's interest in safety and its ability to invest resources in safety practices and policies. More specifically, analysts have traced the declining fatality rate to a handful of key factors in highway design, vehicular design, and medical practice.

Perhaps the single most important factor acting to depress the traffic fatality rate was the rapid construction and use of the Interstate Highway System (16, 25, 39). Miles driven on interstates now account for almost one third of total miles driven on US roads and highways (107). Modern interstate highways are extremely safe because they were built with divided traffic streams, controlled access (with entrance and exit ramps), few dangerous curves, highly visible traffic signs, wide roadside shoulders, and forgiving roadside fixtures, such as breakaway sign posts and crash-absorbing barriers. The rural two-lane highways built before World War II were designed with few of these safety features.

Together, these design factors help explain why the mileage fatality rate on interstate highways is only one-third the rate observed on rural highways (107). Drivers have traded some of the improved safety of interstate highways for more travel at higher speeds, but the net effect has been a sharp decline in the traffic fatality rate.

Among highway variables, another significant factor depressing the traffic fatality rate was the urbanization of the American population. The fraction of miles driven in urban areas increased from 47% in 1950 to 60% in 1990 (107). Fatality rates on rural roads and highways are higher than on urban roads and highways, in part because the congestion in urban areas reduces travel speeds and the lethality of crashes.

The traffic fatality rate has also declined because of the enhanced safety of motor vehicle designs. In the 1950s and 1960s, a small community of engineers and clinicians asserted that cars could be better designed to protect occupants when crashes occur. New vehicle safety regulations were spawned by the writings of Daniel Patrick Moynihan and the advocacy of Nader. The resulting improvements in the probability of occupants surviving crashes without serious injuries are well documented (39). Although it is difficult to isolate and quantify the effects of individual safety features, studies indicate that cars meeting the initial federal motor vehicle safety standards of the late 1960s had 20–40% fewer fatalities in crashes than cars that did not meet these standards (16, 39, 36, 87). Whether cars meeting minimum federal safety standards had lower collision rates than unregulated cars is uncertain, although some reduction in collisions may have occurred because of enhanced braking, better tires, and extended visibility from improved lighting. Some studies suggest that drivers responded to enhanced vehicle safety with more risky driving behaviors, but the evidence for this hypothesis is weak and inconsistent (40, 78, 87).

The specific vehicle safety features believed to be responsible for improved occupant safety include interior padding schemes, collapsible steering columns, lap and shoulder belts, improved roof and door strength, and head restraints. Although these features were offered voluntarily to consumers by some vehicle manufacturers from 1955 to 1965, state and federal policies spurred the introduction of safety features as standard equipment by 1966 (35).

Improvements in the delivery of emergency medical services have reduced the lethality of traffic crashes by assuring motorists prompt medical attention (3, 75). Progress in response time (shorter transport times to the crash location and to the receipt of proper care) has been dramatic in both urban and suburban populations, although more progress is needed in rural areas (68). Although the regionalization of trauma systems is a topic beyond the scope of this chapter, progress in the medical treatment of the injured since World War II has contributed to the impressive decline in the traffic fatality rate.

The hypothesis that motorists drive more safely in 1990 than they did in 1950 has been advanced. Some analysts point to favorable changes in social norms about driving (e.g. less acceptance of risky driving as recreation), whereas others emphasize the improvements in the level of education and economic well-being of drivers (25). Although such speculation is plausible, there is no direct empirical evidence on these important behavioral questions.

A final point worth noting is the distinction between the vehicle and passenger fatality rates. As the number of vehicles per capita in the United States has proliferated, the average occupancy rate per trip has been declining (73, 107). Direct data on occupancy rates are unavailable, but some of the sharp decline in the fatality rate per vehicle mile is probably attributable to a decline in the average number of passengers in the vehicle when crashes occur. Thus, some of the alleged improvement in the vehicle fatality rate may be an artifact of unmeasured declines in rates of vehicle occupancy.

MISSED OPPORTUNITIES, 1965–1985

One of the major obstacles to more dramatic safety progress during 1965–1985 was an increasingly adversarial relationship between the federal government and the automotive industry. The leadership of the domestic auto industry contributed to the problem by refusing to implement promising safety innovations advanced by auto engineers (13, 88). The disinterest in safety among auto executives reflected a rather sluggish consumer demand for safety compared with the strong consumer interests in vehicle performance, appearance, and reliability (35, 36).

Spurred by Nader, officials of the National Highway Traffic Safety Administration (NHTSA) promulgated unrealistic safety rules and schedules, questioned the motives of industry officials who called for more realistic safety rules, and neglected promising safety policies that did not entail regulation of new vehicles (35). Consumer advocates saw ambitious rule-making tactics as necessary to overcome the disinterest and recalcitrance of automakers on safety questions (13).

One can point to evidence of the culpability of either side in this struggle, but the important lesson is that traffic safety progress was retarded by an excessively adversarial relationship between the public and private sectors. The fate of air bags and mandatory safety-belt use laws in the 1970s illustrates this perverse phenomenon. Consumer advocates and insurance interests saw air bags (and other automatic restraints) as the key solution to low rates of voluntary safety-belt use. Vehicle manufacturers advocated education and later legislation as means to increase usage. With little effort to forge a reasonable compromise, the opposing parties battled in Congress, the federal courts, and the White House from 1970 to 1985.

During the stalemate that ensued, few new vehicles were equipped with air bags and automatic safety belts. Voluntary rates of manual belt use actually declined from roughly 20% in 1970 to a low of 10% in 1980 (39). Meanwhile, nations as diverse as Australia and Sweden achieved belt-wearing rates of 60–80% with mandatory belt use laws (32, 35). Cars with air bags were first offered by Mercedes throughout Europe by the early 1980s, even though the technology was invented in the 1960s by engineers employed by suppliers to General Motors Corporation and Ford Motor Company (35).

The stalemate was broken in the mid-1980s by a fascinating and fortunate combination of circumstances. The US Supreme Court blocked the Reagan Administration's "arbitrary and capricious" attempt to repeal the automatic-restraint standard. In response to the Court's remand, Secretary of Transportation Elizabeth Dole crafted a creative policy in 1984 that permitted repeal of the automatic restraint standard only if enough states were persuaded to pass strong mandatory belt use laws by 1989. Working through the organization Traffic Safety Now, automotive interests lobbied for mandatory belt use laws in state capitals throughout the nation. Meanwhile, Ford Motor Company worked to build its pro-safety reputation by advancing the air bag technology and working with the insurance industry to propose a revision in Dole's plan that encouraged manufacturers to install air bags. By the end of the 1980s, America had achieved what had been impossible more than a decade earlier: widespread implementation of both mandatory safety-belt use laws and air bag technology.

TRAFFIC SAFETY PROGRESS IN THE 1980s

From an actuarial perspective, the safety progress of the 1980s exceeded the progress achieved in each of the three previous decades. As Table 2 indicates, from 1981 to 1990, the number of traffic fatalities declined 10%, while the traffic fatality rate (per mile of travel) declined 35%.

Some of this apparent progress is an artifact of the business cycle. Traffic fatality counts and rates tend to fall in recessions and climb during economic upturns (76, 112). This association reflects decreased motor vehicle travel during recessions, especially relatively hazardous discretionary driving (27, 49). The perverse effects of upturns in the business cycle, which tend to increase fatality counts and rates, should not be confused with the well-established, long-term safety improvements associated with rising levels of real per capita income (27, 38).

The deep recession of 1981–1983 accounted for most of the absolute decline in fatality counts observed in the 1980s. Remarkably, traffic fatality counts increased only slightly in the remainder of the 1980s, when the economy experienced its most robust and sustained recovery since World War II. Despite the fact that the economic upturn increased vehicle miles driven 35% from 1982 to 1990, there was virtually no change in the number of traffic fatalities (73). Powerful forces were at work to suppress the traffic fatality

Table 2 Percentage changes in US traffic fatality counts and rates by decade[a]

Fatality measures	1951–1960	1961–1970	1971–1980	1981–1990
Fatality counts	+ 3.08%	+43.43%	− 2.22%	− 9.89%
Fatality rates	−29.48%	− 5.43%	−23.41%	−34.85%

[a] From Ref. 73.

count, which is indicated by the substantial decline in the traffic fatality rate reported in Table 2. Although the reasons for the progress of the 1980s are not yet understood completely, the following factors played an important role.

THE AMERICAN CAMPAIGN AGAINST DRUNK DRIVING

Despite the widely cited statistic that a majority of traffic fatalities involve alcohol (24, 105), the scientific literature before 1980 indicated that few public policies had achieved a significant and sustained decline in alcohol-related fatalities. Some police crackdowns on drunk driving achieved short-term reductions in traffic crashes and fatalities, but these gains tended to be short-lived (91, 92).

The prevailing wisdom in the traffic safety community was that, because driver behaviors are highly resistant to change, policymakers should emphasize policies that improve safety through technological modifications in vehicle and highway design (35, 46, 88). In the 1980s, the United States disregarded this pessimism about behavioral strategies, in part because of the tenacious efforts of grass-roots organizations, such as Mothers Against Drunk Driving (MADD) (48, 122).

Much to the surprise of many skeptics, the American campaign against drunk driving achieved measurable success. The number of alcohol-related fatalities in the 1980s was 10–25% less than the number that might have occurred without the concerted campaign to discourage drunk driving (4, 29, 66, 104, 105, 123). Survey evidence confirms the changing social norms about drinking and driving, as reflected in the growing public conviction that drunk driving is a crime that should be punished (43, 51, 56). These changes may also be responsible, to some extent, for the gradual decline in per capita rates of alcohol consumption reported in the 1980s (104, 118). Throughout the 1980s, the changes in laws and social norms about drinking and driving were mutually reinforcing.

Although the progress against drunk driving is amply documented, it is less clear which public policies (if any) are responsible for the behavioral changes. A wide variety of public policies have been adopted or proposed to curtail the problem (31). Interestingly, there is some confusion about whether the policy objective should be to reduce drunk driving, reduce drinking and driving (regardless of drunkenness), reduce drinking per se, or accomplish all of these outcomes.

Some public policies are intended simply to curtail the consumption of alcoholic beverages, in the hopes that the various adverse consequences of alcohol abuse, such as drunk driving, will be reduced. Such policies include increased taxation of alcohol, increases in the minimum legal drinking age, and restrictions on the advertising of alcoholic beverages. Other policies are designed to separate drinking and driving, without necessarily reducing the amount of alcohol consumed by the public. Such policies include increased criminalization of drunk driving, greater liability for bartenders who serve drunk drivers, information and education campaigns to promote the "designated driver," and laws to prohibit open liquid containers in motor vehicles. The policies discussed below have dominated the deliberations of policymakers in the 1980s.

Raising the Minimum Legal Drinking Age

The only consumption-oriented policy that achieved widespread political support in the United States in the 1980s was an increase in the minimum legal drinking age from 18 or 19 to 21 years of age. Legal drinking ages were actually lowered in the 1970s in response to the urgings of young people, who were not reluctant to remind politicians that 18-year-olds were considered mature enough to be drafted and killed in the Vietnam War (110). Relaxation of the minimum legal drinking age in the 1970s was associated with significant increases in the number of traffic fatalities among drivers under the age of 21 (14, 120). This evidence formed the basis of a legislative campaign in the 1980s to return the minimum legal drinking age to 21, which virtually all states have done (94).

The higher minimum drinking age has been associated with lower rates of serious traffic crashes among young people (17, 74). The precise magnitude of the decline varies from study to study and from state to state, in part according to how well the old and new drinking ages were enforced and in part according to whether border states had also raised their drinking age (14). By reducing access to alcohol among 18-year-olds, access was also expected to be reduced among 15–17-year-olds, and some evidence supports this hypothesis (110, 121). More progress could be made through better enforcement of laws against underage drinking (17, 31, 57, 111, 121).

The trends in national fatality statistics provide some circumstantial evidence of policy effectiveness. The rate of alcohol involvement in fatal crashes declined in every age group throughout the 1980s, but the largest percentage declines have been observed among drivers in the youngest age group (ages 15–20). However, the declining rates of alcohol involvement among drivers aged 21 and older suggest that policies other than the minimum legal drinking age were also playing a significant role (66).

The fundamental question that has been raised about the higher drinking age is whether it simply delays the hazardous synergism of drinking and driving from age 18 to 21. According to this view, the crashes due to drinking and driving among young people are delayed, rather than prevented (4, 54,

59). If the key problem for young drivers is inexperience with drinking, other policy solutions, such as early or later licensure, may be preferable (80). Introducing young people to alcohol before the onset of driving is an alternative strategy. In several European countries, adolescents regularly consume alcohol before the onset of driving privileges. The suggestion, as yet unproven, is that the harmful effects of drinking and driving among young people might be reduced by increasing experience with alcohol consumption in the years before onset of driving. In light of the broader social concerns about the adverse consequences of alcohol abuse, American policy will unlikely become more permissive of alcohol consumption at younger ages (110).

Punishing the Drunken Driver

The major focus of American policy against drunk driving in the 1980s has been to increase the likelihood, swiftness, and severity of punishment (48, 51, 117). A primary objective of this punitive approach is to deter drivers from operating a motor vehicle while under the influence of alcohol. Interestingly, this policy approach has been questioned by an international literature, which suggests that general deterrence can achieve, at best, only a temporary reduction in the frequency of alcohol-related crashes (61, 91).

The cornerstone of America's punitive campaign was a new law that defines driving with an elevated blood alcohol concentration (BAC) as a crime (i.e. a threshold of legal intoxication), regardless of whether driving behavior is detectably influenced. In drafting this "illegal per se" legislation, most states have placed the BAC limit at 0.10% although there is considerable pressure to lower the limit to 0.08 or 0.05%, especially for younger drivers (42, 45, 106).

The purpose of illegal per se laws is to make it easier for law enforcement officials to apprehend and convict drunk drivers. Police use a variety of techniques to strengthen the enforcement of illegal per se laws. Roadside sobriety checkpoints are increasingly employed to increase the probability that drunk drivers will be detected and apprehended (55). Preliminary breath test devices, which provide some chemical evidence of alcohol, are increasingly used in normal highway patrols and at checkpoints to determine which drivers should be apprehended and taken to the police station for conclusive blood tests (29, 55). Despite the utility of new technologies to detect alcohol in the breath, their use by police is under scrutiny in state and federal courts (51).

Swiftness of punishment has been enhanced by new state legislation and judicial doctrines that authorize police to suspend a driver's license before conviction on the basis of evidence that the driver has exceeded the legal BAC limit. Under these "administrative per se" laws, drivers who flunk breath tests and/or blood tests may have their licenses suspended immediately. The suspension periods range from 30 to 90 days and are typically accompanied with threats of severe sanctions if offenders are caught driving with a suspended license. Recent studies of license suspension have reported positive results for the deterrence of drunk driving (44, 60, 77, 116).

Historically, many citizens apprehended for driving under the influence (DUI) of alcohol have escaped punishment. New legislation calls for mandatory, 48-hour jail terms or community service for first offenders. Repeat offenders face more severe sentencing prospects. New state legislation also restricts the freedom of police, prosecutors, and judges to plea bargain DUI offenses to charges with less severe penalties (29, 60).

Administrative and judicial proceedings that involve DUI charges are also being taken more seriously, in part because of the court monitoring programs launched by citizen groups. Some evidence indicates that these monitoring programs influence adjudicatory outcomes, especially in cases involving drivers who refused to submit to a BAC test (95).

The preponderance of evidence suggests that the punitive approach to drunk driving has contributed to the observed declines in alcohol-related fatal crashes in the 1980s. However, it is uncertain which punitive policies are the most effective (29). Many of the studies in the literature examine one change in punitive policy (e.g. authorization of police to use preliminary breath test devices) without controlling for the influences of other changes in punitive policies (e.g. use of roadside sobriety checkpoints). Because some of these punitive policies were simultaneously adopted by states, it is difficult to isolate the deterrent effects of each individual policy. There may be synergistic deterrent effects when two or more punitive policies are adopted together. The evaluation task is further complicated by the fact that enforcement and sentencing practices are stricter in some states than others, even when the provisions of new state laws appear similar on paper. Further research is needed to determine which punitive strategies offer the most promise in the prevention of alcohol-related traffic fatalities.

Although it is tempting to interpret punitive legislation as the primary cause of changing social norms about drunk driving, it is also important to see punitive legislation as a manifestation of changing social norms (43, 51). In either case, changes in social norms, in part spurred by such citizen activist groups as MADD, have apparently achieved what many traffic safety professionals believed was virtually impossible: a meaningful change in driver attitudes and behaviors resulting in a reduction of traffic fatalities. It is less clear, however, whether the punitive strategy can deter the hard-core drinking drivers, who are now responsible for a majority of the fatal crashes attributed to alcohol (96).

THE AMERICAN CAMPAIGN TO INCREASE OCCUPANT-RESTRAINT USE

In most countries around the world, efforts to increase safety-belt use began with adult populations and were later extended to young children. In the United States, the order of the campaign was reversed; it focused on young children in the late 1970s and has only recently begun to influence the behaviors of most adults. Although more progress is urgently required, the 1980s must be considered a decade of accomplishment in occupant protection through restraint use. As was the case with the campaign against drunk driving, this campaign achieved considerable success, despite the prevailing belief that strategies aimed at changing human behaviors are unlikely to succeed.

In 1978, in response to the urgings of pediatrician Robert Sanders, Tennessee became the first state in the nation to require parents to restrain their infants and toddlers during motor vehicle travel (35, 115). Similar legislation followed in other states, and by 1985 all 50 states had enacted some form of child-restraint use legislation. Laws were often preceded and/or accompanied by educational programs targeted at pregnant women, with hospital-based loaner programs to insure parental access to approved child-restraint devices from birth onward.

Observational surveys at shopping centers in 19 cities have documented the dramatic changes in parental practices regarding the restraint of young children. The rate of child restraint use increased from roughly 20% in 1980 to 80% in 1990 (35). It is too early to discern whether the new protective behaviors of young children will translate into habitual belt-wearing behaviors later in life. Misuse of child-restraint systems, which can reduce system effectiveness, has emerged as a significant problem, as has continued nonuse of restraints by parents and children from low-income and minority communities (1, 2).

Recent estimates suggest that the numbers of infant and toddler fatalities in motor vehicle crashes are 25–40% less than they might have been if child-restraint use laws had not been adopted (28). The national fatality statistics, reported in Table 3, also indicate that progress has been made in

Table 3 Percentage changes in US traffic fatality rates (per 100,000 population) by age group, 1980–1990[a]

All Ages	Under 5	5–14	15–24	25–44	45–64	65–74	75+
−21%	−33%	−28%	−25%	−22%	−12%	+1%	+11%

[a] From Ref. 73.

reducing traffic fatalities among young children. Whereas the crude mortality rate (per 100,000 population) has declined 21% among passengers of all ages, the age-specific mortality rate for kids under 5 has declined 33% from 1980 to 1990.

Restraining adults in the United States has proven to be much more difficult than restraining children. Informational and educational programs improved public knowledge and attitudes about safety belts, but did little to change belt-wearing behaviors. While consumer interest groups criticized vehicle manufacturers for marketing uncomfortable belt designs, vehicle manufacturers criticized government, insurers, and consumer advocates for neglecting to promote belt use.

In 1974, an effort was made to coerce belt use by requiring manufacturers to install ignition interlock devices in all new cars. This device prevented the car from starting unless belts were fastened. The interlock quickly became so unpopular that it was no longer required. Although Australia and other nations required belt use, highway funding incentives for American states that mandated adult restraint use were terminated in the midst of anti-interlock sentiments. Indeed, the interlock fiasco triggered political opposition to mandatory automatic restraints. On the one hand, conservatives lumped air bags and interlocks together in their legislative campaign to terminate Big Brother's regulatory powers. On the other hand, some insurers and consumer advocates began to oppose belt-promotion efforts actively, because they saw them as political substitutes for mandatory automatic restraint regulation (35).

It was not until 1984 that New York became the first state in the nation to require safety belt use (50, 98). Moving cautiously, the New York legislature began by requiring older children to wear restraints and later expanded the law to cover adults. Other states followed New York's lead, particularly when the Department of Transportation offered to repeal the automatic-restraint standard if two thirds of the nation were covered with belt-use laws by April 1989. Much to the dismay of insurers and consumer advocates, automotive interests financed lobbying efforts in numerous states to pave the way for belt-use laws. Although the April 1989 goal was not achieved (allowing the automatic restraint standard to take effect), many states continued to enact mandatory belt use laws (35). At latest count, 41 states have some form of adult restraint-use legislation.

State belt-use laws vary dramatically in their strength and comprehensiveness. The most significant flaw in these laws is that only eight states permit primary police enforcement (30). The other states restrict highway patrols to secondary enforcement, which means that an unbelted driver or passenger must be issued a ticket for another offense (e.g. speeding) before a fine for nonuse of belts may be assessed.

Observational studies indicate that belt-use rates increase significantly following enactment of adult restraint use legislation. Compared with pre-law usage rates of 10–20%, states with weak laws achieve compliance rates of 30–40%, whereas states with strong laws achieve compliance rates of 45–65% (8, 30). Specialized police enforcement campaigns can increase compliance rates under legislation that permits either primary or secondary police enforcement, but the gains from such campaigns are difficult to sustain over time. Belt-use rates have also increased modestly in those states that are not covered by belt-use legislation, which suggests a changing social norm toward belt use (30).

Because lap/shoulder belts are known to be about 40% effective in reducing an occupant's chance of crash-related fatality (22), one might expect recent laws to reduce occupant fatalities by 5–20%, depending upon the degree of compliance with the law (30). Although primary enforcement states have achieved fatality reductions within this range, it is difficult to detect any safety benefits in states that permit only secondary police enforcement (8, 9, 12, 30, 50, 82, 98, 113). The most prominent explanation for this discrepancy is the "selective recruitment" hypothesis, which posits that the first drivers to buckle up are those least likely to be involved in crashes (25, 81). If correct, this hypothesis suggests that far fewer lives are saved by increasing belt use from 10 to 40% than would be saved by increasing belt use from 40 to 70% or from 70 to 100%.

The introduction of automatic belt systems into new cars has also contributed to increasing rates of safety-belt use. Automatic safety belts are available in three basic designs that have achieved varying degrees of use.

Volkswagen (VW) pioneered the earliest design, which consists of a shoulder belt attached to the upper rear of the front door and connected to a take-up reel located between the front seats. Lower body restraint is provided by a knee bolster that prevents the occupant from submarining the shoulder belt. More recent VW designs include a manual lap belt. Although the VW belt design is detachable, it was originally guarded by an ignition-interlock system. Roadside observational surveys indicate that this system is used by about 80% of motorists, although the rate of use among motorists in crashes is reported to be as low as 40–50% (11, 83). The system's effectiveness in preventing fatalities (when used) has been demonstrated to be comparable to the effectiveness of manual lap/shoulder belts (when used) (11).

With the 1981 Cressida, Toyota introduced the first motorized automatic belt system, which was later modified by Ford and several other manufacturers. The shoulder belt is motor-driven and nondetachable. Both a knee bolster and manual lap belt are also provided with the system. Roadside observational surveys reveal that about 95% of motorists are restrained by the motorized shoulder belt, although only about 30% of motorists make the effort to fasten the manual lap belt (83). The effectiveness of the motorized system in reducing fatalities is not firmly established, but the results of the only published study are encouraging (64).

The third type of automatic belt design, used extensively by General Motors and Honda, is a lap/shoulder belt mounted near the upper and lower rear edge of the front door of the vehicle. This design is readily disconnected and is not guarded by an ignition-interlock system. Some motorists choose to use this system manually by disconnecting it at the end of a trip and reconnecting it at the beginning of the next trip (119). Observational surveys indicate that the rates of use achieved by this system in new cars approach 75%, although similar rates are achieved in new cars where manual lap/shoulder belt use is required by law (83). There is no reason to expect the effectiveness of this system (when used) to differ greatly from the effectiveness of manual lap/shoulder belts (when used).

In the future, manufacturers have indicated their intentions to replace automatic belt systems with manual lap/shoulder belt systems that are supplemented by driver and passenger air bags. Moreover, recent legislation passed by Congress mandates air bags and manual lap belts. Fears have been expressed that the presence of air bag protection might discourage motorists from buckling up, but early observations of cars equipped with air bags suggest that such fears may be groundless. One study found that 73.5% of motorists in new cars equipped with air bags were restrained by manual safety belts in a state (North Carolina) that requires belt use (83). Policymakers have not yet determined whether it makes sense to require manufacturers to install both air bags and automatic belt systems.

COST-EFFECTIVENESS COMPARISONS OF TRAFFIC SAFETY POLICIES

Although numerous traffic safety policies are being advocated and implemented in the United States, not all policy options are equally cost effective. Some preliminary cost-effectiveness ratios for traffic safety policies are presented in Figure 1.

The cost-effectiveness ratio is the estimated net cost of the policy divided by the estimated number of years of life saved (41). Net costs are equal to the gross resource costs of the policy minus any resource savings (e.g. reduced health care costs resulting from fewer injuries) attributable to the policy. Costs are calculated from a societal perspective, regardless of who bears the costs and savings. The ratios exclude various cost savings that are often included in complete benefit-cost analyses. Also excluded are intangible consumer inconveniences or dislikes of safety equipment. The estimated number of life years saved reflects the estimated number of premature deaths avoided by the policy and the average number of life years gained for each premature death

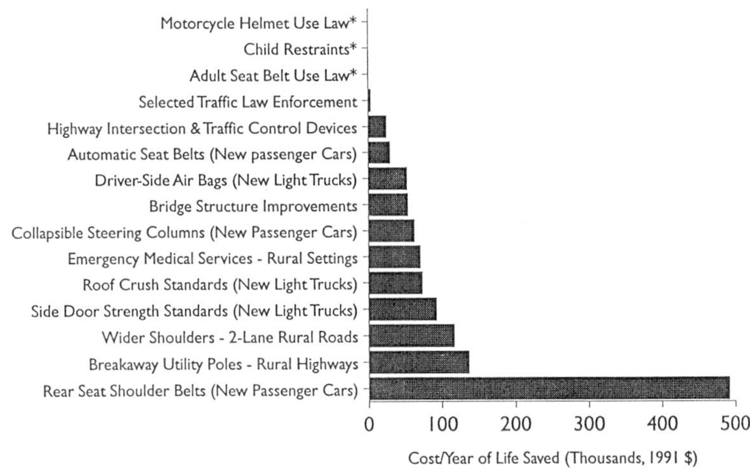

Figure 1 Cost-effectiveness ratios for selected traffic safety programs in the United States.

avoided. By using life years saved as the measure of policy effectiveness (instead of lives saved), more weight is given to policies that avert deaths in younger populations. Future costs, savings, and longevity gains are discounted at a real rate of 5% per year. All costs are expressed in dollars of 1991 purchasing power.

The ratios in Figure 1 demonstrate that traffic safety policy options vary widely in cost-effectiveness. Interestingly, motorcycle helmet-wearing laws are so attractive that the resources saved by reducing head trauma more than compensate for the resources consumed by the laws. Most of the cost-effectiveness ratios for traffic safety policies are less than $100,000 per life year saved.

When gauging the magnitude of cost-effectiveness ratios, it is useful to have some benchmarks from other fields of public health and medicine. The estimated costs of programs to prevent and treat coronary heart disease rarely exceed $100,000 per life year saved (41). Many occupational and environmental health regulations have cost-effectiveness ratios that exceed $100,000 per life year saved, although such rules are coming under increasing scrutiny by economists in the federal government (103).

Another sense of perspective is provided by economic studies of marketplace decisions involving risks to life by workers and consumers. These studies suggest that many citizens behave as if they are willing to pay at least $5 million to prevent an anonymous statistical death (108, 109). At a rate of 20 discounted life years per life saved, the willingness of citizens to pay for saving a statistical life year may exceed $250,000. This benchmark suggests that relatively few of the traffic safety policies under consideration represent poor economic investments. Although no one is advocating a strict, uniform cost-effectiveness criterion as social policy, good reasons should be offered to explain why cost-effective safety policies are not implemented.

OMINOUS TRENDS FOR THE FUTURE

Looking toward the year 2000, traffic safety policymakers will confront new challenges to the historical record of progress in reducing the fatality rate. Particularly important challenges are posed by the following trends: the rapidly growing number of older drivers, increasing travel speeds, the declining size and weight of passenger cars, the rapidly growing fleet of light trucks, and the exploration of intelligent vehicle and highway system (IVHS) technology.

More Older Drivers

From 1985 to 2020, the percentage of the US population over age 65 is predicted to increase from 10 to 17%, which may translate into a population of 50 million older drivers. Almost half of these drivers are predicted to be over the age of 75. Policymakers are only beginning to consider the implications of these demographic trends for occupant and pedestrian safety (100).

The number of motor vehicle fatalities per 100,000 population is higher for those aged 75 and older than for all other age groups, except 15–24-year-olds (73). This disparity is growing over time. From 1975 to 1990, the motor vehicle occupant fatality rate (per 100,000 population) declined in all age groups, except for those over the age of 80 who experienced a 20% increase (73). Although older drivers travel less frequently and at safer times than younger drivers, their rates of collision and fatality per mile of travel are elevated (15, 62). When collision rates per mile of travel are plotted by driver age, a U-shape curve emerges, with the youngest and oldest drivers exhibiting the highest collision rates. There is also good biomedical evidence that older drivers and pedestrians suffer more severe injuries than younger drivers and pedestrians for the same physical impact, which explains some of the elevated risks faced by older drivers (23, 100). Figure 2 reports estimated driver fatality rates per million miles of travel by driver age, thus revealing the sharply increasing mileage fatality rate for those persons over age 75.

State licensing authorities are already struggling with the implications of the changing age distribution of the population, but the scientific basis for new licensing policies is weak. Special driver education classes aimed at senior citizens are increasingly common in the effort to improve driving safety.

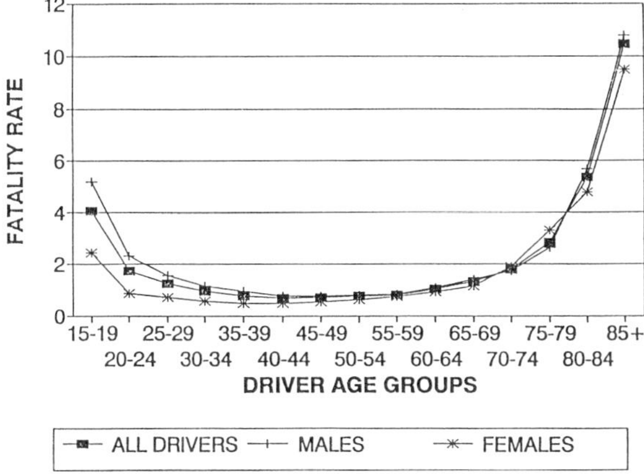

Figure 2 Driver fatality rate, 1990 (per 100 million vehicle miles traveled).

Although graduates are sometimes offered lower insurance premiums, the effectiveness of the classes in reducing traffic crashes has not been established. Some state licensing authorities are inclined to tighten licensing standards for senior citizens, but there is no indication that advanced age, per se, is a risk factor for traffic crashes. Certain medical impairments, such as decreased vision and dementia, are thought to contribute to the elevated fatality risks. There are no well-accepted tests that identify medically impaired elderly drivers (100, 101).

A case can be made for replacing standard road and knowledge testing with vision screening tests that detect impairment of nighttime and dynamic visual acuity. Further research is required to assess the reliability and validity of the assorted vision screening tests that have been proposed. Support is growing for graduated restrictions in the driving privileges of the elderly that might stipulate particular times of the day and/or roads where driving is permissable. Although such schemes already exist for youth with driving permits (80), a strong empirical basis does not yet exist for establishing a graduated licensing scheme for the elderly.

Physicians are also faced with the challenge of advising patients and their families about whether a patient should curtail or quit driving. Because many communities lack alternative transportation for senior citizens, a physician recommendation against driving can have profound effect on the patient's mobility and quality of life. Prescription drug use among the elderly may also impair driving performance, but more definitive research in this area is needed. Some states now require that physicians report to licensing authorities patients with medical conditions that may contraindicate driving, such as dementia. Such requirements complicate the physician-patient relationship, and evolving standards of medical negligence place physicians who refuse to report at greater liability. Although patients and families may be inclined to trust clinical judgments about traffic safety, no clinical guidelines in this area have a strong empirical basis.

Although much progress has been made in traffic safety, the efficacy of safety measures for elderly drivers are often unknown. Air bag systems, for example, may need to be redesigned to account for the frailty of the elderly. Traffic signs and electronic displays need to be understood by senior citizens. Given the growing size of the elderly population, progress in this area is urgently needed.

Faster Travel Speeds

The 55 MPH national maximum speed limit of 1974 was an historical aberration from the perspective of long-term trends in vehicle travel speeds (71). With that one major exception, travel speeds have increased steadily on all road and highway systems since World War II. During the last ten years, speeds have been rising steadily, even on highways that did not relax their speed limits (107).

In 1987, Congress permitted states to increase maximum speed limits from 55 to 65 miles per hour on selected portions of the rural Interstate Highway System. Roughly two thirds of the states elected this option, which has caused significant increases in average speeds on these segments of the interstates. Time series studies of individual states and highways, as well as national data, indicate that the higher speed limit has tended to increase average travel speeds and the number of traffic fatalities by 5–20% (6, 33). Some states, however, have managed to relax their speed limit to 65 MPH on rural interstate highways without experiencing significant increases in highway fatalities (34). The explanation for this phenomenon may lie in a decline in speed variance that can result from a more permissive, yet strictly enforced, speed limit (52).

Climbing travel speeds have been facilitated by increasing consumer interest in engine horsepower. The average horsepower of new cars per pound of vehicle weight has increased markedly in the 1980s, and this ratio now exceeds the ratio observed in the 1960s, the era of "muscle cars" (37, 72). Engine horsepower permits faster acceleration times and higher mean speeds, which can increase the probability of collisions and increase the severity of injuries when collisions occur. Cars with more powerful engines are associated with higher fatality rates, but it is unclear whether this association reflects differences in drivers, differences in engines, or both (90). Unless fuel prices increase significantly in the future, there is little reason to expect that consumer desires for increasing engine horsepower will fade.

Declining Size and Weight of Passenger Cars

In response to gasoline shortages in the 1970s and intensified regulatory pressures for improved fuel economy, vehicle manufacturers have reduced both the size (exterior dimensions) and weight of new passenger cars. From 1974 to 1990, average new car fuel economy doubled from 14 to 28 miles per gallon. During the same period, the average weight of new cars declined 25%, while average vehicle shadow (weight times width) declined 16% (37). The recent Persian Gulf crisis and concerns about global warming have led to legislative proposals to increase average new car fuel economy to 40 or more miles per gallon by the year 2000.

Other things being equal, reducing vehicle size and weight increases the probability that vehicle occupants will experience serious or fatal injuries in crashes (19, 53, 69, 70). This effect occurs in both single- and multivehicle crashes, although it is stronger in single-vehicle crashes, which account for the majority of occupant fatalities (25). Car mass is so important to occupant safety that driving unbelted in a larger car is about as safe as driving restrained in a small car (20). Because vehicle weight and size have subtly different effects on occupant protection, they need to be considered separately.

If two vehicles of comparable size, weight, and integrity collide at equal speeds, occupant injury risks should be comparable in the two vehicles. If one of the two vehicles is heavier (without being larger), its occupants will be safer, but only at the expense of increasing danger to occupants of the other vehicle. For this reason, it is not clear whether reduction of vehicle weight, per se, results in a net increase in safety risks for occupants in the two vehicles (37). If one of the two vehicles is made heavier by providing larger exterior dimensions and energy-absorbing structure, the safety impacts for the occupants of both vehicles may be favorable. Not only are the occupants of the larger vehicle better off, but the occupants in the smaller vehicle are safer because the improved management of crash forces in the larger vehicle reduces transfer of energy to the occupants of the smaller vehicle. Empirical studies of real-world crash data suggest that the crashworthiness benefits of larger vehicles more than offset the aggressivity risks that heavier vehicles create in multivehicle crashes (26, 37).

In the single-vehicle crash, both vehicle size and vehicle weight operate to protect occupants (25). Larger exterior dimensions provide more room for buckling as the occupant rides down the crash (47). Vehicle mass would be irrelevant to crash injury risk if the roadside object was absolutely immovable and impenetrable, but most roadside objects are somewhat movable and penetrable. Hence, single-vehicle crashes are more dangerous to light cars than to heavy cars, even if vehicles sizes are comparable (69, 70).

There is considerable interest in whether vehicle dimensions influence the probability of collision, but reliable empirical evidence is scant (21). The fundamental problem is that the drivers of large and small vehicles behave differently in ways that influence collision risks, and driver behavior is the dominant factor in determining collision frequency. The only clear result has been that vehicle dimensions influence the probability of a rollover crash, which is known to cause serious injuries and fatalities. Smaller cars have less directional stability than larger cars, and they are less likely to remain upright if the vehicle is tripped during an off-road excursion. Thus, some combination of vehicle height, weight, and width causes large cars to have fewer fatal rollover crashes than small cars, adjusting for differences in driver behavior (37, 69).

Growth of the Light Truck Fleet

While the passenger car fleet grows smaller and lighter, consumers are buying increasing numbers of light trucks, such as pick-ups, minivans, and multipurpose vehicles. The introduction of light trucks has reduced the market for large cars (e.g. station wagons), as many light trucks are used regularly for passenger-carrying purposes. About one third of all new vehicle sales are comprised of various types of light trucks (37). The relative growth of the light truck fleet is apparent in crude fatality counts. From 1975 to 1990, while occupant fatalities in passenger cars declined 7%, occupant fatalities in light trucks increased 77% (66).

Although light trucks are not necessarily more dangerous than large cars, they pose new safety questions that have not been studied adequately. Some light trucks have elevated rates of rollover crashes, which has led to interest in new designs that might improve vehicle stability. Unlike cars built with unibody construction, some light trucks are designed with frame construction (i.e. the body rests on a rectangular frame). Some analysts hypothesize that the stiffness of the frame construction causes these vehicles to be more aggressive in multivehicle crashes than vehicles designed with unibody construction (46). Finally, the federal government has only recently begun to insist that federal motor vehicle safety standards applicable to passenger cars (e.g. automatic restraint protection) are also applied to the light-truck fleet.

Intelligent Vehicle and Highway Systems

Recent advances in technology have stimulated the development and testing of IVHS, which utilizes computer and communications technology to provide information to motorists about road and travel conditions and to monitor and/or control the operation of vehicles (102). Although the primary purpose of IVHS technology is improved traffic flow and communications, the technology may have important consequences for traffic safety. For example, innovative applications of radar and computer technology may be used to prevent motor vehicle collisions on the highway.

The implementation of "smart" vehicles and highways, if not designed with the entire driving population in mind, could create new safety problems. For instance, elaborate instrument panels need to be designed for use by elderly drivers with slow reaction times and significant visual impairments. Some IVHS technologies, however, can provide early warnings to drivers of dangerous conditions, which might be particularly valuable to elderly drivers. The US Department of Transportation is launching a major research and development program to advance IVHS concepts. This program needs to give significant attention to the safety benefits and risks of IVHS technology (101).

THE NEGLECTED ROAD-USERS

Although motor vehicle occupants account for two thirds of traffic fatalities each year, other road-users are also endangered and have tended to be neglected by traffic safety policymakers. Pedestrians, motorcyclists, and bicyclists are the most important categories of other road-users.

Pedestrians

In 1990, about 6500 pedestrians were killed in motor vehicle crashes (66). Persons under age 10 or over age 65 are at increased risk of pedestrian fatalities (79, 85). Poor urban communities exhibit higher rates of pedestrian injury than wealthier suburban communities, presumably because of higher traffic densities, greater population densities, higher average vehicle speeds, and fewer alternatives for street play (63). The "dart-out" type of injury, in which a child darts out into the street in midblock, accounts for 60–70% of pedestrian injuries among children under age 5 and 50–60% for those aged 5–9 (85).

Childhood training programs have been initiated to reduce the incidence of pedestrian injuries (58). The evaluations have been mixed and of varying technical quality. At present, there is no well-developed curriculum that can be readily transferred to the school setting with the promise of producing large increases in correct pedestrian behavior by children (85, 86).

The effects of new traffic laws on pedestrian safety have been mixed. Popular "right-turn-on-red" laws have been associated with a 30% increase in child pedestrian injuries (85). Where laws exist to protect pedestrians, their enforcement receives little emphasis by police or support by elected officials. Few programs aimed at changing driver behavior to protect pedestrians have demonstrated effectiveness (58).

Modification of the roadway environment offers some promise of pedestrian protection. Sidewalks, pedestrian paths, and off-street playgrounds reduce pedestrian exposure to traffic. Greater use of one-way streets and parking restrictions can make it easier for both drivers and pedestrians to avoid collisions (65, 85).

Vehicles can be redesigned to reduce the severity of pedestrian injury. When pedestrians are injured by motor vehicles, a majority of the injuries are attributable to the pedestrian being "run under" and thrown up on to the car, rather than being "run over" and contacted only by the wheels and pavement. The exterior of the vehicle, particularly the front hood, can be redesigned to reduce significantly the severity of pedestrian injury. Recent studies suggest significant variation in the pedestrian protection offered by various cars in the fleet (85, 89). Any design changes proposed to protect pedestrians may need to be refined to avoid unexpected increases in crash risks to drivers and passengers.

Bicyclists and Motorcyclists

Each year, about 1000 bicyclists are killed, primarily because of collisions with motor vehicles (73). Another 500,000 bicyclists suffer nonfatal injuries of varying degrees of severity, although most of these injuries are attributable to falls that are not caused by collisions with motor vehicles (65, 67). Children and young adults account for the majority of bicycle injuries and fatalities.

In 1990, 3238 motorcyclists died in crashes, or about 27% fewer than the 4453 motorcyclists who were killed in 1982 (66). This decline reflects primarily the sharp drop in the popularity of motorcycling that occurred in the 1980s, which is reflected in the dwindling number of registered motorcycles and the estimated decline in vehicle miles traveled by motorcyclists (73).

The patterns of bicycle and motorcycle injuries differ significantly (5). The ratio of nonfatal injuries to fatalities is much smaller for motorcyclists than bicyclists. Whereas injured bicyclists are most likely to be in the 5–14-year age group, motorcyclists are most likely to be in the 15–24-year age group. A majority of fatally injured motorcyclists exhibit elevated blood alcohol concentrations, yet few bicyclists had been drinking alcohol before their accidents (66). Despite these differences, the principal cause of serious trauma among both types of cyclists is head injury.

In the 1966 Highway Safety Act, Congress required states to adopt motorcycle helmet-wearing laws as a condition for receiving federal highway funds. By 1974, all but three states had adopted such laws, and the Department of Transportation was moving to reduce their highway funding allocations. In 1975, at the insistence of the state of California, which had not adopted a helmet law, Congress removed the federal government's power to rescind highway funds from states without helmet laws. This legislative change not only protected California, but induced two dozen other states to repeal or weaken their helmet-wearing laws.

Numerous studies have traced the public health consequences of adopting and repealing motorcycle helmet-wearing laws. Helmet-wearing rates increase from less than 50% to almost 100% following enactment of helmet laws. Wearing rates decline to almost 50% when laws are repealed or applied only to younger motorcyclists (40). The immediate and large changes in head protection have been linked directly to changes in the numbers of motorcyclists killed in motorcycle crashes (40, 114).

Recent studies demonstrate that head injuries, which are a major cause of serious trauma among bicyclists, can also be prevented by wearing approved bicycle helmets (10). Current rates of bicycle helmet use are quite low, but community demonstration projects have shown that voluntary rates of bicycle helmet use among children can be increased through information and education. In Australia, bicycle helmet-wearing rates among children of 60–80% have been achieved through legal requirements. The Centers for Disease Control (CDC), through its Injury Prevention Centers, has recently played an increasingly effective role in promoting bicycle helmet use among children (10).

CRISIS IN TRAFFIC SAFETY RESEARCH?

Despite the track record of progress in traffic safety and the new challenges that lie ahead, investments in traffic safety research declined in the 1980s. For example, the amount of real research dollars expended by the NHTSA declined 30% in the 1980s (101). The number of university-based research teams is declining, and few young scientists are entering the field. A panel of the Transportation Research Board recently called for the federal government to reverse this trend by making peer-reviewed, investigator-initiated research a funding priority at the US Department of Transportation (101). The insurance industry recently made a multimillion dollar commitment to a new crash testing facility that should provide independent data on the relative safety of motor vehicle designs. The major domestic and foreign vehicle manufacturers also need to make greater investments in traffic safety research. Yet, private sector investments in safety research are quite vulnerable to the vagaries of the business cycle.

SAFETY IN THE ECONOMIC AND POLITICAL MARKETPLACES

The early years of the 1990s suggest that trauma from traffic crashes may emerge again as one of the nation's major health priorities. Growing public concern about traffic safety is apparent in both the economic and political marketplaces.

In dealer showrooms, consumers are demanding more information about which vehicle safety features are available and which models offer the best safety protection. Vehicle manufacturers are beginning to compete on the basis of safety in their advertising campaigns, despite the conventional wisdom that "safety doesn't sell." The competition among manufacturers for the pro-safety image has become so intense that manufacturers frequently install safety features (e.g. rear-seat shoulder belts) before they are required to do so by the federal government (36). The growing threat of product liability may also be motivating manufacturers to install safety features, but in some cases the incentives induced by liability have perverse effects on safety (36, 99). For instance, manufacturers may be reluctant to correct design defects promptly out of fear that plaintiffs' attorneys will use such actions as evidence of prior negligence in product liability suits (36).

The interest of elected officials in traffic safety is increasing as the public health community portrays injury as a major health issue. Citizen activist groups at the federal, state, and local levels are building grass-roots constituencies to place motor vehicle trauma on the agenda of policymakers (7). In 1987, with support from the Institute of Medicine and Congress, CDC launched a major new program of research and intervention to control all forms of intentional and unintentional injury. A national agenda for the 1990s has been established (10). CDC is working with states to forge coalitions between transportation officials, public safety officers, and public health professionals (18). CDC is also working with NHTSA and other federal agencies to coordinate the federal government's multifaceted effort to improve the safety of drivers, vehicles, and highways. One of the keys to achieving success in the 1990s is to foster constructive partnerships between both different government agencies and organizations in the public and private sectors.

CONCLUSION

Traffic injuries remain a large public health problem, even though major progress has been made in reducing the rate of fatal injury from highway travel. Pro-safety programs have not been as balanced and comprehensive as they should have been. Vehicle occupants are much safer in crashes today than they were 20 years ago, yet less attention has been given to the safety of bicyclists and pedestrians. Technological improvements in vehicle and highway design dominated the attention of policymakers in the 1960s and 1970s, but the recent trends toward safety-belt use and sober driving suggest that the behavioral strategy also has an important role to play.

Progress in traffic safety has taken a long time, which reflects the necessity of changing the attitudes and social norms of elected officials, corporate executives, consumer interests, and the public. The new generation of safety leaders will face a different mix of safety challenges spawned by an aging population of drivers, smart vehicles and highways, more small cars and light trucks, and more powerful engines and permissive speed limits.

To meet these challenges, traffic safety professionals need a richer knowledge base, more appreciation of cost-effectiveness in use of scarce resources, and a collaborative approach to organizing the efforts of traditional adversaries in the public and private sectors. The growing consumer and public interest in vehicle and highway safety is an encouraging sign, because it will help attract resources to a field that is paradoxically rich in public health success yet poor in resources.

ACKNOWLEDGEMENTS

Helpful comments on this article were provided by Bei-Hung Chang, Joshua Cohen, Bruce Kennedy, Lester Lave, Ilana Lescohier, Nancy Isaac, Deborah Servi, and Constance Williams.

Literature Cited

1. Agran, P., Castillo, D., Winn, D. 1990. Childhood motor vehicle occupant injuries. *Am. J. Dis. Child.* 144:653–62
2. Agran, P., Winn, D. G., Castillo, D. N. 1992. On-lap travel: still a problem in motor vehicles. *Pediatrics* 90:27–29
3. Alexander, R. H., Pons, P. T., Krischer, J., Hunt, P. 1986. The effect of advanced life support and sophisticated hospital systems on motor vehicle mortality. *J. Trauma* 24:486
4. Asch, P., Levy, D. T. 1982. Does the minimum drinking age affect traffic fatalities? *J. Policy Anal. Manage.* 6:180–92
5. Baker, S. P., O'Neill, B., Ginsburg, M. J., Li, G. 1992. *The Injury Fact Book.* New York: Oxford Univ. Press. 2nd ed.
6. Baum, H. M., Wells, J. K., Lund, A. K. 1991. The fatality consequences of the 65 mph speed limits, 1989. *J. Saf. Res.* 22:171–77
7. Bergman, A. B., ed. 1992. *Political Approaches to Injury Control at the State Level.* Seattle: Univ. Washington Press
8. Campbell, B. J., Campbell, F. A. 1988. Injury reduction and belt use associated with occupant restraint laws. In *Preventing Automobile Injury: Recent Findings from Evaluation Research,* ed. J. D. Graham, pp. 24–50. Dover, Mass: Auburn
9. Campbell, B. J., Stewart, J. R., Reinfurt, D. W. 1991. Change in injuries associated with safety belt laws. *Accid. Anal. Prev.* 23:87–93
10. Cent. Dis. Control. Apr. 1992. *Setting the National Agenda for Injury Control in the 1990's.* Position papers from the 3rd Natl. Injury Control Conf. US Public Health Serv.
11. Chi, G. Y. H., Reinfurt, D. 1981. *A Comparison of the Automatic Shoulder Belt/Knee Bolster Restraint System with the Lap and Shoulder Belt System in VW Rabbits.* Chapel Hill, NC: Highway Saf. Res. Cent., Univ. North Carolina
12. Chorba, T., Reinfurt, D., Hulka, B. S. 1988. Efficacy of mandatory seatbelt legislation. *J. Am Med. Assoc.* 260:3593–97
13. Claybrook, J. 1984. *Retreat from Safety,* Public Citizen, Washington, DC
14. Cook P., Tauchen, G. 1984. The effects of minimum drinking age legislation on youthful auto fatalities, 1970–77. *J. Legal Stud.* 13:169–88
15. Copper, P. J. 1990. Differences in accident characteristics among elderly drivers and between elderly and middle-aged drivers. *Accid. Anal. Prev.* 22:499–508
16. Crandall, R., Graham, J. D. 1989. The effect of fuel economy standards on automobile safety. *J. Law Econ.* 32:97–118
17. Decker, M. D., Graitcer, P. L., Schaf-

fer, W. 1988. Reduction in motor vehicle fatalities associated with an increase in the minimum drinking age. *J. Am. Med. Assoc.* 260:3604–10

18. Educ. Dev. Cent. 1991. *Building Bridges Between Traffic Safety and Public Health.* Newton, Mass: Educ. Dev. Cent.
19. Evans, L. 1984. Driver fatalities versus car mass using a new exposure approach. *Accid. Anal. Prev.* 16:19–36
20. Evans, L. 1985. Fatality risk for belted drivers versus car mass. *Accid. Anal. Prev.* 17:251
21. Evans, L. 1985. Driver age, car mass and accident exposure—a synthesis of available data. *Accid. Anal. Prev.* 17: 439–48
22. Evans, L. 1986. The effectiveness of safety belts in preventing fatalities. *Accid. Anal. Prev.* 18:229–41
23. Evans, L. 1988. Older driver involvement in fatal severe traffic crashes. *J. Gerontol.* 43:5186–93
24. Evans, L. 1990. The fraction of traffic fatalities attributable to alcohol. *Accid. Anal. Prev.* 22:587–602
25. Evans, L. 1991. *Traffic Safety and the Driver.* New York: Van Norstrand Reinhold
26. Evans, L., Frick, M. C. 1992. Car size and car mass: which has greater influence on fatality risk? *Am. J. Public Health* 82:1105–12
27. Evans, W., Graham, J. D. 1988. Traffic safety and the business cycle. *Alcohol Drugs Driving* 4:31–38
28. Evans, W., Graham, J. D. 1990. An estimate of the lifesaving benefit of child restraint use legislation. *J. Health Econ.* 9:121–42
29. Evans, W., Neville D., Graham, J. D. 1991. General deterrence of drunk driving: Evaluation of recent American policies. *Risk Anal.* 11:279–89
30. Evans, W., Graham, J. D. 1991. Risk reduction or risk compensation? The case of mandatory safety belt use laws. *J Risk Uncertainty,* pp. 61–73
31. Farrell, S. 1989. Policy alternatives for alcohol-impaired driving. *Health Educ. Q.* 16:413–27
32. Foldary, L. A. Lane, J. C. 1974. The effectiveness of compulsory wearing of seat belts in casualty reduction. *Accid. Anal. Prev.* 6:59–81
33. Freedman, M., Williams, A. F. 1991 Speeds associated with 55-mph and 65-mph speed limits in Northeastern states. *ITE J.,* pp. 17–21
34. Garber, S., Graham, J. D. 1990. The effects of the new 65 mile-per-hour speed limit on rural highway fatalities: a state-by-state analysis. *Accid. Anal. Prev.* 22:137–49
35. Graham, J. D. 1989. *Auto Safety: Assessing America's Performance.* Dover, Mass: Auburn. 253 pp.
36. Graham, J. D. 1991. Product liability and motor vehicle safety. In *The Liability Maze,* ed. P. W. Huber, R. Litan, pp. 120–90. Washington, DC: Brookings Inst. 513 pp.
37. Graham, J. D. 1992. The safety risks of new fuel economy legislation. *Risk: Issues Health Saf.* 3:95–126
38. Graham, J. D., Chang, B.-H., Evans, J. S. 1992. Poorer is riskier. *Risk Anal.* 12:333–37
39. Graham, J. D., Garber, S. 1984. Evaluating the effects of automobile safety regulation. *J. Policy Anal. Manage.* 3:206–24
40. Graham, J. D., Lee, Y. 1986. Behavioral responses to safety regulation: the case of motorcycle helmet-wearing legislation. *Policy Sci.* 19:253–73
41. Graham, J. D., Vaupel, J. W. 1981. The value of a life: what difference does it make? *Risk Anal.* 1:89–95
42. Howat, P., Sleet, D., Smith, I. 1991. Alcohol and driving: is the 0.05% blood alcohol concentration limit justified? *Drug Alcohol Rev.* 10:151–66
43. Howland, J. 1988. Social norms and drunk driving countermeasures. In *Preventing Automobile Injury: New Findings from Evaluation Research,* ed. J. D. Graham, pp. 163–80. Dover, Mass: Auburn. 287 pp.
44. Hingson, R., Howland, J, Levenson, S. 1988. Effects of legislative reform to reduce drunken driving and alcohol-related traffic fatalities. *Public Health Rep.* 103:659–67
45. Hingson, R., Heeren, T., Howland, J., Winter, M. 1991. Reduced BAC limits for young people. *Alcohol Drugs Driving* 7:117–27
46. Insur. Inst. for Highway Saf. 1981. *Policy Options for Reducing the Motor Vehicle Crash Injury Cost Burden,* Alexandria, Va: Insur. Inst. Highway Saf.
47. Insur. Inst. for Highway Saf. 1990. *Status Report: Highway Loss Reduction* 25(8):1–12
48. Jacobs, J. B. 1989. *Drunk Driving: An American Dilemma,* Chicago: Univ. Chicago Press
49. Joksch, H. C. 1984. The relation between motor vehicle accident deaths and economic activity. *Accid. Anal. Prev.* 16:207–10
50. Latimer, E., Lave, L. B. 1987. Initial effects of the New York state auto

safety belt use law. *Am. J. Public Health* 77:183–86
51. Laurence, M. D., Snortum, J. R., Zimring, F., eds. 1988. *Social Control of the Drinking Driver*. Chicago: Univ. Chicago Press
52. Lave, C. 1985. Speeding, coordination, and the 55-mph limit. *Am. Econ. Rev.* 75:1159–64
53. Lave, L. B. 1981. Conflicting objectives in regulating the automobile. *Science* 212:893–99
54. Levy, D. 1990. Youth and traffic safety: The effects of driving age, experience, and education. *Accident Anal. & Prev.* 22:327–334
55. Levy, D., Shea, D., Asch, P. 1989. Traffic safety effects of sobriety checkpoints and other local DWI programs in New Jersey. *Am. J. Public Health,* 79:291–293
56. Lund, A. K., Wolfe, A. C. 1991. Changes in the incidence of alcohol-impaired driving in the United States, 1973–86. *J. Stud. Alcohol* 52:293–310
57. MacKinnon, D. P., Woodward, J. A. 1986. The impact of raising the minimum drinking age on driver fatalities. *Int. J. Addict.* 21:131
58. Malek, M., Guyer, B., Lescohier, I. 1990. The epidemiology and prevention of child pedestrian injury. *Accid. Anal. Prev.* 22:301–13
59. Males, M. 1986. The minimum purchase age for alcohol and young-driver fatal crashes: a longterm view. *J. Legal Stud.* 15:181–209
60. Mann, R. E., Vingilis, E. R., Gavin, D., Adlaf, E., Anglin, L. 1991. Sentence severity and the drinking driver: relationships with traffic safety outcome. *Accid. Anal. Prev.* 23:483–91
61. Masher, J. F. 1985. Alcohol policy and the Presidential Commission on Drunk Driving: the paths not taken. *Accid. Anal. Prev.* 17:239
62. Mortimer, R. G., Fell, J. C. 1989. Older drivers: their night fatal crash involvement and risk. *Accid. Anal. Prev.* 21:273–82
63. Mueller, B. A., Rivaa, F. P. 1990. Environmental factors and the risk for childhood pedestrian-motor vehicle collision occurrence. *Am. J. Epidemiol.* 132:550–60
64. Nash, C. 1989. The effectiveness of automatic belts in reducing fatality rates in Toyota Cressidas. *Accid. Anal. Prev.* 21:517–27
65. Natl. Comm. for Injury Prev. and Control. 1989. *Injury Prevention: Meeting the Challenge*. New York: Oxford Univ. Press
66. Natl. Highway Traffic Saf. Adm. *Fatal Accident Reporting System*. Washington, DC (annual)
67. Natl. Highway Traffic Saf. Adm. *General Estimates System*. Washington, DC (annual)
68. Natl. Highway Traffic Saf. Adm. 1985. *Emergency Medical Services Program and its Relationship to Highway Safety*. Washington, DC: Natl. Highway Traffic Saf. Adm.
69. Natl. Highway Traffic Saf. Adm. 1991. *A Collection of Recent Analyses of Vehicle Weight and Safety*. Washington, DC: Natl. Highway Traffic Saf. Adm.
70. Natl. Highway Traffic Saf. Adm. 1990. *Effect of Car Size on Fatality and Injury Risk in Single-Vehicle Crashes*. Washington, DC: Natl. Highway Traffic Saf. Adm.
71. Natl. Res. Counc. 1984. *55: A Decade of Experience,* Washington, DC: Natl. Acad. Press
72. Natl. Res. Counc. 1992. *Automotive Fuel Economy: How Far Should We Go?* Washington, DC: Natl. Acad. Press
73. Natl. Saf. Counc. 1992. *Accident Facts 1991 Edition*. Chicago: Natl. Saf. Counc.
74. O'Malley, P. M., Wagenaar, A. C. 1991. Effects of minimum drinking age laws on alcohol use, related behaviors, and traffic crash involvement among American youth: 1976–1987. *J. Stud. Alcohol* 52:478–91
75. Onato, J. P., Craren, E. J., Nelson, N. M., Kimball, K. F. 1985. Impact of improved emergency medical services and emergency trauma care on the reduction of mortality from trauma. *J. Trauma* 25:575–79
76. Partyka, S. 1984. Simple models of fatality trends using employment and population data. *Accid. Anal. Prev.* 16:211–22
77. Peck, R. 1991. The general and specific deterrent effects of DUI sanctions: a review of California's experience. *Alcohol Drugs Driving* 7:13–42
78. Peltzman, S. 1975. *Regulation of Automobile Safety*. Washington, DC: Am. Enterp. Inst.
79. Pitt, R., Guyer, B., Hsieh, C., Malek, M. 1990, The severity of pedestrian injuries in children: an analysis of the pedestrian injury causation study. *Accid. Anal. Prev.* 22:549–59
80. Preusser, D. 1988. Delaying teenage licensure. *Alcohol Drugs Driving: Rev. Abstr.* 4:283–95
81. Preusser, D. F., Williams, A. F. 1991.

Characteristics of belted and unbelted drivers. *Accid. Anal. Prev.* 23:475–82
82. Reinfurt, D. W., Campbell, B. J., Stewart, J. R., Stutts, J. C. 1990. Evaluating the North Carolina safety belt wearing law. *Accid. Anal. Prev.* 22:197–210
83. Reinfurt, D. W., St. Cyr, C. L., Hunter, W. W. 1991. Usage patterns and misuse rates of automatic seat belts by system type. *Accid. Anal. Prev.* 23:521–30
84. Rice, D. P., MacKenzie, E. J. 1989. *Cost of Injury in the United States: A Report to Congress.* San Francisco: Univ. Calif.
85. Rivara, F. P. 1991. Prevention of pedestrian injuries to children: effectiveness of a school training program. *Pediatrics* 88:770–775
86. Rivara, F. P. 1990. Child pedestrian injuries in the United States. *Am. J. Dis. Child.* 144:692–96
87. Robertson, L. S. 1981. Automobile safety regulations and death reductions in the United States. *Am. J. Public Health,* 71:818–22
88. Robertson, L. S. 1983. *Injuries: Causes, Control Strategies, and Public Policy.* Lexington, Mass: Heath
89. Robertson, L. S. 1990. Car design and risk of pedestrian deaths. *Am. J. Public Health* 80:609–10
90. Robertson, L. S. 1991. How to save fuel and reduce injuries in automobiles. *J. Trauma* 31:107–9
91. Ross, H. L. 1982. *Deterring the Drinking Driver: Legal Policy and Social Context,* Lexington, Mass: Heath
92. Ross, H. L., Klette, H., McCleary, R. 1984. Liberalization and rationalization of drunk driving laws in Scandinavia. *Accid. Anal. Prev.* 16:471–87
93. Saffer, H., Gorssman, M. 1987. Beer taxes, the legal drinking age, and youth motor vehicle fatalities. *J. Legal Stud.* 26:351–74
94. Saffer, H., Grossman, M. 1987. Drinking age laws and highway mortality rates: cause and effect. *Econ. Inq.* 25:403–17
95. Shinar, D. 1992. Impact of court monitoring on the adjudication of driving while intoxicated. *Accid. Anal. Prev.* 24:167–79
96. Simpson, H. M., Mayhew, D. R. 1991. *The Hard Core Drinking Driver.* Ottawa: Traffic Injury Res. Found. of Canada. 110pp.
97. Deleted in proof.
98. States, J. D. 1990. A time comparison study of the New York State Safety Belt Use Law utilizing hospital admission and police accident report information. *Accid. Anal. Prev.* 22:509–21
99. Teret, S. 1981. Injury control and product liability. *J. Public Health Policy* 2:49–57
100. Transp. Res. Board. 1988. *Transportation in an Aging Society.* Washington, DC: Transp. Res. Board
101. Transp. Res. Board. 1990. *Safety Research for a Changing Highway Environment.* Washington, DC: Transp. Res. Board
102. Transp. Res. Board. 1991. *Advanced Vehicle and Highway Technologies.* Washington, DC: Transp. Res. Board
103. Travis, C. C., Pack, S. R., Fisher, A. 1987. Cost-effectiveness as a factor in cancer risk management. *Environ. Int.* 13:469–74
104. US Public Health Serv. 1990. *Alcohol and Health.* 7th Special Rep. to the Congress. Rockville, Md.
105. US Public Health Serv. 1988. *Surgeon General's Workshop on Drunk Driving,* Washington, DC:
106. US Dep. of Transp. 1991. *Alcohol Limits for Drivers: A Report on the Effects of Alcohol and Expected Institutional Responses to New Limits.* Rep. to Congress
107. US Dep. of Transp. *Highway Statistics Annual,* Washington, DC (annual)
108. Viscusi, W. K. 1986. The valuation of risks to life and health. In *Benefit Assessment: The State of the Art,* ed. J Bentkover, pp. 193–210. Boston: Reidel
109. Viscusi, W. K. 1983. *Risk by Choice,* Cambridge, Mass: Harvard Univ. Press
110. Wagenaar, A. 1983. *Alcohol, Young Drivers, and Traffic Accidents.* Dover, Mass: Heath
111. Wagenaar, A., 1983. Raising the legal drinking age in Maine: impact on traffic accidents among young drivers. *Int. J. Addict.* 18:365–77
112. Wagenaar, A. C. 1984. Effects of macroeconomic conditions on the incidence of motor vehicle accidents. *Accid. Anal. Prev.* 16:191–205
113. Wagenaar, A. 1987. Mandatory seat belt laws in eight states: a time-series evaluation. *J. Saf. Res.* 19:243–49
114. Watson, G. S., Zador, P. L., Wilks, A. 1980. The repeal of helmet use laws and increased motorcyclist mortality in the United States, 1975–78. *Am. J. Public Health* 70:579–85
115. Williams, A. F. 1979. Evaluation of the Tennessee Child Restraint Law. *Am. J. Public Health* 69:455–58
116. Williams, A. F. 1991. The effectiveness of administrative license suspen-

sion laws. *Alcohol Drugs Driving* 7: 55–62

117. Williams, A. F. 1992. Decline in alcohol-impaired driving and crashes and why it occurred. *Alcohol Drugs Driving* 8:71–76
118. Williams, A. F., Lund, A. K. 1990. Alcohol-impaired driving and crashes involving alcohol in the United States during the 1970s and 1980s. *Proc. of 11th Int. Conf. on Alcohol, Drugs, and Traffic Saf.* (T89), pp. 109–5. Chicago: Natl. Saf. Counc.
119. Williams, A. F., Wells, J. K., Lund, A. K., Teed, N. 1989. Observed use of automatic seat belts in 1987 cars. *Accid. Anal. Prev.* 21:427–33
120. Williams, A. F., Zador, P. L., Harris, S. S., Karpf, R. S. 1983. The effect of raising the legal minimum drinking age on alcohol involvement in fatal crashes. *J. Legal Stud.* 12:169–79
121. Williams, T. P., Lillis, R. P. 1986. Change in alcohol consumption by 18-year olds following an increase in New York's purchase age to nineteen. *J. Stud. Alcohol* 47:290–96
122. Wilson, R. J., Mann R., eds. 1990. *Drinking and Driving: Advances in Research and Prevention.* New York: Guilford
123. Zobeck, T. S., Elliott, S. D., Bertolucci, D. 1991. Trends in alcohol-related fatal crashes, United States. *Surveillance Report,* No. 19. Washington, DC: US Dep. of Health and Hum. Serv.

Annu. Rev. Publ. Health 1993. 14:545–84

RESTRAINING RESTRAINTS: Changes in a Standard of Care

Robert L. Kane
School of Public Health, University of Minnesota, Minneapolis, Minnesota 55455

Carter C. Williams
287 Dartmouth Street, Rochester, New York 14607

T. Franklin Williams
Department of Preventive Medicine and Community Health, University of Rochester, Rochester, New York 14627

Rosalie A. Kane
School of Public Health, University of Minnesota, Minneapolis, Minnesota 55455

KEY WORDS: psychoactive drugs, nursing homes, elderly, regulations

INTRODUCTION

Societal views about the appropriate role of physical and chemical restraints have long been an issue. The last decade has witnessed a remarkable change in American social philosophy and concomitant nursing and medical practice, which has led to a repudiation of indiscriminate use of restraints to control patients' behavior. Strumpf & Tomes (52) trace the accepting attitudes that permitted the use of physical restraints, which predominated until the 1980s, back to nineteenth century ideas about how to manage mentally ill persons. The authors distinguish between the moral treatment practiced in England, which viewed restraints as a last resort, with the treatment practiced by American asylum superintendents, who viewed security and restraint as critical aspects of responsible patient management. The mantle of responsibility for implementing physical restraint use was quietly shifted to nursing, which was emerging as a profession.

Restraint use is a metaphor for society's approach to care. This century has seen a dramatic shift from a model of professional dominance to one in which

0163-7525/93/0510-0545$02.00

the patient has a substantial role. Attention has shifted, to at least some degree, from simply performing technical acts on or for the patient to a philosophy of person-centered care, in which the autonomous functioning of the client becomes a major goal. As emphasis shifts from examining only the individual elements of care to appreciating the importance of how those elements fit into a full system of care delivery, so too does the importance of the total effect of all parts of caring (both intended and not) on the patient. New strategies for care that involve the patient, rather than act on the patient, are being incorporated in nursing and other disciplines.

CONVERGING INTELLECTUAL STREAMS

Although there are threads of concern about the use of physical restraints in the nursing literature dating back to the nineteenth century, the recent change in thinking seems to reflect the confluence of at least three intellectual streams: a general questioning of medical precepts, the rise of geriatrics, and a press for patient autonomy. The pressure to reexamine long-held beliefs about common care practices and a general skepticism about orthodox practices with unproven outcomes are the most recent phenomena. In many ways, the recent history of restraint use reflects what is happening in many areas of health care. Practices that had long been assumed to be appropriate are now coming under closer scrutiny. A new spirit of empiricism, which questions the unproven assumptions that have guided many of our professional activities for some time, is being applied (10, 14, 54, 55).

The recognition of changing demographics has prompted a growing appreciation for the need for more attention to the care of older persons, especially those who are dependent. This awareness opened the way for the establishment of a geriatric specialty area within several health-care professions, including medicine and nursing, and greater scrutiny of how the needs of frail older patients are met. Finally, the growth of bioethics over the past 20 years has brought an emphasis on the importance of the individual and the centrality of patient autonomy. Although much of this concern has focused on the rights of the individual to forego treatment, as reflected statutorily in the recent federal Patient Self-Determination Act, it has also involved a more general renegotiation of the decision-making relationship between the patient and the doctor, and a respect for the dignity of the individual patient (5, 45).

Important contributions from the emerging field of geriatric medicine have included the development of comprehensive geriatric assessment, which emphasized the functioning of older persons and identifying their medical problems (46, 47, 61), and the focus on rehabilitation.

Collopy (11) notes the "growing emphasis on the autonomy of patients, their right to be fully informed, to make their own health care decisions, to take risks, to withhold consent, to define their own 'quality of life' outcomes, to have their preferences and values ensured by surrogates who act for them in the face of mental incapacity." A new moral climate has arisen that reflects "a growing consensus that in terms of patient choice and self-determination, the routine use of restraints is an invasive, unjustified, and therefore unethically acceptable practice."

The work of the National Citizens Coalition for Nursing Home Reform (NCCNHR) and its constituent groups has provided increasingly strong and effective consumer advocacy. In the late 1970s and through the 1980s, the Coalition worked continuously, though unsuccessfully, to get enforcement teeth into the regulations on the resident rights provisions of the federal nursing home code, which included, even in those pre-OBRA (Omnibus Budget Reconciliation Act) days, the right to be "free from chemical and (except in emergencies) physical restraints except as authorized in writing by a physician for a specified and limited period of time, or when necessary to protect the patient from injury to himself and to others."

The role of the Congress and its passage of nursing home reform legislation (OBRA 87) was vital in changing practice in regard to both chemical and physical restraints. The practice of restraining persons who lived in nursing homes has been decried in congressional hearings over the years, one of which captured in its title the essence of the situation: "The Rights of America's Institutionalized Aged: Lost in Confinement" (Hearing before the Subcommittee on Health and Long-Term Care of the Select Committee on Aging, House of Representatives, September 18, 1985). Congressional concern about restraining practices culminated, largely through the efforts of the Kendal Corporation, in a symposium before the Special Committee on Aging, United States Senate, December 4, 1989, entitled "Untie the Elderly: Quality Care Without Restraints."

The statutory and professional forces for change were given momentum by strong public opinion against restraints. A sense of moral certitude on the part of lay and professional people pervades discussions about the matter. "Tying people up is treating them like animals," or "It's such a relief to hear that there are other ways of caring for people" are the kinds of comments heard from laypeople. More than one nurse assistant has said, "You'll never get me in a nursing home—I can't stand the thought of being tied up; I'd go crazy." (Quotes are comments made to C. C. Williams in presentations around the country 1987–1992.) Strumpf & Evans (51) have documented the conflicting feelings of nurses in the acute care setting about the use of restraints.

Several investigative reports on the devastating consequences of using restraints stirred public ire. Beginning with a series by Fried (20) in the Long Beach *Press-Telegram* in June 1987 entitled "Care That Kills," investigative reporters across the United States have examined restraint use. In December

1987, Nohlgren (38) ended his series in the *St. Petersburg Times* with an editorial entitled "Punishment Without Crime." In December 1990, Rigert & Lerner (43), investigative reporters for the Minneapolis *Star Tribune,* published a four-part series entitled "Safeguards that Kill." With the help of physicians who examined many reports of restraint associated deaths, they produced an estimate of 200 such deaths in this country annually.

In addition, many participants in the change believe that, as restraining devices are reduced or eliminated, a new energy for creative ways of giving care is generated (30). Manuals and workshops constantly note that individualized care, which must be developed in removing restraints, calls for the creativity of all involved: staff at all levels, the resident, and the family. [See manuals by Burger (9) and Rader (42) and presentations in workshops by the Kendal Corporation (39)].

Although there were occasional notices about the dangers of restraints as early as 1968, it was not until the late 1980s that the articles by Evans & Strumpf (16, 17) raised the consciousness of American health professionals to the possibility that restraining patients was often not only unnecessary but harmful. Methods of restraint-free care in other countries were cited as examples of the art of the possible. Evans & Strumpf (16) described virtually restraint-free care in Scotland, and Williams (58, 59) reported it in a Scandinavian nursing home. The fact that severely confused and disabled patients could be cared for without the use of restraints and with less resultant disruption stood as an important lesson to those who would theorize about the need for such control devices.

There were a few pre-OBRA 87 examples of restraint-free environments in the United States. Kendal at Longwood in Kennett Square, Pennsylvania, a continuing care community of Quaker sponsorship that opened in 1973, has never used restraints in its skilled care facility or in any other level of care. This practice was first formally described at a meeting of the American Homes for the Aged in 1986. Since then, the Kendal staff have actively offered a training program, "Untie the Elderly," which describes their approach to providing quality care without restraints.

The freeing of the American nursing home resident has occurred in the context of a general shift in attitudes toward care. As noted earlier, our society is gradually moving from a position of professional dominance (18) to one that acknowledges a central role for the recipient of care. This paradigm shift has been urged for some time (53), but has been slow in coming. A commitment to the strong belief in autonomy, which is at least as old as the country's founding, is patients' rights, especially the right to choose treatments. These rights have been only titularly promoted until recently (with the exception of the previously noted rights advocacy work of NCCNHR). The last decade has seen a dramatic change in attitude, which reflects both a growing skepticism about the efficacy of various clinical practices (8, 27) and genuine efforts to involve patients meaningfully in clinical decisions (13).

The restraint control movement was assisted by the Institute of Medicine's report on *Improving the Quality of Care in Nursing Homes* (34), which called for more resident-centered approaches to overseeing care and a stronger focus on the outcomes of care. The report urged that residents be studied directly, rather than having the inspectors rely on the nursing home records. These recommendations were translated into legislation appearing as OBRA 87. Specific sections of OBRA 87 speak to both physical and chemical restraints:

> Residents have the right to be free from . . . any physical or chemical restraint imposed for purposes of discipline or convenience and not required to treat the resident's medical symptoms . . . Restraints may be only imposed (I) to ensure the physical safety of the resident or other residents, and (II) only upon the written order of a physician that specifies the duration and circumstances under which the restraints are to be used.

The proposed regulations (published in the Federal Register as recently as February 1992) go on to prohibit standing or blanket orders for restraints. They describe procedures for emergency and nonemergency use of restraints. Emergencies are limited to a 12-hour period. For nonemergencies, the use of restraints must be explained to the resident (or his/her guardian if the resident is not competent or cannot understand) and written consent for their use be obtained before using them.

The same proposed regulations contain explicit directions for the use of psychopharmaceutical agents in nursing homes, which parallel those for physical restraints. In addition to demanding proper justification for their use, especially a calculation of the risk-benefit ratio, and clear, informed resident consent for any use of such medications, the resident must be closely monitored for both desired and adverse consequences. At least semiannually, a therapeutic trial is mandated wherein the drug is gradually withdrawn to test for signs of clinical effectiveness. At least annually, the medication regimen must be reviewed by an appropriately trained physician with no ties to the facility.

THE EVIDENCE BASE FOR REFORM

There is no precise turning point when definitive data were presented to demonstrate that the management of restraints was inappropriate. Table 1 summarizes the available studies, including some summarized in the review by Evans & Strumpf (17). The table is separated into studies on the risk factors associated with using restraints and the evidence of adverse events from using them. Although there is a good deal of documentation about the adverse

Table 1 Use of physical restraints in nursing homes

Authors	Sample	Restraint rate	Risk factors	Adverse effects
Risk factors and adverse effects				
Dietsche & Pollmann (11b)	Alzheimer's patients no sample		•agitation •hostile behavior •akathisias, and/or parkinsonian reaction	Chemical restraints •dystonias, dyskinesias
Frengley & Mion (19)	Acute care, 1292 adults on 4 medical units	Overall rate = 7.4% age > 70 = 20.3% age 40–50 = 2.9%	•over age 70	•higher death rate •longer length of stay
Lofgren et al (30b) Macpherson et al (32)	VA hospital, acute care 1661 patients	102 patients; rate was 6% (mean age = 75.4)	•cognitively impaired •infectious diseases •CNS disorders •cancer •reasons for restraints: -prevent falls -prevent wandering -prevent devices -subdue agitation	•more likely to be discharged to chronic care facilities •nosocomial infections •new pressure sores
Mion et al (36a)	hospital: 278 from medical ward; 143 from rehab-medical ward	13% for medical ward 34% for rehab-medical ward	•physical dependency •poor cognition •high severity of illness •white •admitted from NH •psychiatric diagnosis •gender (male)	•high mortality rate •higher morbidity rate •psychological distress •longer length of hospital stay

Robbins et al (44)	VA hospital 137 med-sug patients ≥70 years old and 85 patients < 70 years old	18% > 70 years old 14% > 70 years old total rate = 17%	•abnormal mental status on admission •organic brain syndrome/ dementia •surgery •monitoring and support devices (e.g. IV lines)	•longer length of stay •higher death rate •increasing NH replace-ment
Strumpf & Evans (52a)	20 NH residents mean age = 88.6 years old	25%	•impaired physical func-tion •impaired orientation	•physical •behavioral •emotional
Tinetti et al (53a)	12 SNFs; 397 residents mean age = 83.6 years old 78% were women	31%	•unsteadiness •concern about falls •maintenance of position •disoriented •female	•high risk of serious fall related injuries

Table 1 (*Continued*)

Authors	Sample	Restraint rate	Risk factors	Adverse effects
Tinetti et al (53b)	12 SNFs (bed size 60–360); 1756 residents > 60 years old	66%	•older age •female •disorientation •wandering •a diagnosis of dementia •use of neuroleptics •dependence with regard to activities of daily living •incontinence of urine and stool •history of falls in the previous six months •greater participation in social activities •lack of use of anti-depressants	•increased agitation •withdrawal or depression •sedatives
Adverse Effects				
Cape (9d)	Acute care in Canada/Britain	restraint use in Canada greater by 8 : 1		•higher accident rate

Covert et al (11a)	no specific sample	Mechanical— •impair circulation or compress nerves •increase agitation •skin abrasions •fatal in someone with compromised cardiac or respiratory function Chemical— •produce paradoxic agitation •depraving someone of freedom of movement •clouding a person's consciousness •bring on a state of relative sensory •deprivation with secondary payshosis
Miles & Irvine (36)	Hennepin County nursing home deaths national death register	•strangulation deaths •other fatal complications

Table 1 *(Continued)*

Authors	Sample	Restraint rate	Risk factors	Adverse effects
Powell et al (41a)	acute care hospital geriatric department	Use of physical restraints*		
		Fiscal year / No. of cases per 1000 patient days		Number of falls per 1000 patient-days
		1980–81 / 52		7.3
		1981–82 / 53		8.8
		1982–83 / 2		12.5
		1983–84 / 1.5		12.6
		1984–85 / 1		7.1
		1985–86 / 0.5		7.1
		1986–87 / 0.3		8.7
		*No specific data on chemical restraints. There was a 40% reduction in use of chemical restraints during study period.		
Strumpf & Evans (51)	acute care, 20 medical patients			•physical •behavioral •emotional
Werner et al (55a)	24 agitated residents in 3 units of a 550-bed long-term care facility	22/24 (92%)		•no reduction in agitation •after restrained
Burton et al (9c)	8 nursing homes 431 admissions	after one year, 31% restrained at least once, 9% get neuroleptics, 30% get both		•restraint with or without neuroleptics associated with lower cognitive score

Risk factors			
Appelbaum & Roth (2b)	14 med-sug patients acute care	1.17 incidents per 100 patient day	•age over (60 ($\bar{x}$ = 74) •impaired mental status
Berland et al (6a)	a 719-bed university affiliated teaching hospital 80 patients had a restraint 80 unrestrained controls		•disruptive behaviors •nursing assessment of risk of falling •cognitive impairment
Folmar & Wilson (17b)	112 SNF patients age over 55	53 had restraint orders only 21 (19%) restrained	•lower level of social and ritual behavior
Morrison et al (36c)	acute and extended care	13.2%	•older age •hospitalized in general medicine or neurology
Ray et al (42a)	173 nursing homes 5902 Medicaid residents	74% patients use CNS drugs; 43% were antipsychotic	•large NHs •family practitioners •use of dominant MD •rural practice

Table 1 (*Continued*)

Authors	Sample	Restraint rate	Risk factors	Adverse effects
Sloane et al (50c)	nursing homes 31 specialized dementia units and 32 traditional units	Physical—dementia unit = 18.1% trad. unit = 51.6% Pharmacologic—dementia unit = 45.3% trad. unit = 43.4%	Physical— •residence in a nonspecialized NH unit •nonambulatory status •transfer dependency •mental status impairment •hip fracture history •high nursing staff-to-patient ratio Pharmacologic— •physical abusive behavior •severe mental status impairment •frequent family visitation	
Evans & Strumpf (17)	summary paper	7.4—22% (hospital) 25—84.6% (NH)		
Farnsworth (17a)	random sample of 500 US NHs (36.6% response rate)	restraints used in 99% of NHs		
Mitchell-Pedersen et al (36b)	acute care, 180-bed medical department	1570 incidents in first 6 months 45 incidents in last 6 months		

effects of restraint use, neither this list nor the earlier review contains many rigorous studies. Few prospective studies have been reported from which one might obtain evidence to distinguish potential causation from associations. To date, there has not been a scientifically strong study documenting a dramatic reduction in untoward events from discontinuing restraints or an increase when they are imposed. Most of the studies described patients in acute hospitals, rather than nursing homes. There is not always a clear statement about how often or how long the restraints were applied.

Nor is there a consistent definition of what constitutes a physical restraint. The simplest, and perhaps most useful, definition is "any device that restricts voluntary movement" (28). The regulatory definition of a physical restraint is "any manual method or physical or mechanical device, material, or equipment attached or adjacent to the resident's body that the resident cannot remove easily, which restricts freedom of movement or access to his or her body" [Federal Register, Vol. 57, No. 24, February 6, 1992, §483.13 (a) (1) (i)]. Restraints include formal devices, like vests and arm restraints, and special equipment, like the gerichairs, which include a locked-in-place table to prevent exit. Some people also include as restraints bed rails and belts used either to tie patients into chairs or to hold them up while walking. Sometimes sheets or other common equipment can be used for restraining purposes.

The use of restraints on patients in acute hospitals has been a long-standing practice and, as is true of many nursing home practices, has probably been carried over to the residents of nursing homes with little further thought. However, even in hospitals, the documentation of restraint use and its perceived rationale and liabilities has only recently received attention. Several reports from 1986 through 1990 indicate that at any time up to 20% of older hospitalized patients have been found to be restrained (19, 44). Reasons offered include the use of monitoring or support devices, disruptive behavior, dementia, and nursing assessment of risk of falling. One study (32) in the Minneapolis VA Medical Center found that in many instances of restraint use, the physician was not aware of or had not participated in the decision to use restraints and thought there may have been other alternative approaches. Reported complications of restraint use in hospitals have included compromised vascular flow, skin breakdown, musculoskeletal injury, aspiration pneumonia, increased cardiac stress, and "emotional desolation" (44). With the increased attention in nursing homes to minimizing the use of restraints, nursing home staff are registering concern about the use of restraints on their residents when they are hospitalized.

Despite the absence of a strong empirical literature, there has been a dramatic change in beliefs about the right way to care for frail older persons in nursing homes. Previous thinking argued that patients who were a risk to themselves or others were better treated by being restrained in the name of protecting them from falling, from removing needed equipment (like nasogastric feeding tubes or intravenous lines), or from harming others. To caregivers of that era, it made sense that a person who was at risk from sliding out of a chair should be tied into it. The benefit of the therapy was thought to outweigh the indignity experienced by persons who were tied down to prevent them from pulling out tubes. Generally, such treatment was directed at persons who were confused, but even mentally active persons were harnessed into place.

The use of restraints, developed first in the mental hospital and subsequently in the acute hospital, came with a philosophy of practice that placed the control firmly in the hands of the professionals. Physical restraints may be viewed as the embodiment of that control; professionals literally had the ability and they assumed the right to tie patients up in the name of protecting them. As with many medical concepts, the use of restraints as a management tool spread easily to the nursing home, where labor was in even shorter supply and most operators and directors of nursing believed that it was more efficient to tie someone down than to have to keep them under constant supervision, although findings now suggest that significantly more nurse aide time must be spent delivering care to restrained patients (41). Somehow, behaviors that had become acceptable to manage short-term, often very acute bouts of delirium and agitation became the basis for the management of chronic symptoms.

Despite occasional concerns expressed about the iatrogenic sequelae of restraints, such as bed sores and induced urinary and fecal incontinence, there was virtually universal agreement that such measures were necessary for many patients who, it was thought, simply could not be cared for efficiently any other way. Moreover, there was a belief that using such measures reflected a genuine concern for the patient's safety. Evans & Strumpf (17) report an increase in the use of restraints from 25% to 41% nationwide between 1977 and 1988. Occasional reports of strangulation and induced trauma brought cautions about the best ways to manage the use of restraints and even led to management guidelines for how to apply and periodically release them and how to turn patients to avoid bed sores.

Although family members might initially shrink from the thought of tying up a family member, as the need for presumed safety precautions was explained to them, restraints became viewed as a necessary precaution. Many could transform their horror into a sense of doing the right thing to protect the patient from herself. Somehow, the increased agitation that often resulted was overlooked, or psychoactive drugs were used to control it.

Just as with Philippe Pinel's unchaining the asylum inmates in the late eighteenth century and Dorothea Dix's campaign for reform of the treatment of the mentally ill in the latter part of the nineteenth century, the change in attitude toward restraints in the 1980s was based less on science than on philosophy. Although there was no evidence of the original efficacy of restraint use, changing the dominant practice pattern required a combination of a changing ethos about the goals of long-term care and a demonstration that not using restraints did not pose a major risk to society. The latter was especially important in what have become increasingly litigious times. Even though there have been few suits over the damages done to frail nursing home residents, who are seen as having little human capital value and hence whose damages and shortened life spans have lesser value, there was still great concern about moving against tradition. Or, perhaps, there was no strong incentive to the risk of alienating society by innovating. The generally conservative values were strongly reinforced by an active regulatory system that punished deviation from established standards of practice (23).

MOVEMENT TOWARD REFORM

The philosophic revolution with regard to the use of restraints was built on the fundamental American value for autonomy, but was catapulted to new heights in a concern for patients' rights, especially about terminal events, which gained prominence a little more than a decade ago. The right to refuse care quickly became a major ethical issue, centered around the rights of those no longer able to communicate their wishes. Ironically, the concern for patient control of care was exercised through advance directives and substitute judgments for those who had lost the capacity to implement their autonomy—all persons who could no longer communicate their wishes effectively. Meanwhile, discussions about long-term care took on a new vocabulary as people started talking about quality of life, not simply survival (6, 24, 40). A series of studies showed how nursing home residents' sense of well-being could benefit significantly from very modest techniques to give them greater control over even small portions of their daily lives (4, 26, 50).

During this time, case reports from settings in which residents were being cared for without restraints suggested that such care could be provided safely and with great gains in quality of life (59). This "art of the possible" lent credence to the campaign to humanize nursing home care.

By the time of the codification of the recommendations of the Institute of Medicine Committee on Improving the Quality of Care in Nursing Homes (34), which spoke directly to issues of quality of life and residents' rights into OBRA 87, restraints had become a very visible and specific topic in the parlance of nursing home reform. The new criteria for caring for nursing home residents discouraged using restraints and indicated that any use needed the resident's (or guardian's) permission. The law explicitly prohibits the use of restraints "imposed for purposes of discipline or convenience and not required to treat the resident's medical symptoms." Moreover, "Restraints (physical or chemical) may only be imposed (I) to ensure the physical safety of the resident or other residents, and (II) only upon the written order of a physician that specifies the duration and circumstances under which the restraints are to be used . . . [PL 100-103 §1919 (c) (1) (A) (ii)]." The restraint prohibition is further buttressed by other provisions requiring "accurate assessment" and the facility's responsibility to bring about "the highest practicable" levels of physical, mental, and social functioning of each resident.

The operational step in implementing changes in nursing home behavior with regard to restraint use has come through the regulations and the interpretive guidelines that guide the surveyors in their examination of nursing home performance. Although final regulations seem as elusive as the Holy Grail, much has happened under the aegis of draft regulations, which seem to have the durability of a Quonset hut. OBRA 87 began implementation on October 1, 1990. Proposed final regulations were issued in August 1992, but as of that date, definitive enforcement regulations had not been published.

The proposed rules dealing with the use of restraints published in the Federal Register, February 5, 1992, go to some length to specify the steps necessary before a decision to restrain a resident is acceptable. They suggest that "the decision to apply physical restriants would come only after assessing each resident's capabilities, evaluating less restrictive alternatives, ruling out their use for each resident, and identifying within the plan of care rehabilitative training to enable progressive removal of restraints or progressive use of less restrictive means."

VARIATIONS IN RESPONSE

The response to the proposed regulations has varied dramatically among the states. Some states saw the attention to restraints as a means to effect a new approach to care. Others chose to resist change, arguing that the costs of the new regulations would stress an already overwhelmed Medicaid program. Thus, while New Hampshire and Vermont nursing homes worked to make themselves restraint free, California took to the courts and the back rooms to negotiate deals that would eventually emasculate the implementation program for restraint regulation.

New Hampshire and Vermont stand as models of states that seized the opportunity to improve care. Under the leadership of the state nursing home association, the New Hampshire Health Care Association (NHHCA), a program of consciousness raising and active education was undertaken. Beyond urging reduced use of restraints, the sessions demonstrated alternative ways to respond to the symptoms for which residents might otherwise be restrained. The repeated message was that restraints should be the last choice.

The program worked. The NHHCA reports that restraints use has dropped impressively. They cite Health Care Financing Administration (HCFA) data that show that the proportion of residents requiring restraints in New Hampshire in 1987–1988 was 34.8% and 43.8% in Intermediate Care Facilities (ICFs) and Skilled Nursing Facilities (SNFs), respectively, compared with a national average of 41.3%. In 1988–1989, the reported rates were 33.3% and 37.2%, compared with a national rate of 40.4%. In a special 1992 survey of its membership, NHHCA found that only 11% of residents had any orders for physical restraints (V. Wisdom 1992, personal communication). Neighboring Vermont, with leadership from state agencies, conducted numerous workshops that challenged the nursing homes to change their patterns of care. Vermont, too, now reports only about 11% of nursing home residents in restraints (P. Flood 1992, personal communication).

By contrast, California determined that the costs of implementing OBRA 87 was prohibitive and chose to fight the process. It first sought to be exempted from the national program on the basis of having an equivalent system. A lawsuit was filed by nursing home residents and Congressman Stark to compel California to participate in the national program. This led to a court order for participation. Various political maneuvers, including withholding HCFA funds because of nonparticipation and lobbying by California representatives within the executive branch, and a counter suit by California challenging the legality of the guidelines, particularly those addressing restraint use, led eventually to a political compromise whereby the survey interpretative guidelines were revised to permit surveyors to use more individual judgment in determining whether a facility was in compliance with a particular law or regulation. Many saw the relaxation of rigor in applying the guidelines as a major setback for an effort to develop more consistency and meaning to the regulation process. For many states, the new OBRA standards represented a major step forward (toward more structure and consistency). Relaxing standards or permitting individual interpretation threatened the very cause for which Nursing Home Reform Amendments of OBRA 87 were passed (1).

The American Health Care Association, which represents most of the nation's nursing homes, responded to the changing environment by developing guidelines for the use of physical restraints (2). These guidelines tend to codify quite general statements that reflect the regulations, but they add legitimacy to the effort to move away from restraint use. They emphasize efforts to find other means of managing resident problems and reinforce the need to act continuously to reduce the use of restraints among those for whom they are used. The level of their doctrine, as reflected in the following statement, does not suggest a restraint-free standard, but rather clings to a benevolent control mode of an earlier era:

> AHCA believes that to promote the dignity and highest practicable physical, mental, and psychosocial well-being of residents of nursing facilities, restraints should only be considered when the protocol of the interdisciplinary health care team determines that restraint use will enhance the resident's quality of care and quality of life or when the need for restraints clearly outweighs the resident's right to be free from restraints and the risks of restraint use (2).

The response to the changing regulatory climate has also taken on some uniquely American characteristics. In response to a strict reading of the regulations, new approaches to care have sprung up that proposed alternative modes, just outside the bounds of those formally labeled as restraints. Thus, at least some parts of the industry have addressed the letter, rather than the spirit, of the law. They have adopted devices that avoid the regulatory definition of a restraint; but, these devices nonetheless pose the same threats to dignity and autonomy as do their formal counterparts. For example, residents may have neither the strength nor the understanding to unfasten belts with Velcro fasteners. Others have developed sophisticated behavioral training programs for staff to assure that they reposition restrained residents regularly and check their restraints (49).

MOMENTUM OF CHANGE

One of the things that makes the story of restraint use so remarkable is the rapidity (but not necessarily universality) with which the movement to reduce or remove restraints occurred. In stark contrast with the repeated difficulty experienced in trying to introduce change based on the pronouncements of prestigious scientific groups, such as the National Institutes of Health consensus statements (25) or similar groups in Canada (31), the advocacy on behalf of restraint reduction seems to have fallen on receptive ears despite no stronger (and perhaps even weaker) evidence of the efficacy for that position. An alternative interpretation is that less evidence for the benefit of removing restraints is needed because the burden of evidence originally belongs with those who would impose the restraints in the first place. Nonetheless, as an example of how practices change, the use (or disuse) of restraints raises interesting questions.

Although no formal data are available to assess the effects of the changing climate for restraints, there are indications, beyond anecdotes, that substantial change is afoot. Table 2, derived from HCFA's Online Survey Certification and Reporting System, shows the percentage of residents within a nursing home that were physically restrained during different time points before and after the October 1990 implementation of the OBRA 87 regulations. Each point in time includes a different set of nursing homes, depending on which ones were surveyed during that month. Overall, the rate of restraint use fell

Table 2 Percentage of residents physically restrained by region for surveys conducted pre- and post-OBRA

Region	3/90	6/90	9/90	10/90	12/90	2/91	4/91	9/91	1/92
CT, MA, ME, NH, RI, VT	35	27	23	23	17	18	18	19	16
NJ, NY, PR, VI	31	34	30	22	27	24	16	22	15
DC, DL, MD, PA, VA, WV	41	37	36	28	29	27	22	24	26
AL, FL, GA, KY, MS, NC, SC, TN	31	30	30	28	25	26	24	23	23
IL, IN, MI, MN, OH, WI	37	32	29	28	25	23	26	21	21
AR, LA, OK, NM, TX	26	25	21	23	19	20	17	20	20
IA, KS, MO, NE	33	30	26	26	22	22	19	20	18
CO, MT, ND, SD, UT, WY	37	27	22	24	23	19	17	17	19
AZ, CA, HI, NV	44	34	41	33[a]	29	27	36	31	25
AK, ID, OR, WA	31	34	28	32	28	27	23	22	25
National	36.3	30.9	30.2	26.6	23.8	23.0	22.5	22.0	21.0
Total residents[b]	44,225	111,586	116,640	102,615	87,982	104,507	53,306	114,032	112,272

[a] This total was affected by the absence of any surveys by California. The number of surveys upon which this percentage is based was only 15.
[b] Total residents is the total number of residents in all the facilities surveyed in each time period.
Source: OSCAR data received from Alan Friedlob.

by about one-third in the first year after OBRA, but the pattern of change varies from region to region.

In 1992, the American Association of Homes for the Aging, an organization representing nonprofit nursing homes, released the results of a survey it commissioned on restraint use in nursing homes. The results from 481 homes indicate that the use of physical restraints declined from 43% in 1989 to 23% in 1991. In that year, the larger the facility, the greater the use of restraints. Respondents suggested that although the rate of falls increased, there was no increase in the rate of serious falls. The cost of introducing the changed policy was modest, from $70 to $1500, depending on the size of the facility. The leading obstacles to reducing restraints were resistance from staff, resistance from residents' family members, and problems interpreting the regulations. The study also points to the problem that, other than making a basic change in the philosophy toward increasingly individualized care, other physical measures were being used in lieu of restraints with the same potential psychological and even physical dangers. For example, about 60% of the homes utilized postural supports and adaptive furniture, whereas only 40% involved residents in activities programs in an effort to avoid the behaviors that would require restraints.

McKnight's *Long-Term Care News* conducted a poll by fax machine of all state affiliates of the American Health Care Facilities Association (which also represents the for-profit nursing homes) and the American Association of Homes for the Aging with a response rate of 42%. Among the responding organizations, 24% were not sure by what percent restraints had been reduced in their state in the past year; 6% reported 75% or more; 9%, 50–74%; 12%, 40–49%; 15%, 30–39%; 15%, 20–29%; 15%, 10–19%; and only 4% less than 4%.

Another, less representative, glimpse into the effects of the OBRA regulations comes from an informal survey taken during the recent meeting of the American Medical Directors Association (AMDA), which represents the medical directors of nursing homes. Of the 240 members attending the 1992 annual conference, 99 (41%) completed a short questionnaire. The medical directors, who had served an average of 6.3 years, cover both proprietary (73%) and nonprofit homes from 28 states. The average home had 148 beds. Almost 80% (79%) reported that their nursing homes had a formal policy regarding the use of physical restraints. In 85% of these cases, the policy was developed in response to the OBRA regulations. In 43%, it was developed by an interdisciplinary team. In over half the cases, the policy requires a specific order for restraint use (75%); actively discourages restraint use (64%); specifies the length of time a restraint may be applied, how often the restraint must be checked, and when it must be removed (60%); and specifies alternatives that must be tried before a restraint is used (54%). Only

42% specified the conditions under which a restraint may not be used, and a like number prohibited as-needed (prn) orders for restraints and required that family members must agree to any restraint use; only 72% required a written agreement by the resident or his/her legal guardian to any restraint use. This level of performance can be viewed in two ways. It is encouraging to see such specificity in internal rules, but it is frustrating to see only this proportion of homes responding affirmatively, because all of these items are required under current regulations. On the other hand, half of the policies require that any restraint use must be formally evaluated by the nursing supervisor, a step not mandated by regulation. Two thirds of the medical directors indicated that they had observed a decrease in the numbers of persons physically restrained since the new regulations went into effect in October 1990. Only 12% reported that their facility had adopted a completely restraint-free policy.

RESTRAINT USE AS A SPECIAL CASE

Several factors distinguish the restraint issue from others involving defining appropriate standards of care. First, the use of restraints was specifically incorporated into regulations that affected an industry with a long history of responding to such requirements. Second the use of restraints is more a social issue than a medical one. Miles (35) argues that restraints are not medical care. Restraint use addresses questions of lifestyle, dignity, and potential psychological harm, and involves questions about physical risk. But, as we discuss below, the challenge to more medical aspects, such as the use of psychoactive medications, produced an equally dramatic response. Finally, despite the wide prevalence of restraints, there was an underlying discomfort about their use.

When this tendency to change was reinforced by regulations that mandated such behavior change, the tide quickly turned. Indeed, Kapp (23) has argued that, in aspects of care like restraint use, the burden of proof is on the user. Because restraints represent an assault on a person's dignity, they should not be used without great prior efforts to find better solutions. That is the gist of the regulatory language now incorporated. However, it is easy to lose sight of the fact that, just a decade earlier, restraints were viewed as the logical and effective way to respond to residents who posed a threat to themselves or others. Physical safety, presumed to be assured by physical restraint, was the predominant value.

Over the years, persons who have been restrained have been expressing their intense dislike, pain, fear, discomfort, and shame, but their feelings and opinions have not been heard. Not only can caregivers testify to the negative reactions of residents, which include the struggles to free themselves that have instead led to their deaths, but anyone who visits a nursing home with any degree of frequency will have encountered pleas from a resident for help in securing release from the binding device (51, 59).

The change in attitudes toward restraint use also shares traits with other movements that are going on in health care. There is a general tendency to challenge concepts that have been formerly accepted as the litany of practice. This new cry for empiricism extends to reassessing commonplace practices and questioning their benefit. In part, at least, it reflects a shift in emphasis in medical care from a focus exclusively on the technical aspects of care to one that is more centered on the effects on the person with the problem, with more attention paid to psychological well-being. This recentering extends not just to considering outcomes of care that incorporate the effects of care on the whole person (e.g. functional status, general well-being, and perceived health status); it also redirects the distribution of power in decision-making to give the consumer of care more of a voice in the decisions being made and, hence, a greater responsibility for their consequences.

The presumed dichotomy of trading safety for autonomy, often posed as a nursing dilemma (33), erroneously frames the question, because, as noted above, restraint use is associated with very real and substantial risks, including functional loss, "emotional desolation," and death, whether or not the device was properly applied (36).

The appropriate framing of the question has to do with choosing from among risks, and, significantly, those risks must be broadened to include overall risks to psychological as well as physical well-being. The reframing of the question comes with the recognition that in truth all life, including daily living in a nursing home, involves risks (57, 60). Whenever families talk in terms of total saftey for their relatives, the new standard of care calls for staff to educate about the hazards of restraint, as well as nonrestraint, of voluntary movement and to help the family see the total picture. Scottish and Swedish caregiving in long-term care settings reveals an acceptance of risk taking and value placed on personal choice about what risks one will take as a mark of individuality and adulthood (56). The restoration of this choice to the nursing home resident is a giant step toward dignity and maintenance of identity (59). Choice is possible for those who are victims of dementia, as well as the cognitively unimpaired, because there are many clues in body language, as well as in the history and context of the individual's earlier life. The importance of the maintenance of self-identity in advanced old age is reported in the studies of Lieberman & Tobin (29) who conclude that "The core task, maintenance of self, represents the psychological survival of the elderly and may be usefully seen as analogous to physical survival."

The balance between risk-taking and safety, though erroneous, underpins much, but not all, of the dialogue about the use of restraint. The other critical piece of information is the growing awareness that other approaches to care, which substitute individual attention for the use of restraints, can achieve the same ends without the need to sacrifice independence and dignity. Some have challenged these approaches as too expensive. They are dismissed as impractical in a setting like the typical nursing home, where costs are closely monitored. Here again, thinking is changing. Much of the management philosophy of the past has been driven by a limited concept of task accomplishment and efficiency. As long as the productivity of caring was measured in terms of carrying out needed tasks, then the fastest way to get the job done was usually considered the best. However, an appreciation is developing slowly that the goal of long-term care is not simply task accomplishment but enabling people to live fuller, more meaningful lives. As the goals become more firmly focused on maintaining function and enhancing quality of life, the relative value of alternative management strategies changes. A philosophy of more individualized care encourages caregivers to search for ways by which to meet the clients' needs without resorting to physical control.

When evidence suggests that better care may even be cheaper care, the appeal is that much stronger. One such study used data collected for another purpose to compare the costs of personnel time for similar residents who were and were not restrained. In contrast to popular belief, the costs of caring for restrained residents was greater than that for similar unrestrained residents. Much of the added cost came from the need to attend those restrained to release the restraints, to move the residents, and to observe for complications (41).

CHEMICAL RESTRAINTS

The same enthusiasm that has attended releasing physical restraints has also been applied to chemical restraints. Ironically, the introduction of psychoactive drugs was hailed as a mechanism to release the mentally ill. Largely because behaviors could be controlled with medications, millions of mentally ill persons were discharged from institutions in a tidal wave of community-based treatment that began in the 1960s. For the purposes of deinstitutionalizing the mentally ill, however, the nursing home was considered part of the community. A substantial number of mentally ill persons, especially those who were elderly, were transferred to nursing homes (48). Over time, the use of psychoactive drugs was applied to nursing home residents to control disruptive or disturbing behaviors.

Reports of adverse side effects from these drugs, especially excess sedation and increased risk of falls, prompted widespread concerns. The efforts to reduce physical restraint use were extended to chemical restraints, as well. Moreover, some feared that unilaterally reducing the use of physical restraints could prompt even wider use of chemicals to replace them.

Concern over misuse of psychoactive medications is reflected in the hearings of the Senate Subcommittee on Aging, chaired by Frank Moss, in the mid-1970s (37). They heard testimony about nursing home residents reduced to stupor because of drugs and created vivid images of flagrant misuse. (One of the reports is entitled *Nursing Home Drugs: Pharmaceutical Roulette*.) This same theme was reflected in subsequent hearings in the House Subcommittee on Aging chaired by Claude Pepper.

This raised consciousness was associated with the issuance of regulations in 1974 that mandated reviews by licensed pharmacists of all medications received by nursing home residents. By 1980, indicators had been developed for appropriate drug-diagnoses relationships and dosages, drawn heavily from a project to develop screening criteria for psychoactive drugs conducted by the American Psychiatric Society (12). The Institute of Medicine report on *Improving the Quality of Care in Nursing Homes* suggested that excessive use of tranquilizers and antipsychotic drugs represented evidence of poor quality of care in nursing homes (34), but offered few specifics on how to use this indicator.

The potential for harm from misuse or overzealous use of psychoactive medications is greater than that for physical restraints. This potential is borne out by the literature on drug misuse summarized in Table 3. The table is organized like the review table for physical restraints, with a summary of the information on the risk factors associated with their use and the evidence for adverse effects from using them. There is more documentation that implicates psychoactive drugs in producing disability than is the case for physical restraints. The side effects of psychoactive drugs have been well recognized in general. But, at the level of broader measures of functional impairment, as with the use of physical restraints, there are few well-designed longitudinal studies to demonstrate conclusively the causal linkages. Much of the risk imputed to drug use is based on clinical judgments about side effects, only some of which is substantiated in controlled studies.

The concern about the excessive use of psychoactive drugs prompted a set of regulations that extended the government's dictation about the practice of medicine further than it had ever gone before. Although there had previously existed laws mandating bodies to be formed to assure quality of care, these bodies were left in the hands of the medical profession. Professional Standards Review Organizations and their successors, Peer Review Organizations, were chartered from medically sponsored organizations, However, OBRA 87 represents the first time that legislation specifically dictated the terms under which a segment of medicine in nursing homes was to be practiced by requiring documentation of the reasons for the use of specified psychoactive medications.

Table 3 Use of psychoactive drugs in nursing homes

Authors	Sample	Drug use rate	Risk factors	Adverse effects
Risk factors and adverse effects				
Avorn et al (3a)	First phase— •50 free-standing rest homes and 5 additional rest homes from the multilevel facilities total 1201 residents Second phase— •44 rest homes all in Massachusetts total 837 residents	—First phase •55% psychoactive drugs •39% antipsychotic drugs •9% antidepressants •8% minor tranquilizers •3% lithium •3% lithium •antipsychotic: 41% in free standing homes and 12% in multilevel homes —Second phase •82% antipsychotic	free-standing nursing homes	moderate or severe tardive dyskinesia
Hulisz et al (22a)	788 patients in 7 skilled and intermediate nursing care centers	25.9%	•senility and dementia •rural facility	tardive dyskinesia
Rovner et al (45a)	8 Baltimore area proprietary nursing homes	antidepressant—13.4%	major depressive disorder	increased mortality
Adverse effects				
Burgio et al (19a)	3 elderly nursing home residents who received psychotric medications			•decreasing aberrant behaviors •decreased performance on motor assessments

Table 3 (*Continued*)

Authors	Sample	Drug use rate	Risk factors	Adverse effects
Covert et al (11a)	summary paper			•produce paradoxic agitation •depraving someone of freedom of movement •clouding a person's consciousness •bring on a state of relative sensory deprivation with secondary payshosis
Larson et al (26b)	380 patients, 60 or older, global cognitive impairment suspected			
Lipsitz et al (30a)	2 long-term care facilities 70 recurrent fallers and 56 nonfallers, mean age = 87 year	•antidepressant—24% in fallers vs. 5% in nonfallers •neuroleptic agents—9% in fallers vs. 4% in nonfallers •sedative—37% in fallers vs. 23% in nonfallers		falls
Ray et al (42b)	Michigan Medicaid program, from 1980–1982			increased risk of hip fracture
Sherman (50b)	summary paper			•cognitive impairment •risk of falling •two or three times more likely to experience a hip fracture •tradive dyskinsia •confusion or agitation

Sobel & McCart (50d)	an intermediate care facility 45 patients who had fallen and 30 matched control patients who had not fallen	•antidepressants 17.8% for the fall group vs. 13.3 for the control group •antipsychotics 11.1% for the fall group vs. 10.0% for the control •sedatives/hypnotics 53.3% for the fall group vs. 33.3% for the control group •overall, 57.8% of fall group vs. 40% of the control group had a neuroactive drug in the past 24 hours		sedatives/hypnotics are associated with falls
Risk Factors				
Anderson (2a)	191 NH patients and 42 medical home care (MHC) patients in south-western Sweden	•NH—54%, 39% had more than one prescriptions •MHC—48%, 20% had more than one prescriptions •by type, 24% of NH patients and 14% of MHC patients had neuroleptic drugs; 18% in NH and 19% in MHC used anxiolytic drugs; 18% in NH and 14% in MHC had antidepressants	•psychoactive drugs in general demented patients •neuroleptic drugs—women in NH •anxiolytic drugs—non-demented patients	

Table 3 (*Continued*)

Authors	Sample	Drug use rate	Risk factors	Adverse effects
Billig et al (6b)	a 550-bed nursing home		•demented and agitated were more likely to receive neuroleptic •non-demented agitated patients to receive benzodiazepine	
Blazer et al (7a)	5902 continuous NH residents and 4161 ambulatory patients All the patients were 65 or older in Tennessee Medicaid program	•NH—59% had anticholinergic drugs •ambulatory group—23% had anticholinergic drugs anticholinergic drugs (include: antipsychotic agents; antidepressants; antiparkinsonian agents; belladonna alkaloids; and antihistamines)	reside in NHs	
Buck (8a)	33,351 Medicaid recipients from NHs	•60% had at least one psychtropic drugs •by type, 74% of patients who on medications had antipsychotic; 25% had antiparkinson; 22% had sedatives/hypnotics; 19% received antidepressant; and 12% had antianxiety	•diagnosis of functional mental illness •age	

Garrard et al (21)	5752 randomly sampled admissions and 3191 residents in 60 nursing homes	on admission—17% of patients were on neuroleptics residents—21%	•physical restraints •age (younger, patients <75 were more likely to take drugs)
Nolan & O'Mally (38a)	301 residents (mean age = 83) in 11 nursing homes in Ireland	65%	smaller size of nursing home
Sloane et al (50c)	31 specialized dementia NH units and 32 traditional NH units	dementia unit = 45.3% trad. unit = 43.4%	•physical abusive behavior •severe mental status •impairment •frequent family visitation
Svarstad & Mount (52b)	7 skilled nursing facilities	38% patients had an order for an antipsychotic or antianxiety agent 28% actually received a tranquilizer	NHs have less adequate staffing and other resources
Beardsley et al (5a)	526 patients from 112 NHs, 65 or older who had active psychotropic drug orders	34.6% on psychotropics medications (45% used antipsychotic agents; 21% on antianxiety; 32% on antidepressants; and 20 on sedative/hypnotics	

Table 3 (*Continued*)

Authors	Sample	Drug use rate	Risk factors	Adverse effects
Beers et al (5b)	12 intermediate-care facilities in Massachusetts	•65% of the patients had orders for psychoactive drugs, 53% of patients actually used psychoactive drugs on five or more days •32% of patients had orders for antipsychotic, and 26% actually used it •40% had order for sedative/hypnotic drugs, 28% actually used these drugs		
Buck & Sprague (8b)	long-term care facilities in Illinois 5,766 Medicaid patients	•28.9% had psychotropic medication •by type: 88% of patients who were on medications had antipsychotic; 22% had antiparkinson; 11% had antianxiety; and 8% had sedative/hypnotics		
Burns & Kamerow (9b)	112 nursing homes 526 patients	32.7% of patients had a psychotropic medication		

Lantz et al (26a)	200-bed, voluntary, non-profit, teaching nursing home 91 patients who lived in NH from 1983 through 1987; mean age = 87	•70% of the patients were exposed to at least one psychotropic drug at some during the 5-year study period •depending on the period, from 42% to 51% of patients received at least one psychotropic drug •46% had episodic treatment, and 24% were on psychotropic drug during every consecutive period studied	
Ray et al (42a)	5902 Medicaid patients in a NH, 65 or older	•74% patients had at least a psychotropic medication •43% had antipsychotic	•large nursing home •dominant physician •family practitioners •rural practice
Seifert et al (50a)	83 NH patients mean age = 83	34.5% received at least one anticholinergic drug by type, 24% had antipsychotics drugs	
Zawadski et al (61a)	361,000 aged patients from California Medicaid program in fiscal year 1975–76	8% used psychotropic medication	

OBRA 87 addresses the use of psychoactive drugs in two separate places, once as psychopharmacologic drugs and elsewhere as chemical restraints.

> Psychoharmacologic drugs may be administered only on the orders of a physician and only as part of a plan . . . designed to eliminate or modify the symptoms for which the drugs are prescribed and only if at least annually an independent external consultant reviews the appropriateness of the drug plan of each resident receiving such drugs [PL 100-103 §1919 (c) (1) (D)].

The regulations clarify that a chemical restraint means a psychopharmacologic drug, and that

> [Except in emergency situations] a facility may not use a chemical restraint [defined as any drug prescribed with the intent of controlling mood, mental status or behavior] that is used for the purpose of discipline or convenience and not required to treat the resident's medical symptoms, including one or more of the following ways:
> (i) In excessive dose (including duplicate therapy);
> (ii) For excessive duration;
> (iii) Without adequate monitoring;
> (iv) Without adequate indications for its use;
> (v) In the presence of adverse consequences which indicate the dose should be reduced or discontinued; and
> (vi) In a manner that results in a decline in the resident's functional status. (Federal Register vol. 57 No 24, February 5, 1992).

These regulations have, in turn, been translated into interpretive guidelines that suggest standards of practice more specific than most clinical guidelines. The initial guidelines addressed specific classes of drugs, including neuroleptics, sedatives, and antidepressants. Because this left other drug classes (e.g. benzodiazapines) uncovered, there was concern that physicians might begin to prescribe drugs from the uncovered classes to avoïd the scrutiny of the regulators.

The new guidelines, issued in April 1992, cover a larger range of drugs, including benzodiazapines. They require trying short-acting drugs before long-acting ones and limiting the use of both to four continuous months unless gradual dose reduction was unsuccessful. Their use is limited to four conditions, which do not appear to be terribly restrictive, but which must meet *Diagnostic Statistical Manual III* diagnostic criteria:

1. generalized anxiety disorder
2. organic mental syndromes, including dementia, with associated agitated states that constitute sources of distress or dysfunction to the resident or represent a danger to the resident or others
3. panic disorder

4. symptomatic anxiety in a resident with another psychiatric disorder, including adjustment disorder

The second allusion to chemical restraints in OBRA 87 addresses the general limitations on the use of any type of restraint noted above [PL 100-103 §1919 (c) (1) (A) (ii)] with the specific prohibition against using them for purposes of discipline or convenience. This aspect has proven a better basis for developing regulations than the first approach, because it is more concrete than simply a restatement of the definition of good care.

The regulations for using psychopharmacologic drugs not only call for appropriate indications, but require that efforts be made at least semiannually to withdraw the drug unless there are clear contraindications. They also call for annual review of drug regimens by an independent physician with training or experience in geriatrics and psychopharmacology (given the small number of trained geriatricians, to say nothing of those with both types of training, experience will have to be quite broadly defined) to determine whether

(A) The drug has an appropriate indication for use;
(B) The dose is appropriate;
(C) The duration of therapy is appropriate;
(D) Valid justification exists for the use of chemical restraints;
(F) (sic) The benefits of using the drug outweigh the risk to the resident; and
(G) Nondrug therapy approaches have failed [Federal Register vol. 57 No 24, §483.13 (a) (5) (i)].

Before using a psychopharmacologic drug in an nonemergency situation, the facility must

(i) Explain the use of the drug to the resident, or, if the resident has been declared to be legally incompetent or cannot understand his or her rights, to the resident's legal representative;
(ii) Explain the resident's right to refuse the drug;
(iii) Obtain written consent of the resident or the resident's legal representative. [Federal Register, Vol. 57, No 24, §483.13 (a) (4) (ii)].

A study examining the use of psychoactive drugs in nursing homes during the years before OBRA 87 suggests that there is a substantial basis for concern. A large proportion of residents receiving such medications lacked the justifying diagnosis (21).

Although no scientific studies have yet been published to document the changes wrought by the new regulations, the anecdotal data suggest that the impact has been profound. Table 4 presents data from a large pharmacy consulting corporation that works in California and several other states. They

Table 4 Psychoactive medication usage

Month	Number of patients	Neuroleptic Routine %	Neuroleptic PRN %	Antidepressant Routine %	Antidepressant PRN %	Benzodiazepine Routine %	Benzodiazepine PRN %	Sedative/Hypnotics Routine %	Sedative/Hypnotics PRN %
June 1989	6,114	17.81	11.68	18.56	.16	5.25	7.75	3.63	6.02
Oct. 1990	5,692	11.86	3.30	17.52	.46	5.31	7.52	2.44	4.15
Nov. 1991	11,362	12.5	2.4	16.0	.2	7.6	7.4	1.7	2.9

Source: Pharmacy Corporation of America.

have tracked the changes in the rate of use for psychoactive medications from the period before (June 1989), just around (October 1990), and subsequent to (November 1991) the implementation of the OBRA regulations. The changes in use preceded the effective date of the regulations, which suggests that the nursing homes may have anticipated the regulations. Routine use of neuroleptic drugs fell by almost one-third, and the drop in prn use was especially remarkable. Viewed as a proportion of the baseline rate, routine use of sedatives declined even more, again with a dramatic drop in prn use. As might be anticipated, antidepressants, which are likely underused and are not specifically covered by the regulations, showed little effect (22). The concerns about compensatory use of benzodiazapines seem to be borne out to some extent, with an increase of about 50% in their routine use, but no change in their prn use rate.

The size of the reductions is impressive, especially in light of a report from a experiment designed specifically to reduce use of psychoactive drugs in nursing homes. An active educational program for all levels of staff produced an 18% reduction in antipsychotic medications and a 36% reduction in nonbenzodiazepine hypnotics, compared with a 3% reduction in antipsychotics and a 2% reduction in nonbenzodiazepine hypnotics in the control group (3). The apparently greater effects seen in the data from the consulting pharmacist group may speak to the power of direct intervention. Active efforts by well-prepared consulting pharmacists may produce greater results than even aggressive educational programs.

The 1992 survey of nursing homes done by the American Association of Homes for the Aging also asked about the use of chemical restraints. The reported decline was less than that for physical restraints. In 1989, 29% of residents were chemically restrained; by 1991, the proportion had fallen to 21%. Once again, larger homes were more likely to use restraints than were smaller ones.

The AMDA medical directors surveyed about restraint use were also queried about the use of chemical restraints. About 80% reported that their facility had changed its formal policy with regard to the use of psychoactive medications; in almost every case, the change was prompted by the OBRA regulations. An interdisciplinary team authored the policies in about 42% of cases. Some 72% of the policies required that psychoactive medication orders be reviewed by a pharmacist, but only 18% had to be reviewed by the medical director. In 63% of policies, use of psychoactive medications is actively discouraged. Some 56% of policies specified conditions for which a psychoactive medication may not be used, and 52% specified alternatives that must be tried before a psychoactive medication is used; 42% prohibit prn orders for psychoactive medications. Only 10% require a written agreement signed by the resident or his/her legal guardian for any psychoactive medication. Once again, these requirements are built into the regulations currently in force.

COMMON GROUND

The movement to reduce, or even eliminate, restraints appeats to be affecting the use of both physical and chemical restraints. Although some feared that releasing residents from physical restraints might lead to greater reliance on chemical approaches, this does not seem to be happening. A positive interpretation of this still only anecdotal observation is that the basic change in care is driven by a common recognition of the centrality of personhood in nursing home residents. An alternative reading suggests that heavy regulation of both forms of restraints has prevented any such shift.

It will likely be impossible to interpret with confidence the meaning of the impressive change in practice patterns we are currently witnessing with regard to the use of both types of restraints. Those who favor a more holistic approach will view this transformation as long-delayed appreciation of the dehumanizing of institutionalized persons and the psychological brutality to which they have been inappropriately subjected. On a broader plane, the discontinuance of restraints is part of a larger movement toward person-centered care, an approach that emphasizes individualized care plans designed to minimize the trauma of institutions.

Those more given to regulatory policy will point to the success of the nursing home regulations and question whether less stringent approaches, such as the use of guidelines for the appropriateness of medical care, will have as profound an impact. They will point to this experience as an object lesson in the need for strong and specific controls of how care is delivered.

The two interpretations are not necessarily incompatible. In fact, each may lend insight to the other. The success of the regulations, and the relatively mild resistance encountered, may be attributable, at least in part, to the general sense of their moral correctness. Although some railed against specific provisions, the speed with which change occurred suggests a latent belief in the correctness of the mandated change. At the same time, it is much less likely that such change would have occurred simply on the basis of moral suasion, even if better data were available to establish the efficacy of the recommended change.

The two forces appear to be acting synergistically, but they are still not without problems. The American penchant for rule-making carries an equally strong corollary for rule-bending and loophole searching. Ours is a mechanistic society, which looks for precise formulations of problems and solutions. Some portion of the society will emphasize the mortar rather than the bricks and search for chinks. At least some providers of care and merchants of services have responded to the new mandate in a narrower way. They test the letter and not the spirit of the effort by promoting new approaches to restraining residents that evade the regulatory definitions. It thus becomes clear that any successful transformation in approaches to care must be able to define the outcomes that are sought rather than relying exclusively on specifications of the processes of care. The more the goals are defined as the maximization of resident functioning and autonomy and the opportunity for personal satisfaction, the easier it will be to press for better ways to deliver care to frail elderly persons.

The term "individualized care" is used to describe the conceptual framework of restraint-free care (7, 15, 58). In this approach, the focus shifts to the person, the care recipient. No longer is the accomplishment of task given priority; it takes second place after response to the needs of the resident. This shift in priority, if its implications are fully absorbed, has potential for profound change in the way in which long-term care is experienced by both resident and staff.

Individualized care rests on a thorough knowledge of the person who is the resident and, therefore, necessitates the building of relationship between caregiver and resident. Communication becomes of primary importance. Individualized care uses every possible aspect of daily life to help the resident shape a way of life that responds to her/his individual preferences and values. Daily routines and schedules, the physical environment, staff-resident interactions, meals and manner of their serving, individual seating arrangements, incontinence equipment, and many more aspects of daily life are seen as tools for individualizing care. Thus, more opportunities for choice are introduced into the resident's life, individually, and coping abilities are strengthened, rather than assaulted by demands of uniformity and conformity, and the right to resident decision making about risk taking is recognized.

ACKNOWLEDGMENTS

The authors thank numerous people for their assistance in compiling information for this paper. Mary Parker of the American Medical Directors Association coordinated the survey of its members. Alan Friedlob provided HCFA data on restraint use. Thomas Lackner supplied data on psychoactive drug use in nursing homes. Patrick Flood, Mary Jane Koren, and Vivienne Wisdom provided information on specific state activities. The staff of the National Citizen's Coalition for Nursing Home Reform provided an array of helpful information.

Literature Cited

1. Subcomm on Aging. 1991. *Nursing Home Residents rights: Has the Administration Set a Land Mine for the Landmark OBRA 1987 Nursing Home Reform Law?* Washington, DC: GPO
2. Am. Health Care Assoc. *Clinical Practice Guidelines for the Use of Restraints.*

2a. Anderson, M. 1989. Drugs prescribed for elderly patients in nursing homes or under medical home care. *Compr. Gerontol. A+B* 3:8–15

2b. Appelbaum, P. S., Roth, L. H. 1984. Involuntary treatment in medicine and psychiatry. *Am. J. Psychiatry* 141:202

3. Avorn, J., Soumerai, S. B., Everitt, D. E., Ross-Degan, D., Beers, M. H., et al. 1992. A randomized trial of a program to reduce the use of psychoactive drugs in nursing homes. *N. Engl. J. Med.* 327(3):168–73

3a. Avorn, J., Dreyer, P., Connelly, K., Soumerai, S. B. 1989. Use of psychoactive medications and quality of care in rest homes. *N. Engl. J. Med.* 320(4):227–32

4. Banziger, G., Roush, S. 1983. Nursing homes for the birds: a control-relevant intervention with bird feeders. *Gerontologist* 23:527–31

5. Barry, M. J., Mulley, A. G. Jr., Fowler, F. J., Wennberg, J. W. 1988. Watchful waiting vs. immediate transurethral resection for symptomatic prostatism: the importance of patients' preferences. *J. Am. Med. Assoc.* 259: 3010–17

5a. Beardsley, R. S., Larson, D. B., Burns, B. J., Thompson, J. W., Kamerow, D. B. 1989. Prescribing of psychotropics in elderly nursing home patients. *J. Am. Geriatr. Soc.* 37:327–30

5b. Beers, M., Avorn, J., Soumerai, S. B., Everitt, D. E. 1988. Psychoactive medication use in intermediate-care facility residents. *J. Am. Med. Assoc.* 260(20): 3016–20

6. Bergner, M., Bobbitt, R. A., Kressel, S., Pollard, W. E., Gilson, B. S., et al. 1976. The sickness impact profiile: conceptual formulation and methodology for the development of a health status measure. *Int. J. Health Serv.* 6:393–415

6a. Berland, B., Cohen-Mansfield, J., Lipson, S. 1990. Patient characteristics associated with the use of mechanical restraints. *J. Gen. Intern. Med.* 5:480–85

6b. Billig, N., Cohen-Mansfield, J., Lipson, S. 1991. Pharmacological treatment of agitation in a nursing home. *J. Am. Geriatr. Soc.* 39(10):1002–5

7. Blakeslee, J. 1989. *Untie the elderly: quality care without restraints.* Symp. before Special Comm. on Aging, US Senate, Washington, DC

7a. Blazer, D. G., Federspiel, C. F., Ray, W., Schaffner, W. 1983. The risk of anticholinergic toxicity in the elderly: a study of prescribing practices in two populations. *J. Gerontol.* 38(1):31–35

8. Brook, R. H., Park, R. E., Chassin, M. R., Solomon, D. H., Keesey, J., et al. 1990. Predicting the appropriate use of carotid endarterectomy, upper gastrointestinal endoscopy, and coronary angiography. *N. Engl. J. Med.* 323(17):1173–77

8a. Buck, J. A. 1988. Psychotropic drug practice in nursing homes. *J. Am. Geriatr. Soc.* 36:409–18

8b. Buck, J. A., Sprague, R. L. 1989. Psychotropic medication of mentally retarded residents in community long-term care facilities. *Am. J. Ment. Retard.* 1989. 93(6):618–23

9. Burger, S. G. 1989. *Inappropriate use of chemical and physical restraints.* Nat. Cent. for State Long-Term Care. Ombudsmen and Nat. Citiz. Coalit. for Nursing Home Reform, Washington, DC

9a. Burgio, L. D., Hawkins, A. M. 1991. Behavioral assessment of the effects of psychotropic medications on demented nursing home residents. *Behav. Modif.* 15(2):194–212

9b. Burns, B. J., Kamerow, D. G. 1988. Psychotropic drug prescriptions for nursing home residents. *J. Fam. Pract.* 26(2):155–60

9c. Burton, L. C., German, P. S., Rovner, B. W., Brant, L. J. 1992. Physical restraint use and cognitive decline among nursing home residents. *J. Am. Geriatr. Soc.* 40(8):811–16

9d. Cape, R. D. T. 1983. Freedom from restraint. *Gerontologist* 23(special issue):217

10. Chassin, M. R., Kosecoff, J., Park, R. E., Winslow, C. M., Kahn, K. L., et al. 1987. Does inappropriate use explain geographic variations in the use of health care services? A study of three procedures. *J. Am. Med. Assoc.* 258:2533–37

11. Collopy, B. 1992. The use of restraints in long-term care: the ethical issues. White Paperl Third Age Cent., Fordham Univ.

11a. Covert, A. B., Rodrigues, T., Solomon, K. 1977. The use of mechanical and chemical restraints in nursing homes. *J. Am. Geriatr. Soc.* 25:85–89

11b. Dietsche, L. M., Pollmann, J. 1982. Alzheimer's diseases: advances in clinical nursing. *J. Gerontol. Nursing* 8:97–99

12. Dorsey, R., Ayd, F. J., Cole, J., Klein, D., Simpson, G., et al. 1979. Psychopharmacological screening criteria development project. *J. Am. Med. Assoc.* 241(10):1021–31

13. Dubler, N. 1992. *Ethics on Call.* New York: Humana

14. Ellwood, P. M. 1988. Outcomes management: a technology of patient experience. *N. Engl. J. Med.* 318: 1549–56

15. Evans, L., Strumpf, N. Williams, C. 1991. Redefining a standard of care for frail older people: alternatives to routine physical restraint. In *Advances in Long Term Care,* ed. P. Katz, R. L. Kane, M. Mezey, pp. 81–108. New York: Springer

16. Evans, L. K., Strumpf, N. E. 1987. Patterns of restraint use with institutionalized elderly: a cross-cultural view. *Gerontol. Soc. Am.* Washington, DC: Gerontol. Soc. Am.

17. Evans, L. K., Strumpf, N. E. 1989. Tying down the elderly: a review of the literature on physical restraint. *J. Am. Geriatr. Soc.* 37:65–74

17a. Farnsworth, E. L. 1973. Nursing homes use caution when they use restraints. *Mod. Nursing Home* 30(3):4,9–10

17b. Folmar, S., Wilson, H. 1989. Social behavior and physical restraints. *Gerontologist* 29:650–53

18. Freidson, E. 1970. *Professional Dominance: The Social Structure of Medical Care.* New York: Atherton

19. Frengley, J. D., Mion, L. C. 1986. Incidence of physical restraints on acute general medical wards. *J. Am. Geriatr. Soc.* 34:565–68

20. Fried, J. 1987. Care that kills. *Press-Telegram,* June 21–22, pp. C4-5, C7. Long Beach, Calif.

21. Garrard, J., Makris, L., Dunham, T., Heston, L. L., Cooper, S., et al. 1991. Evaluation of neuroleptic drug use by nursing home elderly under proposed Medicare and Medicaid regulations. *J. Am. Med. Assoc.* 265:463–67

22. Heston, L. L., Garrard, J., Makris, L., Kane, R. L., Cooper, S., et al. 1992. Inadequate treatment of depressed nursing home elderly. *J. Am. Geriatr. Soc.* 40:1178–22

22a. Hulisz, D. T., Sumner, E. D., Hodge, F. J., Weart, C. W. 1991. Study of antipsychotic drug use in long-term care facilities. *J. Pharmacy Technol.* 7:13–18

23. Kapp, M. B. 1991. Nursing home restraints and legal liability: merging the standard of care and industry practice. New York: Commonwealth Fund

24. Katz, S. 1987. The science of quality of life. *J. Chron. Dis.* 40(6):459–63

25. Kosecoff, J., Kanouse, D. E., Rogers, W. H., McCloskey, L., Winslow, C. M. et al. 1987. Effects of the National Institutes of Health Consensus Development Program on physician practice. *J. Am. Med. Assoc.* 258:2708–13

26. Langer, E., Rodin, J. 1976. The effects of choice and enhanced personal responsibility for the aged. A field experiment in an institutional setting. *J. Personal. Soc. Psychol.* 34:191–98

26a. Lantz, M. S., Louis, A., Lowenstein, G., Kennedy, G. J. 1990. A longitudinal study of psychotropic prescriptions in a teaching nursing home. *Am. J. Psychiatry* 147(12):1637–39

26b. Larson, E. B., Kukull, W. A., Buchner, D., Reifler, B. V. 1987. Adverse drug reactions associated with global cognitive impairment in elderly persons. *Ann. Intern. Med.* 107:169–73

27. Leape, L. L., Park, R. E., Solomon, D. H., Chassin, M. R., Kosecoff, J., et al. 1990. Does inappropriate use explain small-area variations in the use of health care services. *J. Am. Med. Assoc.* 263:669–72

28. Leverett, M. 1992. Restraint or enabler? *Restraint Rev.* 1(1):2

29. Lieberman, M. A., Tobin, S. S. 1983. *The Experience of Old Age*. New York: Basic Books

30. Liebow, L. 1992. Statement before the Oversight Comm. of the Commonwealth Fund Restraint Minimization Project, April 14

30a. Lipsitz, L. A., Jonsson, P. V., Kelley, M. M., Koestner, J. S. 1991. Causes and correlates of recurrent falls in ambulatory frail elderly. *J. Gerontol.* 46(4):M114–22

30b. Lofgren, R. P., MacPherson, D. S., Granieri, R., Myllenbeck, S., Sprafka, J. M. 1989. Mechanical restraints on the medical wards: are protective devices safe. *Am. Public Health* 79:735–38

31. Lomas, J., Anderson, G. M., Domnick-Pierre, K., Vayda, E., Enkin, M. W., et al. 1989. Do practice guidelines guide practice? The effect of a consensus statement on the practice of physicians. *N. Engl. J. Med.* 321(19):1306–11

32. Macpherson, D. S., Lofgren, R. P., Cranieri, R., Myllenbeck, S. 1990. Deciding to restrain medical patients. *J. Am. Geriatr. Soc.* 38:516–20

33. McHutchion, E., Morse, J. M. 1989. Releasing restraints: a nursing dilemma. *J. Gerontol. Nursing* 15(2):16–21

34. Inst. of Med. 1986. *Improving the Quality of Care in Nursing Homes.* Washington, D.C.: Nat. Acad. Press

35. Miles, S. H. 1990. *Restraints: Controlling a Symptom or a Symptom of Control*. Atlanta: Am. Geriatr. Soc.

36. Miles, S. H., Irvine, P. 1992. Deaths caused by physical restraints. *Gerontologist.* 32:762–66

36a. Mion, L. C., Frengley, J. D., Jakovcic, C. A., Marino, J. A. 1989. A further exploration of the use of physical restraints in hospitalized patients. *J. Am. Geriatr. Soc.* 37:949–56

36b. Mitchell-Pedersen, L., Edmund, L., Fingerote, E., Powell, C. 1985. Let's untie the elderly. *CAHA Q.* 21(10):10–14

36c. Morrison, J., Crinklaw-Wiancko, D., King, D. 1987. Formulating a restraint use policy for adults based on the research process. *J. Nursing Adm.* 17:39–42

37. Moss, F. E., Halamandaris, V. J. 1977. *Too Old, Too Sick, Too Bad: Nursing Homes in America.* Germantown, Md: Aspen Syst. Corp.

38. Nohlgren, S. 1987. Restraints: critics search for better way. *St. Petersburg Times,* Dec. 13, 14, 16, pp. B1, 16; B1, 8; A18

38a. Nolan, L., O'Malley, K. 1989. The need for a more rational approach to drug prescribing for elderly people in nursing homes. *Age Ageing* 18:52–56

39. Papongenis, D., ed. 1989–1992. *Untie the Elderly,* Vols. 1–4. 1989–1992. Kennett Square, Penn: Kendal Corp.

40. Patrick, D., Erickson, P. 1992. *Health Status and Health Policy.* New York: Oxford Univ. Press

41. Phillips, C. D., Hawes, M. C., Fried, B. E. 1992. *Does It Cost Less to Care for Physically Restrained Nursing Home Residents?* Nat. Inst. of Mental Health and Nursing Home Commun. Coalition of NY State

41a. Powell, C., Mitchell-Pedersen, L., Fingerote, E., Edmund, L. 1989. Freedom from restraint: consequences of reducing physical restraints in the management of the elderly. *Calif. Med. Assoc. J.* 141:561–64

42. Rader, J. 1991. *Magic, Mystery, Modification, and Mirth: The Joyful Road to Restraint Free Care.* Mt. Angel, Oreg: Benedictine Inst. for Long-Term Care

42a. Ray, W. A., Federspiel, C. F., Schaffner, W. 1980. A study of antipsychotic drug use in nursing homes: epidemiologic evidence suggesting misuse. *Am. J. Public Health* 70(5):485–91

42b. Ray, W. A., Griffin, M. R., Schaffner, W., Baugh, D. K., Melton, L. T. III. 1987. Psychotropic drug use and the risk of hip fracture. *N. Engl. J. Med.* 316:363–69

43. Rigert, J., Lerner, M. 1990. Safeguards that kill. *Star Tribune,* Dec. 2–5, pp. A1, 16, 17, 19, 20–22; A1, 10, 11; A1, 18–20, A1, 18–20. Minneapolis

44. Robbins, L. J., Boyko, E., Lane, J., Cooper, D., Jahnigen, D. W. 1987. Binding the elderly: a prospective study of the use of mechanical restraints in an acute care hospital. *J. Am. Geriatr. Soc.* 35:290–96

45. Rothman, D. J. 1991. *Strangers at the Bedside: A History of How Law and Bioethics Transformed Medical Decision Making.* New York:Basic Books

45a. Rovner, B. W., German, P. S., Brant, L. J., Clark, R., Burton, L., et al. 1991. Depression and mortality in nursing homes. *J. Am. Med. Assoc.* 265(8): 993–96

46. Rubenstein, L. Z., Campbell, L. J., Kane, R. L., eds. 1987. *Geriatric Assessment: An Overview of Its Impacts, in Clinics in Geriatric Medicine.* Philadelphia: Saunders

47. Rubenstein, L. Z., Stuck, A. E., Siu, A. L., Wieland, D. 1991. Impacts of geriatric evaluation and management programs on defined outcomes: overview of the evidence. *J. Am. Geriatr. Soc.* 39S:8S–16S

48. Schmidt, L., Reinhardt, A. M., Kane, R. L., Olsen, D. M. 1977. The mentally ill in nursing homes: New back wards in the community. *Arch Gen Psych,* 34:687–691

49. Schnelle, J. F., Newman, D. R., White, M., Volner, T. R., Burnett, J., et al. 1992. Reducing and managing restraints in long-term care facilities. *J. Am. Geriatr. Soc.* 40:381–85

50. Schultz, R. 1976. Effects of control and predictability on the physical and psychological well-being of the institutionalized aged. *J. Personal. Soc. Psychol.* 33:563–73

50a. Seifert, R., Jamieson, J., Gardner, R. J. 1983. Use of anticholinergics in the nursing home: an empirical study and review. *Drug Intell. Clin. Pharm.* 17(6):470 73

50b. Sherman, D. S. 1988. Paychoactive drug misuse in long-term care: some contributing factors. *J. Pharm. Pract.* 1(3):41–46

50c. Sloane, P. D., Matthew, L. J., Scarborough, M., Desai, J. R., Koch, G. G., et al. 1991. Physical and pharmacologic restraint of nursing home patients with dementia: impact of specialized units. *J. Am. Med. Assoc.* 265:1278–82

50d. Sobel, K. G., McCart, G. M. 1983. Drug use and accidental falls in an intermediate care facility. *Drug Intell. Clin. Pharm.* 17(7-8):539–42

51. Strumpf, N. E., Evans, L. K. 1988. Physical restraint of the hospitalized elderly: perceptions of patients and nurses. *Nursing Res.* 37:132–37

52. Strumpf, N. E., Tomes, N. 1993. Restraining the troublesome patient: an historical perspective on a contemporary debate/ *Nursing Hist. Rev.* In press

52a. Strumpf, N. E., Evans, L. K. 1987. Patterns of restraint use in a nursing home (abstr.). In *Nursing Advances in Health,* Proc. of Am. Nurses' Assoc. Counc. of Nurse Res. Meet. Washington, DC

52b. Svarstad, B. L., Mount, J. K. 1991. Nursing home resources and tranquilizer use among the institutionalized elderly. *J. Am. Geriatr. Soc.* 39(9):869–75

53. Szasz, T. S., Hollander, M. H. 1956. A contribution to the philosophy of medicine: the basic models of the doctor-patient relationship. *Arch. Intern. Med.* 97:585–92

53a. Tinetti, M. E., Liu, W., Ginter, S. F. 1992. Mechanical restraint use and fall-related injuries among residents of skilled nursing facilities. *Ann. Intern. Med.* 116:369–74

53b. Tinetti, M. E., Wen-Liang, L., Marottoli, R. A., Ginter, S. P. 1991. Mechanical restraint use among residents of skilled nursing facilities. *J. Am. Med. Assoc.* 265:468

54. Wennberg, J. E. 1990. Outcomes research, cost containment, and the fear of health care rationing. *N. Engl. J. Med.* 323(17):1202–4

55. Wennberg, J. E., Freeman, J. L., Culp, W. J. 1987. Are hospital services rationed in New Haven or over-utilized in Boston? *Lancet* 1:1185–89

55a. Werner, P., Cohen-Mansfield, J., Braun, J., Marx, M. 1989. Physical restraints and agitation in nursing home residents. *J. Am. Geriatr. Soc.* 37: 1122–26

56. Williams, C. C. 1991. *Daily Life of Residents in Restraint-Free Nursing Homes in Scotland and Sweden.* San Francisco: Gerontol. Soc. of Am.

57. Williams, C. C. 1991. *Elders: Experienced Risk Takers.* Durham, NC: Duke Univ. Cent. for the Study of Aging and Hum. Dev.

58. Williams, C. C. 1989. The experience of long-term care in the future. *J. Gerontol. Soc. Work* 14:3–18

59. Williams, C. C. 1990. Long-term care and the human spirit. *Generations* 14(4):25–28

60. Williams, C. C. 1991. *Negotiated risk: liability or liberty?* Panel presentation, Am. Soc. on Aging, New Orleams

61. Williams, T. F., Hill, J. G., Fairbank, M. E. 1973. Appropriate placement of the chronically ill and aged: s successful approach by evaluation. *J. Am. Med. Assoc.* 226:1332–35

61a. Zawadski, R. T., Glazer, G. B., Lurie, E. 1978. Psychotropic drug use among institutionalized and noninstitutionalized Medicaid aged in California. *J. Gerontol.* 33(6):825–34

Annu. Rev. Publ. Health. 1993. 14:585–604

CALIFORNIA'S PROPOSITION 99 ON TOBACCO, AND ITS IMPACT

Lester Breslow
School of Public Health and Division of Cancer Control, University of California, Los Angeles, Los Angeles, California 90024

Michael Johnson
Tobacco Control Section, California Department of Health Services, Sacramento, California 94234

KEY WORDS: smoking, tobacco tax, trends in smoking, prevention program

---

PUBLIC HEALTH SIGNIFICANCE OF TOBACCO

Tobacco consumption, especially in the form of cigarette smoking, continues toward the year 2000 as the great pestilence of the twentieth century. For people in the United States, it is the largest single preventable cause of mortality, now responsible for shortening about 400,000 lives each year, i.e. about one sixth of all deaths in the nation. Approximately one third of these deaths are from coronary heart disease; one third from lung cancer; and the remaining third mainly from other types of cancer, chronic lung disease, and stroke (32–42).

Roughly the same situation prevails throughout the developed world and is spreading rapidly through the developing world (23).

Recognition of the health devastation from tobacco use began in the 1930s. The biostatistician Raymond Pearl demonstrated that smoking was "statistically associated with an impairment of life duration" (18). Only in the late 1940s, however, did epidemiologists and other health scientists initiate the many substantial studies that led to the 1964 publication of the Surgeon-General's Report, *Smoking and Health* (25).

Even before that landmark document appeared, public health agencies had begun to accept tobacco consumption as a major public health problem and to advocate action. In one early such endeavor, the California Department of Public Health published a review of its own studies, which emphasized "the substantial public health significance of the problem" and a proposal for action (28). The latter included education, stricter enforcement of the law against sale of cigarettes to minors, removal of vending machines from public health and other health facilities, smoking cessation clinics, consideration of a tax increase on cigarettes, and restrictions on the advertising and distribution of cigarettes and places where they can be smoked. Although links between that proposal and Proposition 99 cannot be traced, Californians have for some years been using tobacco less than people in the country as a whole.

PATTERNS AND TRENDS IN TOBACCO USE

Native Americans were smoking tobacco when Europeans arrived in the Americas. It was carried thereafter to other parts of the world, but remained a rare product until about 1900. Then, the introduction of cigarette manufacturing machines and the "safety match" led to vast spread of tobacco consumption. Facilitating this expansion were linkage of the tobacco and advertising industries with nicotine's great addictive power.

The United States

The rise and beginning fall of the cigarette scourge in the United States during this century is shown in Figure 1 (27). In 1900, annual consumption was only

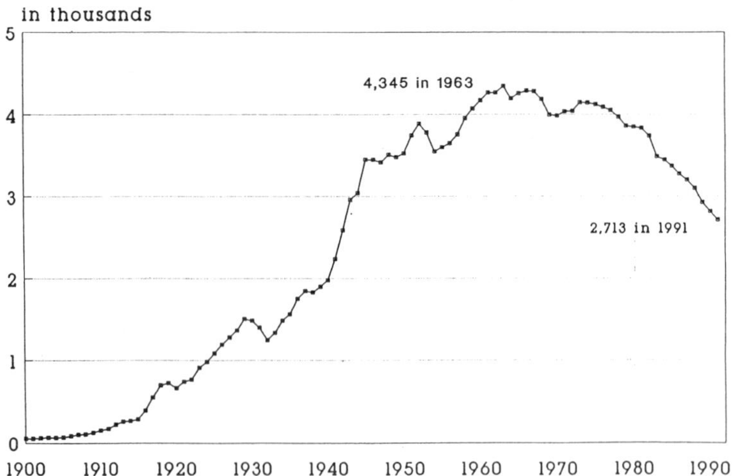

Figure 1 US per capita cigarette consumption, 1900–1991. (Source: US Department of Agriculture, courtesy of Donald Shopland.)

54 cigarettes per capita. That increased fairly steadily, reaching a peak of 4345 in 1963, and declining thereafter. Since 1985, consumption has been dropping about 3% per year.

Because different segments of the population use cigarettes (the principal form of tobacco use) in considerably varying amounts, control efforts require monitoring smoking's demographic profile. Men in the United States born between 1910 and 1930 smoked the most, with a peak prevalence of 60–65% during the 1940s and 1950s (8, 33). Subsequent cohorts of men have been smoking less; for example, cigarette smoking by men born in 1951–1960 reached a high point of only 40%. Women in the United States began smoking later than, and not as heavily as, men; their 1921–1940 cohorts smoked the maximum, 40–45%, in the 1950s and 1960s. These time relationships account for the fact that the lung cancer epidemic became apparent among women only in the 1960s.

Tobacco use typically starts during the teen years and is most prevalent in the early adult years. Thereafter, smokers increasingly quit. Although cigarette smoking became popular among women some years after men developed the habit, in recent years teenage smoking among girls has been almost as high as that among boys. Black females have experienced smoking rates similar to those of white females. Smoking by black males in the United States started to climb some decades after white males and has been persisting longer; the peak prevalence rates are somewhat lower but last longer.

Smoking in the United States is increasingly concentrated among persons of lower socio-economic status, as measured by nature of employment and levels of income and education (20). Thus, a 1986 survey disclosed that 34–43% of craftsmen, operatives, and laborers smoked cigarettes, but only 21–28% of managers, professional/technical workers, and sales/clerical workers did so (30). Prevalence among college graduates was down to 21%, but it remained at 37% among persons who did not complete high school. Those in the upper socio-economic levels had also tended to start smoking later in life and had quit smoking to a greater extent.

California

California's cigarette smoking rates as far back as 1974 have been slightly lower than in the United States as a whole, and the gap has been slowly growing (3). Generally, the same socio-economic gradients and trends that have been noted for the nation prevail in California.

The racial-ethnic mix in California is both different and changing more rapidly than elsewhere in the country, with important implications for tobacco consumption and its control. As recently as 1960, Caucasians constituted 78% of the population; African-Americans, 7%; Latinos, 12%; and Asians, only

3%. The 1990 census showed Caucasians, 57%; Latinos, 26%; African-Americans 7%; and Asians, 10%.

It seems clear that, in California, tobacco control efforts should concentrate on restraining the initiation of smoking among teenagers, especially by those who do not complete high school or enter college; on minimizing the use of tobacco among Latinos and Asian/Pacific Islanders (particularly the women) before they are drawn into the tobacco habits of their new neighbors; and facilitating cessation of smoking among young people who have taken up the habit (Table 1).

Although this review focuses on California, with the United States as background (14, 18, 20, 37), it should be noted that as tobacco consumption comes under control in North America, the nation's tobacco industry is marketing heavily in South America, Asia, and other parts of the world. Because of California's racial/ethnic composition, the state's tobacco control experience may be useful in other regions of the world where the tobacco industry is marketing intensively among corresponding demographic groups.

Table 1 Current smoking status, Californians, 1990–1991[1]

	Current smoker %	Former smoker %	Never smoker %
Total	22	27	51
Men	25	32	44
Women	19	23	58
Age			
18–24	22	12	65
25–44	24	23	54
45–64	22	38	41
65+	12	42	46
Hispanic	18	21	61
Non-Hispanic	23	29	48
Race			
White	21	28	50
Af.-Amer.	29	25	46
Asian	16	19	66
Other	32	22	46
Education			
<12 years	26	28	47
12 yrs	25	27	49
13–15 yrs	21	27	52
16+ yrs	13	29	58

[1]From Ref. 3.

ACTIONS AGAINST TOBACCO USE

Since the recognition of tobacco's hazard to health, proposals for comprehensive approaches to its control have come from numerous agencies (1, 2, 11, 13, 16, 29, 45). In general, the aim is to create a total social milieu that discourages the use of tobacco. In the words of the World Health Organization, "the application of whatever downward pressures on smoking rates that are practical" should be sought (46).

Initial efforts were directed toward informing people of the dangers and encouraging smokers to quit and persuading nonsmokers, especially youth, to avoid the habit. Recently, a trend toward establishing overall living circumstances that restrain smoking has taken root. Education, for example assisting young people to develop skills to resist peer and other pressures to smoke, remains an important element of the campaign. Creating an all-inclusive environmental situation adverse to smoking, however, is now seen as necessary.

The latter involves mobilizing community forces, including government, to join the effort (7). Until the past decade or two, the tobacco and advertising industries had a free hand, aided by the addictive properties of tobacco, to spread its use. If tobacco were proposed for introduction in the United States now, the Food and Drug Administration might well prohibit its use on the grounds of its known carcinogenic and other harmful properties. Several steps to combat its consumption are under way:

1. Enlisting mass media against, instead of for, tobacco use: prohibiting advertising of smoking and other forms of tobacco use; social marketing of tobacco avoidance.
2. Making cigarettes more difficult to obtain, especially by young people: increasing the price through higher taxation at time of purchase; eliminating, or at least severely restricting, vending machine sales; enforcing bans on sales to minors.
3. Requiring warning labels on cigarette packages.
4. Encouraging physicians to advise patients against tobacco use.
5. Prohibiting smoking in public places where others can be exposed, such as in public buildings, public vehicles, work places, and restaurants.
6. Offering assistance to smokers who want to quit.
7. Stopping government support of the tobacco industry: domestically, e.g. subsidies for growing tobacco and allowing the cost of tobacco promotion as a "business expense"; in foreign trade.

In the United States, voluntary health agencies concerned with tobacco-related diseases, such as cancer, heart, and lung associations, have been devoting substantial effort toward smoking control. They have been joined by other voluntary organizations formed specifically to combat smoking. Besides activating millions of individuals and groups throughout the country in the struggle against tobacco use, these organizations have been pressing federal, state, and local governments to adopt moves that will curtail it. Effectiveness in the latter regard can be seen in reports of widespread action toward the objectives listed above (23, 24, 27). Thus, a comprehensive strategy is being realized.

CALIFORNIA'S PROPOSITION 99

In 1988, the citizens of California succeeded in placing a powerful tax initiative on the November ballot. Proposition 99, as the measure was called, raised the surtax on cigarettes and other tobacco products and specified that the new revenues both fund health-care services for the medically indigent and support statewide antitobacco health education efforts. Supporters of the measure resorted to the initiative process after the tobacco industry had succeeded for 20 years in staving off any tobacco tax increase by the California legislature.

Tobacco companies viewed Proposition 99 as a serious threat and mounted a $20 million advertising and public relations effort to defeat it. However, supports of the measure, with less than $1.6 million at their disposal, fought and won by a three to two margin.

Specifically, Proposition 99 added a 25-cent tax per pack on cigarettes (to the existing 10-cent tax) and a proportional tax increase on other tobacco products. The new law earmarked the added revenues for the following uses:

1. 20% for antitobacco education in schools and communities;
2. 35% for hospitals and 10% for physicians, for treatment of patients who could not afford to pay and for whom payment would not otherwise be made;
3. 5% for research on tobacco-related disease;
4. 5% for public resources; and
5. the final 25% to be allocated by the legislature among the preceding categories.

Proposition 99 prohibited use of the funds to supplant existing funding of services.

The Proposition 99 campaign unfolded in four stages: formation of the core coalition and writing of the initiative, the petition phase, the campaign phase, and, once successful, the appropriation phase.

Formation of the Core Coalition/Writing the Initiative

Early proponents included the American Lung Association, the American Cancer Society, the American Heart Association, the California Association of Hospitals and Health Services, the California Medical Association, the Services Employees' International Union, the California Dental Association, and the Planning and Conservation League. Supporters estimated that the tax would raise approximately $600 million annually.

The Petition Phase

A total of 600,000 signatures were required to qualify the proposition for the ballot. With the assistance of a professional signature-gathering firm, over 1,000,000 signatures were obtained.

The Campaign Phase

Proposition 99 proponents formed a coalition and sought to portray the campaign as a "David-Goliath" struggle with the tobacco industry. The latter's obviously expensive advertising facilitated that effort. However, while recognizing the underdog appeal, the "Yes on 99" forces kept the health issue as their central theme. Spokespersons were trained and encouraged to use the facts about control of tobacco-related disease and its cost to society. The campaign was never against smokers and avoided mudslinging with the tobacco industry.

Coalition staff came together late in the struggle, with little coordination of resources. In contrast, the tobacco industry had well-versed public relations spokespersons who visited many, even small, county boards for endorsements of their positions. They employed minority lobbyists to influence minority organizations against the Proposition. The Coalition also initiated a substantial effort to involve minority groups, especially prominent members of such groups, in talk shows, editorial action, and a speaker's bureau.

An initial tactic of the tobacco industry's campaign was to emphasize the alleged greed of doctors who would profit from Proposition 99's allocation of funds for medical services, but the main strategy of the "No on 99" forces centered around the crime and bootlegging theme. Media spots claimed that Proposition 99 would cause crime, especially bootlegging of cigarettes, and billboards reinforced that theme. In one television advertisement paid for by "Californians Against Unfair Tax Increases," but sponsored by the Tobacco Institute, a character identified himself as an undercover cop at a supposed crime scene, with police car lights flashing near a huge truck pulled over into an alley. Proposition 99 was the culprit in causing this "crime wave involving gangs and bootlegging."

This crime strategy apparently had influence. Polls showed a drop from an early high of 73% favoring Proposition 99 to 58% in September, and the undecided increased. Then, three fortuitous events occurred within about a week. California's Attorney General held a press briefing to refute the crime allegations. Peace officers' and sheriffs' organizations, embarrassed that their endorsements had been used prominently by the tobacco industry, announced that they were dropping their "No on 99" endorsement. Finally, the undercover cop in the "No on 99" spots was revealed as a police officer with a desk job who had also played a cop killer in a movie. The "undercover cop" apparently became the symbol of a misleading campaign. The "Yes on 99" slide in the polls stopped at 58% positive for the election vote.

The Appropriation Phase

With passage of Proposition 99, the State Legislature began to implement the initiative. Some factional differences within the Coalition emerged during this phase: Voluntary health organizations focused on the health education account, whereas the physician and hospital groups emphasized treatment services.

Faculty from several universities in the state formed a "Committee on Expertise for Tobacco Use Control" and proposed specific allocation of funds to various elements of the tobacco control program that would be funded by the health education account. Representatives of the Committee and the Coalition testified on behalf of the health education account at the public hearing on AB 75, the implementing legislation.

During this period, literally dozens of lobbyists under contract to the tobacco industry worked to subvert constructive use of the health education account. They fought particularly hard against inclusion of a media component that was designed to complement school and community-based education activities, and in favor of redirecting most of the education funds to health care.

High visibility of the tobacco industry's furiously stepped-up lobbying efforts appear to have backfired. The press began to focus on their presence and watch for their influence. AB 75 was passed by the Assembly and Senate in the last 48 hours of the legislative session, and the Governor signed the bill on October 2, 1989.

SMOKING INITIATION AND CESSATION AS A DYNAMIC PROCESS

Becoming a smoker usually involves several identifiable stages; similarly, quitting the habit typically entails gradual change that can be broken into stages (3, 21). Both initiation and cessation can thus be understood as processes involving movement from one status to another (12, 21).

Exploration and initiation of cigarette smoking is largely confined to adolescence, with the transition from regular use to dependence occurring in late adolescence and early adulthood (3). Experimentation with cigarettes and initial use are subject to influences that particularly affect adolescents, whereas dependent use develops when the personal and social utility of smoking is incorporated into how the smoker functions and copes in the adult world. Many adolescents who experiment with tobacco never become regular smokers; they stop before developing dependence on cigarette use.

The vast majority of smokers would like to quit smoking. The process of stopping is often a cyclical one, with the smoker usually making multiple attempts to quit before finally becoming successful. Eighty percent of attempts lapse before a full year passes (3).

Cessation is best understood as a process in which smokers cycle through stages of cessation. Each time they go around the cycle, more of them become successful in their efforts. Tobacco control strategy aims, therefore, to move smokers from one stage of the cessation cycle (precontemplation, contemplation, quitting) to the next. Correspondingly, one can use movement on the cessation cycle as a short-term measure of program impact.

Influences on Initiation

As children move into their teen years, some change from believing that they will never use cigarettes to considering experimenting with cigarette smoking. The images from tobacco advertising of the smoker as an attractive, secure individual, as well as the example of adults and older siblings who smoke, are powerful factors in children's perception of smoking as an entry into adulthood. Counter-advertising that creates a negative image of the smoker may help repel these influences.

Having the first cigarette may not lead irreversibly to becoming a smoker, but is clearly an important milestone in that passage. The widespread availability of cigarettes, and particularly the promotional free distribution of cigarettes into the hands of teenagers, clearly facilitate experimentation with cigarette use. Assertiveness training of teens and modeling of refusal responses can block acceptance of cigarettes offered by peers and others. Access to cigarettes can also be reduced through merchant education.

With movement from occasional experimentation to regular use of cigarettes, the adolescent experiences smoking as psychologically and socially useful, as well as physically addicting. Images created by advertisements of smokers as physically and sexually attractive adults may resonate strongly in adolescents who are desperately attempting to achieve and project exactly these images. This advertising effect on self-image may explain why adolescents who have the least external validation of their self-worth are also the most likely to take up smoking.

Health education and other programs that raise adolescent self-worth and self-esteem, as well as restrict advertising and promotional activities, are directed especially at the move to regular smoking. Raising the price of cigarettes and increasing the social unacceptability of smoking are also barriers to this transition, especially among teens.

Moving from regular use to socially and physically dependent use requires that the utility of tobacco use persist after maturity is reached. For that to happen, cigarette smoking must be allowed in those situations where the adult wants to smoke. For example, if worksite smoking is banned, smokers cannot learn to use cigarettes to cope with stress at work; they are also obligated to develop alternative mechanisms to handle stress, and the latter may be substituted for smoking in nonworkplace settings (22).

Influences on Cessation

Tobacco control efforts currently under way in California are intended to influence smokers at various points in the cessation cycle. Public information campaigns emphasizing the risks of smoking are intended to move smokers from the precontemplation to the contemplation stage, as is personalization of the risk to the smoker through physician warnings (44). Other reasons smokers think about quitting include concerns about being dependent on cigarettes, interest in being a good example, and, recently, the negative image of the smoker and the social unacceptability of smoking. California's tobacco control program aims to intensify these concerns in the smoker.

A variety of environmental stimuli can trigger movement from thinking about quitting to actually attempting to quit. For example, increasing the cost of cigarettes can stimulate cessation attempts. Physician advice to quit, particularly during an acute illness, can also aid cessation (10). Adopting workplace rules to restrict smoking in the worksite likewise facilitates quit attempts by substantial numbers of workers (5).

A major gap in current tobacco control efforts lies in converting quit attempts into long-term successes. Self-help programs, telephone hotlines, and nicotine gum all enhance short-term cessation (19). Clinic-based programs provide substantial help for long-term cessation among those who can be recruited to participate.

The major barriers to long-term success, however, remain difficult to alter. In addition to physical addiction, they are largely in the smoker's environment, including social norms and workplace rules that tolerate and even promote smoking and thus facilitate relapse. Continued smoking of peers and family members and unusual episodes of personal or environmental stress can also lead the smoker to fall back upon the old coping strategy, smoking. Long-term success, therefore, remains the most elusive component of a comprehensive tobacco control strategy. The prospect of continued movement toward nonsmoking as the social norm, coupled with increasing restrictions on where smokers can smoke, offers hope that more smokers will quit and fewer young people will start.

IMMEDIATE IMPACT ON TOBACCO USE IN CALIFORNIA

To assess the initial and ongoing impact of California's Tobacco Control Program, three major sets of evaluation have been undertaken. The first is periodic surveillance of tobacco use among random samples of the population, being conducted by the University of California at San Diego (UCSD). The second, "process evaluation," coordinated by the California State University at San Diego, assesses various program components, such as the efforts of local health departments and other community tobacco control activities, as well as tobacco sales in California. All of these studies serve as primary sources of data on the impact of California's tobacco control program. The third consists of evaluating the tobacco control work of schools in California made possible by Proposition 99. This monitoring for evaluation includes the critical stages in initiation and cessation previously described.

Prevalence of Smoking

The prevalence of smoking disclosed by UCSD's population survey can be compared with both national estimates of smoking and the trend in smoking by Californians during the years preceding the 1989 increase in the tobacco excise tax. Figure 2 shows smoking prevalence in California from 1974 to the time of the most recent survey (1990–1991) based on a series of estimates derived from multiple National Health Interview Surveys (NHIS). The individual NHIS survey estimates for California and for the rest of the United States from 1974 to 1987 are consistent with a linear decline in smoking prevalence, with the average annual rate of decline about three fourths of 1% greater for California than for the rest of the nation. The 1990–1991 prevalence measured in California by the UCSD survey was substantially lower than would have been expected from the 1974–1987 trend. The smoking prevalence

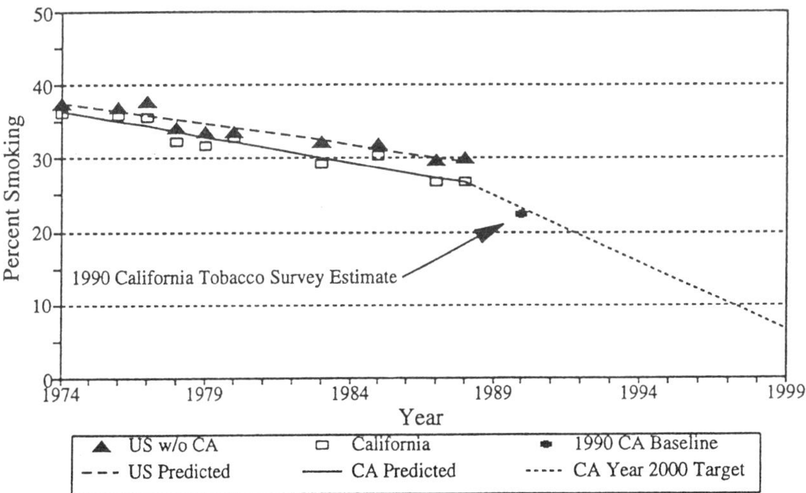

Figure 2 Adult smoking prevalence: California and US without California. (Source: NHIS 1974–1988, 1990 California Tobacco Survey.)

for 1987 was 26.8%, whereas the 1990 UCSD survey estimate was 22.2%. This 17% decline in three years, during which the Proposition 99 campaign (1988), the increase in tax (1989), and the initiation of the program took place, doubles the decline based on the 1974–1987 trend. Thus, the current lower prevalence of smoking in California compared with the rest of the nation resulted from the combination of a very slightly more rapid decline in smoking among Californians preceding the tax increase and a steep decline that coincided with the increase and implementation of the tobacco control effort.

The California legislature has established a target of 75% reduction in the prevalence of smoking among adults in California by the year 1999. Figure 2 shows the smoking prevalence in 1988 on a line that connects with the defined target for the year 1999. By tracking smoking prevalence in relation to this line, it will be possible to determine whether the tobacco control campaign in California is on schedule to achieve the target. The 1990 data indicate that the control program would achieve the 1999 goals if the 1988–1990 rates of decline in smoking are sustained.

Purchase of Cigarettes

A somewhat similar picture is seen when the data on cigarette sales, based on taxes paid, are examined. Plots of quarterly adult per capita purchases (total purchases, by any age person, per person 18 years and over) from January 1980 to September 1991 for California and the United States minus California, as shown in Figure 3, show a general downward trend.

Figure 4 shows quarterly per capita purchases adjusted for real price,

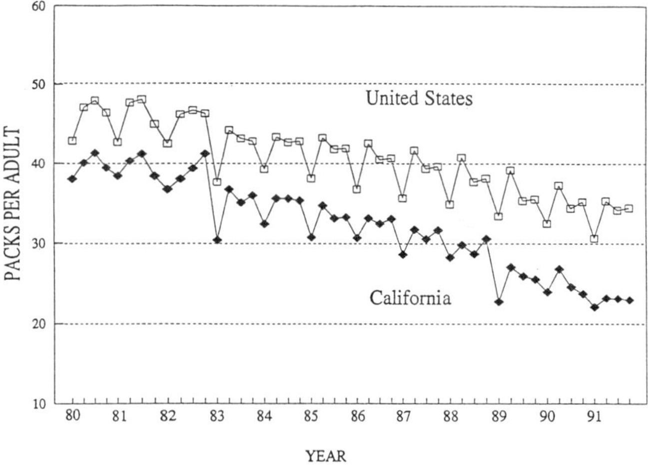

Figure 3 United States and California quarterly adult per capita purchasing (ratio of tobacco sales to adult population). (From Ref. 6.)

seasonal variations, and the federal tax increase for California and the United States. These adjusted data reveal the same overall pattern as that exhibited in Figure 3, that is, California has lower purchases overall and a higher rate of decline than the United States. From 1980 through 1988, per capita cigarette purchases in California were declining at an average annual rate of 3.6%. In 1989, the first year of the tax increase, the rate of decline jumped to 9.4%; in 1990, the rate of decline was 4.4%; and in 1991, it rose again to 7.7% (6). Thus, the rate of decline during the three-year period following implementation of the added tax and health education program averaged 7.2% annually, double what it had been during the preceding eight years. The imposition of the added tax and the corresponding rise in the price of cigarettes apparently influenced the quickened decline in smoking prevalence in California, from 1988 to 1989; California's new educational tobacco control efforts were only in the early stages of implementation in 1990. The fact that the rate of decline in cigarettes purchased accelerated again in 1991 indicates that the health education program was having an effect; other factors, of course, may also have been involved, e.g. the general economic downturn. A time-series regression analysis indicates that the effect of the tax had stabilized by 1991 (3). Further experience and analysis is needed to determine the extent and nature of the impact of Proposition 99 and its various possible influences on cigarette purchases.

Clearly, the California tobacco excise tax sharply accelerated the drop in both sales of cigarettes and in smoking. The data also suggest that the impact of the tax did not continue alone. The state's paid advertising campaign against

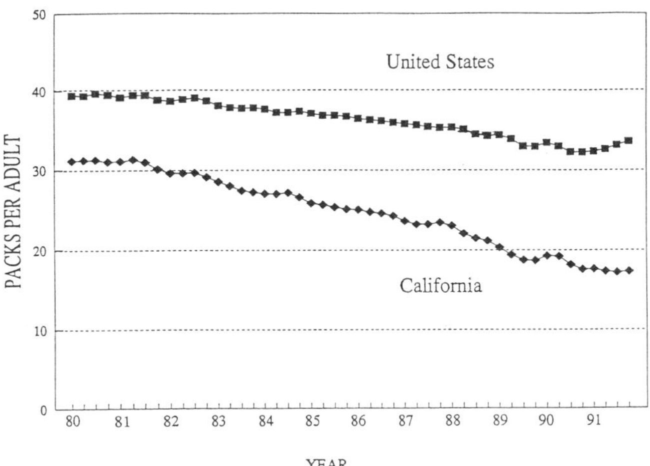

Figure 4 United States and California adjusted quarterly adult per capita purchasing (linear time trends and California excise tax effects). (From Ref. 6.)

tobacco use and its many other statewide, regional, and local tobacco control activities supported by revenues from that tax already seem to be contributing to curtailment of cigarette smoking among Californians.

Smoking Cessation

To achieve the goal of a 75% reduction in smoking prevalence by the year 1999, many current smokers will have to quit smoking permanently. As described previously, quitting smoking is a dynamic process that includes developing interest in and motivation for quitting, actually making the attempt to quit, overcoming smoking withdrawal, achieving short-term success, and resisting relapse to achieve long-term success. Individual components of the current tobacco control effort are designed to influence the various points in the cyclic process of cessation, relapse, and new cessation attempts that mark the progress from smoking to becoming a nonsmoker.

Approximately one half of California smokers made an attempt to quit in the 12 months before the survey. The rate of quit attempts was highest among black smokers of both sexes (Figure 5). However, smokers could not translate their high rate of cessation attempts fully into successful cessation. Only 11.3% of those who were smokers one year previously were nonsmokers at the time of the survey. This high rate of failed cessation attempts is most evident for black males; 60% of those who were smokers one year ago attempted to quit, but only 4% were current nonsmokers (Figure 5). Clearly,

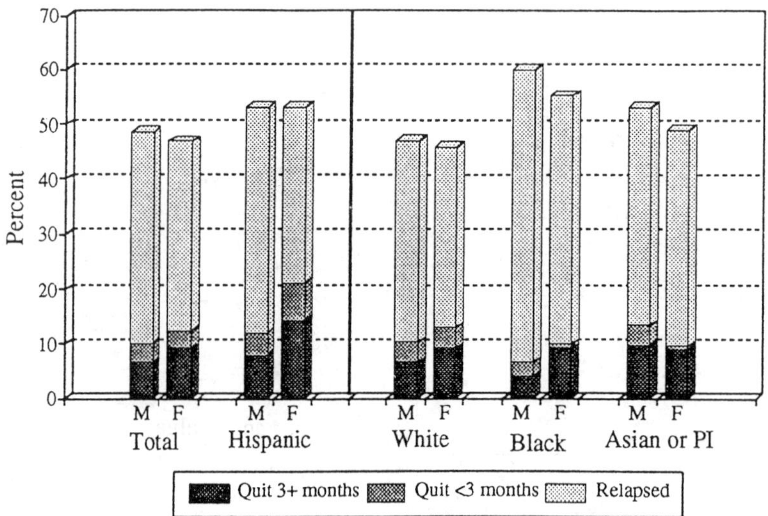

Figure 5 Rates of cessation attempts and their results by gender/race and ethnicity. (From Ref. 3.)

continued program efforts, especially focused on relapse prevention, are needed for California to achieve its goal.

The survey data show not only the decline in smoking and the attempts to quit, both successful and unsuccessful, but also the distribution of smokers along the cycle of cessation. Among those who had ever smoked, about half were no longer smoking; 34% had quit more than five years ago; another 12%, one to five years ago; and 6% had stopped for 0–12 months. Moreover, among those same people who had ever smoked, 8% were smokers preparing to quit, 23% were smokers contemplating quitting, and only 18% were still not even contemplating it. Dropping out of school and other circumstances that affect adolescents make it difficult to assess smoking initiation in California's population. Continuing efforts to determine trends in both initiation and cessation among various segments of the population will help delineate the natural history of cigarette smoking and thus indicate where to focus control activities.

Because the language of Proposition 99 emphasized prevention of tobacco use, and the legislature initially allocated approximately 30% of the health education account to schools through the State Department of Education, the latter has been endeavoring rapidly and equitably to distribute the funds into effective school programs. Because the Department had earlier initiated specific education against drugs and alcohol, with special funds, the Proposition 99 monies were joined in a DATE (Drug, Alcohol, and Tobacco Education) program. Thus, the tobacco revenues made possible a substantial school effort, supported by a total of $27.2 million in fiscal year 1991–1992, toward prevention of a broad range of hazardous behavior by young people. To evaluate the school tobacco control program, the State Department of Education contracted for a study to ascertain "(a) the extent to which tobacco use prevention education programs have been implemented in the schools; (b) the extent to which students—by grade and risk group—have been exposed to programs; (c) the impact of tobacco use prevention programs on knowledge, attitudes, and behaviors of students; and (d) the extent to which funds are translated into relevant programs for students." Results from this effort should be forthcoming in the next year or two.

The third main component of the effort to determine the impact of Proposition 99 has consisted of an independent evaluation conducted by the San Diego State University, including "(1) monitoring of public, institutionally based, centrally funded programs such as local lead agencies (local health departments) and public schools, (2) monitoring and evaluation of innovative community-based programs funded through a competitive grants process, (3) monitoring of secular events that may not be directly funded by the program such as the passage of tobacco control ordinances, voluntary organization activities, tobacco-industry sponsored counter-attacks, and activities of primary health care providers" (directed toward prevention and cessation of smoking).

As of November 1991, within two years of the time the funds became available, 60 of the 61 Local Lead Agencies had formed tobacco control coalitions, usually with a broad scope of activity; 90% were planning to coordinate their services with schools, voluntary agencies, and the like. Considerable new tobacco control activities were under way, including those directed toward prevention and cessation, especially among minority ethnic/racial groups; policy actions, such as local ordinances; technical assistance; and evaluation (4).

OTHER EFFECTS OF PROPOSITION 99

Besides the above immediate impacts on the tobacco situation in California, other important effects should be noted. Passage of Proposition 99 and its implementation have galvanized local communities throughout the state to take action against tobacco use. For example, they have substantially increased the number and strength of ordinances prohibiting smoking in certain places. Since 1989, dozens of cities, including Sacramento, have required that restaurants, work-places, and/or public buildings be 100% smoke-free, i.e. without even designated smoking areas. From three local ordinances prohibiting vending machines for cigarette sales, except in bars, the number has increased as of May 1992 to 26 such ordinances, and seven that do not exempt even bars. Efforts to repeal or vitiate such actions to limit places for smoking or placement of cigarette vending machines have generally been rebuffed by judges, city councils, or, in one case, a special election. (Americans for Nonsmokers Rights, Berkeley. Tobacco Control Section, California Department of Health Services.)

The tobacco industry has launched a vigorous advertising and political counter-offensive in California. The latter is concentrating on state preemption of authority over tobacco access and use to avoid strong local ordinances against tobacco. Thus far, that effort has not been successful. After state legislation prohibiting free distribution of tobacco products passed, a stalemate between pro- and antitobacco forces seems to have developed in the Legislature. The Governor is seeking to divert some of the Proposition 99 health education (prevention) account to medical services, but the first court ruling has denied that proposal. There is some chance that the current severe budget crisis may lead to further increase in the tobacco tax for which the UCSD survey shows popular support (3).

The influence of California's experience with Proposition 99 may have emboldened action beyond California. For example, Maryland has recently increased its tobacco tax 20 cents per package, much beyond the typical increment; citizens in other states are considering the plebescite process for doing so, although Montana has been unsuccessful in that regard.

Early experience with Proposition 99, particularly with state guidelines on tobacco control, proved useful in refining the American Stop Smoking Intervention Study for Cancer Prevention (ASSIST) program, a national $120 million effort now operating in 17 states. The National Cancer Institute-American Cancer Society sponsored Smoking Control Advocacy Resource Network makes the California experience available to thousands of users throughout the country by means of an electronic network.

Responding to the legislation, the California Department of Health Services and the local health departments have devoted substantial attention in tobacco control to racial/ethnic minority groups. The latter's extensive participation in tobacco use prevention, in conjunction with the official agencies, may yield benefit not only in that effort, but also may lead to their greater involvement in other health promotion/disease prevention programs.

Proposition 99 earmarked 5% of the revenues to research on tobacco-related disease. After two (annual) funding cycles, the University of California, which has been responsible for the research program, reported that 281 grants had been made to investigators at 37 California institutions for a total of $92 million (31). Priority areas that were identified for the third funding cycle include environmental tobacco smoke, prevention and cessation of tobacco use, tobacco control, and more traditional biomedical research.

Proposition 99 has also stimulated much closer collaboration between state and local health and education agencies than existed before 1989. For peculiar, historical reasons, the California Departments of Education and Health Services had not previously worked closely together, and that estrangement had adversely affected local cooperation. The Legislature and other forces in Proposition 99's implementation nudged the health and education departments to work cooperatively on this endeavor. Hopefully, that encounter will lead to joint efforts on other health matters.

DISCUSSION

California's Proposition 99 has marked a high point in the growing national and international movements against tobacco use. It has not only inspired hundreds of thousands of residents to quit smoking and, thus, sharply accelerated the decline in recent years, but it also seems to have encouraged similar actions across the country. Inquiries about the campaign have come from tobacco control activists in many countries.

Beyond reducing smoking prevalence, Proposition 99 has stimulated health efforts generally, for example, in greater attention to racial/ethnic minorities and by enhancing collaboration between health and education agencies.

From the start of program planning, much debate has focused on which elements of the program will prove to be most effective: the tax increase itself, the media campaign, school education-health department programs, community agency activities, or some other. Because influences on behavior regarding tobacco are so complex, the answer may never be entirely clear. The tax rise, however, was followed by prompt acceleration of the declining trends of cigarette purchasing and smoking prevalence in California. Early statistical studies indicate, moreover, that the tax impact stabilized within two to three years and that other program elements may subsequently be responsible for the continuing decline. The media campaign has attracted the greatest controversy: A substantial proportion of smokers who quit attribute their action to media influence, and the tobacco industry has directed a major effort to stopping that part of the program. Although it is still too early for thorough analysis of the relative importance of its various components, Proposition 99's impact has significantly accelerated the decline of smoking in California. The very broad action engendered by the Proposition is creating a social milieu that is hastening the trend.

Fortunately for California program guidance and for others' understanding of the situation, a considerable research and evaluation effort is under way, which involves dozens of university and other groups in the state, as well as external advisers. Also, a statutory Tobacco Education Oversight Committee keeps careful tabs on the program and prepares a tobacco control plan annually (29).

Although this review focuses on Proposition 99 and its impact, other factors are no doubt significantly influencing tobacco use during the 1990s. The political feasibility of increasing tobacco taxes, demonstrated in California, may prove particularly attractive in these government-deficit, budget-crunch years; for example, the federal excise tax was increased four cents per cigarette pack in 1992 and again in 1993. Also, with little public notice, cigarette companies have, in recent years, sharply raised their manufacturer pre-tax prices—14% in 1991 alone; however, cheaper brands are gaining market share (4).

Finally, several problems in the implementation of Proposition 99 should be noted. The executive branch of state government has consistently sought to bolster underfunded medical services by diverting funds from the health education account. To some extent, that foray has been successful through insistence that the services are actually devoted to tobacco control. A judge recently decided, however, that Proposition 99 did not permit eliminating the media component of the program in favor of medical services.

In these times of financial duress and corresponding tight restraint on government program staff generally, bureaucratic controls on hiring made it difficult to start the program as rapidly as would have been desirable. To some extent, this problem has been alleviated by contracting out for services. Lack of good baseline data on tobacco use by adolescents has impeded school and out-of-school program development and evaluation. Disjointed efforts in that regard by the Departments of Health Services and Education and by the Attorney General's Office are, hopefully, being resolved.

Overall, California's Proposition 99 has become an important beacon in the growing world-wide struggle against the health devastation caused by tobacco.

Literature Cited

1. Assoc. of State and Territ. Health Off. 1989. *Guide to Public Health Practice: State Health Agency Prevention and Control Plans*. McLean, Va.:Assoc. State Territ. Health Off.
2. Breslow, L. 1982. Control of cigarette smoking from a public policy perspective. *Annu. Rev. Public. Health* 3:129–51
3. Burns, D., Pierce, J. P. 1992. *Tobacco Use In California. 1990–91*. Sacramento: Calif. Dep. Health Serv.
4. Calif. Dep. of Health Serv. 1991. *Independent Evaluation of California Tobacco Control Efforts*. San Diego State Univ. Found.
5. Cent. for Dis. Control. 1985. *A Decision-Maker's Guide to Reducing Smoking at the Worksite*. Washington, DC: US Public Health Serv.
6. Elder, J. P., Kenney, E. 1992. *Independent Evaluation of Efforts to Prevent and Control Tobacco Use in California, Progress Report*. San Diego State Univ./Calif. Dep. Health Serv. Tob. Control Sect., July
7. Farquhar, J. W., Fortmann, S. P., Flora, J. A., Taylor, C. B., Haskell, W. L., et al 1990. Community education of cardiovascular disease risk factors: the Stanford five-city project. *J. Am. Med. Assoc.* 264:350–65
8. Fiore, M. C., Novotny, T. E., Pierce, J. P., Hatziandreu, E. J., Patel, K. M., et al 1989. Trends in cigarette smoking in the United States: the changing influence of gender and race. *J. Am. Med. Assoc.* 261(1):40–55
9. Glynn, T. J., Boyd, G. M., Gruman, J. C. 1990. Essential elements of self-help/minimal intervention strategies for smoking cessation. *Health Educ. Q.* 17:329–45
10. Glynn, T. J., Manely, M. 1989. *How to Help Your Patients Stop Smoking: A National Cancer Institute Manual for Physicians*. Washington, DC: US Dep. Health Hum. Serv. Publ. NIH 89-3046
11. Gov. Advis. Comm. on Cigarette Smoking and Health (Calif.). 1964. *Health vs. Cigarette Smoking*
12. Hatziandreu, E. J., Pierce, J. P., Lefkoloulou, M., Fiore, M. C., Mills, S. L. 1990. Quitting smoking in the United States in 1986. *J. Natl. Cancer Inst.* 82:1402–6
13. Int. Union Against Cancer. *Guidelines for Smoking Control 1980*. ed. N. Gray, M. Daube, UICC Tech. Rep. Ser. Vol. 52. Geneva. 2nd ed.
14. Marconi, K. M., Colborn, J. W. 1990. State tobacco-use prevention and control plans. *Morbid. Mortal. Wkly. Rep.* 39:134–36
15. McGinnis, J. M., Shopland, D., Brown, C. 1987. Tobacco and health: trends in smoking and smokeless tobacco consumption in the United States. *Annu. Rev. Public Health* 8:441–67
16. Novotny, T. E., Romano, R. A., Davis, R. M., Mills, S. L. 1992. The public health practice of tobacco control: lessons learned and directions for the states in the 1990s. *Annu. Rev. Public Health* 13:287–318.
17. Off. on Smoking and Health, Cent. for Dis. Control. 1982. *State and Local Programs on Smoking and Health*. Washington, DC: GPO 1982–361–166: 445
18. Pearl, R. 1933. Tobacco smoking and longevity. *Science* 78:216–17
19. Pertschuk, M., Shopland, D. R., eds. 1989. *Major Local Smoking Ordinances in the United States*. Washington, DC: DHHS (NIH) Publ. No. 90–479
20. Pierce, J. P., Fiore, M. C., Novotny, T. E., Hatziandreu, E. J., Davis, R. 1989. Trends in cigarette consumption

in the United States: educational differences are increasing. *J. Am. Med. Assoc.* 261:56–60
21. Pierce, J. P. 1990. The quitting process. In *Smoking Cessation: The Organization, Delivery and Financing of Services,* ed. Inst. Study of Smoking Behav. and Policy. Cambridge, Mass: Harvard Univ. Press
22. Pierce, J. P., Naquin, M., Gilpin, E., Giovino, G., Mills, S., et al. 1991. Smoking initiation in the United States: a role for worksite and college smoking bans. *J. Natl. Cancer Inst.* 83:1009–13
23. Pierce, J. P. 1991. Progress and problems in international efforts to reduce tobacco use. *Annu. Rev. Public Health* 12:383–400
24. *Post Prop 99 Update: A Public Issues Update on the Disposition of the Funds Created by the Passage of Proposition 99, the Tobacco Tax and Health Promotion Act 1990*. Oakland: Am. Cancer Soc., Calif. Div.
25. Rep. of the Advis. Comm. to the Surgeon Gen. of the Public Health Serv. 1964. *Smoking and Health*. PHS Publ. No. 1103
26. Shopland, D. R. 1992. Toward a tobacco-free society 1990. *Semin. Oncol.* 17:402–12
27. Shopland, D. R., Brown, C. 1985. Changes in cigarette smoking prevalence in the US: 1955 to 1983. *Ann. Behav. Med.* 7:5–8
28. State of Calif. Dep. of Public Health. 1963. *Cigarette Smoking and Health*. Sacramento, Calif.
29. Tob. Educ. Oversight Comm. 1991. *Toward a Tobacco-free California: A Master Plan to Reduce California's Use of Tobacco*. Sacramento, Calif.
30. Type, J. B., Warner, K. E., Glantz, S. A. 1987. Tobacco advertising and consumption: evidence of a causal relationship, *J. Public Health Policy* 8: 492–508
31. Univ. of Calif. 1991. *Tobacco-Related Disease Research Program*. Annu. Rep. to the State of Calif. Legis.
32. US Dep. of Health and Hum. Serv. 1982. *The Health Consequences of Smoking: A Report of the Surgeon General*. DHHS Publ. No. (PHS) 82-50179
33. US Dep. of Health and Hum. Serv. 1986. *Tobacco Use in 1986: Methods and Basic Tabulations from Adult Use of Tobacco Survey*. Rockville, Md: Public Health Serv.
34. US Dep. of Health and Hum. Serv. 1986. *The 1990 Health Objectives for the Nation: A Midcourse Review*. Off. Dis. Prev. Health Promot.
35. US Dep. of Health and Hum. Serv. 1986. *The Health Consequences of Involuntary Smoking*. DHHS Publ. No. (PHS) 87–8398.
36. US Dep. of Health and Hum. Serv. 1988. *The Health Consequences of Smoking: Nicotine Addiction. A Report of the Surgeon General*. DHHS Publ. No. (CDC) 88–8406
37. US Dep. of Health and Hum. Serv. 1988. *State and Local Programs on Smoking and Health*. Washington, DC: US Public Health Serv. Off. Smoking Health
38. US Dep. of Health and Hum. Serv. 1989. *Reducing the Health Consequences of Smoking: 25 Years of Progress. A Report of the Surgeon General*. DHHS Publ. No. (CDC) 89–8411
39. US Dep. of Health and Hum. Serv. 1990. *Smoking, Tobacco, and Cancer Program: 1985–1989 Status Report*. NIH Publ. No. 90–3107
40. US Dep. of Health and Hum. Serv. 1990. *The Health Benefits of Smoking Cessation: A Report of the Surgeon General*. DHHS Publ. No. (CDC) 90–8416
41. US Dep. of Health and Hum. Serv. 1990c. *Preventing the Sale of Tobacco to Minors. Proceedings of the Interagency Committee on Smoking and Health*. Washington, DC
42. US Dep. of Health and Hum. Serv. 1991. *Strategies to Control Tobacco Use in the United States*. NIH Publ. No. 92–3316
43. Warner, K. E. 1989. Effects of antismoking campaign: an update. *Am. J. Public Health* 79:144–51
44. West. Consort. for Public Health 1990. *Proposition 99: The California Tobacco Tax Initiative*
45. Working Group to the Subcomm. on Smoking of the Am. Heart Assoc. 1986. Public policy on smoking and health: toward a smoke free generation by the year 2000. *Circulation* 73:381A–95A
46. World Health Org. 1979. Report of a WHO expert committee: controlling the smoking epidemic. *World Health Org. Tech. Rep.*, Ser. 636

Annu. Rev. Publ. Health. 1993. 14:605–33

MAMMOGRAPHY UTILIZATION, PUBLIC HEALTH IMPACT, AND COST-EFFECTIVENESS IN THE UNITED STATES

Emily White, Nicole Urban, and Victoria Taylor
Cancer Prevention Research Program, Fred Hutchinson Cancer Research Center, Seattle, Washington 98104

KEY WORDS: breast cancer statistics, breast cancer screening

INTRODUCTION

Breast cancer is a major health problem in the United States: An estimated 175,000 women were diagnosed with breast cancer in 1991, and 45,000 died from the disease (2). Among women, breast cancer is the most common form of cancer, and only lung cancer causes more cancer deaths. The lifetime cost of treating a case of breast cancer was estimated to be $37,000 in 1984 dollars (8), equivalent to $61,000 in 1991 dollars, which suggests that breast cancer cost society over $10 billion in 1991. These are only the dollar costs borne by the medical care system, exclusive of the costs of pain, anxiety, and suffering borne by the women and their families.

Recently, the General Accounting Office presented to the US Congress a report reviewing 20 years of progress in the prevention, diagnosis, and treatment of breast cancer (79). The report concluded that, among the advances in these three areas, the best prospect for reducing the number of deaths from breast cancer is increased utilization of screening mammography. This recommendation was based on controlled studies that have demonstrated that screening asymptomatic women for breast cancer can substantially reduce deaths from the disease.

As evidence for the efficacy of mammography accumulated during the last

0163-7525/93/0510-0605$02.00

decade, efforts to increase the proportion of women screened intensified through a variety of methods, including private and public promotional campaigns, professional education, and legislation to make mammography reimbursable by third party payers (5, 11, 20, 74). Successful planning for future activities aimed at promoting the appropriate use of mammography in the United States requires an assessment of the impact of these efforts on the population, as well as the costs and benefits of mammography use. After a brief overview of studies of the effectiveness of mammography and a summary of screening guidelines, we review the present state of adoption of screening mammography in the United States, including the current utilization and factors associated with use, the impact to date of screening on breast cancer morbidity and mortality, and the evidence regarding cost-effectiveness of screening mammography.

Effectiveness of Mammography

Selected literature on the effectiveness of breast cancer screening by mammography is summarized in Table 1. The first important study was a randomized controlled trial conducted in the 1960s by the Health Insurance Plan of Greater New York (HIP) (65). Two-view mammography was performed in combination with clinical breast examination (CBE) annually for four years on more than 30,000 asymptomatic women aged 40–64. A sustained reduction in breast cancer mortality of 30% was found for women aged 50–64, despite compliance with all four screens of only about 50%. No reduction in mortality was found for younger women. This study was significant because it demonstrated conclusively that breast cancer screening reduces mortality among women aged 50–64. However, because the HIP study used mammography in combination with CBE relative to a "no screening" control group, it does not provide an estimate of either the effectiveness of mammography used alone, or of mammography used in combination with CBE relative to CBE alone.

One study that addressed the issue of mammography used alone was a controlled trial conducted in Sweden, in which 38 communities within two counties were randomized (71, 72). In 19 communities allocated to the study arm, approximately 78,000 women aged 40–74 were offered screening by single-view mammography alone. The screening interval varied among women, but averaged about two years among the women aged 40–49 and 33 months among the women aged 50–74. Compliance was high: 88% at the first screen, 83% at the second. At an average of eight years of follow-up, mortality reduction was 38% among the women aged 50–69, with no significant decrease observed for younger women. The authors report that 13% of women in the control group had mammography as part of routine care

Table 1 Studies of breast cancer screening effectiveness[a]

Study/country (reference)	Study design[b]	Year study began	Age group	Screening mammogram	Clinical Breast exam	Screening interval	Compliance[c] (%)	Difference in mortality 5–10 yrs[d] (%)
HIP/USA (65)	RCT	1963	40–49	2 view	yes	12 mos.	67	−5 (ns)
			50–64					−32
Two-county/Sweden (71,72)	RCT	1977	40–49	1 view	no	24 mos.	88	−8 (ns)
			50–69			33 mos.		−38
Malmo/Sweden (6)	RCT	1976	55–70	1–2 view	no	18–24 mos.	74	−20 (ns)
Edinburgh/Scotland (63)	RCT	1979	45–64	2 view	yes	24 mos.	61	−17 (ns)
BCDDP/USA (7,53)	Demonstration[e]	1973	35–49	2 view	yes	12 mos.	100	−11
			50–74					−25
Nijmegen/The Netherlands (83,84)	Case-control	1975	50–64	1 view	no	24 mos.	100	−52
Utrecht/The Netherlands (19)	Case-control	1975	50–64	2 view	yes	12–24 mos.	100	−70
Florence/Italy (57)	Case-control	1979	50–70	2 view	no	30 mos.	100	−76

[a] Adapted from Ref. 80.
[b] RCT = randomized clinical trial.
[c] Compliance with first mammogram in first five studies.
[d] Percent difference in breast cancer mortality: [intervention (screened)—control]/control; ns = not statistically significant.
[e] Results compared with national rates.

during the period, but they do not report the rate at which women received CBE.

Two additional randomized trials (6, 63) and one demonstration project of screening mammography (7, 53) found a 17–25% reduction in mortality from breast cancer among middle aged women (Table 1). Case-control studies conducted in the Netherlands and Italy suggest that mortality reduction attributable to obtaining a mammogram may be even higher (52–76%) (19, 57, 84). These studies differ from the randomized trials in that they measure the effect of having participated in screening versus the effect of a screening program, which includes women with varying degrees of compliance. The results of case-control studies must be interpreted with caution, because it is difficult in these studies to control adequately for self-selection of women to screening and "healthy-screenee" bias (52). Analysts reviewing data from the various trials and other studies have concluded that screening by mammography every one to three years reduces breast cancer mortality among women aged 50–70 by approximately 40% (21, 23, 48).

Screening Guidelines

Published guidelines pertaining to mammographic screening are summarized in Table 2 (3, 4, 31, 81). In an effort to increase the regular use of mammography, 11 organizations, including the American Cancer Society, the American Medical Association, and the National Cancer Institute, issued a consensus statement about breast cancer screening guidelines in 1989 (31). However, because there is a lack of conclusive evidence concerning the benefits of mammography for younger women and appropriate screening frequencies for older women, both the American College of Physicians and

Table 2 Screening mammography recommendations by US organizations

Group or organization (reference)	Age group	Recommendation
US Consensus Statement[a] (31)	40–49	Every 1–2 years
	≥50	Annually
US Preventive Services Task Force (81)	35–49	Consider if family history of breast cancer
	50–75	Every 1–2 years
American College of Physicians (3)	40–49	Consider if family history of breast cancer or otherwise at increased risk
	≥50	Annually
American Geriatrics Society (4)	65–85	Every 2–3 years

[a]American Cancer Society, American Medical Association, National Cancer Institute, and eight other organizations.

the US Preventive Services Task Force (USPSTF) chose not to endorse this statement (3, 40, 81).

The consensus statement supports screening every one to two years for women in their forties (31). This was based on a 25% mortality reduction after 18 years of follow-up among women aged 40–49 at entry into the HIP trial (18), even though, as shown in Table 1, there was no significant mortality reduction within ten years. In contrast, the American College of Physicians and USPSTF maintain that regular screening should be initiated at age 50, and mammography should only be considered among younger women at increased risk of disease (3, 81).

Information on optimal screening frequencies can be obtained through comparisons of the number of interval cancers occurring between screenings in intervention groups with the expected number estimated from control groups. In the Swedish two-county study, relatively few interval cancers were seen within two years of screening among women aged 50 and over (79). Within 11 months of screening, enrolled women had 13% of the breast cancer incidence seen among control women, and only 29% within 12–23 months. Therefore, although the groups participating in the consensus statement recommend annual mammography for women aged 50 and over, the USPSTF feels a one to two year screening interval is sufficient (81), and the American Geriatrics Society recommends an interval of two to three years for women over 65.

UTILIZATION OF SCREENING MAMMOGRAPHY

In this section, we review levels of mammographic screening in the United States in terms of current utilization, secular trends, and geographic variation, as well as patterns of utilization among women in different age, racial, and socioeconomic groups. In addition, predisposing, enabling, and reinforcing factors are systematically considered as predictors of women's use (32). Because mammography participation is rapidly changing (39), cited literature is largely restricted to studies based on data collected after 1985. Additionally, only studies reporting results from a defined US population are included in this review.

Use Over Time and by Geographic Area

Table 3 summarizes the methods and key results of recent population based surveys addressing women's utilization of mammography (15–17, 22, 33, 56, 59). A dramatic increase in participation, over the last 15 years, is demonstrated by comparing these results with earlier national studies. Surveys conducted in the late 1970s suggested that only 15–20% of women, aged 50 and over, had ever obtained the test and that a much smaller proportion were

Table 3 Population studies of mammography use: United States, 1986–1990[a]

Data source (reference)	Geographic area	Year(s) survey conducted	Age group	Survey response rate (%)	Sample size	Ever screened (%)	Screened within last year (%)	≥2 previous mammograms (%)
Access to care survey[b] (33)	US	1986	≥50	76	2071	39	20	—
NHIS[b] (22)	US	1987	≥40	86	6858	38	15	—
Rhode Island BCSP (15,16)	Rhode Island	1987	≥40	78	852	—	37	—
		1989	≥40	79	856	—	46	—
BRFSS (59)	Wisconsin	1987–88	≥40	83[d]	747	54	32	—
BCSC[c] (56)	Suburban Los Angeles	1987–88	50–74	65	277	—	34	42
	Eastern Massachusetts	1987–88	50–74	75	861	—	32	32
	Long Island	1987–88	50–74	74	2180	51	26	26
	Eastern North Carolina	1987–88	50–74	75	735	—	36	25
	Greater Philadelphia	1987–88	50–74	73	788	—	39	34
	Washington state	1989	50–74	72	1473	74	41	37
NKAB[b] (17)	US	1989–90	≥40	—	836	67	—	—
MAUS[b] (17)	US	1990	≥40	64	980	64	—	35

[a] All studies were conducted by telephone except the NHIS (in-person interview) and the Long Island NCI BCSC survey (mailed questionnaire).
[b] Results weighted to be generalizable to the US population.
[c] Restricted to non-Hispanic white women without a history of breast cancer.
[d] Median for 33 states.

being examined with systematic regularity (37). In contrast, the 1987 National Health Interview Survey (NHIS) found 37% of women aged 40 and older had received at least one mammogram (22). By 1990, 64% of women in this age group, who participated in the Mammography Attitudes and Usage Survey (MAUS) and 67% of partipants in the National Knowledge, Attitudes, and Behavior (NKAB) survey reported ever having had the procedure (17). Furthermore, 23% of the MAUS respondents had received their first mammogram in the previous two years (17). However, for screening mammography to achieve long-term public health impact, women must be screened at regular intervals. Less encouraging are reports concerning the proportion of women who are receiving routine mammograms. For example, the MAUS found only 35% of women in the 40-plus age group to have been screened on at least two occasions (17).

As shown in Figure 1, the marked upward trend in mammography use is mirrored by an explosive growth in the installation of dedicated mammography equipment (13; M. Brown 1992, personal communication). This information, based on Food and Drug Administration x-ray assembly forms, shows that installations soared between 1982 and 1988. Kessler et al (39) have commented that the pattern of change in installations demonstrates the fit of a logistic curve often seen in association with the successful diffusion of a new technology.

Geographical variations in levels of mammography use have been investigated by using the 1987 NHIS data. The proportion of women reporting previous mammography was highest in the West (43%) and lowest in the

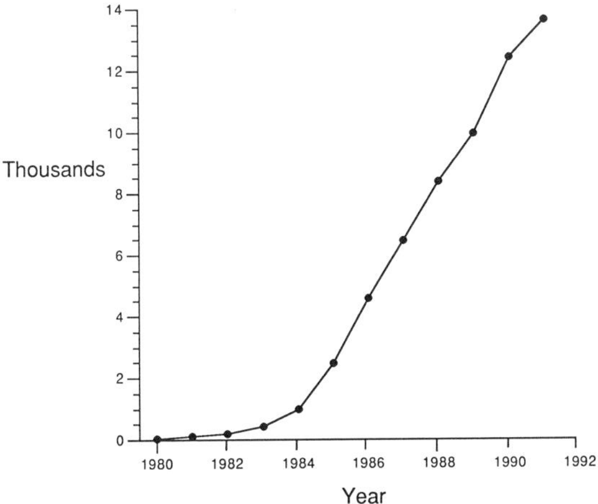

Figure 1 Cumulative installations of dedicated mammography x-ray machines (13; M. Brown 1992, personal communication).

South (35%), with residents of the Northeast (37%) and Midwest (39%) reporting intermediate screening rates (22). A wealth of information about mammographic screening has recently been provided by the National Cancer Institute Breast Cancer Screening Consortium (BCSC) (14, 30, 43, 51, 56, 58, 61, 62, 68, 76, 89, 90). As shown in Table 3, analysis of data from the BCSC also shows some regional differences in utilization patterns (56).

Although population studies clearly demonstrate a strong secular increase in use of mammography, the reported percentages of women receiving screening are probably overestimates. Response rates in surveys addressing breast cancer screening have ranged from approximately 65% to 85% (15–17, 22, 33, 56, 59). Women who obtain breast cancer screening may be more likely to participate in surveys than those who do not. Additionally, most studies were conducted by using random digit dialing methods and are subject to selection bias because of telephone noncoverage. Because of this bias, women from lower income households, who are less likely to be screened, are underrepresented (5). Finally, a proportion of women reporting previous mammography actually received the procedure for diagnostic, rather than screening, purposes (89).

Use by Sociodemographic Characteristics

Findings with respect to sociodemographic characteristics, from the two most recently conducted studies of the US population, are shown in Table 4 (17). Age differences in screening mammography use have been consistently demonstrated. Utilization prevalence has generally been reported to be highest among women in their fifties and then to decrease steadily with advancing age. However, if use is defined in terms of adherence to the widely promoted American Cancer Society guidelines, higher compliance is seen among the 40–49 age group than among women in their fifties (17, 59). An analysis of 1987 and 1988 Wisconsin data found that 42% of asymptomatic women in their forties had received mammography in the previous two years, and were thus in compliance with American Cancer Society guidelines. Among the 50-plus age group, 32% reported mammographic screening in the last year and were therefore adherent (59). These age patterns are particularly disturbing, as the incidence of breast cancer increases with age; therefore, the women at highest risk are those least likely to be appropriately screened (22).

Racial discrepancies in use of mammographic screening have been demonstrated by several investigators. Although earlier reports described wide differences in use by whites and blacks, three more recent national studies have shown participation rates to be only 5–10% lower among black than white women (17, 22). However, appreciably lower use has been found among Hispanic women than either whites or blacks. A 1988 survey of Los Angeles women, in the 35–47 age group, found that whereas 57% of white and 53%

Table 4 Proportion of women aged ≥40 years ever having had mammography by sociodemographic characteristics: United States, 1989–1990[a,b]

Characteristic	*MAUS* (%)	*NKAB* (%)
Age		
40–49	64	68
50–59	71	70
60–69	65	71
≥70	56	59
Race		
White	65	69
Black	58	59
Annual income		
<$25,000	60	65
≥$25,000	71	74
Education		
<High school	58	58
High school	65	67
Some college	72	72
≥College	74	79

[a] Adapted from Centers for Disease Control (17).
[b] Results weighted to reflect the age, education, and race distribution of US women.

of black women had ever received mammography, only 29% of Hispanic respondents had (68). Little information is currently available with respect to use of the test by Asians or Native Americans.

Results from national studies and the BCSC surveys show a pattern of decreased use among women with lower income and less education (17, 22, 56). Furthermore, a recent study found improvements in levels of use over time to be significantly lower, when compared with other groups, among women with less than 12 years education and household incomes of below $10,000 (5). Recent population studies have also suggested that married women are more likely to be screened than those who are single, divorced, or widowed (17, 43, 62).

Predisposing, Enabling, and Reinforcing Factors

Factors relevant to effective intervention planning can be broadly categorized as predisposing, enabling, and reinforcing (32, 51, 62, 89). Reported correlates of mammography participation are summarized, within this conceptual framework, in Table 5. Predisposing factors encompass beliefs, knowledge, and attitudes about both breast cancer and mammography.

Various studies have investigated women's perceptions about the benefits of, and barriers to, mammography. A perception that the procedure is important in the absence of symptoms and a positive belief concerning efficacy of the test have both been reported to be associated with mammography use (43, 61, 62, 89). The BCSC has demonstrated that higher levels of concern about cost, discomfort, embarrassment, inconvenience, and radiation can negatively impact use (43, 51, 61, 62). These results should be interpreted with some caution, however, because most of the cited studies were cross-sectional. Therefore, it is impossible to assess the degree to which beliefs, among screened and unscreened women, are a result of their screening behavior rather than a predictor of behavior. Also, the few studies addressing regular use suggest that the barriers to initial and habitual adoption of mammography may differ (43, 62).

Perceived susceptibility to breast cancer has been shown to be related to mammography use in retrospective and prospective studies (43, 50). Women with known breast cancer risk factors, or previous breast disease, might be expected to have an enhanced perception of vulnerability to breast cancer and the importance of screening mammography. Several investigators have demonstrated an association between a positive family history of breast cancer, as well as prior breast disease, and use of the procedure (58, 73, 76, 89, 90).

The value attached to prevention in general, as reflected by other positive preventive habits, can be considered predisposing. Several studies have demonstrated relationships between primary prevention behaviors and utilization of mammography (5, 50, 62). Surprisingly, findings with respect to breast self-examination have been inconsistent (56).

Enabling factors ae largely related to the health-care system and its use by women. Mammography participation has been shown to be influenced by the woman's type of medical insurance (10, 76, 89, 90). In a 1987 Massachusetts study, women with commercial insurance or health maintenance organization coverage were more likely to have been recently screened than those reporting Medicare, Medicaid, or no coverage (89). However, many states have recently

Table 5 Predisposing, enabling, and reinforcing factors associated with mammography use

Predisposing	Enabling	Reinforcing
Beliefs regarding mammography benefits/ barriers	Regular source of health care	Physician recommendation
Perception of personal vulnerability to breast cancer	Routine gynecologist visits	Support of family/friends
Value attached to prevention	Other preventive care	

mandated third-party reimbursement for screening mammography by private carriers and extended such benefits to Medicaid recipients (11, 20, 74). Additionally, mammography screening has been covered by the Medicare system since 1991 (20).

There is increasing evidence that not only having a regular source of medical care, but more specifically routinely visiting a gynecologist, facilitates completion of mammographic screening (14, 51, 56, 62, 76, 89). Significantly higher utilization rates have been reported among women who receive their primary health care from a gynecologist rather than a general internist or family practitioner (14, 76, 89). Women who choose to obtain care from gynecologists might be inherently more likely to seek screening. However, studies addressing the self-reported mammography referral rates of physicians also indicate that gynecologists are more likely to recommend the procedure actively than other primary care specialists (1, 67).

Not surprisingly, the provision of other preventive services appears to provide a clinical opportunity for physicians to refer women to mammography. The ongoing Behavioral Risk Factor Surveillance System (BRFSS) survey, which is conducted by the Centers for Disease Control, provides information about breast cancer screening in 33 states. In the 1987 survey, 29% of respondents who reported having had a recent physical were screened with mammography during the previous year; however, only 4% of women who had not received a check-up were screened (5). Similarly, a correlation between receiving clinical breast examinations and mammographic screening has been demonstrated (51, 90).

Reinforcing factors include the support of screening mammography by health-care providers, family, and friends (15, 30, 43, 50, 62, 89). In particular, physician advice and referral for mammography has been repeatedly shown to be one of the strongest predictors of participation by women (15, 30, 43, 62). Fox et al (30) found that women were 4–12 times as likely, depending on their age group, to have ever had a mammogram if their physicians had discussed the procedure with them (30).

Summary

Mammographic screening in the United States demonstrates a strong secular increase in use over the last decade. However, the proportion of women who are receiving regular screening remains relatively low. Certain sociodemographic groups, including the elderly, racial minorities, the low income, and the less educated, report meaningfully lower screening rates than the population as a whole. The decision to obtain mammography is a complex process influenced not only by beliefs, attitudes, and perceptions, but also by factors related to the health-care system and physician-patient interactions.

PUBLIC HEALTH IMPACT OF MAMMOGRAPHY

As noted in the introduction, studies of the efficacy of mammography suggest that an approximate 40% reduction in mortality from breast cancer can be achieved if a large proportion of women over age 50 are screened every one to three years (23, 48). However, the magnitude of the reduction in mortality that can be expected in a population may not be that achieved in centrally organized programs. The effectiveness of mammography screening in a population depends on the proportion of women who are screened, the frequency with which they are screened, the quality of the screening process, and the efficacy of treatment of early disease (25). Measures of the quality of the screening process include the ability of mammography to detect asymptomatic cancers and the accuracy of the further diagnostic procedures for those found positive by screening. These parameters related to the efficacy of screening may be diminished in the widespread application of mammography compared with a controlled setting. Therefore, the population effectiveness of mammography screening in the United States needs to be monitored.

Although a decline in breast cancer mortality is the ultimate measure of the effectiveness of the adoption of mammography screening, such a decline may not be expected for many years. In the two-county study conducted in Sweden (72) and the two studies in the Netherlands (19, 83), differences in mortality between the screened and unscreened groups were not significant until approximately seven years after the screening program began (Table 1). Thus, a population-wide effect of mammography on mortality may not be apparent until five to ten years after a majority of women have begun regular screening. For this reason, earlier measures of the effectiveness of screening are needed. Morrison (52) and Miller (46) describe such "intermediate" measures, but discuss the limitations of using these early measures for the evaluation of screening effectiveness.

Day et al (25), however, propose that intermediate measures can and should be used for the evaluation of the introduction of mammography into the regular health-care system of a population. The earliest measure is the proportion of women who are screened, which we discussed in the previous section. A high compliance rate is necessary, but not sufficient for program effectiveness. Day et al propose additional intermediate measures, which we have adapted to reflect the type of data that are available on the US population:

1. Incidence rate (detection rate) of breast cancer. Many screen-detected cases are discovered years earlier than they would otherwise have been. At the beginning of a screening program, these screen-detected cases are in addition to the usual rate of clinically detected cases. This

increased detection of breast cancer leads to an apparent transient increase in the incidence of breast cancer, which would revert to the usual incidence after several years, when a steady state of earlier detection is achieved.
2. Distribution of stage at diagnosis and tumor size. Screening would lead to an increased proportion of breast cancer cases detected at an earlier stage of disease, when the tumor is smaller and disease has not spread.
3. Incidence rate of late stage cancers. A decline in the absolute rate of advanced cancers in the population should occur within three to six years after a screening program has begun (25). Several years are needed to observe this decline because the deficit of late stage cases is due to their detection years earlier by screening.

In this section, we review the time trends in breast cancer mortality and trends in these intermediate measures that would be influenced by increased utilization of mammography. We also discuss issues affecting the interpretation of these data. Specifically, many of the trends may also reflect changes in other modes of early detection (e.g. clinical breast exam) or changes in the underlying risk of breast cancer in the population or changes in treatment.

Sources of Data

Our review of the population impact of mammography on breast cancer morbidity and mortality is limited to the United States. We review published reports, most of which are based on data from the Surveillance, Epidemiology, and End Results (SEER) program of the National Cancer Institute. We also include additional analyses of SEER data from the public access tape. The SEER program collects data on all incident cancers in nine geographic areas of the United States: the states of Connecticut, Hawaii, Iowa, New Mexico, and Utah; the metropolitan areas surrounding Detroit and San Francisco-Oakland; metropolitan Atlanta and ten rural counties in Georgia; and a 13-county areas of western Washington around Seattle (60). The nine areas cover 9.5% of the United States and are reasonably representative of the demographic characteristics of the US population. Information is abstracted on cancer cases, including carcinoma in situ, from all hospitals in which residents of the area may be seen (including hospitals outside the area), from death certificates, pathology laboratories, radiotherapy units, and nursing homes. For each case, information is collected on demographic characteristics and extent of disease at diagnosis and other characteristics, and each patient is followed yearly for vital status. Population data are provided by the US Census Bureau under contract to the SEER program. Mortality data are based on the underlying cause of death from death certificates as reported by the National Center for Health Statistics (54, 55, 60).

Trends in Breast Cancer Mortality

The degree of decline in breast cancer mortality rates is the ultimate measure of the population effectiveness of mammography. As shown in Table 6, the age-adjusted breast cancer death rate for women has not declined; rather a 4% increase was observed between 1979–1980 and 1987–1988 (60). More recent US data through 1990 are available, based on a 10% sample of US death certificates (54, 55) (Table 6). These rates have not been age-adjusted so cannot be compared with the earlier rates. (Age-adjustment yields the rate for a population with the age distribution of the 1970 US population to remove trends due to population aging.) Nonethless, comparing these rates between 1987–1988 and 1989–1990 shows no evidence for a recent decline in breast cancer mortality. The only area in the United States to report a decline in breast cancer mortality is San Francisco (34). However, the decline was uniform over the 1970–1986 period, which suggests that screening mammography was not the cause of the reduction.

The failure to observe a decline in breast cancer mortality is not surprising: The benefits of mammography on mortality would not become apparent until years after a large proportion of women are screened. Furthermore, trends in mortality rates are influenced by trends in incidence and treatment, as well as early detection. The incidence rate of breast cancer has been steadily increasing for decades (38), which, if early detection were held constant, would lead to increasing mortality. Conversely, the efficacy of breast cancer treatment has improved, in part, through the use of tamoxifen (27), which would lead to reduced mortality if incidence and screening were held constant. Nonetheless, mammography use has not had a major impact on breast cancer mortality rates by 1990.

Trends in Breast Cancer Incidence

Although it may be too early to detect any population benefit of mammography in terms of a reduced death rate from breast cancer, other measures relating to breast cancer detection are changing. The earliest population effect of mammography would be an increased incidence rate of breast cancer, which is caused by detection of cases of breast cancer that would not have become clinically apparent for another one to four years (24). Among US women, the incidence of invasive breast cancer increased by 31% between 1979–1980 and 1987–1988 (Table 6).

The difficulty in interpreting this increase is that if mammography is playing the major role by detecting tumors earlier, the increase is encouraging; alternatively, the increase may be due to a true increase in breast cancer risk in the population. Other factors may be playing a role, such as trends in postmenopausal estrogen use (9, 12) in reproductive factors (38, 77, 87), in

Table 6 Time trends in breast cancer morbidity and mortality among US women, 1979–1990

	Year					
	1979–80	81–82	83–84	85–86	87–88	89–90
Mortality rate (per 100,000)						
US[a]	26.2	26.7	27.0	27.3	27.3	—
US—10% sample[b]	—	—	—	—	34.3	35.3
Incidence rate of invasive breast cancer (per 100,000)						
US[c]	84.9	88.4	94.5	104.6	111.0	—
Western Washington[d]	87.0	89.3	97.7	111.1	120.1	113.3
Incidence rate of in situ breast cancer (per 100,000)						
US[e]	3.7	4.1	5.9	10.2	14.0	—
Western Washington[d]	4.0	4.6	6.3	13.1	18.9	16.7
Stage distribution (%)						
US[f]						
local	50.0	50.3	53.1	56.7	60.5	—
advanced	50.0	49.7	46.9	43.3	39.5	—
Western Washington[g]						
local	53.9	53.2	56.8	58.9	64.0	65.0
advanced	46.1	46.8	43.2	41.1	36.0	35.0
Average tumor size (cm.)[h]	3.5	3.3	3.1	3.0	2.6	—
Relative survival (%)[i]						
2-year	89.7	90.7	91.5	92.0	—	—
5-year	75.1	77.0	77.6	—	—	—
Rate of advanced cancer (per 100,000)[j]						
US	42.5	43.9	44.3	45.3	43.8	—
Western Washington	40.2	41.8	42.2	45.7	43.3	39.7

[a] Rate of death with breast cancer as underlying cause of death, entire US population, age-adjusted to 1970 US population (60).
[b] Rate of death with breast cancer as underlying cause (not age-adjusted), based on 10% sample of US death certificates (54,55). Reported rates were divided by .505 to reflect rate among women.
[c] Incidence rate age-adjusted to 1970 US population, based on the nine areas of US in SEER program (60).
[d] Incidence rate age-adjusted to 1970 US population, based on analyses from western Washington SEER data.
[e] Incidence rate age-adjusted to 1970 US population based on analyses from nine area SEER public access tape, 1979–1987.
[f] Stage distribution among women with breast cancer with known stage, based on analyses from the nine area SEER data public access tape 1979–1987. (See text for stage definitions.)
[g] Stage distribution among women with breast cancer with known stage, based on analyses from western Washington SEER area data.
[h] Average tumor size from nine SEER areas (79).
[i] Two- and five-year relative survival from nine areas of US in SEER program, computed as ratio of observed survival to expected two (or five) year survival for women of that age (60). Data for white women only.
[j] Rate of advanced breast cancer computed as percent advanced cancer times incidence of breast cancer.

diet (86), or in unknown factors. Several authors provide evidence that mammography accounts for the majority of the increase. The increase in incidence became particularly steep after 1982 (Table 6), which is consistent with the secular trend in installations of mammography equipment (Figure 1). Miller et al (49) statistically demonstrated this change by fitting a regression model to the SEER incidence data. The model confirmed a significant increase in the slope for the years after 1982 versus the years before. Furthermore, in the San Francisco-Oakland SEER area, the early increase was largely confined to those hospitals with mammography screening units (34).

Although these studies suggest that the increase in breast cancer incidence is consistent with increases in mammography usage, four studies attempted to quantify the proportion of increase due to mammography. McWorter & Eyre (45) found an increased incidence of breast cancer of 30% between 1979–1981 and 1986–1987 in Utah. Through contact with 200 physicians of cases, they found that 30% of the recent cases were discovered by screening. If none of these cases would have become clinically evident in that year, then screening mammography completely accounted for the increase. Liff et al (44) reviewed hospital records of 100 black and 100 white women with breast cancer in Atlanta, in each of two time periods, 1979–1980 and 1985–1986, to determine the mode of diagnosis. The increase between these two time periods in the diagnosis of cancer by screening mammography only accounted for 40% of the increased incidence among whites and 25% of the increase among blacks in the Atlanta area. White and colleagues (88) modeled the expected increase in breast cancer incidence for western Washington state based on estimates of mammography use from a survey of 1212 women and on data from published efficacy studies that reported the impact of mammography on the detection rate of breast cancer. When the predicted rates were compared with the observed increases between 1974–1978 and 1986–1987, all of the increase for women aged 45–64 could be explained by increased use of mammography. However, for women aged 65–74 only half of the observed increase appeared to result from mammography. Lantz et al (42) modeled the breast cancer incidence in Wisconsin in relation to mammography use estimated from surveys of x-ray facilities and surveys of women. They found that 74% of the incidence increase was explained by the amount of mammography screening. Thus, there is substantial evidence that mammography has had a population impact, and that most, but not all, of the rising incidence of breast cancer is a favorable indication of earlier detection of breast cancer.

Finally, any increase in breast cancer incidence attributable to mammography would be transitory: After several years, a steady state of early detection would be achieved, and the incidence would return to the prescreening levels. Although the national data show a consistent increase in incidence, data from western Washington, which are available through 1989–1990, suggest that rates may be recently declining (Table 6).

Rates of in situ breast cancer, which reflect preinvasive disease detected primarily through mammography, are also presented in Table 6. These rates increased almost fourfold in the United States, between 1979–1980 and

1987–1988, with the steepest increases after 1982. Some of these lesions would likely have progressed to invasive breast cancer, which is another reason why rates of invasive breast cancer may be expected to decline in the near future.

Stage at Diagnosis, Tumor Size, and Survival

The stage of breast cancer at the time of diagnosis is an important indicator of prognosis. Women whose cancer is diagnosed while it is localized to the breast have a 91% chance of surviving for five years (relative to expected survival), whereas survival for five years among those with advanced disease is 64% (60). (Advanced disease is defined here as lymph node involvement or tumor invasion of muscle or more distant sites.) The proportion of US women with breast cancer whose tumors were diagnosed while still localized has risen dramatically from 50% in 1979–1980 to 60% in 1987 (Table 6). Western Washington data are also presented in Table 6 to show that the trend toward earlier detection has continued through 1990. Several researchers have reported similar changes in early measures of screening effectiveness across the United States and in specific geographic areas (35, 36, 44, 49, 69, 88). The 60% of cancer detected at an early stage in 1987 is a particularly encouraging statistic: If all women were screened, one might expect 70% of breast cancers to be diagnosed before lymph node invasion, based on breast cancer cases with known nodal status in the Breast Cancer Detection Demonstration Project (BCDDP) (7). Although these trends are promising, the increase in the proportion of tumors detected at a local stage mostly reflects additional numbers of cancers being detected early, rather than a decline in the number of late stage cancers.

Tumor size is another prognostic indicator that is also used to stage breast cancer. The average tumor size at diagnosis has declined steadily between 1979–1980 and 1987–1988, from 3.5 cm to 2.6 cm (Table 6) (79).

Survival from cancer is not a good measure of effectiveness of screening (52), but for completeness we present trends in breast cancer survival in Table 6. Survival is a poor measure of screening effectiveness, because survival can be lengthened by moving the diagnosis backward in time, even if screening has no effect on lengthening survival to a point forward in time. The most recently available five-year relative survival rates are for women diagnosed in 1983, which encompass survival until 1988. Thus, these data refer to a diagnosis year too early to expect to see any impact of mammography. Two-year relative survival, on the other hand, is available up to diagnosis years 1985–1986. Both five-year and two-year survival rates have been slowly increasing (Table 6). These increases may be attributable to improvements in treatment for breast cancer (27) in addition to screening. Miller et al (49) modeled the trend in two-year survival for the years before 1982 versus the trend after 1982. Although not apparent in the table, they found a small but significantly greater slope for the survival trend since 1982. This suggests that the trend in improvement in survival has been accelerating beginning at a time coincident with increases in screening.

Trends in Rate of Advanced Breast Cancer

As discussed above, certain biases limit the interpretation of most intermediate measures of the population effectiveness of breast cancer screening. The least biased measure that would be expected to change earlier than mortality is a reduction in the incidence rate of advanced breast cancer, i.e. the occurrence of advanced cancers in the population. Day et al (25) noted that in the Swedish two-county study, a decline in the incidence of advanced cancers was similar in magnitude to the decline in mortality, but began two years earlier.

In the US, the incidence rate of advanced disease slowly increased between 1979–1980 to 1985–1986 with a small decline in 1987–1988 (Table 6). The increase is probably due to increases in the underlying risk of breast cancer in the population. The decline in 1987–1988, however, suggests that a population benefit of screening has begun. Based on the most recent western Washington data, the decline continued into 1989–1990, for a substantial 15% decline in advanced breast cancer since 1985–1986.

Trends by Race

A major public health concern is the difference between black and white women in breast cancer detection. Although black women have an incidence of breast cancer somewhat lower than white women (93.9 per 100,000 versus 114.7 for 1987–1988), black women are diagnosed at a later stage than white women and experience poorer survival (five-year relative survival rates of 63% and 78%, respectively) (60). However, the trend over time toward earlier detection of breast cancer appears to be similar for black and white women. In 1979–1980, 41% of invasive tumors diagnosed among black women were localized, which increased to 51% by 1987 (Figure 2). For white women, these figures were 50% in 1979–1980 and 61% in 1987. A study in metropolitan Detroit, however, found that the improvement toward earlier diagnosis was less among black women than white (69).

Summary

The anticipated benefit of mammography on breast cancer mortality has not yet been reported. Although this has led some researchers to question the population effectiveness of mammography (66), the potential reduction in mortality would not be expected to occur until five to ten years after a large majority of women have been regularly screened. Beneficial trends have been seen in the percentage of breast cancers diagnosed at an early stage;

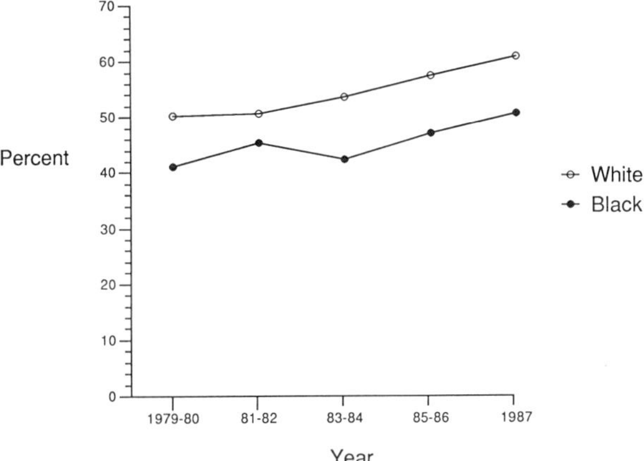

Figure 2 Time trends for white and black women in the proportion of breast cancer cases detected while localized to the breast.

importantly, there is evidence of a decline in the incidence rate of advanced stage breast cancer. These are promising signs that mortality from breast cancer will decline in the near future.

COST-EFFECTIVENESS OF SCREENING FOR BREAST CANCER BY MAMMOGRAPHY

The benefits of mammography cannot be achieved without monetary costs. The purpose of cost-effectiveness analysis is to judge the relative efficiency of various ways to achieve a benefit in order to guide resource allocation. Strategies to reduce disease incidence, mortality, and morbidity can be compared when analyses use the same measure of cost-effectiveness and comparable methods. The measure most frequently recommended is the cost per year of life saved, adjusted for quality of life (64, 85). In practice, because measurement of quality of life is seldom performed, the simpler cost per year of life saved is often used to compare strategies to reduce disease mortality, such as screening for breast cancer by mammography.

A new strategy is said to be cost-effective if it yields an additional benefit worth the additional cost, relative to a defined baseline. The additional benefit (effectiveness) is measured as the change in expected years of life attributable to the strategy. It is calculated from age-specific rates of disease mortality and life expectancies, and estimates of the reduction in mortality associated with the strategy. The latter is usually estimated by a randomized controlled trial or a case-control study. The additional cost is measured as the change in expected costs over the period of the analysis, including the direct costs of the strategy, the costs attributable to any side effects of the strategy, and the savings in treatment costs attributable to prevention of morbidity attributable to the strategy. The ratio of the attributable cost to the attributable benefit measures the marginal cost per additional unit of benefit of the new strategy, relative to some standard of comparison, or baseline. These basic relationships can be summarized as:

Cost-effectiveness = additional costs/additional benefits

where costs = costs of screening
+ costs associated with false positives
– savings in treatment costs,

and benefits = years of life saved.

In estimating the cost-effectiveness of screening for breast cancer by mammography, assumptions must be made about three critical factors. The first is the effectiveness of screening by mammography, which depends on its application (one-view or two-view, alone or in combination with CBE, and the screening interval) and the baseline with which it was compared (no screening or CBE alone). The second factor is the cost of screening by mammography, including the costs of diagnostic work-up of the false-positives, which depend on the rate of false-positive in the screening program. The third is the savings in treatment costs that can be expected as a result of screening by mammography, which depend directly on the effectiveness of the screening: the greater the reduction in late stage cases and mortality, the greater the savings in treatment costs. The baseline for the analysis is important. If CBE is effective, and there is some redundancy between the two modes of detection, the effectiveness of mammography screening is expected to be less compared with screening by CBE than compared with no screening at all. Also, in general, programs that save more years of life cost more per year of life saved.

Selection of Studies

This review was limited to studies with comparable methods addressing the issue of cost-effectiveness of screening by mammography. No studies were identified that reported costs per quality-adjusted year of life saved. It has recently been estimated that quality adjustment reduces the estimated effectiveness of a breast cancer screening program by about 8%, which is considered too small an effect to influence decision-making (26). Studies were included in the review only if costs per year of life saved were reported; costs were defined to include screening costs, the costs associated with the diagnostic work-up of false-positives, and the savings in treatment costs; and both costs and benefits occurring in the future were discounted to reflect societal time preference. In the four studies that met these criteria, a discount rate of 5% was employed. Because there is no firm economic basis for the choice of a discount rate, Russell (64) has recommended that a 5% discount rate be used by analysts of prevention interventions for the sake of consistency. Using a discount rate of 0% in the breast cancer screening analyses would reduce the cost per year of life saved by about 20% (80).

The studies vary considerably in their assumptions regarding the screening strategies to be evaluated and the target populations to which they are applied, and regarding their assumptions about effectiveness. They also vary in their assumptions about the costs associated with screening, diagnostic work-up, and treatment. In addition, each reports cost-effectiveness in different currencies or year's dollars. Accordingly, the most significant assumptions affecting estimates of cost-effectiveness were identified so that the studies can be compared meaningfully. For the same reason, all costs and cost-effectiveness ratios were converted to 1991 dollars (78).

Estimates of Cost-Effectiveness

Results of the four selected studies on the cost-effectiveness of mammography are summarized in Table 7. The earliest of the studies was done in 1987 by the US Office of Technology Assessment to evaluate the cost-effectiveness of breast cancer screening, defined as annual mammography in combination with CBE, in the Medicare population (80). As shown in Table 7, the cost per year of life saved of breast cancer screening was an estimated $57,300 for women aged 65–74 who receive annual mammography in combination with a physical examination of the breasts. The estimate was calculated over the 33-year period 1899–2020, based on the assumptions that 30% of women offered screening would accept and that among those accepting, screening would reduce mortality by 50% at five years, gradually falling to 30% mortality reduction at 20 years.

The analysts assumed that mammography, including a physical examination of the breasts, cost $83 and that a diagnostic work-up for a false-positive cost about $1500 and would be required in 2% of the women screened. Assumptions about savings in treatment costs attributable to screening were based on analysis of Medicare claims data. They estimated that early-stage breast cancer cost $2000 less to treat than late-stage disease during the initial three months of treatment and that the cost attributable to continuing care for survivors was about $300 per month. The cost of terminal care for breast cancer was estimated to be about $18,000, whereas the cost of terminal care for other conditions was estimated to be $12,500. Although the results of the Swedish two-county trial and the BCDDP, as well as the European case-control studies, were considered in the analyses, estimates of effectiveness were based

Table 7 Estimates of cost-effectiveness of screening by mammography

Mammography screening strategy (reference)	Screening interval	Age of target population	Cost per screen[a]	Biopsy rate	Source of effectiveness assumptions	Cost per year of life saved in 1991 dollars[a]
Two-view with CBE (80)	Annual	65–74	$83	2% of women screened	HIP, two-county, BCDDP, and case-control studies	$57,300
Single-view (41)	Every three years	50–65	—	—	HIP & two-county	$5,400
Single-view (82)	Biennial	50–70	$46	Less than 2 per cancer found	Two county & Dutch trials	$6,200
Two-view relative to CBE alone (28)	Annual	55–65	$124 ($41 for CBE)	2% of women screened	BCDDP	$35,900
					HIP	$138,700
CBE alone (28)	Annual	55–65	$41		BCDDP	$13,400
					HIP	$25,700
Two-view relative to CBE (28)	Annual	40–50	$124 ($41 for CBE)	2% of women screened	BCDDP	$48,700
					HIP	$222,000
CBE alone (28)	Annual	40–50	$41		BCDDP	$24,000
					HIP	$54,600

[a]Converted from reported currency to 1991 US dollars using the Medical Care Price Index (78).

primarily on long-term follow-up of the women who participated in the HIP study. Cost-effectiveness of annual mammography in combination with CBE was assessed in this study, rather than the cost-effectiveness of mammography either used alone or relative to the use of CBE alone.

Estimates of the cost-effectiveness of mammography used alone come from studies conducted in the UK and the Netherlands. The Forrest working group produced a report in 1986 that recommended that women in the UK aged 50–65 be offered single-view screening mammography once every three years, a total of six screens per woman (29). In 1988, Knox (41) published an evaluation of that recommendation with respect to its cost-effectiveness, taking into account savings in treatment costs attributable to avoidance of mortality. Knox employed a simulation model in which he assumed that the disease progresses faster among young women than among older women. He assumed that the disease duration is about 7.0 years at age 55, 5.4 years at age 25, and 8.6 years at age 85. Based on the results of the Swedish two-county study, he further assumed that mammography detects 70% of presymptomatic disease. Compliance was set at 60%, 50%, and 40% for women aged 40, 60, and 80, respectively. His model permitted assessment of alternative screening strategies, such as a shorter screening interval, as well as the one recommended by the Forrest working group. He estimated that the cost per year of life saved of the recommended strategy was about $5400. Although increased expenditure yielded diminishing returns in years of life saved, he reported that at least twice as much could be invested before efficiency was seriously reduced.

In the United States, screening is generally recommended annually or biennially, rather than every three years. The cost-effectiveness of a screening program in which biennial (single-view) mammography is used alone among women aged 50–70 has been assessed by van der Maas and colleagues (82), based on results of the Swedish two-county trial and the Dutch trials. Like Knox, they employed a simulation model and assumed that the mean duration of the presymptomatic phase of the disease increases from below two years among women under age 45 to more than four years among women over age 65. They assumed that screening would detect 70% of early stage disease, and based their estimate of improved prognosis attributable to earlier detection on the 29% mortality reduction in the early reports of the Swedish study. The attendance rate was assumed to decrease with age from 75% at age 50 to 65% at age 70. The cost of a screen was assumed to be $46, and one false-positive was expected for each cancer detected. Analysis of screening over the 28-year period 1988–2015 yielded a cost-effectiveness estimate of about $6200 for biennial screening by mammography alone.

Because most women in the United States probably receive regular CBE (56), the cost-effectiveness of mammography, when added to CBE, is a particularly relevant consideration. Unfortunately, the results of the only effectiveness trial that has addressed this question have not yet been published (47). However, Eddy (28) has reported the cost-effectiveness of annual mammography relative to a baseline of annual CBE, based on the assumptions that half the benefit of screening in the BCDDP, and one third of the benefit of screening in the HIP study, was attributable to the mammography alone, rather than to CBE. Assuming that mammography alone costs $124, whereas CBE alone costs $41, Eddy estimated that the cost per year of life saved attributable to mammography relative to a baseline of CBE alone was about $36,000 for women aged 55–65, based on the results of the BCDDP study. Using the results of the HIP study instead, cost-effectiveness for the same age group was estimated to be $138,700. However this latter figure is probably not relevant to screening in the 1990s, because mammography quality has improved considerably since the HIP study was conducted in the 1970s.

The effectiveness of screening women under 50 years of age is still being debated in the literature. Nevertheless, in his study of the marginal cost-effectiveness of mammography relative to a baseline of screening by CBE alone, Eddy estimated the cost-effectiveness of screening by mammography for women in the 40–50 age group. Based on the results of the BCDDP study, he estimated that the cost per year of life saved attributable to mammography relative to a baseline of CBE alone was $48,700 for women aged 40–50. Using the results of the HIP study instead, cost-effectiveness for the same age group was estimated to be $222,000. Table 7 presents Eddy's estimates, including estimates of the cost-effectiveness of screening by CBE alone for each age group, for purposes of comparison.

Summary

It is generally agreed that breast cancer screening by mammography is not cost-saving, because the savings in treatment costs are not sufficient to offset the costs of screening and diagnosis. However, this does not mean that it is not cost-effective. Screening for breast cancer using mammography is cost-effective if it saves additional years of life at a cost that society is willing to pay. Mammography cost-effectiveness remains a subject of debate, in part because the most cost-effective programs use a three-year interval for screening, but these programs save fewer years of life than programs with annual screening. Estimates of the cost-effectiveness of mammography in screening for breast cancer in women over age 50 range from $5400 to nearly $140,000 in 1991 dollars per year of life saved, depending on the screening strategy employed and the baseline used. Although these estimates seem to cover a very broad range, their variation can be explained by differences in the assumptions employed.

The most relevant figure may be the estimate of $36,000 for the cost-effectiveness of annual mammography relative to a baseline of CBE alone, using the effectiveness estimates from the BCDDP and false-positive rates consistent with experience in the United States. This compares favorably to figures that have been reported for standard procedures, such as interventions commonly used to prevent coronary heart disease mortality. For example, in 1991 dollars, estimates of the cost-effectiveness of treating hypertension range from $15,000 to $98,000, depending on the particular drug involved; estimates of the cost-effectiveness of treating hypercholesterolemia range from $7000 to $208,000, depending on the cholesterol level and risk status of the patient; and estimates of the cost-effectiveness of coronary artery bypass surgery range from $6500 for left-main disease to over $900,000 for single-vessel disease, depending on the risk factors of the patient (75). As in the breast cancer analyses, a discount rate of 5% was used in the heart disease analyses.

CONCLUSION

To achieve the magnitude of decline in breast cancer mortality that was observed in the controlled trials, a large proportion of American women over age 50 would need to be screened at regular intervals by high quality mammography and with appropriate follow-up of abnormal exams. There is clear evidence that the proportion of women who have ever received screening mammography has been rapidly increasing. However, regular use of the procedure remains far from widespread, and screening prevalence remains unacceptably low among certain population subgroups. As the focus of efforts to maximize the public health impact of mammography moves to routine screening, the greatest potential may lie with activities targeting the health-care sector, such as the design and implementation of office-based reminder systems. Innovative interventions will be needed to reach those women who are apparently least ready or able to participate: senior citizens, racial minority groups, and the socioeconomically disadvantaged.

Although US breast cancer mortality has not declined to date, there is evidence of a trend toward earlier detection of breast cancer. There has been a dramatic increase over the last decade in the proportion of breast cancers detected at an early stage, and the incidence of late stage disease in the population appears to have begun to decline. These statistics, which are the most promising to date, suggest that the anticipated decrease in US breast cancer mortality will begin to occur within the next several years. Monitoring of breast cancer morbidity and mortality should continue on a regional and national basis to measure the effectiveness of public health programs aimed at increasing mammography use.

The estimated cost of annual mammography relative to clinical breast exam alone is $36,000 per year of life saved. It should be remembered, in discussions of the cost-effectiveness of mammography, that the criterion for cost-effectiveness is that the strategy must yield a benefit worth its cost (64). Just as society expects to spend money on surgery and chemotherapy to save lives, so society should expect to spend money on screening to save lives. In the future, the relative cost-effectiveness of various strategies to reduce breast cancer mortality should be considered, and strategies that maximize benefits in the context of other competing uses of health-care funds should be selected.

ACKNOWLEDGMENTS

The authors thank Leslie Dennis for data analyses and Shelly Sestak and Teri Platt for manuscript preparation. This work was supported by grant CA 34847 from the National Cancer Institute.

Literature Cited

1. Albanes, D., Weinberg, G. B., Boss, L., Taylor, P. R. 1988. A survey of physician's breast cancer early detection practices. *Prev. Med.* 17:643–52
2. Am. Cancer Soc. 1991 *Cancer Facts & Figures—1991*. New York: Am Cancer Soc.
3. Am. College of Physicians. 1985. The use of diagnostic tests for screening and evaluating breast lesions. *Ann. Intern. Med.* 103:143–46
4. Am. Geriatr. Soc. 1989. Screening for breast cancer in elderly women. *J. Am. Geriatr. Soc.* 37:883–84
5. Anda, R. F., Sienko, D. G., Remington, P. L., Gentry, E. M., Marks, J. S. 1990. Screening mammography for women 50 years of age and older: practices and trends 1987. *Am. J. Prev. Med.* 6:123–29
6. Andersson, I., Aspegren, K., Janzon, L., Landberg, T., Lindholm, K. et al. 1988. Mammographic screening and mortality from breast cancer: the Malmo mammographic screening trial. *Br. Med. J.* 297:943–48
7. Baker, L. H. 1982. Breast cancer detection demonstration project: five-year summary report. *CA Cancer J. Clin.* 32:194–225
8. Baker, M. S., Kessler, L. G., Urban, N., Smucker, R. C. 1991. Estimating the treatment costs of breast and lung cancer. *Med. Care* 29:40–49
9. Bergkvist, L., Adami, H. O., Persson, I., Hoover, R., Schairer, C. 1989. The risk of breast cancer after estrogen and estrogen-progestin replacement. *N. Engl. J. Med.* 321:293–97
10. Bernstein, A. B., Thompson, G. B., Harlan, L. C. 1991. Differences in rates of cancer screening by usual source of medical care: data from the 1987 National Health Interview Survey. *Med. Care* 29:196–209
11. Boss, L. P., Guckes, F. H. 1992. Medicaid coverage of screening tests for breast and cervical cancer. *Am. J. Public Health* 82:252–53
12. Brinton, L. A., Hoover, R., Fraumeni, J. F. Jr. 1986. Menopausal oestrogen and breast cancer risk: an expanded case-control study. *Br. J. Cancer* 54: 825–32
13. Brown, M. L., Kessler, L. G., Rueter, F. G. 1990. Is the supply of mammography x-ray machines outstripping need and demand? An economic analysis. *Ann. Intern. Med.* 113:547–52
14. Burg, M. A., Lane, D. S., Polednak, A. P. 1990. Age group differences in the use of breast cancer screening tests: the effects of health care utilization and socieconomic variables. *J. Aging Health* 2:514–30
15. Cent. for Dis. Control. 1988. Use of mammography for breast cancer screening—Rhode Island 1987. *Morbid. Mortal. Wkly. Rep.* 37:357–60
16. Cent. for Dis. Control. 1990. Trends in breast cancer screening—Rhode Island 1987–1989. *Morbid. Mortal. Wkly. Rep.* 39:569–71
17. Cent. for Dis. Control. 1990. Use of mammography-United States, 1990. *Morbid. Mortal. Wkly. Rep.* 39:621–30
18. Chu, K. C., Smart, C. R., Tarone, R. E. 1988. Analysis of breast cancer

mortality and stage distribution by age for the Health Insurance Plan clinical trial. *J. Natl. Cancer Inst.* 80:1125–32

19. Collette, J. H. A., Day, N. E., Rombach, J. J., de Waard, F. 1984. Evaluation of screening for breast cancer in a non-randomized study (the DOM Project) by means of a case-control study. *Lancet* 1:1224–26
20. Costanza, M. E., D'Orsi, C. J., Greene, H. L., Gaw, V. P., Karellas, A., Zapka, J. G. 1991. Feasibility of universal screening: lessons from a community intervention. *Arch. Int. Med.* 151:1851–56
21. Counc. on Sci. Aff. 1989. Mammographic screening in asymptomatic women aged 40 years and older. *J. Am. Med. Assoc.* 261:2535–42
22. Dawson, D. A., Thompson, G. B. 1990. *Breast Cancer Risk Factors and Screening: United States 1987*. Hyatsville, Md: DHHS
23. Day, N. E. 1991. Screening for breast cancer. *Br. Med. Bull.* 47:400–15
24. Day, N. E., Walter, S. D., Tabar, L., Fagerberg, C. J. G., Collette, H. J. A. 1988. The sensitivity and lead time of breast cancer screening: a comparison of the results of different studies. In *Screening for Breast Cancer,* ed. N. E. Day, A. B. Miller, pp. 105–110. Toronto: Huber
25. Day, N. E., Williams, D. R. R., Khaw, K. T. 1989. Breast cancer screening programmes: the development of a monitoring and evaluation system. *Br. J. Cancer* 59:954–58
26. de Haes, J. C. J. M., de Koning, H. J., von Oortmarssen, G. J., van Agt, H. M. E., de Bruyn, A. E., von der Maas, P. J., 1991. The impact of a breast cancer screening programme on quality-adjusted life-years. *Int. J. Cancer* 49:538–44
27. Early Breast Cancer Trialists' Collaborative Group. 1992. Systematic treatment of early breast cancer by hormonal, cytotoxic, or immune therapy. *Lancet* 339:1–15
28. Eddy, D. M. 1989. Screening for breast cancer. *Ann. Intern. Med.* 111:389–99
29. Forrest, P. 1987. *Breast Cancer Screening*. Rep. to Health Ministers of Engl., Wales, Scotl. and North. Ireland by a work. group chaired by Prof. Sir P. Forrest. London: Her Majesty's Stationery Off.
30. Fox, S. A., Murata, P. J., Stein, J. A. 1991. The impact of physician compliance on screening mammography for older women. *Arch. Intern. Med.* 51:50–56
31. Godillo, C. 1989. Breast cancer screening guidelines agreed on by AMA, other medically related organizations. *J. Am. Med. Assoc.* 262:1155
32. Greene, L. W., Eriksen, M. P., Schor, E. L. 1988. Preventive practices by physicians: behavioral determinants and potential interventions. *Am. J. Prev. Med.* 4(Suppl.):101–7
33. Hayward, R. A., Shapiro, M. F., Freeman, H. E., Corey, C. R. 1988. Who gets screened for cervical and breast cancer? *Arch. Intern. Med.* 148: 1177–81
34. Henson, D. E., Ries, L. A. 1990. Progress in early breast cancer detection. *Cancer* 65:2155–58
35. Hiatt, R. A., Tekawa, I. S. 1990. Mammography utilization in relation to stage at diagnosis for breast cancer. In *Advances in Cancer Control: Screening and Prevention Research,* ed. P. F. Engstron, B. Rimer, L. E. Mortenson, pp. 227–38. New York: Wiley Liss
36. Horm, J. W. 1990. An overview of female breast cancer. In *Advances in Cancer Control: Screening and Prevention Research,* ed. P. F. Engstron, B. Rimer, L. E. Mortenson, pp. 217–26. New York: Wiley Liss
37. Howard, J. 1987. Using mammography for cancer control: an unrealized potential. *CA Cancer J. Clin.* 37:33–48
38. Kelsey, J. L., Gammon, M. D. 1991. The epidemiology of breast cancer. *CA Cancer J. Clin.* 41:146–65
39. Kessler, L. G., Feuer, E. J., Brown, M. L. 1991. Projections of the breast cancer burden to US women: 1990–2000. *Prev. Med.* 20:170–82
40. King, A. 1989. Not everyone agrees with new mammographic screening guidelines designed to end confusion. *J. Am. Med. Assoc.* 262:1154–55
41. Knox, E. G. 1988. Evaluation of a proposed breast cancer screening regimen. *Br. Med. J.* 297:650–54
42. Lantz, P. M., Remington, P. L., Newcomb, P. A. 1991. Mammography screening and increased incidence of breast cancer in Wisconsin. *J. Natl. Cancer Inst.* 83:1540–96
43. Lerman, C., Rimer, B., Trock, B., Balshem, A., Engstrom, P. F. 1990. Factors associated with repeat adherence to breast cancer screening. *Prev. Med.* 19:279–90
44. Liff, J. M., Sung, J. F. C., Chow, W.-H., Greenberg, R. S., Flanders, W. D. 1991. Does increased detection account for the rising incidence of

breast cancer? *Am. J. Public Health* 81:462–65
45. McWorter, W. P., Eyre, H. J. 1990. Impact of mammographic screening on breast cancer diagnosis. *J. Natl. Cancer Inst.* 83:153
46. Miller, A. B. 1985. Principles of screening and of evaluation of screening programs. In *Screening for Cancer,* ed. A. B. Miller, pp. 3–24. Orlando: Academic
47. Miller, A. B. 1988. The Canadian National Breast Cancer Screening Study. In *Screening for Breast Cancer,* ed. N. E. Day, A. B. Miller, pp. 51–58. Toronto: Huber
48. Miller, A. B., Chamberlain, J., Day, N. E., Hakama, M., Prorok, P. C. 1990. Report on a workshop of the UICC Project on Evaluation of Screening for Cancer. *Int. J. Cancer* 46:761–69
49. Miller, A. B., Feuer, E. J., Hankey, B. F. 1991. The increasing incidence of breast cancer since 1982: relevance of early detection. *Cancer Causes Control* 2:67–74
50. Montano, D. E., Taplin, S. H. 1991. A test of an expanded theory of reasoned action to predict mammography participation. *Soc. Sci. Med.* 32:733–41
51. Morisky, D. E., Fox, S. A., Murata, P. J., Stein, J. A. 1989. The role of the needs assessment in designing a community-based mammography education program for urban women. *Health Educ. Res.* 4:469–78
52. Morrison, A. S. 1985. *Screening in Chronic Disease*. New York: Oxford Univ. Press
53. Morrison, A. S., Brisson, J., Khalid, N. 1988. Breast cancer incidence and mortality in the Breast Cancer Detection Demonstration Project. *J. Natl. Cancer Inst.* 80:1540–47
54. Nat. Cent. for Health Stat. 1989. Births, marriages, divorces and deaths for December 1988. *Mon. Vital Stat. Rep.* 38(1):10
55. Nat. Cent. for Health Stat. 1991. Births, marriages, divorces and deaths for December 1990. *Mon. Vital Stat. Rep.* 39(13):20
56. NCI Breast Cancer Screen. Consort. 1990. Screening mammography: a missed clinical opportunity? *J. Am. Med. Assoc.* 264:54–58
57. Palli, D., Del Turco, M. R., Buiatti, E., Carli, S., Ciatto, S., et al. 1986. A case-control study of the efficacy of a non-randomized breast cancer screening program in Florence (Italy). *Int. J. Cancer* 38:501–4
58. Polednak, A. P., Lane, D. S., Burg, M. A. 1991. Risk perception, family history, and use of breast cancer screening tests. *Cancer Detect. Prev.* 15:257–63
59. Remington, P. L., Lantz, P. 1989. Mammography guidelines and practices in Wisconsin. *Wisc. Med. J.* 9:38–42
60. Ries, L. A. G., Hankey, B. F., Miller, B. A., Hartman, A. M., Edwards, B. K. 1991. *Cancer Stat. Rev. 1973–88 (NIH Publ. No. 91-2789).* Bethesda, Md: Natl. Cancer Inst.
61. Rimer, B. K., Keintz, M. K., Kessler, H. B., Engstom, P. F., Rosan, J. R. 1989. Why women resist screening mammography: patient-related barriers. *Radiology* 172:243–46
62. Rimer, B. K., Trock, B., Lerman, C., King, E., Engstrom, P. F. 1991. Why do some women get regular mammograms? *Am. J. Prev. Med.* 7:69–74
63. Roberts, M. M., Alexander, F. E., Anderson, T. J., Chetty, U., Donnan, P. T., et al. 1990. Edinburgh trial of screening for breast cancer: mortality at seven years. *Lancet* 355:241–46
64. Russell, L. B. 1986. *Is Prevention Better Than Cure?* Washington, DC: Brookings Inst.
65. Shapiro, S., Venet, W., Strax, P., Venet, L., Roeser, R. 1985. Selection, follow-up and analysis in the Health Insurance Plan study: a randomized trial with breast cancer screening. *Natl. Cancer Inst. Monogr.* 67:65–74
66. Skrabanek, P. 1985. False premises and false promises of breast cancer screening. *Lancet* 2:316
67. Slenker, S. E., Wright, J. M. 1988. A survey of physician beliefs and practices concerning routine mammography. *Ohio Med.* 84:476–80
68. Stein, J. A., Fox, S. A., Murata, P. J. 1991. The influence of ethnicity, socio-economic status, and psychological barriers in usage of mammography. *J. Health Soc. Behav.* 32:101–13
69. Swanson, G. M., Satariano, E. R., Satariano, W. A., Threatt, B. A. 1990. Racial differences in the early detection of breast cancer in Metropolitan Detroit, 1978 to 1987. *Cancer* 66:1297–1301
70. Tabar, L., Fagerberg, G., Day, N. E., Holmberg, L. 1987. What is the optimum interval between mammographic screening examinations? An analysis based on the latest results of the Swedish two-county breast cancer screening trial. *Br. J. Cancer* 55:547–51

71. Tabar, L., Fagerberg, G., Duffy, S. W., Day, N. E. 1989. The Swedish two-county trial of mammographic screening for breast cancer: recent results and calculation of benefit. *J. Epidemiol. Commun. Health* 43:107–14
72. Tabar, L., Fagerberg, G., Gad, A., Baldetorp, L., Holmberg, L. H., et al. 1985. Reduction in mortality from breast cancer after mass screening with mammography: randomized trial from the Breast Cancer Screening Working Group of the Swedish National Board of Health and Welfare. *Lancet* 1:829–32
73. Taplin, S. H., Anderman, C., Grothaus, L. 1989. Breast cancer risk and participation in mammographic screening. *Am. J. Public Health* 79: 1494–98
74. Thompson, G. B., Kessler, L. G., Boss, L. P. 1989. Breast cancer screening legislation in the United States: a commentary. *Am. J. Public Health* 79:1541–43
75. Urban, N. 1992. Cost effectiveness. In *Prevention of Coronary Heart Disease,* ed. I. Ockene, J. Ockene. Boston: Little, Brown
76. Urban, N., Anderson, G., Peacock, S. 1993. Screening mammography: how important is cost as a barrier to use? *Am. J. Public Health.* In press
77. US Bur. of Census. 1984. Fertility of American women: June 1983. In *Current Population Reports (Ser. P-20, No. 395).* Washington, DC: GPO
78. US Bur. of Census, 1990. *Statistical Abstract of the United States: 1990,* Table No. 761. Washiongton, DC: GPO. 110th ed.
79. US Gen. Account. Off. 1991. *Breast Cancer, 1971–91: Prevention, Treatment, and Research.* (GAO No. PEMD-92–12). Washington, DC: GAO
80. US Off. of Technol. Assess. 1987. *Breast Cancer Screening for Medicare Beneficiaries: Effectiveness, Costs of Medicare and Medical Resources Required.* Washington, DC: US Congress Off. of Technol. Assess. Health Progr.
81. US Prev. Serv. Task Force. 1989. *Guide to Clinical Preventive Services.* Baltimore: Williams & Wilkins
82. van der Maas, P. J., de Koning, H. J., van Ineveld, B. M., van Oortmarssen, G. J., Habbema, J. D. F., et al. 1989. The cost-effectiveness of breast cancer screening. *Int. J. Cancer* 43:1055–60
83. Verbeek, A. L. M., Hendricks, J. H. C. L., Holland, R., Mravunac, M., Sturmans, F., Day, N. E. 1984. Reduction of breast cancer mortality through mass screening with modern mammography: first results of the Nijmegen project 1975–1981. *Lancet* 1:1222–24
84. Verbeek, A. L. M., Hendricks, J. H. C. L., Holland, R., Mravunac, M., Sturmans, F., Day, N. E. 1985. Mammographic screening and breast cancer mortality: age-specific effects in Nijmegen Project, 1975–82. *Lancet* 1: 865–66
85. Weinstein, M. C., Stason, W. B. 1977. Foundations of cost-effectiveness analysis for health and medical practice. *New Engl. J. Med.* 296:716–21
86. Welch, S., Marston, R. M. 1982. Review of trends in food use in the United States: 1890–1980. *J. Am. Diet. Assoc.* 81:120–25
87. White, E. 1987. Projected changes in breast cancer incidence due to the trend toward delayed childbearing. *Am. J. Public Health* 77:495–97
88. White, E., Lee, C. Y., Kristal, A. R. 1990. Evaluation of the increase in breast cancer incidence in relation to mammography use. *J. Natl. Cancer Inst.* 82:1546–55
89. Zapka, J. G., Stoddard, A. M., Costanza, M. E., Greene, H. L. 1989. Breast cancer screening by mammography: utilization and associated factors. *Am. J. Public Health* 79:1499–1502
90. Zapka, J. G., Stoddard, A. M., Maul, L., Costanza, M. E. 1991. Interval adherence to mammography screening guidelines. *Med. Care* 29:697–707

Annu. Rev. Publ. Health 1993. 14:635–48

TEMPLES OF THE FUTURE: An Historical Overview of the Laboratory's Role in Public Health Practice[1]

Ronald O. Valdiserri
National Center for Prevention Services, Centers for Disease Control, Atlanta, Georgia 30333

KEY WORDS: public health laboratory, laboratory history, bacteriology, sanitation, state laboratory

ANTECEDENTS OF THE PUBLIC HEALTH LABORATORY

Public health practice predates the development of the public health laboratory. But, with the birth of modern laboratory science, especially microbiology and serology, disease prevention and control activities developed a more rational scientific basis and, hence, more effective outcomes. However, before the public health laboratory could exist, two prerequisites were necessary: a firm knowledge base that supported laboratory practice as a routine component of scientific inquiry, and a stable and administratively sound organization devoted to public health, into which the laboratory could be integrated. Both elements were lacking in America's early years. Several American cities established boards of health in the late eighteenth and early nineteenth centuries (26); however, these boards tended to be poorly organized and often lay dormant until "an epidemic knocked at the gates of the city" (25).

Urbanization and rapid population growth, both consequences of industrialization, created health problems that, unlike epidemics, were not cyclical in nature. The persistently negative health consequences of poor housing, overcrowding, and inadequate sanitation were difficult to ignore and raised public health issues to a level that demanded permanent action. In the years following the American Civil War, improved methods in the collection of statistics, which showed alarming rates of morbidity and mortality in large cities, coalesced public opinion in support of sanitary reform, thus paving the way for legislative changes (15). Beginning with New York City in 1866, many larger American cities implemented improved public health laws that permitted a "stable administrative foundation" for public health activities by creating independent boards of health composed of physicians and sanitarians (36). In 1869, the Massachusetts legislature passed a bill to create a state board of health (26). As Rosen indicates, this change "from a haphazard to an efficient administration" made it easier "to incorporate new scientific knowledge into public health practice" (36).

Other municipal and state governments followed the examples of New York City and Massachusetts. By 1890, 292 of 345 (85%) American cities with populations in excess of 10,000 reported that they had municipal boards of health—the majority of which met regularly and had physician members (3). In 1870, California created a state health department and was soon joined by Minnesota and Virginia in 1872 and by Michigan in 1873 (36). By 1900, "all but eight of the states had state boards of health, and by 1907 this was accomplished for all states" (48).

With the development of an adequate infrastructure, the stage was set for the institutional birth of the public health laboratory. But, a stable, permanent public health department was not the only ingredient required for its debut. Because the laboratory is the place where scientific methods are applied to solve problems, its birth was delayed until science and technology had reached a level of development that permitted the practical application of this knowledge.

Like most human knowledge, laboratory science did not arise de novo. It evolved over time, and its precursors are evident throughout history. Today, when we think of a public health laboratory, we envision a place where specimens, often derived from the human body, are tested for various analytes or microorganisms. However, the practice of studying material from the human body to learn more about disease is probably as old as human consciousness. Urine, no doubt because of its accessibility, was examined by physicians throughout antiquity (8). But, because of an inadequate knowledge base, these ancient observations were often explained by incorrect theoretical constructs. Nevertheless, these early examinations did establish the practice of searching for clues, within human excretions and discharges, to discover the cause or course of an illness.

The adoption of the scientific method, i.e. posing a hypothesis to explain a phenomenon and testing the veracity of that hypothesis through the systematic collection of data, did much to advance the knowledge base and pave the way for laboratory investigation as an integral component of disease prevention and treatment activities. Medical historians often cite William Harvey's work in elucidating the circulation of blood as one of the major milestones in the use of the scientific method to answer a medical question (46).

As new discoveries were added to the scientific knowledge base, laboratory investigation slowly moved from the realm of the alchemist to the scientist and eventually became recognized as an essential component in the process of scientific problem solving. When Wilhelm von Humboldt founded the University of Berlin in 1810, he foresaw the necessity of linking the academic institution to laboratories, where students could receive practical instruction (37). In 1826, Justus von Liebig, a pioneer in metabolic physiology, persuaded the Hessian government to build and support a chemistry laboratory at the University of Giessen. And, in 1839, the Prussian government constructed an institute of physiology for Johann E. Purkinje—the man who described the purkinje cells of the cerebellar cortex (37). According to Rosen, these events signaled the transition from "the situation in which laboratories had existed as private studies in which scientists did their work to that where the research laboratory was accepted as an integral element in the university and, more specifically, of the medical school" (37).

The appearance of research laboratories as institutional components of centers of higher education marked the acceptance of laboratory study as a legitimate and necessary tool in scientific inquiry. Soon, the European concept that "a thorougly equipped laboratory for the scientific investigation of clinical problems should be an integral part of a teaching hospital" was adopted in America (37), often popularized by Americans who had studied in European laboratories (35). Training in scientific laboratory methods become an accepted part of the academic curriculum, and subsequent generations of graduates ultimately helped move the laboratory from a strictly experimental realm into routine clinical and public health practice.

BIRTH OF THE PUBLIC HEALTH LABORATORY

In America, even before the germ theory became widely accepted, scientists began to use laboratory investigations in their studies of hygiene and sanitation. In 1870, the Massachusetts State Board of Health invited William Ripley Nichols "to investigate the sanitary conditions of water supplies by laboratory methods" (57). However, the public health laboratory truly came into being with the incontrovertible proof of the germ theory.

In the late 1850s, Louis Pasteur's seminal work on fermentation disproved the theory of spontaneous generation and brought science to the brink of accepting the germ theory (36). However, it was not until 1876 that Robert Koch proved, for the first time, that a specific microorganism, *Bacillus anthracis,* was the definite cause of a specific disease, anthrax (41). Before this indisputable proof of the germ theory, epidemic outbreaks of infectious disease were explained by one of three schools of throught: the miasmatic theory, the strict contagionist theory, or the contingent contagionist theory (36).

Proponents of the miasmatic theory believed that disease resulted from the inhalation of putrid air, tainted by decaying organic matter. The contagionists believed that epidemics were caused by "an animated particle invisible to the naked eye" (20). The contingent contagionist theory represented an amalgam of the other two; supporters of this view believed that infectious diseases were caused by contagia that acted "in conjunction with other elements such as the state of the atmosphere, condition of the soil, or social factors" (36). By the mid-1800s, it was the miasmatic theory that predominated in explaining epidemics of infectious disease (36).

With Koch's discovery in 1876, the theory of miasma was all but discarded. In rapid succession, the causative organisms for leprosy (1880), typhoid fever (1880), tuberculosis (1882), cholera (1883), and diphtheria (1883) were discovered (36). Equally impressive was Pasteur's work in the early 1880s in the field of immunization. Working with chicken cholera, Pasteur demonstrated that hens inoculated with attenuated organisms could subsequently withstand a challenge of virulent organisms without becoming ill (36).

As America approached the end of the nineteenth century, the appearance of laboratories within institutions and organizations concerned with public health and hygiene reflected the dramatic effect of these discoveries on the world of science. In 1887, Joseph Kinyoun established one of the first American research laboratories of bacteriology at the Marine Hospital in Stapleton, Staten Island; in 1892, the laboratory was moved to Washington, DC, where nearly 40 years later it would become the National Institutes of Health (37). Under the guidance of Charles V. Chapin, a municipal public health laboratory was established in Providence, Rhode Island, in 1888 (48). That same year, Michigan opened a hygienic laboratory at Ann Arbor (57).

According to Rosen (36), the primary purpose of these early public health laboratories was to perform microbiological analyses of water and food. In Providence, the bacteriology laboratory was under the immediate supervision of Gardner T. Swarts, who "purchased the equipment for the laboratory and ran it largely at his own expense for several years" (9). Exemplifying the work of these early laboratories was Swarts' 1888 analysis of household water filters. He detected typhoid bacilli in several of these filters, thus proving that they were "not only useless but actually dangerous because of their tendency in heated rooms to act as incubators for germs" (9). The bacteriology laboratory in Providence continued to perform routine bacteriologic testing of commercial water, spring water, ice, and water filters for several years (9). Diagnostic testing of human specimens did not routinely occur in these early public health laboratories until several years later, after the practice had been introduced by the New York City Health Department (3, 36, 50).

In 1892, in response to the threat that a European cholera epidemic might spread to the eastern seaboard, the New York City Health Department established a division of bacteriology and disinfection (16, 36). Herman Michael Biggs, a physician who taught bacteriology at Bellevue Hospital, was recruited to take charge of this newly established division and its associated laboratory (47). Shortly thereafter, Biggs recruited William H. Park to work in the laboratory on the problem of diphtheria (36).

Diphtheria, long a major cause of childhood mortality, had come under intense study using the new scientific techniques pioneered by the early microbiologists. Soon after Klebs described the causative organism responsible for diphtheria in 1883 (23), Loeffler successfully cultivated it and reproduced its characteristic pseudomembrane by swabbing the mucous membranes of various animals with pure cultures of the bacillus (29). Beginning in 1888, Roux & Yersin (40) confirmed Loeffler's findings and demonstrated the exotoxin of *Corynebacterium diphtheriae,* by showing that bacillus-free culture filtrates would kill guinea pigs. Their work paved the way for von Behring. Working with Kitasato at the Hygienic Institute at the University of Berlin, he discovered diphtheria antitoxin (2), which was later shown by Roux and Martin to be beneficial in the treatment of human diphtheria (39).

In 1893, these findings were put to practical use by Biggs and Park. By culturing throat swabs for the presence of *Corynebacterium diphtheriae,* Park demonstrated that, at one New York City hospital, many persons diagnosed with diphtheria did not actually have the disease and that "placing these patients in contact with the real disease endangered their lives" (50). In his 1893 annual report to Biggs, Park presented the results of "bacteriological examination of 5611 cases of suspected diphtheria" (34) and noted that the bacillus could be recovered from the throats of convalescents, as well as from healthy persons who were in contact with infected individuals (47).

To encourage the use of the diagnostic diphtheria tests, the New York City Health Department offered the tests free of charge to the medical community; "a doctor could pick up a 'culture outfit' left by the health department at a local pharmacy, inoculate and return it, and receive the laboratory verdict by mail within 24 hours" (50). In the year following its introduction of diphtheria diagnostic services, New York City began to aid physicians in treating the disease. While traveling in Europe in 1894, Biggs "heard Roux and von Behring describe the effects of antitoxin in diphtheria" and cabled Park "to start production of antitoxin at once" (47). Park's laboratory became the first in America to make the antitoxin, which was sold in drugstores and "made available to physicians for free for patients in hardship" (50).

Other laboratories quickly followed New York's example. Massachusetts organized a laboratory to produce diphtheria antitoxin in 1894. And, early in 1895, a laboratory for the diagnosis and control of diphtheria was established in Philadelphia (36). Chapin's laboratory in Providence began culturing throat swabs for *Corynebacterium diphtheria* in January 1895 (12). Soon, "almost every state and practically all large cities in the United States had established a diagnostic bacteriological laboratory" (36). These laboratory-supported diagnostic and therapeutic efforts paid off in significant reductions in diphtheria mortality. Spink cites that New York City's 1894 death rates from diphtheria and croup were 105 per 100,000, but that by 1905 this rate had decreased to 38 per 100,000 (49).

Expansion of the public health laboratory's diagnostic ability had a direct and significant impact on public health practice. Culture methods permitted the discovery of previously unrecognized cases of infection in asymptomatic persons. Proof that carriers did exist eventually led to a reexamination of the age-old practice of isolation, i.e. separating diseased persons from the nondiseased population to prevent further spread of illness. In his seminal work, *The Sources and Modes of Infection,* Chapin (12) advised that "the effectiveness of isolation varies inversely as the number of missed cases and carriers" and that when large numbers of unrecognized carriers remained in the population, the isolation of persons with symptomatic illness would have little overall benefit.

Laboratory science's contribution to the study of epidemics of infectious disease permitted more rational and focused interventions to prevent and control them. By 1894, when the New York City Health Department laboratory began examining sputum for *Mycobacterium tuberculosis* (57), tuberculosis (TB) had moved from being a "constitutional, hereditary disease related in some vague way to deleterious environmental conditions" (36) to a communicable infection caused by a specific microbe. Public health departments began to use the information provided by the laboratory to shape TB control efforts by developing public education campaigns that stressed the importance of personal hygiene in preventing the spread of infection (3). The laboratory's ability to confirm clinical diagnoses also bolstered both surveillance and reporting practices, although not without some opposition, especially from the medical community who believed that these health department activities were encroaching upon the traditional role of the physician in treatment and diagnosis (17, 38, 50). In general, however, the functions of assessment, policy development, and assurance, which are now recognized as core activities of public health agencies at all levels of government (14), were significantly strengthened as a result of information provided by the burgeoning public health laboratory.

EARLY YEARS OF THE PUBLIC HEALTH LABORATORY

In many respects, the annals of the early years of the public health laboratory are indistinguishable from the history of bacteriology. In 1897, when Henry B. Horlbeck addressed the twenty-fifth Annual Meeting of the American Public Health Association, he opined that "bacteriology is now a part and parcel of our science. It is one of the foundation stones of all progress in the opening of our knowledge of sanitary science" (52).

The new science of bacteriology added a dimension to public health activities that had been previously lacking, such that the prevention of illness became more than minimizing filth in the environment. The ability to visualize, isolate, and culture the causative agents of disease proved a powerful boon to prevention and control activities. In rapid succession, scientists built upon the findings of their colleagues, and soon the impact of these early discoveries spread into other disciplines. Gruber & Durham's (21) discovery that sera from patients with typhoid fever would agglutinate with typhoid bacillus led to the application of testing patient sera with bacteria of known type to diagnose or confirm infectious diseases (55). In 1901, Bordet & Gengou (15) demonstrated that bacteriolysis by immune serum required a heat-labile serum component, which is today known as complement; their complement-fixation reaction served as the basis for diagnostic tests for many infectious diseases, including the Wassermann test for syphilis (54). It is no wonder that laboratories, the facilities where microbes were studied so that their secrets might be revealed, were so effustively described by Pasteur (4):

> Take interest, I implore you, in those sacred dwellings which are designated by the expressive term: Laboratories. Demand that they be multiplied; that they be adorned. These are the temples of the future. . . . Temples of well being and happiness. There it is that humanity grows greater, stronger, better.

Winslow's 1914 survey of state health department laboratories provides an excellent overview of the activities of the early public health laboratory (57). Among his other achievements, Winslow was a founding editor of the *Journal of Bacteriology* and served as the Chairman of the Committee on Administrative Practice for the American Public Health Association (47). In 1914, as part of his American Public Health Association activities, he surveyed secretaries of state departments of health and asked for information about the variety of work performed in their laboratories. Although his questionnaire did not attempt to quantify testing volume, it did document a remarkable complexity of services, considering the relatively young age of the public health laboratory at the time of his survey.

Table 1 summarizes Winslow's findings. Of 48 states, 47 responded to the survey. New Mexico, which did not have a state health department at the time, established one in 1919 (10). Almost all of the laboratories surveyed performed diagnostic tests for diphtheria, typhoid fever, and tuberculosis. A majority performed diagnostic tests for malaria, rabies, gonorrhea, glanders *(Malleomyces mallei),* and syphilis. Other activities reported with a high

Table 1 Activities of state health department laboratories in 1914 (57)

Number of states performing diagnostic tests for	
Diphtheria	45/47 (96%)
Typhoid fever	45/47 (96%)
Tuberculosis	44/47 (94%)
Malaria	41/47 (87%)
Rabies	37/47 (79%)
Gonorrhea	36/47 (77%)
Glanders *(Malleomyces mallei)*	30/47 (64%)
Syphilis	27/47 (57%)
Cancer	19/47 (40%)
Number of states performing tests on water supply	
Bacteriological tests	44/47 (94%)
Chemical tests	36/47 (77%)
Number of states performing tests on milk	
Bacteriological tests	30/47 (64%)
Chemical tests	26/47 (55%)
Number of states performing tests on food/drugs	
Bacteriological tests	24/47 (51%)
Chemical tests	20/47 (42%)
Number of states manufacturing antitoxin for	
Diphtheria	5/47 (11%)
Tetanus	1/47 (2%)
Number of states manufacturing "vaccines" for	
Typhoid	19/47 (40%)
Rabies	7/47 (15%)
Tuberculosis	3/47 (6%)
Smallpox	1/47 (2%)
Number of states reporting research activities	20/47 (42%)

frequency included examination of water, milk, and food/drugs; research; and manufacture of "vaccine" for typhoid.

While Winslow was conducting his survey, Chapin, at the request of the Council on Health and Public Instruction of the American Medical Association, was conducting a comprehensive study of the activities of state health departments. His findings on the scope of state health department laboratory activities are essentially identical to Winslow's. Unlike Winslow's survey, however, Chapin sought quantitative data on testing volume, which demonstrated that tests for diphtheria, tuberculosis, typhoid fever, and malaria were among the most commonly performed (13). Chapin also documented that fecal examination for intestinal parasites, especially hookworm, was performed by 18 of the 48 state laboratories (13). Perhaps the most important contribution of his report, from a laboratory perspective, was his evaluation of the role of the laboratory in public health programs, for it provides additional documentation of the speed with which laboratory services had become an integrated and indispensable component of the public health system (13):

> The diagnostic laboratory is the most essential part of the machinery for the control of communicable diseases. Without it municipality and state can do nothing. It has been well said that 'the laboratory is the handmaid of epidemiology.' The laboratory has a threefold function. It discovers cases of communicable diseases. It keeps the physician acquainted with scientific methods of diagnosis. It teaches that the mild, atypical case is more common that the typical case of the textbooks.

DEVELOPMENT OF THE MODERN PUBLIC HEALTH LABORATORY

Tracking the evolution of the public health laboratory from its early years to the present day reveals the continued influence of two major variables: science and public policy. Throughout the twentieth century, advances in scientific technology have been manifested in new and improved tests for disease surveillance and diagnosis within the public health laboratory. Public policy decisions, especially those with funding ramifications, have also had a major impact on shaping the configuration of public health laboratories and in refining their role in the overall public health system. Both of these influences are evident in the results of a 1940 survey conducted by Mountin and Flook.

To provide the Public Health Service with "a general inclusive picture of health work at the state level," Mountin & Flook (31–33) surveyed the 48 states; the District of Columbia; and the territories of Alaska, Hawaii, Puerto Rico, and the Virgin Islands. They collected information on the scope of public health work at the state level and on which state agencies were involved in providing services, state health expenditures, and staffing patterns.

Regarding laboratory services, Mountin & Flook (32) identified three major reasons why public health laboratories were maintained by the state:

> First, they make available to physicians, hospitals, and public health personnel diagnostic facilities which would otherwise be unavailable. Second, certain biologicals to be distributed for preventive or therapeutic purposes are prepared therein. Third, the personnel of such laboratories act in a supervisory capacity with regard to practices and procedures of private laboratories.

Mountin & Flook (32) found that most laboratory services provided by the state supported the control of communicable disease programs and that "serologic tests for syphilis represent approximately two thirds of the entire diagnostic laboratory work of state health departments for all communicable diseases." Laboratory testing in support of noncommunicable disease control was less common. Chemical and bacteriologic testing of drinking water samples, milk, foods, and drugs were performed by most of the laboratories surveyed.

One of the major differences between Mountin & Flook's findings and those of Chapin and Winslow, who had surveyed essentially the same target audience 26 years earlier, was the large increase in publicly supported testing for syphilis. This development was the result of both scientific advances and changes in public policy.

In 1905, Schaudinn & Hofmann (43) identified the causative organism of syphilis by examining serum obtained from a genital lesion. In the following year, Landsteiner (27) described the use of dark field microscopy for detecting the presence of *Treponema pallidum*. However, von Wassermann's (54) modification of the complement-fixation reaction of Bordet & Gengou produced the first specific blood test for syphilis. And, in 1909, Ehrlich, working with Hata, discovered Salvarsan, the first effective treatment for syphilis (6).

With the discovery of a laboratory test to diagnose syphilis and an effective treatment to halt the course of infection and render the patient noninfectious, public health practitioners were provided with two essential ingredients for prevention and control programs. But, despite the public health benefit heralded by these advances, this new technology was slow to move into public health practice. According to Brandt (6), "as late as 1912, few physicians had the necessary laboratory and technical facilities to conduct these tests." When Winslow surveyed state health department laboratories in 1914, more than half reported offering tests for syphilis, but he believed "that in a number of instances only a microscopic examination for spirochaetes is relied upon" (57). However, Chapins's 1914 survey documented that only one third of state health department laboratories were actually performing Wasserman tests on human sera (13).

Several factors impeded the development of public health programs for the control of syphilis, and thereby the full-scale implementation of syphilis testing in the public health laboratory. Brandt (6), Duffy (17), and Starr (50) all cite the sentiment expressed by organized medicine that public health efforts to diagnose and treat syphilis were unwelcomed forays into medical practice. According to Brandt, opposing moral values about sexuality and sexually transmitted diseases (STDs) also contributed to the delay in broad-based public support for syphilis control programs.

Although the exigencies of World War I induced the federal government to take a more proactive interest in the control of STDs, including syphilis (16), it was not until the passage of the Social Security Act of 1935 that the federal government "established a permanent machinery for distributing Federal funds for health purposes and recognized special needs in allocating these funds" (16). Title VI of the Act was administered by the US Public Health Service and authorized grants-in-aid to the states for strengthening state and local health departments (56). A significant portion of Title VI monies were used by states to develop STD control programs, including "diagnostic facilities, clinics, and epidemiological programs" (7). The signing of the National Venereal Disease Control Act on May 24, 1938, brought even more resources to bear on this important public health problem, such that the number of laboratory tests performed to detect syphilis "increased 300 percent between 1936 and 1940" (7). The influence of these changes in public policy, especially in terms of funding initiatives, is evident in the large numbers of serologic tests for syphilis documented by Mountin & Flook's survey (32).

Advances in the scientific knowledge base and changes in public policy continue to exert their influence on the public health laboratory. In the Association of State and Territorial Public Health Laboratory Directors 1989 Annual Report, which summarizes the services offered by public health laboratories for that year, the largest number of tests is reported in the category of newborn screening—40% of nearly 36 million (1). This category of testing was not present on either of the two earlier surveys discussed, because the scientific knowledge needed to understand and ultimately diagnose these disorders was not yet available. Phenylketonuria (PKU), one of the first metabolic disorders proven to be a cause of mental deficiency, was not discovered until 1934 (19). And, an effective neonatal screening test for PKU, which facilitated mass newborn screening programs, was not developed until the early 1960s (22, 51).

Just as advances in technology will continue to shape the future of the public health laboratory, so too will policy issues. One of the more significant issues currently facing policy makers relates to the overall distribution of laboratory services in this country. When the American College of Surgeons surveyed hospitals in the early decades of the twentieth century, they found that "many institutions did not yet possess laboratories" (45). Yet, by 1957, more than 90% of all US hospitals maintained clinical laboratories (28). This increase in national laboratory capacity means that the performance of tests that support public health surveillance, prevention, and control efforts may not be limited exclusively to public health laboratory settings (18).

Expansion of the availability of laboratory services has raised policy issues about duplication of effort, thus forcing many to consider the questions of privatization of public health laboratory services (24, 30). Some have suggested that public health laboratories should concentrate on assuring the quality of testing, rather than on duplicating tests that are available elsewhere (42, 44).

THE FUTURE OF THE PUBLIC HEALTH LABORATORY

Reviewing the history of the public health laboratory helps us not only to understand its contribution to public health practice, but also to anticipate how it will continue to evolve in the future, along lines discussed in the accompanying article by Dowdle (14a). This historical overview has demonstrated that technologic advances in testing for diseases of public health significance have ultimately been incorporated into the repertoire of public health laboratories.

More than anything else, this overview reminds us that public health laboratory practice is not static. As our knowledge base increases, our understanding of how to prevent and control disease also expands. Changes in program direction will be mirrored by changes in the services provided by the public health laboratory. Newer, more sophisticated laboratory techniques will result in early diagnosis, earlier intervention, and more complete surveillance. Perhaps Pasteur's description of laboratories as "temples of well being and happiness" was not so extravagant after all.

Acknowledgements

The author wishes to acknowledge the secretarial assistance of Eleanor Herren and Lynn Clemons.

Literature Cited

1. Assoc. State Territ. Public Health Lab. Direct. 1990. *Consolidated Annual Report on State and Territorial Public Health Laboratories, Fiscal Year 1989*. Washington, DC: Assoc. State Territ. Public Health Lab. Direct.
2. Behring, A. E., Kitasato, S. 1890. Ueber das Zustandekommen der Diphtherie-Immunitat und der Tetanus-Immunitat bei Thieren. *Dtsch. Med. Wochenschr.* 16:1113–14
3. Blake, J. B. 1948. The origins of

public health in the United States. *Am. J. Public Health* 38:1539–50
4. Bodily, H. L. 1973. The first section: laboratory. *Am. J. Public Health* 63(8): 667–68
5. Bordet, J. J., Gengou, O. 1901. Sur l'existence de substances sensibilisatrices dans la plupart des serums antimicrobiens. *Ann. Inst. Pasteur* 15: 289–302
6. Brandt, A. M. 1985. Damaged goods: progressive medicine and social hygiene. In *No Magic Bullet, A Social History of Venereal Disease in the United States Since 1880,* pp. 7–51. New York/Oxford: Oxford Univ. Press. 245 pp.
7. Brandt, A. M. 1985. Shadow on the land: Thomas Parran and the New Deal. See Ref. 6, pp. 122–60
8. Caraway, W. T., 1973. The scientific development of clinical chemistry to 1948. *Clin. Chem.* 19:373–78
9. Cassedy, J. H. 1962. Environment sanitation. In *Charles V. Chapin and the Public Health Movement,* 4:44–60. Cambridge, Mass: Harvard Univ. Press. 310 pp.
10. Cassedy, J. H. 1962. New forms and old techniques: public health appraisal and epidemiology. See Ref. 9, pp. 194–212
11. Deleted in proof
12. Chapin, C. V. 1910. Limitations to the value of isolation. In *The Sources and Modes of Infection,* pp. 91–121. New York: Wiley. 399 pp.
13. Chapin, C. V. 1916. *A Report on State Public Health Work Based on a Survey of State Boards of Health.* Reprinted 1977 by the Am. Med. Assoc. New York: Arno. 219 pp.
14. Comm. Study Future Public Health. 1988. A vision of public health in America: an attainable ideal. In *The Future of Public Health,* Comm. Study Future Public Health, 2:35–55. Washington, DC: Natl. Acad. Press. 225 pp.
14a. Dowdle, W. R. 1993. The future of the public health laboratory. *Annu. Rev. Public Health* 14:649–64
15. Duffy, J. 1971. Social impact of disease in the late 19th century. *Bull. NY Acad. Med.* 47:797–811
16. Duffy, J. 1976. The public's health. In *The Healers, A History of American Medicine,* pp. 307–19. Urbana, Ill: Univ. Ill. Press. 385 pp.
17. Duffy, J. 1979. The American medical profession and public health: from support to ambivalence. *Bull. Hist. Med.* 53:1–22
18. Felman, Y. M., Corsaro, M. C., Jones, J. R. 1980. Laboratory compliance with syphilis reporting laws: the New York City experience, 1972–1977.
19. Folling, I. A. 1934. Utskillelse av fenylpyrodruesyre i urinen som stoffskifteanomali i forbindelse med imbecilletet. *Nord. Med. Tidskr* 8:1054–59
20. Goudsblom, J. 1986. Public health and the civilizing process. *Millbank Q.* 64(2):161–88
21. Gruber, M., Durham, H. E. 1896. Eine neue Methode zur raschen Erkennung des Choleravibrio und des Typhusbacillus. *Mürnch. Med. Wochenschr.* 43:285–86
22. Guthrie, R., Susi, A. 1963. A simple phenylalanine method for detecting phenylketonuria in large populations of newborn infants. *Pediatrics* 32:338–43
23. Klebs, T. A. 1883. Ueber Diphtherie. *Vehr. Congr. inn. Med.* 2:139–54
24. Kolderie, T. 1986. The two different concepts of privatization. *Public Adm. Rev.* 46 (July/Aug.):285–91
25. Kramer, H. D. 1947. The beginnings of the public health movement in the United States. *Bull. Hist. Med.* 21:352–76
26. Kramer, H. D. 1950. Early municipal and state boards of health. *Bull. Hist. Med.* 24:503–29
27. Landsteiner, K. 1906. Zur Technik der Spirochaetenuntersuchung. *Wien. Klin. Wochenschr.* 19:1349–50
28. Levitt, J. 1984. The growth of technology and corporate profit making in the clinical laboratories. *J. Health Polit. Policy Law* 8:732–42
29. Loeffler, F. 1884. Untersuchungen uber die Bedeutung der Mikroorganismen fur die Entstehung der Diphtherie beim Menschen, bei der Taube und beim Kalbe. *Mitt. K. GesundhAmte, Berlin* 2:421–99
30. Moe, R. C. 1987. Exploring the limits of privatization. *Public Adm. Rev.* 47 (Nov./Dec.):453–60
31. Mountin, J. W., Flook, E. 1941. Distribution of health services in the structure of state government. Chap. 1. The composite pattern of state health services. *Public Health Rep.* 56:1673–94
32. Mountin, J. W., Flook, E. 1943. Distribution of health services in the structure of state government. Chap. 9. Central state services affecting all branches of public health work. *Public Health Rep.* 58:249–78
33. Mountin, J. W., Flook, E. 1943. Distribution of health services in the structure of state government. Chapter 10.

State health department organization. *Public Health Rep.* 58:541–77
34. Park, W. H., Beebe, A. L. 1894. Annual report of the Board of Health of the Health Department of the City of New York for the year ending December 31, 1893. *Med. Rec.* 46:385–401.
35. Rosen, G. 1936. Carl Ludwig and his American students. *Bull. Inst. Hist. Med.* 4:609–50
36. Rosen, G. 1958. Industrialism and the sanitary movement. In *A History of Public Health,* pp. 192–293. New York: MD Publica. 551 pp.
37. Rosen, G. 1965. Patterns of health research in the United States, 1900–1960. *Bull. Hist. Med.* 39:201–21
38. Rosenkrantz, B. G. 1974. Cart before horse: theory, practice and professional image in American public health, 1870–1920. *J. Hist. Med.* 29:55–73
39. Roux, P. P., Martin, A. L. 1894. Contribution a l'etude de la diphtherie (serum therapie). *Ann. Inst. Pasteur* 8:609–39
40. Roux, P. P., Yersin, A. E. 1888. Contribution a l'etude de la diphtherie. *Ann. Inst. Pasteur* 2:629–61
41. Sakula, A. 1982. Robert Koch: centenary of the discovery of the tubercle bacillus, 1882. *Thorax* 37:246–51
42. Schaeffer, M. 1966. Health department's role in improving operations of clinical laboratories. *Public Health Rep.* 81:71–74
43. Schaudinn, F. R., Hoffmann, E. 1905. Vorlaufiger Bericht uber das Vorkommen von Spirochaeten in syphilitischen Krankheitsprodukten und bei Papillomen. *Arb. k. GesundhAmte* 22:527–34
44. Schmidt, R. M., Madoff, M. A. 1977. The state and territorial public health laboratory: program activities, organization, and prospects for the future. *Am. J. Public Health* 67:433–38
45. Shryock, R. H. 1947. Public confidence regained. In *The Development of Modern Medicine,* pp. 336–55. New York: Knopf. 457 pp.
46. Sigerist, H. E. 1960. William Harvey's position in the history of European thought. In *Henry E. Sigerist on the History of Medicine,* ed. F. Marti-Ibanez, pp. 184–92. New York: MD Publicat. 313 pp.
47. Snyder, J. C. 1976. Public health and preventive medicine. In *Advances in American Medicine: Essays at the Bicentennial,* ed. J. Z. Bowers, E. F. Purcell, pp. 384–457. Baltimore: Port City Press. 457 pp.
48. Spink, W. W. 1978. The evolution of public health at national and international levels. In *Infectious Diseases, Prevention and Treatment in the Nineteenth and Twentieth Centuries,* pp. 28–58. Minneapolis: Univ. Minn. Press. 577 pp.
49. Spink, W. W. 1978. Communicable diseases of childhood. In Ref. 48, pp. 168–206
50. Starr, P. 1982. The boundaries of public health. In *The Social Transformation of American Medicine,* pp. 180–97. New York: Basic Books. 514 pp.
51. Stevens, M. B., Rigilano, J. C., Wilson, C. C. 1988. State screening of metabolic disorders in newborns. *Am. Fam. Physician* 37:223–28
52. Terris, M. 1975. Evolution of public health and preventive medicine in the United States. *Am. J. Public Health* 65:161–69
53. Deleted in proof
54. von Wasserman, A. 1906. Eine serodiagnostische Reaktion bei Syphilis. *Dtsch. Med. Wochenschr.* 32:745–46
55. Widal, G. F., Sicard, A. 1896. Recherches de la reaction agglutinante dans le sang et le serum desseches des typhiques et dans la serosite des vesicatoires. *Bull. Mem. Soc. Med. Hop. Paris* 13:681–82
56. Wilson, F. A., Neuhauser D. 1982. The federal government and health. In *Health Services in the United States,* ed. F. A. Wilson, D. Neuhauser, pp. 137–228. Cambridge, Mass: Ballinger. 339 pp. 2nd ed.
57. Winslow, C. E. 1915. The laboratory in the service of the state. *Am. J. Public Health* 6:222–33. Reprinted 1972 in *Health. Lab. Sci.* 9:5–15

Annu. Rev. Publ. Health 1993. 14:649–64

THE FUTURE OF THE PUBLIC HEALTH LABORATORY[1]

Walter R. Dowdle
Centers for Disease Control, Atlanta, Georgia 30333

KEY WORDS: local health department laboratories, state health department laboratories

INTRODUCTION

The widely quoted Institute of Medicine (IOM) report, "The Future of Public Health" (9), only refers to the functions of the public health laboratory indirectly or in an historical context. The current role of the laboratory is not described, nor does the word "laboratory" appear in the index. And, a review of recent strategic planning documents prepared by officials of state and local public health agencies did not mention the public health laboratory.

These findings are not unusual. Today's laboratory is too often taken for granted, in stark contrast to the public health laboratory of the early twentieth century. Pasteur described laboratories as the "temples of the future" [see the accompanying article by Valdiserri (14)]. In 1914, Charles Chapin wrote that "... the diagnostic laboratory is the most essential part of the machinery for the control of communicable disease." Public health laboratories still are essential for the control of communicable (and environmental) diseases. But, times have changed.

Public health laboratories long ago demonstrated the importance of clean food and water. Environmental microbiology testing has become routine. Vaccines are available for many communicable diseases, and more vaccines are on the way. Many antibiotics are available, although clinicians usually shoot first and ask questions only in the event of failure. Today, many competent laboratories operated by hospitals, universities, group medical practices, and private corporations offer wide-ranging services. Medical and environmental laboratories have become big business. Simple test kits for small laboratories and physicians' offices are widely available and aggressively marketed. Against this backdrop is the reality in public health practice of shrinking state and local revenues, increasing costs of laboratory operations, and a frequently negative public perception of government.

Some of today's state or local administrators, when faced with swelling deficits, burgeoning numbers of employees, and public criticism, are questioning the need for publicly supported laboratories. Contracting with the private sector for public health laboratory services is tempting. Other administrators have experienced considerable political pressure in the name of "private enterprise" to limit the activities of public health laboratories. For some public health laboratories, the future does not look bright.

However, the future continues to look bright for other public health laboratories, in spite of today's crises and adversities. Why? What accounts for the difference between the most and least successful laboratories? In this review, I examine the functions, practices, and apparent success factors of today's public health laboratories. There are two underlying assumptions: Public health laboratories are essential resources for the public health of the country. And, with aggressive effort, those resources can grow in strength and effectiveness.

FUNCTIONS OF THE PUBLIC HEALTH LABORATORY

According to the above-mentioned IOM report, the core functions of public health agencies at all levels of government are described as assessment, policy development, and assurance (9). The Centers for Disease Control (CDC) has gone a step further and identified ten organizational practices or processes that must be carried out under these functions (Table 1) (5). I discuss each of these major functions as they relate to the laboratory.

Assessment

The IOM report recommends "...that every public health agency regularly and systematically collect, assemble, analyze, and make available information on the health of the community, including statistics on health status, community health needs, and epidemiologic and other studies of health problems." Of all the functions of public health, the public health laboratory is vital for assessing, investigating, and analyzing the health needs, effects, and health in the community, the state, and the nation.

Consider tuberculosis. In the last few years, the United States has experienced an increase in tuberculosis unprecedented since the introduction of effective antimycobacterial drugs in the early 1950s (8). Control, certainly

Table 1 Functions and practices of public health agencies (5)

Assessment
Assess the health needs of the community.
Investigate the occurrence of health effects and health hazards in the community.
Analyze the determinants of identified health needs.
Policy development
Advocate for public health, build constituencies, and identify resources in the community.
Set priorities among health needs.
Develop plans and policies to address priority health needs.
Assurance
Manage resources and develop organizational structure.
Implement programs.
Evaluate programs and provide quality assurance.
Inform and educate the public.

the elimination, of tuberculosis has been further complicated by the increasing recognition of multidrug-resistant tuberculosis. The prevention and control of no other infectious disease depends so much on laboratory assessment, for rapid diagnosis, for determination of susceptibility of the bacillus to antimycobacterial drugs, and for application of newer technology to epidemiologic investigations. These are not personal health services.

In many ways, the recent increase in tuberculosis, particularly multidrug-resistant tuberculosis, is an indictment of our public health system, especially as it applies to the control of infectious diseases. As such diseases come close to disappearing, public health budgets are cut, interest wanes, research stops, expertise grows thin, and the disease reemerges. The experience with tuberculosis is not unlike the experience with measles. With the advent of the live vaccine, there were decreasing funds for research, monitoring of measles infections, and laboratory capacities for diagnosis. The result was a serious measles epidemic in 1989 and 1990, with more than 45,000 cases and 130 deaths that should never have occurred (6). As measles infections become fewer, the role of the public health laboratory in measles control becomes even greater through the need for early diagnosis of suspected cases.

Other vital assessment functions of the public health laboratory include the detection or documentation of food- and water-borne infections. The public health laboratory is needed to recognize trends, detect clusters of infection, recognize unusual subtypes of etiologic agents, and provide surveillance for antimicrobial resistance. The benefits of a national network for laboratory surveillance are best illustrated by the knowledge gained over the past few years about the emerging problems with food-borne infections. Through the joint efforts of public health laboratories at local, state, and federal levels, we have recognized the health problems associated with antibiotic-resistant salmonella isolates from food sources and *Salmonella enteritides* infections associated with grade A eggs (3). We now recognize the public health impact of listeriosis and better understand its natural history (7). Hemolytic uremic syndrome, a cause of renal failure in children, is now known to be associated with *Escherichia coli* (2). Individual laboratories may recognize only a few cases of uncommon food-borne infection, but collectively those few cases may reveal a regional or national outbreak of major importance.

This interactive network of assessment by individual public health laboratories has been further enhanced through the introduction of the National Public Health Laboratory Information System, which provides direct reporting to CDC and feedback of results to all contributing states. Such data provide an early warning system that permits each state to look outside its borders, gear up for rapid response, and gain perspective on a national problem.

Environmental testing is an equally crucial assessment function. During the last decade, the number of emergency responses to environmental health crises have continued to increase. Assessment is required when a community suddenly finds barrels of toxic waste in a wooded area where children play, or when a train derailment discharges thousands of gallons of benzene into a reservoir.

Only the laboratory measurement of a toxicant in human samples can conclusively demonstrate exposure in environmental health. The Arkansas State Laboratory responded rapidly to an environmental health assessment when it discovered that grain, heavily contaminated with the pesticide heptachlor, had been fed to cattle and that the dairy products derived from the cattle had been widely distributed in neighboring states. State laboratories in Louisiana and Iowa collaborated with Arkansas on large-scale measurements of heptachlor in dairy products and in breast milk and blood specimens from persons at highest risk of exposure. These public health laboratories demonstrated very quickly that potentially exposed persons had only low levels of heptachlor, and a major public health emergency was averted (13).

Research is also a component of assessment. Such research may include epidemiologic studies in partnership with programs, development and improvement of laboratory tests for more effective disease surveillance, and development of rapid methods for laboratory diagnosis.

Policy Development

The IOM report recommends "...that every public health agency exercise responsibility to serve the public interest in the development of comprehensive public health policies promoting use of the scientific knowledge base in decision making in public health by leading and developing public health policy." Ideally, the public health laboratory is a partner in the development of policy related to any issue that has a laboratory component. The public health laboratory director or experts in specific laboratory disciplines can provide valuable advice on the requirements for laboratory tests and the selection of tests based on cost effectiveness, sensitivity and specificity, appropriateness, and technical interpretation. Laboratory personnel can serve as consultants in advance of program development for input into technology application and research opportunities, capabilities, needs, and strategies. Laboratory input is particularly required for development of policy on such matters as sexually transmitted diseases, human immunodeficiency virus (HIV), and the environment. The public health laboratory is a valuable first source of information for all such policy development; it provides the data or information itself, convenes appropriate consultants, or seeks possible solutions from appropriate research institutions.

A major opportunity for the laboratory to influence policy development is in the area of environmental health. The abundance of hazardous waste sites, commercially available products containing hazardous chemicals, contaminated drinking water supplies, and industrial sources of pollution provides opportunities for the public health laboratory to influence environmental health policies directly. One recent example involved commercially available indoor paint that caused acrodynia among children in Michigan. The laboratory finding of mercury in the children's blood not only provided the key to resolving the etiology of the problem, but also led the Environmental Protection Agency to reduce substantially the amount of mercury permitted in household paint (4).

In many states, however, opportunities are limited for the influence of state laboratories on environmental health policy. In several state laboratories, the technology to measure toxicant levels in human samples (i.e. gaschromatography, mass spectroscopy) is exclusively used to measure contaminants in water and soil samples. In addition, sometimes the technical resource resides in another department or agency outside the public health department, which limits access to the technology for public health purposes. Ample data have shown that measurements of toxicants in environmental specimens often bear little relation to measurements of the same toxicants in specimens obtained from persons living near a particular source of exposure. The measurement of toxicant in human tissues is the key for deciding whether epidemiologic studies or public health interventions are necessary. Every state has problems with major environmental hazardous sites. Public health laboratories can help make crucial public health decisions and policies by providing the appropriate expertise for measuring toxicants in human samples.

Assurance

The IOM report recommends "...that public health agencies assure their constituents that services necessary to achieve agreed upon goals are provided, either by encouraging actions by other entities (private or public sector), by requiring such action through regulation, or by providing service directly." The public health laboratory role in assurance ranges from operating or participating in clinical and environmental laboratory improvement and regulatory programs to directly providing, in many states, clinical laboratory tests (services) to publicly supported community-wide programs for those unable to afford other health services.

One of the most visible and successful assurance programs involving the public health laboratories is infant screening for treatable inherited metabolic diseases. Effective infant screening programs in which state laboratories use dried blood spots collected at birth, combined with follow-up diagnostic studies, counseling, and treatment, help prevent mental retardation and premature death. The newborn screening programs have an impressive battery of tests that are performed on each child born in the US, including tests for congenital hypothyroidism, phenylketonuria, galactosemia, maple syrup urine disease, and, most recently, sickle cell disease. This important public health program is largely driven by laboratory measurements. Screening has achieved a high degree of technical proficiency, while maintaining the high-volume specimen throughput that is required.

Another aspect of assurance with a possible role for the public health laboratory is in measuring the effectiveness of intervention programs. Once a major public health intervention has occurred, such as lead poisoning prevention, laboratory data are required to assure that the program is achieving its goal.

The cost of the test in the public health laboratory pays for more than a test result. It provides public health benefits to the local population and the nation as a whole.

A PROFILE OF THE PUBLIC HEALTH LABORATORY

Public health laboratories are operated by states, regions, counties, and cities. All are different in some respects. Each is shaped by its own particular history, governance, health department policies, funding, population served, public health interest and leadership, and political will. Public health laboratories are not easy to describe, but we may begin by dividing the laboratories into those operated by local, city, and/or county health departments and those operated by the states.

Local Health Departments

Local health departments are primarily city and/or county health departments. According to the National Profile of Local Health Departments, prepared by the National Association of County Health Officials (10), there were 2932 local health departments in 1989. A local health department was defined as "...an administrative or service unit of local or state government, concerned with health, and carrying some responsibility for the health of a jurisdiction smaller than a state." This definition excludes district or satellite laboratories of state or local health departments. Of the 2263 health departments responding to a 1989 survey, 65% served populations of less than 50,000. Of the 403 local health departments serving populations of more than 100,000, 69% reported providing laboratory services. Some of these laboratories serve large population centers, such as New York City, Los Angeles, and Chicago. In the US, 20 counties have populations that are larger than the ten smallest states. No further details on laboratory services are available, but from personal observations, such functions at the local level would include, at various degrees of complexity, tests for the laboratory diagnoses of tuberculosis, syphilis, gonorrhea, and HIV; clinical laboratory tests in support of personal health services; environmental tests to sample of milk and water and, to a lesser extent, air quality, radiation control, and hazardous waste. Some of the larger laboratories also provide for laboratory diagnosis of parasitic diseases and enteric bacteria.

Most local health departments have limited capabilities for disease assessment. Only 11% reported having a full- or part-time epidemiologist/statistician on staff.

Of the 1860 responding local health departments serving populations of less than 100,000, 38% reported providing laboratory services (10). Nearly all of these smaller local health departments and many of the 403 serving populations greater than 100,000 rely on contract laboratories (often hospital or commercial laboratories) or state health department laboratories for assistance. In the event of a disease outbreak or environmental hazard investigation that requires specialized tests, equipment, leadership, or knowledge, most of the local health departments turn to the state for assistance.

State Health Departments

In all states and in the District of Columbia, state health departments operate public health laboratories. Four laboratories (California, New York, Texas, Florida) serve nearly one third of the nation's population. Fifteen laboratories serve the next one third of the population. Thirty-two laboratories serve the remaining one-third, with 18 of these laboratories serving populations of less than 2 million each (1). In 1989, the number of laboratory employees ranged from a low of 18 in Wyoming to a high of 495 in California. New York did not report. Only eight laboratories (16%) reported more than 200 employees; 29 of the laboratories (57%) reported less than 100 employees. Although the size of the laboratory staff generally correlated with the size of the state population, there were numerous exceptions. Pennsylvania, with a population of 11 million, reported a laboratory staff of 70. Rhode Island, with a population of approximately 1 million, reported a staff of 90 (1).

The sources of funds, as listed in the Consolidated Annual Report for operation of the state public health laboratories, were as follows: state funds, 80%; fees and reimbursement, 8%; federal funds, 8%; and local and other funds, 3%. The source of funds varies widely with the state. Many state health laboratories receive no federal funds, and some state laboratories depend on fees and reimbursements for more than half of their annual budgets. In the aggregate, 3.3% of the total state health agencies' 1988 budgets were allocated to their public health laboratories (11).

In a recent survey by the Association of State and Territorial Public Health Laboratory Directors (ASTPHLD), with 23 states reporting, all except one reported a personnel hiring freeze or loss of positions in 1992. Nearly half of the laboratories indicated that privatization of some or all of the laboratory activities was under discussion. Virtually every state laboratory charges user fees and accepts Medicare fees and third-party reimbursement for some of its services.

The bulk of the specimens tested by state health laboratories is categorized in the 1990 report as public health chemistry, followed by immunology, public health pathogenic microbiology, environmental microbiology, virology, environmental chemistry, and toxicology (1). But, individual laboratories vary widely. State health laboratories in the larger states with major local or regional laboratories serve primarily as reference sources for specialized or more complex tests. CDC serves the same role for state health laboratories.

Eighteen state laboratories reported at least one project described as research or technical development (1). If New York is included, based on other information, 19 laboratories perform research. Eight of the 19 laboratories received federal support for the projects through grants or contracts. The laboratories with largest research and development commitments were California, New York, and Iowa.

Of the 50 reporting laboratories in 1989, 42 (84%) reported either operating or participating in a state-wide laboratory improvement program that may range from providing continuing education and training for laboratory personnel to fully regulating clinical and environmental laboratories.

FACTORS OF SUCCESS

Considering the clear laboratory missions of assessment, policy development, and assurance, it is a paradox that so many public health laboratories find themselves with such precarious futures. The contributing factors are as many as there are public health laboratories whose futures are in doubt.

In some states, the concept of public health is still little understood or appreciated. Public health is equated with welfare, not health, and welfare is seen as an ever-increasing drain on the budget. The public health laboratory provides many services for those whose medical care is provided by the public sector; therefore, the laboratory is viewed as one more service that needs to be carefully scrutinized as budgets get tighter. States or localities that curtail or discontinue laboratory activities because the results do not justify the costs create self-fulfilling prophesies. If no mechanism exists to assess the health of the population, then policy makers can only conclude that no problem exists.

In other states, policy makers, including legislators, have pushed to curtail public health laboratory functions in the name of private enterprise. The arguments run that private laboratories can meet the state's needs more cheaply than the existing public health laboratories and that the government should not provide services that can be provided by the private sector. There is merit to such continuing sensitivity and debate about government services. However, the one element missing in these arguments relative to laboratories is that, once privatized, where is the advocacy for the public's health? Where is the concern for the public's interest? Who will be alert to solving a previously unrecognized problem? Privatization cannot buy the mission of advocacy that is at the heart of the public health laboratory. The primary purpose of the public health laboratory is to improve public health. Strong private laboratories are an important component of the medical delivery system in this country, and specialized private laboratories play critical support roles at times in public health. However, private laboratories cannot be expected to perform additional tests and uncompensated investigations because of this concern for the public's health or to fulfill the mission of the public health laboratory. The state's responsibility for the health of its citizens cannot be delegated.

Some public health laboratories have severe financial difficulties. A sudden infusion of funds is unlikely, given the ever-present economic pressures at all levels of government, as well as the general reluctance of many legislators to reverse political positions. Money often must come at the expense of other programs that can make equally strong claims for their importance. Recent programs, such as those for chronic diseases, injury, and drug abuse, have come under the purview of the public health department. All of these programs are important. Efforts to stem the erosion of our national laboratory network, so crucial to the health of this country, must be made independently of other needed public health programs.

Despite this dismal picture, a number of state health laboratories not only continue to survive, but have increased in stature and competence and in their contributions to the health of the people. They are doing something right. Interestingly, the strength of the public health laboratory and the strength of the state or local health department do not seem to be directly correlated. In some instances, the laboratory is perceived to be strong and the health department weak. There are numerous perceptions of the reverse. Furthermore, strength can be relative. Some of the public health laboratories in the smaller states are strong within the resources available to them.

Several factors appear to be common among the laboratories that seem to be most successful in carrying out their public health functions. Every factor is not necessarily found in each successful laboratory. A constellation of some of these factors may be sufficient to compensate for the absence of others. The following factors appear to be characteristic of success.

Mission

One striking characteristic among successful laboratories is a sense of mission consistent with the concept of assessment, policy development, and assurance. Too many public health laboratory directors view their mission as providing only a service or support function. Service is an important function of government. All public health departments provide services, and proudly so. But, care must be taken that the provision of personal health services does not overshadow the public health obligations of assessment, policy development, and assurance. This is particularly true for the laboratory. Providing services is passive. Doing assessment is aggressive. Assessment must be foremost in the laboratory mission. Microbiological and environmental testing, outbreak investigations, and surveillance are vital assessment functions. Every specimen tested by the laboratory should represent some carefully planned aspect of assessment. Service not in the context of assessment is a mind set that public health laboratories can ill afford. We need to conceptualize the primary mission of the public health laboratory as assessment.

Image

Another factor associated with successful laboratories is a strong reputation built on high standards, quick responses, wide-ranging capabilities, close working relationships with the medical community, and protection of the public's health. However, a reputation of good work among a small circle is not always good enough. Legislators and the public must also know what the laboratory does. In one state plan for improving the public health system, the very first recommendation was to institute a statewide marketing campaign (12). A formal campaign may not be the best solution for every public health laboratory, but each laboratory can take advantage of every opportunity to make its activities known through promotional efforts, individual contacts, briefings of public officials, carefully planned publications and reports, and involvement in public health activities at the state or local areas.

Partnership with Epidemiology

In successful laboratories, epidemiology and laboratory personnel operate together to provide a quality and quantity of assessment that is not otherwise possible. Full integration of these activities has a profound effect on how the laboratory perceives its public health mission and how it develops assessment strategies. Integration does not mean that epidemiology is subsumed by the laboratory or the laboratory by epidemiology. Numerous opportunities exist for integrating these two core functions. Not all of these opportunities require reorganization, and none of them requires that one function be subservient to the other. Full integration of epidemiology and laboratory activities is crucial to meet that first commandment: assessment.

Organizational Location

A visible location in the public health organization is a feature characteristic of most successful laboratories. Although organizational prominence does not guarantee success, it helps. The presence of a visible organizational position increases effectiveness and enhances the opportunity to work in partnership with other public health programs.

Public health laboratories encounter major collaboration barriers when they are organizationally far removed from the programs to which they most closely relate (such as epidemiology, sexually transmitted disease, tuberculosis, HIV, and environmental health). Bureaucratic layers discourage and often outright prevent working relationships. Organizational distance reinforces the perception of the laboratory as only a service unit. The successful laboratory must be viewed by other programs as a full partner, on an equal organizational footing.

Flexibility of Resources

Ten years ago, few public health laboratories were permitted to charge fees for services. Now, most public health laboratories do so. The hallmark of the more successful laboratories is to charge fees for more routine tests, or to charge for tests that pertain to personal health needs, while continuing public health activities without charge. In some cases, the income from personal health services underwrites the public health mission. Under the best arrangements, the laboratory has the flexibility to use the income as it sees fit: for equipment, supplies, training of personnel, new services, and, above all, hiring. But, this amount of flexibility is rare. Such financial arrangements are in effect in very few laboratories, but could be applied beneficially by others.

Far too often, fees for services have a negative effect on the laboratory. In many states, the income is directed to the state or local general revenue. Although the fee-for-service activities that generate general revenues are usually considered when budgets are determined, the overriding budget decisions are often made regardless of the income generated. Decisions, such as state-wide or department-wide budget cuts and personnel hiring freezes or reductions, are frequently made without regard to specific laboratory situations. In many laboratories, technical positions and equipment purchases have been frozen for two years or more, without regard to the income generated or the service provided, and with no relief in sight.

Without adequate staff or equipment, the types and volume of tests offered by the laboratory are reduced, the remaining staff are overworked, morale drops, user confidence erodes, and the downward spiral of the laboratory's capabilities, reputation, and public health relevance accelerates. This pattern is hardly a recipe for success. Many budgetary practices that adversely affect the future of the laboratory are typically embedded in state laws. Successful laboratories identify the obstacles to flexibility of resources and seek action for relief.

Research

One feature that is common to all top public health laboratories is research, whether it is federally, state, or privately funded, or performed independently or jointly with other programs. Research opportunities attract top-flight scientists, hone expertise, assure a cutting-edge in laboratory capabilities, and stimulate mission-related goals and objectives.

For many laboratories, the flexibility to seek grants and contracts is limited. State laws often prohibit it. Although research, including assessment, should be an activity of every state public health laboratory, it realistically requires a separate stream of funding. Research does not compete well with services. Where budgets are integrated, any activity resembling research is the first to go when funds become short. For many state laboratories, the ability to accept and administer research grants and contracts independently will require legislative action.

Critical Mass

The nation's top public health laboratories are not necessarily found in the nation's most populous states. But, the top quality laboratory operations have the necessary critical mass to maintain the requisite scientific momentum.

In 1989, ten state laboratories reported a staff of less than 50 each. Today, with personnel freezes and budgetary cuts, the number of such laboratories has undoubtedly increased. Although many of these small laboratories have managed to maintain high-quality performance for the tests they provide, the tests are often limited in scope and complexity. Public health could be further served by combining forces with other laboratories (regionalization) in other states or with other state-supported institutions.

Regionalization is not a new concept. For some time, several of the smaller state laboratories have had informal agreements to provide specialized testing for another state, usually in one direction. In some areas, these informal agreements have worked well. However, regionalization based on formal reciprocal agreements between state laboratories is less common. On the surface, formal regionalization has merit, but the concept has yet to undergo the test of state regulations, budgetary realities, and personalities. Each laboratory must also carefully weigh the effect of regionalization on its growth potential.

Academic Ties

Another option, too rarely considered, has been combining forces with other state institutions, such as a school of medicine, school of public health, or state university. The smaller states should find such an arrangement an effective use of scarce resources and a mechanism for assuring critical mass. Furthermore, having the public health laboratory operate under the rules and regulations that govern a university is worth considering for many states and local health departments. Where this arrangement has been instituted, regardless of the size of the laboratory, public health has been the beneficiary.

Under university rules and regulations, the public health laboratory would be able to use fee-for-service income and research opportunities, and to hire staff on "soft" money. This arrangement offers the laboratory the added advantage of participating in the university's educational program and attracting high-quality staff and graduate students. The environment is also conducive to performing the critical assessment functions, including research.

The university benefits through more efficient use of resources, strengthening of educational and research opportunities, and supporting a strong public health laboratory. State-funded university research laboratories in many states already undertake federally supported public health-related surveys and studies that may be defined as public health assessment. University affiliation provides the flexibility of resources, so badly lacking in most state governments, to support a first-class, technically and scientifically sound public health laboratory.

THE CHALLENGE

These days, when funds for state and local health departments have not kept pace with their increased public health responsibilities, elected and appointed officials are understandably seeking ways to cut their losses. In this effort to balance the budget, some of the hard questions have focused on the public health laboratory. Is a publicly supported laboratory essential for the service it provides? For those public health laboratories that primarily provide only personal health services, whether by default or design, the answer would have to be no. Personal health services can be provided by any reputable contract laboratory. Whether such services can be provided in the private sector at a cost that is actually less than that in the public sector is quite another matter.

But, to ask whether a public health laboratory is needed to perform personal clinical services is the wrong question. The right question to ask is whether a public health laboratory is essential to protect the public's health. The answer here is a resounding yes.

The sequence of events around HIV infections is a good example of the important role that public health laboratories play in protecting the public's health. Within days of the approval of the serologic test for HIV, directors and appropriate staff from state and large local public health laboratories convened at CDC for discussions and training. As implementation of the test expanded to other laboratories, the public health laboratories were crucial in providing leadership, training, and quality assurance. In many states, the public health laboratories provided the only testing capabilities and were the only source, other than the blood banks, for the confirmatory Western blot test. The public health laboratories continue to be the primary sources for confidential testing and for data on HIV incidence and prevalence, by providing assessment at a state and local level and, through CDC, for the nation.

HIV will not be the last infectious disease. Other new, as well as re-emerging, infectious diseases will appear in the US, reflecting new discoveries (pneumonia due to chlamydia) and changes in the environment (Lyme disease), technology (Legionnaires' disease), personal behavior (herpes 2, human papilloma virus, and other sexually transmitted diseases), age of population (pneumonia, influenza), food production practices (salmonella, small particle viruses), poverty (tuberculosis), and the microbial world (antibiotic resistance, virulence). Increased travel, immigration, and translocation of populations increasingly expose US citizens to malaria, dengue, parasitic diseases, hemorrhagic fevers, and enteric diseases, such as the current epidemic of cholera spreading throughout South and Central America. Reestablishment of malaria and dengue in vulnerable areas of the southeastern United States is now a possibility. In all these instances, the first point of contact, and often the only source of expertise, is the public health laboratory.

Environmental health will continue to be a burgeoning area for the public health laboratory. The extent and level to which people are exposed to harmful chemicals in their environment (except in cases of high levels of acute exposures) cannot be easily described in terms of physical symptoms, morbidity, or mortality. The laboratory measurement of toxicants in blood and urine specimens will become the standard of practice for establishing whether an individual or community has been excessively exposed to hazardous substances. It is the laboratory measurement of blood lead, not the resulting loss of IQ or neurologic function, that first identifies a child as having lead poisoning, an environmental disease. The public health laboratory will increasingly be called upon to classify human exposure to a wide array of priority toxicant, including toxic elements (e.g. cadmium), pesticides, polychlorinated biphenyls, volatile organic compounds (e.g. benzene), and polyaromatic hydrocarbons.

The potential rapidity, sensitivity, and specificity of microbiological and environmental techniques now under evaluation provide the laboratories and their epidemiology and program partners a degree of sophistication undreamed of only a few years ago. Newer techniques promise to revolutionize methodology in both the microbiology and environmental laboratories, thus widely expanding the capabilities of even the smallest public health laboratory.

Assuring a bright future for state health laboratories requires strong leadership by CDC and ASTPHLD. ASTPHLD has proven to be a highly effective forum for the discussion of common management problems, public health issues, surveillance programs, technical advances, and training needs. In cooperation with CDC, ASTPHLD has established both a national network for training laboratory personnel and a mechanism for establishing priorities for health laboratory practice. The latter project, Laboratory Initiatives for the Year 2000, was designed to integrate planning among laboratory professionals in both the public and private sectors to focus on the National Health Promotion and Disease Prevention Objectives for the Year 2000.

In such planning, public health laboratories also need to consider their roles in the event that some form of universal health care is implemented in the US within the next few years. If, as desired, health care reform fills many health care gaps, public health laboratories may no longer be required to provide personal clinical services. The health department may no longer be the health care provider of last resort. Health care reform may enable state and local health departments to devote full time to public health—to leadership and coordination, surveillance, investigation, prevention, outbreak control health education, and research.

The future of the public health laboratory depends heavily on the ability of current and future health department personnel, appointed and elected officials, and the general public to understand and appreciate the meaning of public health and the functions of the public health laboratory. We have a long way to go. To meet this challenge, the laboratories and their parent organizations must strongly believe in and clearly focus on their functions of assessment, policy development, and assurance. And, they must be able to articulate these functions at every opportunity. Of these three functions, assessment is the first commandment for the public health laboratory.

I am indebted to the following for their advice, suggestions, and critical review of the manuscript: David F. Carpenter, Division of Laboratories, Illinois Department of Public Health; Jon M. Counts, DSHS-Office of Public Health, Seattle, Washington; Elizabeth Franko, Georgia Department of Human Resources; W. J. Hausler, Jr., University Hygienic Laboratory, University of Iowa; Elvin R. Hilyer, Centers for Disease Control; James M. Hughes, National Center for Infectious Diseases, Centers for Disease Control; J. Mehsen Joseph, Department of Health & Mental Hygiene, Baltimore, Maryland; Eric Sampson, Division of Environmental Health Laboratory Sciences, National Center for Environmental Health and Injury Control, Centers for Disease Control; Charles E. Sweet, Bureau of Laboratories, Texas Department of Health; Ronald O. Valdiserri, National Center for Prevention Services, Centers for Disease Control

Literature Cited

1. Assoc. State Territ. Public Health Lab. Dir. 1990. *Consolidated Annual Report on State and Territorial Public Health Laboratories, Fiscal Year 1989*. Washington, DC: Assoc. State Territ. Public Health Lab. Dir.
2. Cent. Dis. Cont. 1985. Hemolytic-Uremic syndrome associated with *Escherichia coli* 0157;H7 enteric infection—United States, 1984. *Morbid. Mortal. Wkly. Rep.* 34:20–21
3. Cent. Dis. Cont. 1988. Update: *Salmonella enteritidis* infections and grade A shell eggs—United States. *Morbid. Mortal. Wkly. Rep.* 37:490–96
4. Cent. Dis. Cont. 1990. Update: mercury exposure from interior latex paint—United States. *Morbid. Mortal. Wkly. Rep.* 39:125–26
5. Cent. Dis. Cont. 1991. Profile of state and territorial public health systems: United States 1990. Atlanta: Public Health Pract. Progr. Off.
6. Cent. Dis. Cont. 1991. Measles—United States, 1990. *Morbid. Mortal. Wkly. Rep.* 40:369–72
7. Cent. Dis. Cont. 1992. Update: food borne listeriosis—United States, 1988–1990. *Morbid. Mortal. Wkly. Rep.* 41: 251–58
8. Cent. Dis. Cont. 1992. Prevention and control of tuberculosis in US communities with at-risk minority populations and prevention and control of tuberculosis among homeless persons. *Morbid. Mortal. Wkly. Rep.* 41:RR-5
9. Comm. Study Future Public Health. 1988. A vision of public health in America: an attainable ideal. In *The Future of Public Health*. Washington, DC: Natl. Acad. Press
10. Natl. Assoc. County Health Off. 1990. *National Profile of Local Health Departments*. Washington, DC: Natl. Assoc. County Health Off.
11. Public Health Found. 1990. *Public Health Agencies 1990: an Inventory of Programs and Block Grant Expenditures*. Washington, DC: Public Health Found.
12. Road Map Implement. Task Force. 1990. *The Road to Better Health for all of Illinois: Improving the Public Health System*. Springfield, Ill: Ill. Dep. Public Health
13. Stehr-Green, P. A., Schilling, R. J., Burse, V. W., Steinberg,K. K., Royce, W., et al. 1986. Evaluation of persons exposed to dairy products contaminated with heptachlor. *J. Am. Med. Assoc.* 245:3350–51
14. Valdiserri, R. O. 1992. Temples of the future: an historical overview of the laboratory's role in public health practice. *Annu. Rev. Public Health* 14:635–48

SUBJECT INDEX

S

CUMULATIVE INDEXES

CONTRIBUTING AUTHORS, VOLUMES 5–14

Z

CHAPTER TITLES, VOLUMES 5–14